A Practical Approach to Transesophageal Echocardiography

Second Edition

A Practical Approach to Transesophageal Echocardiography

Second Edition

Editors

Albert C. Perrino, Jr., MD
Professor
Department of Anesthesiology
Yale University School of Medicine
New Haven, Connecticut

Scott T. Reeves, MD, MBA, FACC, FASE
Professor and Chair
Department of Anesthesiology and Perioperative Medicine
Medical University of South Carolina
Charleston, South Carolina

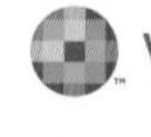
Wolters Kluwer | Lippincott
Health | Williams & Wilkins

Philadelphia • Baltimore • New York • London
Buenos Aires • Hong Kong • Sydney • Tokyo

Acquisitions Editor: Brian Brown
Developmental Editor: Keith Donnellan
Managing Editor: Nicole T. Dernoski
Project Manager: Rosanne Hallowell
Manufacturing Manager: Kathleen Brown
Marketing Manager: Angela Panetta
Creative Director: Doug Smock
Cover Designer: Larry Didona
Production Services: Laserwords Private Limited, Chennai, India

Second Edition

530 Walnut Street
Philadelphia, PA 19106
LWW.com

Printed in China

Library of Congress Cataloging-in-Publication Data

A practical approach to transesophageal echocardiography / editors, Albert C. Perrino Jr., Scott T. Reeves.—2nd ed.
p. ; cm.
Includes bibliographical references and index.
ISBN 978-0-7817-7329-4
1. Transesophageal echocardiography. I. Perrino, Albert C. II. Reeves, Scott T.
[DNLM: 1. Echocardiography, Transesophageal—methods. 2. Heart Diseases—ultrasonography. WG 141.5.E2 P894 2008]
RC683.5.T83P73 2008
616.1′207543—dc22

2007030480

---

10 9 8 7 6 5

RRS1010

❖

To Anita, Mary, Isabella, and Juliana for sustaining another of my adventures and to Winston Churchill whose keen observation also served as a source of support.

Writing is an adventure. To begin with, it is a toy and an amusement. Then it becomes a mistress, then it becomes a master, then it becomes a tyrant. The last phase is that just as you are about to be reconciled to your servitude, you kill the monster and fling him to the public.

—Winston Churchill
ACP

To
My Savior, Jesus Christ, who gives me strength. . .
My wife, Cathy, who loves and puts up with me. . .
My children, Catherine, Carolyn, and Townsend, who give me great joy. . .
My patients, who inspire me to do my best daily!

STR

Contributors

John G. Augoustides, MD, FASE
Assistant Professor, Department of Anesthesiology and Critical Care, University of Pennsylvania; Attending Cardiothoracic Anesthesiologist, Department of Anesthesiology and Critical Care, Hospital of the University of Pennsylvania, Philadelphia, Pennsylvania

Albert T. Cheung, MD
Professor, Department of Anesthiology and Critical Care Medicine, University of Pennsylvania; Faculty, University of Pennsylvania Health System, Department of Anesthesiology and Critical Care, Hospital of the University of Pennsylvania, Presbyterian Medical Center, Philadelphia, Pennsylvania

Ira S. Cohen, MD, FACC
Clinical Professor, Department of Cardiology, Thomas Jefferson Medical College, Jefferson Heart Institute; Director of Echocardiography, Department of Cardiology, Thomas Jefferson University Hospital, Philadelphia, Pennsylvania

Herbert W. Dyal II, BHS, RDCS, RDMS
Eastern Region Applications Manager, Department of Cardiovascular Ultrasound, General Electric Healthcare, Wauwatosa, Wisconsin

Michael D. Frith, BS, RDCS, RDMS
Account Executive, Cardiovascular Ultrasound, General Electric Company, Milwaukee, Wisconsin

Susan Garwood, MB, Ch B
Associate Professor, Department of Anesthesiology, Yale University School of Medicine New Haven, Connecticut

Zak Hillel, MD
Professor, Department of Anesthesiology, Columbia University College of Physicians and Surgeons; Director of Cardiac Anesthesia, Department of Anesthesiology, St. Lukes-Roosevelt Hospital, New York, New York

Gregory M. Hirsch, MD, FRCPS
Associate Professor, Department of Surgery, Dalhousie University; Head, Division of Cardiac Surgery, Queen Elizabeth II Health Sciences Centre, Halifax, Nova Scotia, Canada

Kristine Johnson Hirsch, MD, FRCP
Assistant Professor, Department of Anesthesia, Dalhousie University; Staff Anesthesiologist, Director of Perioperative Transesophageal Echocardiography, Department of Anesthesia, Queen Elizabeth II Health Sciences Centre, Halifax, Nova Scotia, Canada

John S. Ikonomidis, MD, PhD
Associate Professor, CT Surgery, Department of Surgery, Medical University of South Carolina, Charleston, South Carolina

Farid Jadbabaie, MD
Assistant Professor, Department of Internal Medicine and Section of Cardiology and Administration, Yale University School of Medicine, New Haven, Connecticut

Colleen Gorman Koch, MD, MS
Staff Anesthesiologist, Department of Cardiothoracic Anesthesia (G-3), The Cleveland Clinic Foundation, Cleveland, Ohio

A. Stephane Lambert, MD, FRCPC
Assistant Professor, Department of Anesthesia, University of Ottawa, Ottawa, Ontario, Canada; Attending Anesthesiologist, Division of Cardiac Anesthesia, University of Ottawa Heart Institute, Ottawa, Ontario, Canada

Emilio B. Lobato, MD
Professor, Department of Anesthesiology, University of Florida College of Medicine, Gainesville, Florida

Martin J. London, MD
Professor of Clinical Anesthesia, Department of Anesthesia and Perioperative Care, University of California, Attending Anesthesiologist, San Francisco Veterans Affairs Medical Center, San Francisco, California

Jonathan B. Mark, MD
Professor and Vice Chairman, Department of Anesthesiology, Duke University Medical Center, Chief, Anesthesiology Service, Veterans Affairs Medical Center, Durham, North Carolina

Andrew Maslow, MD
Associate Professor, Department of Anesthesiology, Brown Medical School; Department of Anesthesiology, Rhode Island Hospital, Providence, Rhode Island

Joseph P. Miller, MD
Assistant Professor, Department of Anesthesiology, Uniformed Services University, Bethesda, Maryland; Staff Anesthesiologist, Department of Anesthesia and Operative Services Madigan Army Medical Center, Tacoma, Washington

Wanda C. Miller-Hance, MD
Associate Professor, Pediatrics and Anesthesiology, Baylor College of Medicine; Attending Physician in Anesthesiology and Pediatric Cardiology, Department of Pediatrics and Anesthesiology, Texas Children's Hospital, Houston, Texas

Jochen D. Muehlschlegel, MD
Fellow in Cardiothoracic Anesthesiology, Department of Anesthesiology, Perioperative and Pain Medicine, Brigham and Women's Hospital, Harvard Medical School, Boston, Massachusetts

Kim J. Payne, MD
Assistant Professor, Department of Anesthesiology and Perioperative Medicine, Medical University of South Carolina, Charleston, South Carolina

Albert C. Perrino, Jr., MD
Professor, Department of Anesthesiology, Yale University School of Medicine, New Haven, Connecticut

Scott T. Reeves, MD, MBA, FACC
Professor and Chair, Department of Anesthesiology and Perioperative Medicine, Medical University of South Carolina, Charleston, South Carolina

Kathryn Rouine-Rapp, MD
Professor of Clinical Anesthesia, Department of Anesthesia, University of California, San Francisco, California

Rebecca A. Schroeder, MD
Associate Professor, Department of Anesthesiology, Duke University Medical Center, Assistant Chief for Anesthesia Research Administration, Veterans Affairs Medical Center, Durham, North Carolina

Stanton K. Shernan, MD
Associate Professor of Anesthesia, Chief, Division of Cardiac Anesthesia, Brigham and Women's Hospital, Harvard Medical School, Boston, Massachusetts

Gautam M. Sreeram, MD
Assistant Professor, Department of Anesthesiology, Emory University School of Medicine; Anesthesiologist, Department of Anesthesiology, Emory University Hospital, Atlanta, Georgia

Stuart J. Weiss, MD, PhD
Associate Professor, Department of Anesthesia, University of Pennsylvania, Philadelphia, Pennsylvania

Preface

TRANSESOPHAGEAL ECHOCARDIOGRAPHY (TEE) IS THE first imaging technique to enter the mainstream of intraoperative patient monitoring. The dramatic display of detailed cardiac anatomy and physiology provided in real time by two-dimensional (2D) and Doppler techniques quickly convinced the most skeptical among us of the remarkable clinical potential TEE offers to optimize patient management. For clinicians accustomed to invasive hemodynamic monitoring, it is something of a challenge to become an accomplished interpreter of TEE images and Doppler techniques. The multiple views and imaging planes require a readjustment of our orientation to cardiac anatomy. And the quantitative assessments of cardiovascular function, particularly those derived from blood flow velocity, also require new insights for the clinician accustomed to pressure measurements. This second edition of *A Practical Approach to Transesophageal Echocardiography* provides the intraoperative clinician with an updated resource to readily acquire the principles and perspectives underlying the approach used in practice by accomplished intraoperative echocardiographers.

The editors have gathered contributing authors who are internationally renowned and acknowledged for their independent contributions and teaching ability. The authors were given the task of presenting a highly readable and clinically relevant survey of the current practice of perioperative echocardiography. Their enthusiasm, backed with the strong support of the publisher, has produced this book.

Despite the notable comprehensive reference texts and case atlases available on this subject, this book remains the clinicians best resource to acquire the essential skills of TEE practice. The second edition is comprised of up-to-date chapters supported by extensive use of color illustrations and echocardiographic images. The presentation, illustrations, and content create a surprisingly portable text that is conducive to rapid appreciation of the critical elements in the use of TEE for a particular clinical challenge.

The reader is guided through the physics, principles, and applications of 2D imaging and Doppler modalities for assessing ventricular performance and the clinical significance of valvular disease. There is particular emphasis on the use of TEE for valve repair and replacement surgeries. One chapter is dedicated to echocardiographic artifacts and other pitfalls of interpretation that can lead to misdiagnosis, and a complete chapter has been added detailing cardiac masses and sources of emboli. The book concludes with a section on technical issues and echocardiography machine operation. It is our intention that, after an understanding of the imaging modalities has been acquired, the importance and relevance of these somewhat dry but essential concepts will be better appreciated than if they were presented as initial topics. Each chapter concludes with a series of self-assessment test questions to further emphasize important teaching points.

Certainly, the skills required to be an expert echocardiographer cannot be gained from textbooks alone. Extensive clinical training and intraoperative exposure to the application of these techniques remains paramount. In addition, we recommend the excellent educational programs on intraoperative TEE sponsored by the American Society of Echocardiography, the Society for Cardiovascular Anesthesiology, and the American Society of Anesthesiologists. We hope this textbook will become a well-worn and valued asset to your echocardiography practice.

Albert C. Perrino, Jr., MD
Scott T. Reeves, MD, MBA, FACC, FASE

Contents

Essentials of Two-Dimensional Imaging

1 Principles and Technology of Two-Dimensional Echocardiography

Andrew Maslow and Albert C. Perrino, Jr.

Two-dimensional echocardiography generates dynamic images of the heart from reflections of transmitted ultrasound. The echocardiography system transmits a brief pulse of ultrasound that propagates through and is subsequently reflected from the cardiac structures encountered. The sound reflections travel back to the ultrasound transducer, which records the time delay for each returning reflection. Because the speed of sound in tissue is constant, the time delay allows for a precise calculation of the location of the cardiac structures from which the echocardiography system can then create an image map of the heart. Not surprisingly, successful cardiac imaging requires a firm understanding of the interactions of sound and tissue. This chapter reviews the basic principles of ultrasound, its propagation through tissues, and the technologies which create moving images of the heart.

PHYSICAL PROPERTIES OF SOUND WAVES

Vibrations

Sound is vibration of a physical medium. In clinical echocardiography, a mechanical vibrator, known as the *transducer*, is placed in contact with the esophagus [transesophageal echocardiography (TEE)], skin (transthoracic echocardiography), or the heart (epicardial echocardiography) to create tissue vibrations. The resulting tissue vibrations or sound waves consist of areas of **compression** (areas where molecules are tightly packed) and **rarefaction** (areas where molecules are dispersed) resembling a sine wave **(Figure 1.1)**.

AMPLITUDE

The amplitude of a sound wave represents its peak pressure and is appreciated as loudness. The level of sound energy in an area of tissue is referred to as *intensity*. The intensity of the sound signal is proportional to the square of the amplitude and is an important factor regarding the potential for tissue damage with ultrasound. For example, lithotripsy uses high-intensity sound signals to fragment renal stones. In contrast, cardiac ultrasound uses low-intensity signals to image tissue, which produces only limited bioeffects. Because levels of sound pressure vary over a large range, it is convenient to use the logarithmic decibel (dB) scale:

$$\begin{aligned}\text{Decibel (dB)} &= 10\log_{10} I/I_r = 10\log_{10} A^2/A_r^2\\ &= 20\log_{10} A/A_r \end{aligned} \quad [1]$$

where A is the measured sound amplitude of interest and A_r is a standard reference sound level, I is intensity and I_r is a standard reference intensity.

More simply expressed, each doubling of the sound pressure equals a gain of 6 dB. The U.S. Food and Drug Administration (FDA) limits the maximum intensity output of cardiac ultrasound systems to be less than 720 W/cm^2 due to concerns with possible tissue and neurologic damage from mechanical injury (resulting from cavitation or microbubbles caused by rarefaction) and thermal effects. The ALARA principle recommends that clinicians use exposure levels *A*s *L*ittle *A*s *R*easonably *A*chievable to protect patients.

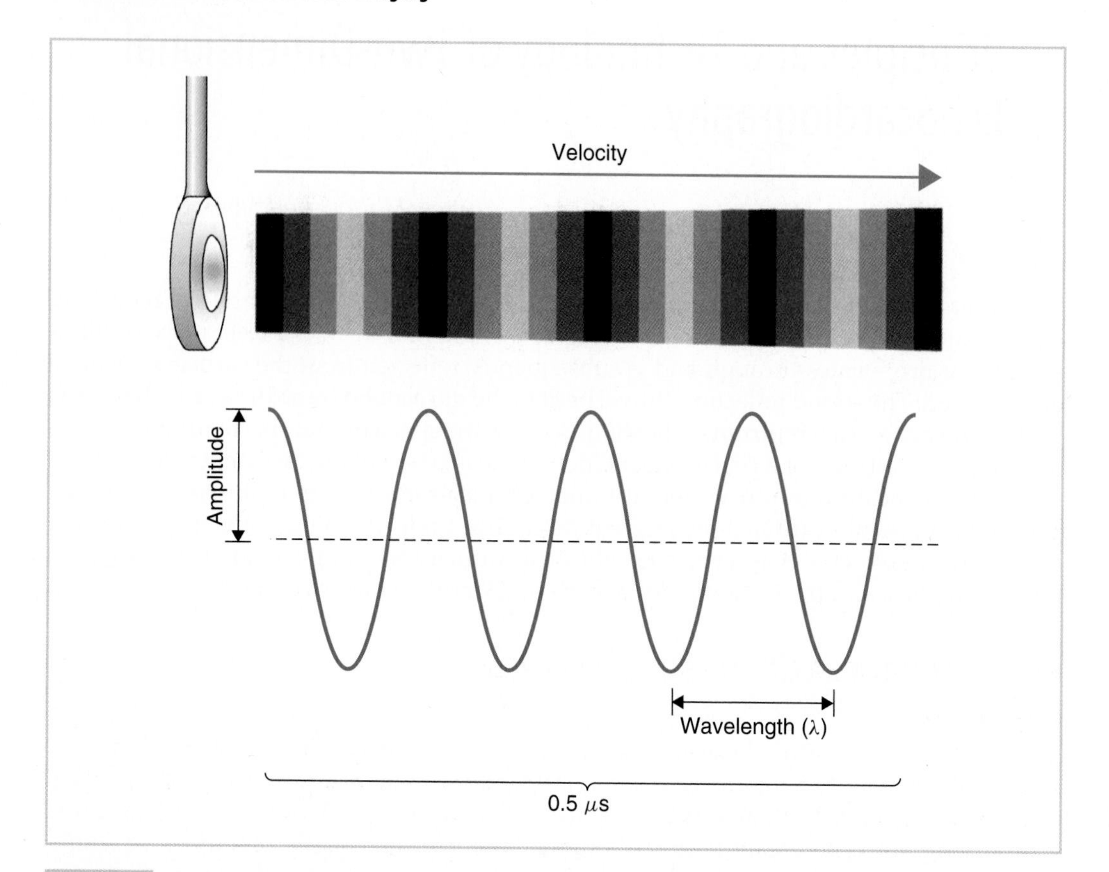

Figure 1.1. Sound wave. Vibrations of the ultrasound transducer create cycles of compression and rarefaction in adjacent tissue. The ultrasound energy is characterized by its amplitude, wavelength, frequency, and propagation velocity. In this example, four sound waves are shown in a period of 0.5 μs. The frequency can be calculated as 4 cycles divided by 0.5 μs and equals 8 MHz.

Frequency and Wavelength

Sound waves are also characterized by their **frequency** (f), or pitch, expressed in cycles per second, or Hertz (Hz), and by their **wavelength** (λ). These attributes have a significant impact on the depth of penetration of a sound wave in tissue and the image resolution of the ultrasound system.

Propagation Velocity

The travel velocity or propagation velocity of sound (v) *is determined solely by the medium through which it passes.* For example, the speed of sound in soft tissue is approximately 1,540 m/s. Velocity can be calculated as the product of wavelength and frequency:

$$\mathrm{v} = \lambda \times \mathrm{f} \qquad [2]$$

It becomes apparent that the wavelength and frequency are necessarily inversely related:

$$\lambda = \mathrm{v} \times 1/\mathrm{f} \qquad [3]$$

$$\lambda = (1{,}500\ \mathrm{m/s})/\mathrm{f} \qquad [4]$$

Table 1.1 lists the corresponding sound wavelengths and frequencies commonly used in clinical ultrasonography.

Table 1.1 Corresponding frequencies and wavelengths in soft tissue

Frequency (MHz)	Wavelength (mm)
1.25	1.20
2.5	0.60
5.0	0.30
7.5	0.20
10	0.15

What's So Special about Ultrasound?

Several favorable physical properties of ultrasound explain its usefulness in clinical imaging. **Ultrasound** is sound with frequencies greater than those of the audible range for humans (20,000 Hz). In clinical echocardiography, frequencies of 2 to 10 MHz are used. The high-frequency, short-wavelength ultrasound beam can be more easily manipulated, focused, and directed to a specific target. Image resolution also increases when higher frequency sound waves are used (see later).

INTERACTIONS OF SOUND AND TISSUE

The propagation, or passage, of a sound wave through the body is markedly affected by its interactions with the various tissues encountered. These interactions result in reflection, refraction, scattering, and attenuation of the ultrasound signal. The exact manner in which sound is affected by the various tissues it encounters determines the resulting appearance of the two-dimensional image **(Figure 1.2)**.

Reflection

Echocardiographic imaging depends on the transmission and subsequent reflection of ultrasound energy back to the transducer. A sound wave propagates through uniform tissue until it reaches another tissue type with different acoustic properties. At the tissue interface, the ultrasound energy undergoes a dramatic alteration, after which it can be reflected back toward the transducer or transmitted into the next tissue, often in a direction that deviates from the original course. Precisely how the ultrasound beam will be affected is predicted by factoring the acoustic properties of the tissues that create the interface and the angle at which the ultrasound beam strikes this interface.

THE TISSUE INTERFACE: ACOUSTIC IMPEDANCE

An important acoustic property of a tissue is its capacity for transmitting sound, known as *acoustic impedance* (Z). This property is largely related to the **density** (ρ) of the material and the speed which ultrasound travel (v):

$$Z = \rho \times \mathrm{v} \qquad [5]$$

As seen in **Table 1.2**, denser materials such as bone and fluids effectively transmit ultrasound, whereas air and lung tissue have a low level of acoustic impedance and are poor transmitters of sound energy. This property explains why an amplification system is required even for a small lecture hall, yet whales can hear sound over great expanses of the ocean.

When sound reaches an interface of two tissues of similar acoustic impedance, the ultrasound beam travels across the interface largely undisturbed. When the tissues differ

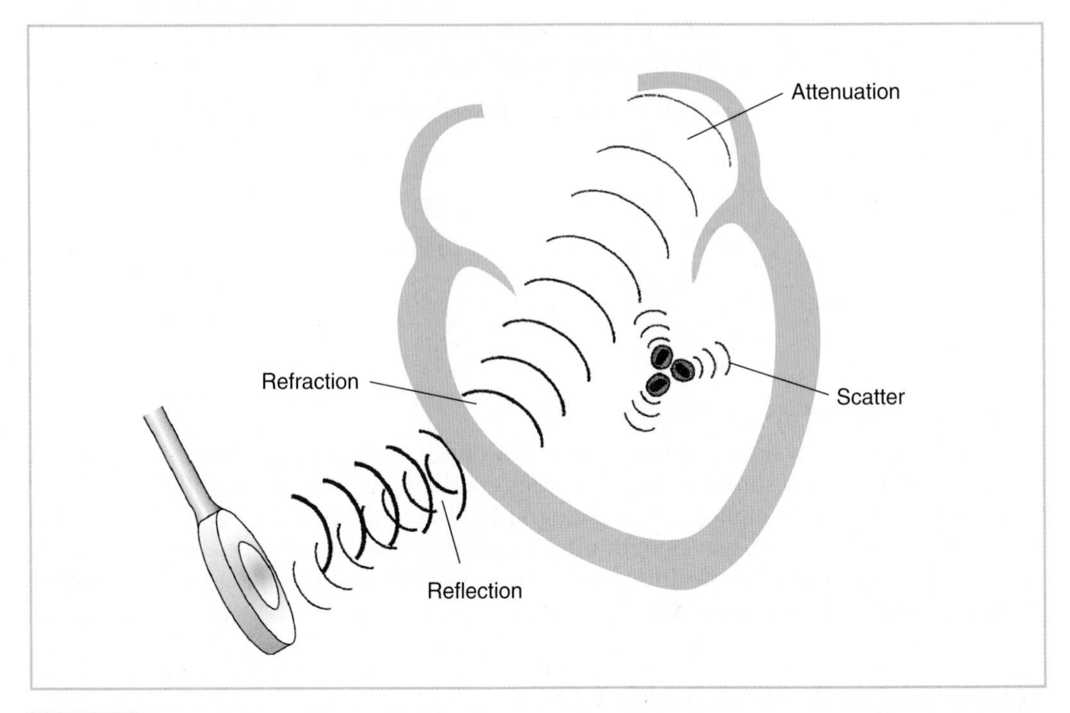

Figure 1.2. Interactions of sound and tissue. Traveling through various tissues, sound energy is altered by four major events. Specular *reflection* creates strong echoes directed back toward the transducer. *Refraction* bends the ultrasound beam, directing it in a new path. As the ultrasound beam travels deeper in tissue, *attenuation* occurs as the beam is dispersed and the sound energy is converted to heat. *Scattering* reflections from small objects such as red cells disperse the sound energy in all directions.

in impedance, a percentage of the ultrasound energy is **reflected** and the remainder is **transmitted.** *The larger the absolute difference in the levels of acoustic impedance across the interface, the greater the percentage of the ultrasound energy that is reflected.* Reflection can be calculated by using the reflection coefficient (R):

$$\text{Reflection coefficient} = \frac{(Z_2 - Z_1)^2}{(Z_1 + Z_2)^2} \quad [6]$$

Table 1.2 Acoustic properties of various tissues

Tissue/medium	Speed of sound (m/s)	Acoustic impedance (kg/m^{2}s x 10^6)	Attenuation coefficient (cm^{-1} at 1 MHz)	Half-power distance (cm at 2.5 MHz)
Air	330	0.00004	—	0.08
Lung	600	0.26	—	0.05
Fat	1,460	1.35	0.04–0.09	—
Water	1,480	1.52	0.0003	380
Blood	1,560	1.62	0.02	15
Muscle	1,600	1.7	0.25–0.35	0.6–1
Bone	4,080	7.80	—	0.7–0.8

The reflective properties of an interface are key factors in the imaged appearance of a structure. *When the absolute difference between the levels of acoustic impedance of the two interfacing media is large, as when soft tissue interfaces with air or bone, more energy is reflected back to the transducer.* These interfaces are represented by echo-dense or bright signals on the echogram. When the absolute difference is small, as when soft tissue interfaces with soft tissue, the interface will not appear as bright and may even be echolucent or dark.

SPECULAR AND SCATTERING REFLECTORS

The reflection of sound is also greatly affected by the size and surface of the tissue. Two types of reflection, specular and scattered, are commonly encountered.

Specular reflection occurs when a sound wave encounters a large object with a smooth surface. Such surfaces act like an acoustic mirror, generating strong reflections that travel away from the interface at an angle equal and opposite to that at which the ultrasound beam traveled to the interface. Reflection is maximal when the angle of incidence is 90 degrees—that is, the ultrasound beam and the object are perpendicular to each another. With an angle of incidence other than 90 degrees, less energy is reflected back to the transducer. Because of the important effect of strong specular reflection on image quality, echocardiographers adjust the position of the TEE transducer so that the direction of its beam is perpendicular to the cardiac structure of interest.

Scattering reflection occurs when an ultrasound beam encounters small or irregularly shaped surfaces. Such small objects, such as red blood cells, scatter ultrasound energy in all directions, so that far less energy is reflected back to the transducer than in the case of a specular reflector. This type of reflection is the basis of the Doppler analysis of red blood cell movement.

Both types of reflection contribute to the two-dimensional image. Although the strongest signals and best images are obtained from interfaces that are perpendicular to the beam orientation, cardiac tissue is to a large extent irregular and nonlinear in shape. Therefore, a significant component of the reflected energy comes from scattering off the smaller irregular components of tissue. An example is imaging of the lateral and septal walls of the left ventricle from esophageal windows. Although the ventricular walls are parallel to the ultrasound beam, they can be imaged as a result of both specular reflection and scattering off the irregular surfaces of the myocardium. However, the total amount of ultrasound returning to the transducer is low, which accounts for the poor quality of images, which often include dark spots called *echo dropout*. Adjusting the transducer angle or using a different echocardiographic window to orient the beam more perpendicular to the structure of interest will often dramatically improve image quality.

Refraction

The portion of the ultrasound beam that is not reflected propagates through the interface, but its direction is often altered, or refracted. Refraction is most pronounced when the difference in sound velocities in the two tissues is large and the angle of incidence is acute. When the angle of incidence is 90 degrees, or when the difference in levels of acoustic impedance is minimal, refraction does not occur because the ultrasound energy either is reflected or continues to travel in the same direction.

Refraction is an important factor in the formation of artifacts. Although the ultrasound beam may proceed in an altered direction, the transducer does not recognize this change.

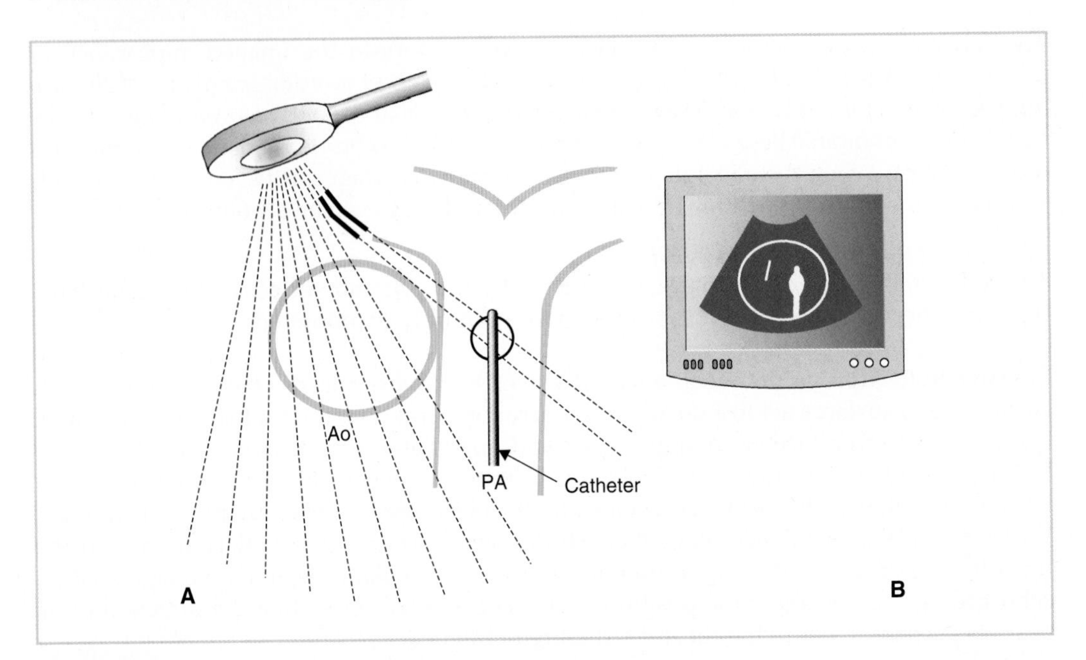

Figure 1.3. Refraction artifact. **A:** Refraction of a portion of the ultrasound beam in the near field (*solid line*) deflects the beam laterally where it interacts with a strong reflector, a pulmonary artery (PA) catheter. **B:** The transducer is unable to recognize that these scan lines have been refracted and incorrectly assumes that the returning reflections have originated from the original course of the beam. Echocardiography display illustrates the resulting artifact as the reflections from the PA catheter are mistakenly positioned within the aorta (Ao).

Consequently, the refracted energy may interface with a cardiac structure outside the *intended* scanning field. The reflected energy from this interface returns to the transducer, which then incorrectly displays the structure alongside structures detected by the beam in its original course **(Figure 1.3)**. Altering the viewing angle so that the ultrasound energy is perpendicular to the area of interest minimizes refraction and any resultant artifact.

Attenuation

In addition to being reflected and refracted from tissue interfaces, the ultrasound signal is altered as it travels through uniform tissue. Most notable is the steady loss (i.e., attenuation) in transmitted intensity as a consequence of dispersion and absorption. The attenuation in ultrasound energy caused by dispersion and absorption result in less energy returning to the transducer, and subsequently a weaker signal on the display with a poor signal to noise ratio.

Dispersion occurs as the ultrasound beam diverges over a greater area in the far field. In addition, because the cellular structure of tissue is irregular, scattering further disperses the ultrasound energy. The amount of scattering varies greatly with tissue type.

Absorption occurs as frictional forces convert ultrasound energy into heat. Because friction is related to the level of tissue movement, it is not surprising that the higher the frequency of the signal and the greater the distance traveled, the greater the absorption **(Figure 1.4)**. The dependence of attenuation on frequency and distance is reflected in the **attenuation coefficient** (dB/cm/MHz), which allows for a comparison of the degree of attenuation

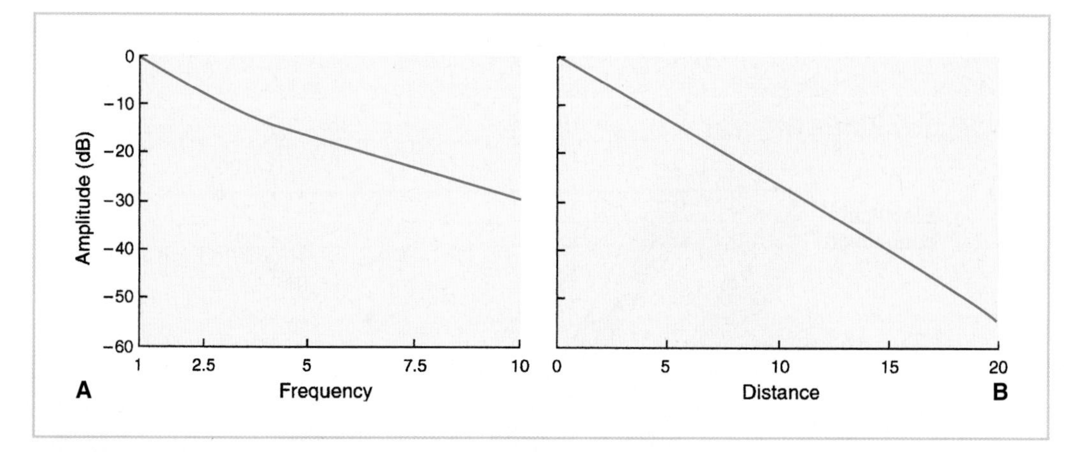

Figure 1.4. Attenuation of ultrasound. The effects of transducer frequency and distance on signal strength are plotted in decibels. **A:** The lower-frequency signals are less attenuated. **B:** The amplitude of a 1-MHz signal traveling through cardiac tissue is plotted. Signals reaching the far field can be more than 60 dB less than those lying close to the transducer. These effects warrant careful selection of the transducer frequency, imaging view, and gain settings to mitigate attenuation.

between tissue types. The penetration of ultrasound can also be expressed by the **half-power distance** specific for each tissue, which expresses the distance sound will travel until half of its original energy is lost. The acoustic properties of various tissues are summarized in **Table 1.2**.

As a result of these phenomena, the returning echoes from deeper structures are weakened. To decrease the negative effects of attenuation during an examination, echocardiographers may choose to use a lower-frequency signal (e.g., a 2.5- instead of a 7.5-MHz transducer frequency) and view the structure from a window either closer to the structure of interest or that avoids a strong near field reflector (e.g., prosthetic valve). In addition, the incoming signal can be enhanced by adjusting the gain controls to amplify the weakened returning signals. These adjustments are discussed in greater detail in Chapter 21.

TRANSDUCER DESIGN AND BEAM FORMATION

Transducer Components

The transducers used in echocardiography systems create a brief pulse of ultrasound that is transmitted into tissue **(Figure 1.5)**. To achieve this goal, most TEE transducer designs use the following components:

1. A *ceramic piezoelectric crystal*, which acts as an ultrasonic vibrator and receiver
2. *Electrodes*, which both conduct electric energy to stimulate the piezoelectric crystal and record the voltage from returning echoes
3. *Backing*, which acts to dampen the vibrations of the crystal rapidly
4. *Insulation*, which prevents unwanted vibration of the transducer from standing waves or extraneous incoming waves
5. A *faceplate*, which optimizes the acoustic contact between the piezoelectric crystal and the esophagus. The faceplate may also include an acoustic lens to focus the beam

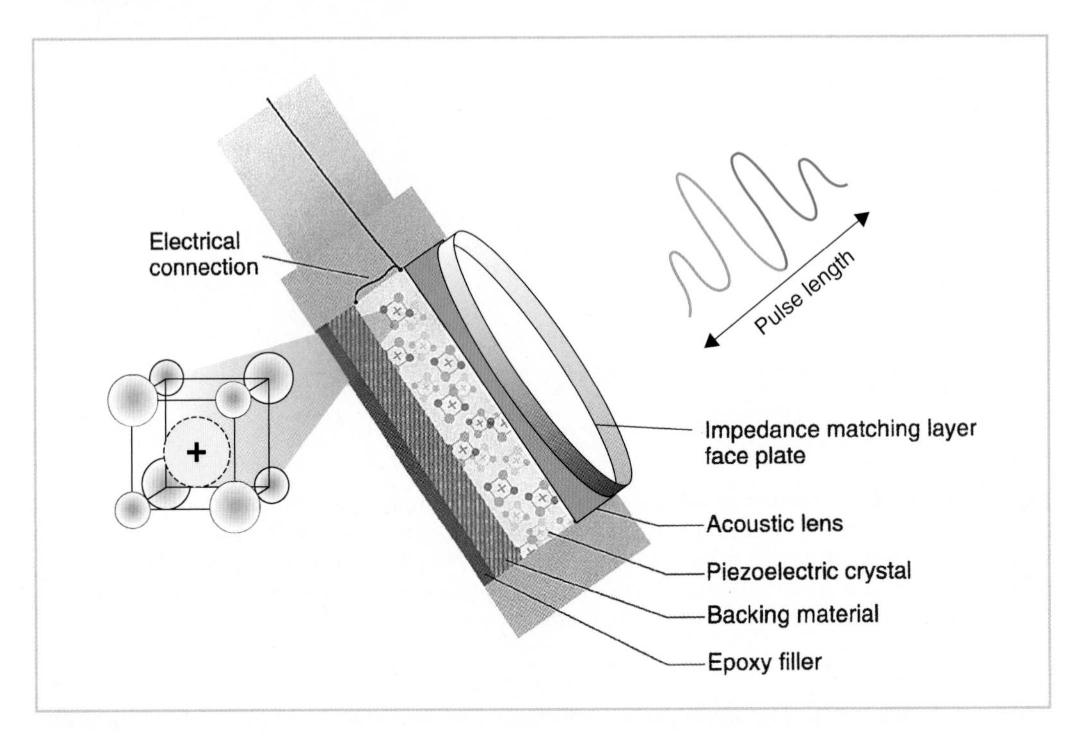

Figure 1.5. Transducer components: creating a sound pulse. A brief transmission of alternating current from the *electric connector* causes charged particles within the matrix of the piezoelectric crystal to vibrate. The *backing material* helps to dampen the crystal vibrations quickly, keeping the pulse length short; in this example, it is four wavelengths. An *acoustic lens* aids in focusing the sound energy. The *faceplate* contains layers of material that match the acoustic impedance of the esophagus, to avoid unwanted reflections and ensure excellent sound transmission. *Epoxy filler* secures the working components to the probe.

The following sections detail the inner workings of the modern ultrasound transducer and their effects on the transmitted sound beam and the echocardiographic image.

Formation of Ultrasound Waves: The Piezoelectric Crystal

The heart of the transducer consists of a piezoelectric crystal, which contains polarized molecules trapped within a matrix. The formation of the sound wave used in echocardiography is based on the principle of **piezoelectricity.** When stimulated by alternating electric current, polarized particles within the crystals matrix vibrate, generating ultrasound. Conversely, when an ultrasound wave strikes the crystal, the resulting vibrations of the polarized particles generate an alternating electric current. Therefore, a piezoelectric crystal can function as both a transmitter and a receiver of ultrasound. This process is the hallmark of piezoelectricity—that is, the transformation of electric energy into mechanical energy and the reverse transformation of mechanical energy into electric energy.

For imaging purposes, the transducer emits a brief burst of ultrasound. Typically, two-dimensional transducers emit a sound pulse of two to four wavelengths. As illustrated in **Figure 1.6**, the shorter the length of the sound pulse, the better the axial resolution of the system. Therefore, the shorter the wavelength, the shorter the resulting pulse length and the greater the axial resolution.

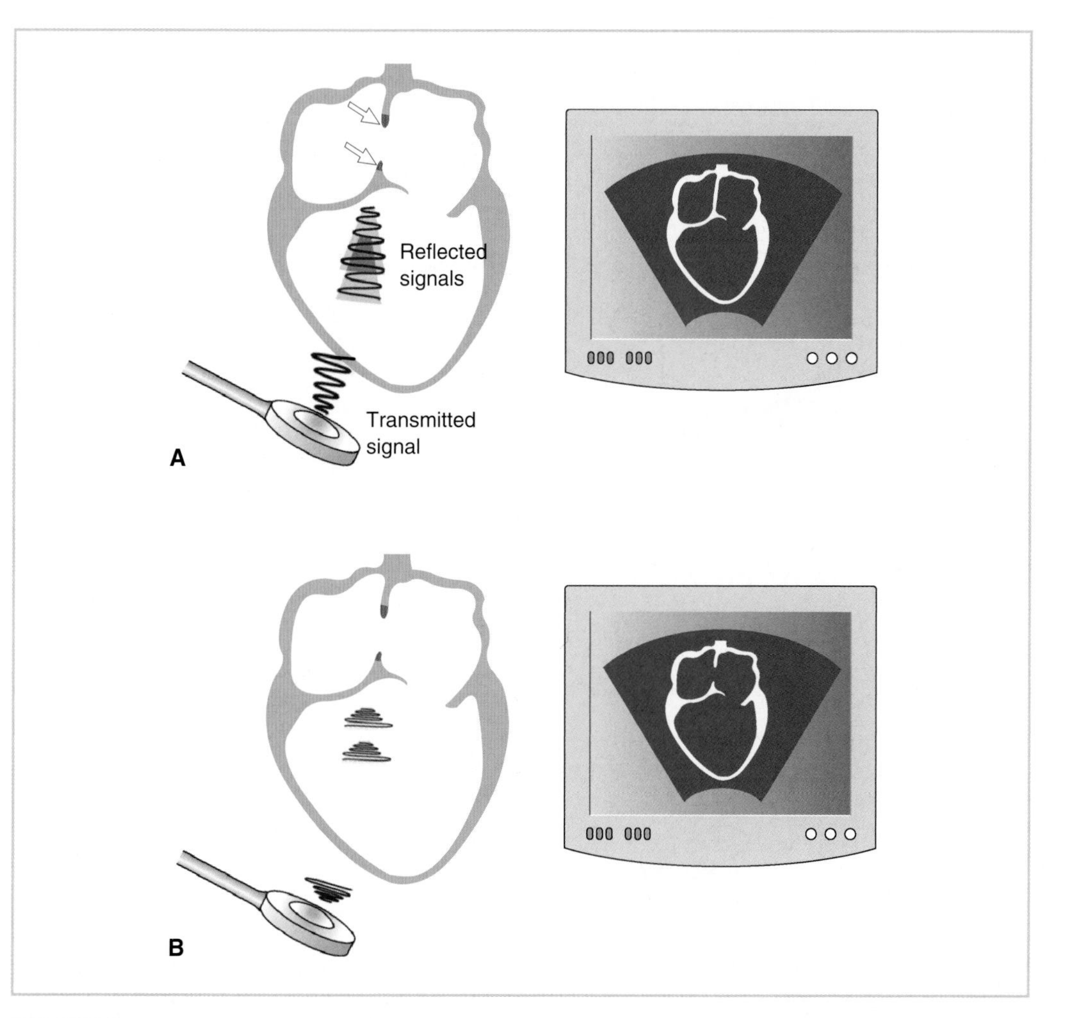

Figure 1.6. Effect of pulse length on axial resolution. **A:** The transducer emits a long sound pulse. Because the length of this pulse is greater than the length of the atrial septal defect (*arrows*), the reflections from the two tips of atrial septum are smeared and the defect cannot be resolved. Consequently, the resulting two-dimensional echocardiographic display (*right*) does not show the abnormality. **B:** The pulse length has been shortened and is now less than the length of the atrial septal defect. The reflections from each interface are clearly identifiable, and the resulting display (*right*) shows the defect.

The Three-Dimensional Ultrasound Beam

NEAR AND FAR FIELDS

The ultrasound transducer emits a three-dimensional ultrasound beam similar to the beam of a flashlight **(Figure 1.7)**. The physical dimensions of this beam determine the following:

1. The specific area of the heart examined
2. The intensity distribution of ultrasound energy
3. The lateral (side-to-side) and elevational (top-to-bottom) resolution of the system

Narrower beams are preferred because they improve resolution, increase the intensity of returning echoes, and reduce artifact. Most commonly, ultrasound beams have either a

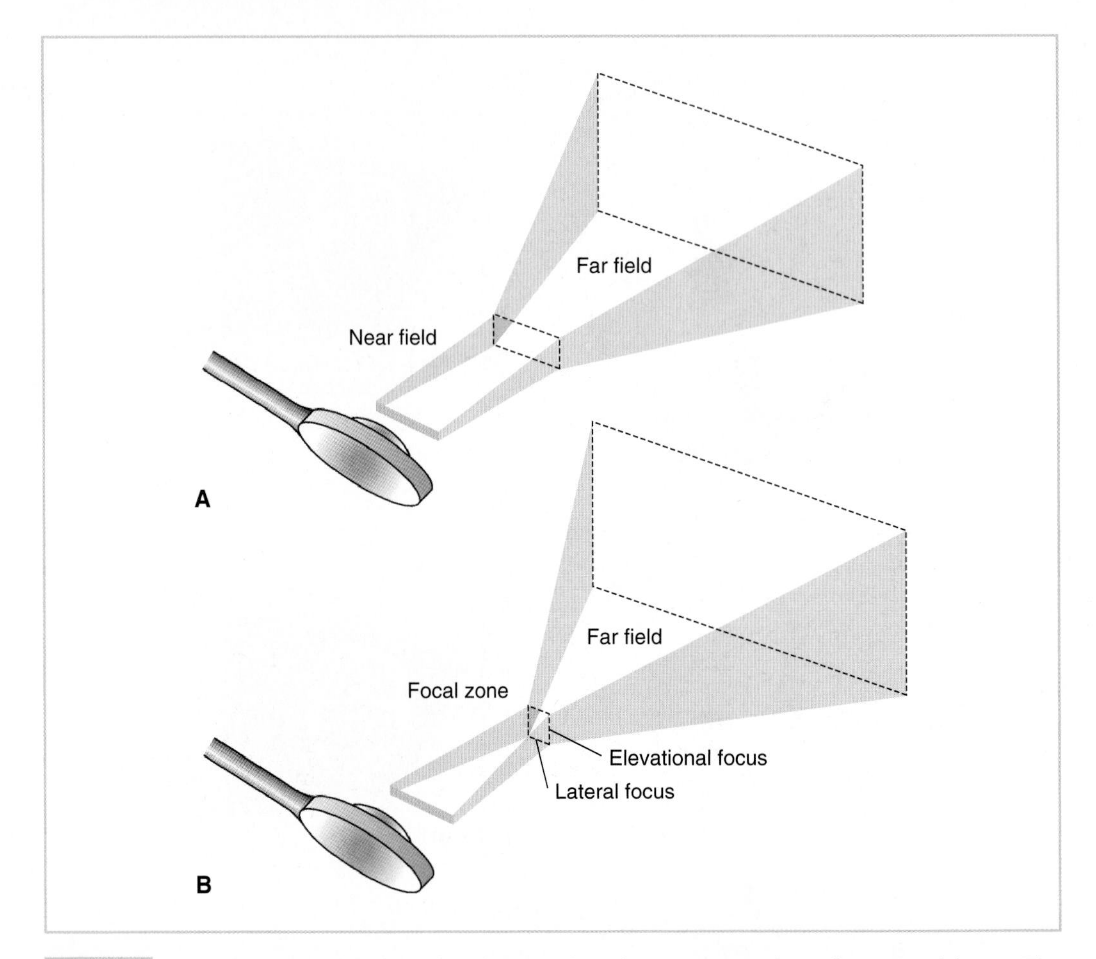

Figure 1.7. Three-dimensional beam. The ultrasound probe projects a three-dimensional beam. The dimensions of this projection have important effects on imaging resolution and artifact. Typically, a narrow profile is preferred. **A:** Unfocused beam. The beam is narrow in the near field and then diverges in the far field. **B:** Focused beam. Focusing has resulted in a narrower beam in both the lateral and elevational planes, so that the imaging resolution of structures in the focal zone is improved. Distal to the focal zone, the beam rapidly diverges, and the images of structures in this area will be of lower quality.

disk or rectangular shape and comprise two main zones: the **near field** (**Fresnel**) and **far field** (**Fraunhofer**) **zones.** Beam manipulation and image resolution are greatest within the near field. Also, ultrasound energy is more concentrated within this zone, yielding stronger echoes and better imaging.

In the near field zone, the ultrasound beam is narrow. The length of the near field zone is proportional to the diameter (D) of the transducer face and inversely proportional to the wavelength:

$$L_{\mathrm{n}} = D^2/4\lambda \qquad [7]$$

Distal to the near field zone, the ultrasound beam diverges, forming the far field zone. The angle of divergence (θ) is inversely related to the diameter (D) of the transducer face:

$$\sin\theta = 1.22\ \lambda/D \qquad [8]$$

Accordingly, larger transducers with high-frequency (small λ) signals produce the most desirable beam profile: a long, narrow near field and a less divergent far field.

FOCUSING

Focusing can further narrow the ultrasound beam. This is accomplished in three ways, as follows:

1. By creating a concave shape in the piezoelectric crystal
2. By gluing an acoustic lens to the front of the crystal
3. Electronically with the use of phased array transducers

The narrow beam at the focal zone enhances imaging at this location. However, the beam diverges widely distal to the focal zone, reducing the intensity of the ultrasound energy and impairing imaging of the far field. The ability of modern echocardiography systems to allow the echocardiographer to adjust the depth of the focal zone selectively provides a means to optimize image quality.

ELECTRONIC BEAM FOCUSING: THE PHASED ARRAY

Modern echocardiography systems allow the echocardiographer to adjust the depth of the focal zone selectively to optimize image quality. A single element transducer emits a wave front that diverges in a hemispheric pattern. By aligning several crystals side by side in a *linear array*, the interaction of the individual sound waves emitted by each crystal creates a narrow, forwardly directed wave front **(Figure 1.8A)**. The beam's shape can be focused further by electrically activating the crystals at the ends of the array before those located at the center creating a concave wave front thereby focusing the beam at a selected distance from the transducer face **(Figure 1.8B)**.

It is important to be cognizant of both the advantages and disadvantages of selecting the focus depth of the beam. As is discussed next, beam shape is of prime importance in determining the resolution of an imaging system.

Resolution

Three parameters are evaluated when assessing the resolution of an ultrasound system: the resolution of objects lying along the axis of the ultrasound beam (axial resolution), the resolution of objects horizontal to the beam's orientation (lateral resolution, and the resolution of objects lying vertical to the beam's orientation (elevational resolution).

AXIAL RESOLUTION

Axial resolution is the ability of the ultrasound system to identify two separate objects that lie along the path of the ultrasound beam axis. Axial resolution is determined by the *bandwidth* of the ultrasound pulse. The bandwidth is the resonant frequencies that are emitted about the center frequency. *High bandwidth pulses are best for axial resolution as they are characterized by high-frequency signals of short duration.* As seen in **Figure 1.6**, short pulses of high-frequency ultrasound offer the greatest axial resolution. A general rule is that the axial resolution of a system is approximately 1.5 times the wavelength of the system. Therefore, for a 7.5 MHz transducer axial resolution is 0.3 mm. Improved axial resolution does not come without a cost. The shorter the pulse, the lower its energy level, so that penetration and returning echoes are weaker. Similarly, high-frequency sound is quickly attenuated. Accordingly, the echocardiographer must select these parameters based on the imaging needs.

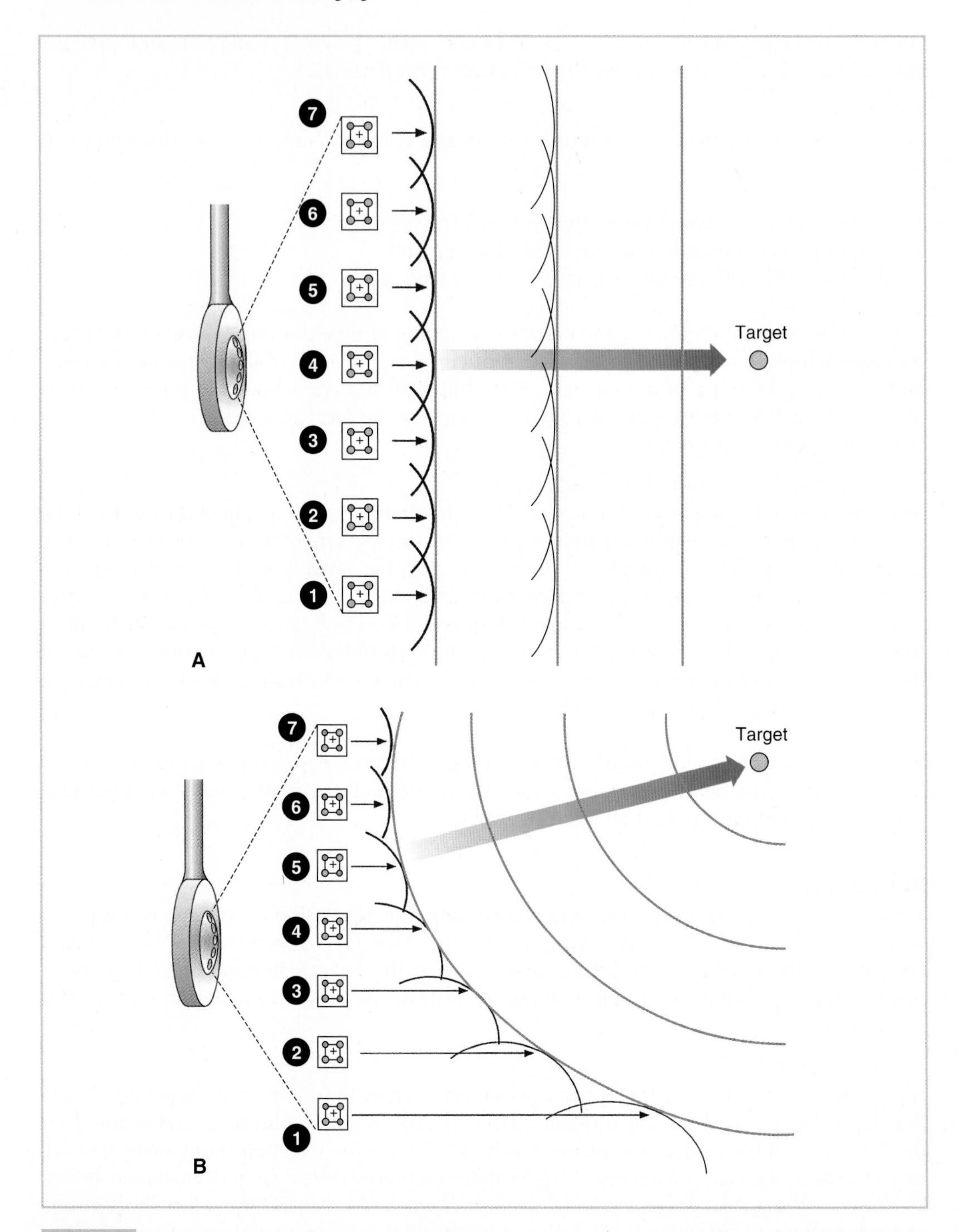

Figure 1.8. Phased array transducers. **A:** This illustration shows seven crystal elements in an array. The interactions of the individual hemispheric wave fronts create a flat, profiled, forward-directed wave front. **B:** Phased array transducer. Here, the crystals have been activated sequentially: crystal 1 first, followed by crystal 2, and so on. This causes the beam to be steered upward toward the target. Note that crystals 7 and 8 have been activated before crystal 6, creating a concave wave front to focus the energy of the beam at the target. The ability to steer electronically and focus the beam is a major advantage of the phased array system.

LATERAL (AZIMUTH) RESOLUTION

Lateral resolution is the ability of the ultrasound system to distinguish between objects that are horizontally aligned perpendicular to the path of the ultrasound beam. Beam width is a primary determinant of lateral resolution. Wide beams produce a "smeared" image of two such objects, whereas narrow beams can identify each object individually. Signal frequency and transducer size impact lateral resolution but for typical cardiac ultrasound transducers the beam width is approximated as depth/50 yielding at 10 cm of depth a beam width of approximately 2 mm.

ELEVATIONAL RESOLUTION

Elevational resolution is the ability of the ultrasound system to distinguish between objects that are vertically aligned and perpendicular to the emitted ultrasound beam. Although two-dimensional images appear to display a thin slice of cardiac anatomy, in actuality the information gathered from the entire thickness of the beam is averaged and displayed. For this reason, the thinner the ultrasound beam, the better the elevational resolution of the system **(Figure 1.7)**. Signal frequency and transducer size impact elevational resolution but a typical cardiac ultrasound transducer has a beam height approximated as depth/30. Accordingly, at 10 cm depth the beam height is approximately 3.3 mm. Note that axial resolution offers fidelity of 50% greater than that achieved in the lateral and elevational planes.

OPTIMIZING RESOLUTION

The interplay of the transducer size, signal frequency, and focal length and the distance of the structure of interest determine beam width and height. The beam is narrowest in the near field or focal zone and divergent in the far field. Resolution is therefore better in the near field and decreases in the far field. Factors that lengthen the near field, such as a higher transducer frequency and a larger transducer radius, improve lateral and elevational resolution. Focusing further decreases the width of the ultrasound beam and improves lateral and elevational resolution at the focal point. However, focusing often increases beam divergence distal to the focal zone, with an associated loss of lateral and elevational resolution. These factors explain why it is preferable to position a transducer with a relatively high frequency (smaller wavelength) close to the target of interest to optimize both lateral and elevational resolution. More precise measurements are made along the axial plane due to the superior resolution in this orientation.

Extraneous Sound Beams

SIDE LOBES

Unfortunately, in addition to the powerful forwardly directed beam of sound energy produced by linear array transducers, additional beams of sound are emitted that travel off axis to the main beam **(Figure 1.9)**. These extraneous beams of sound, called side lobes, significantly affect imaging quality because the transducer incorrectly processes their reflections as reflections of the main beam. Consequently, structures off axis to the imaging plane appear incorrectly located on the two-dimensional image.

GRATING LOBES

Grating lobes are side lobes generated with multielement array transducers. Each crystal of the linear array can be considered a point source of sound emission. When these individual sound waves meet in phase and off axis to the main beam (constructive interference), a grating lobe is created. The position of a grating lobe is predictable as it is related to the spacing of the crystals and the wavelength of the signal.

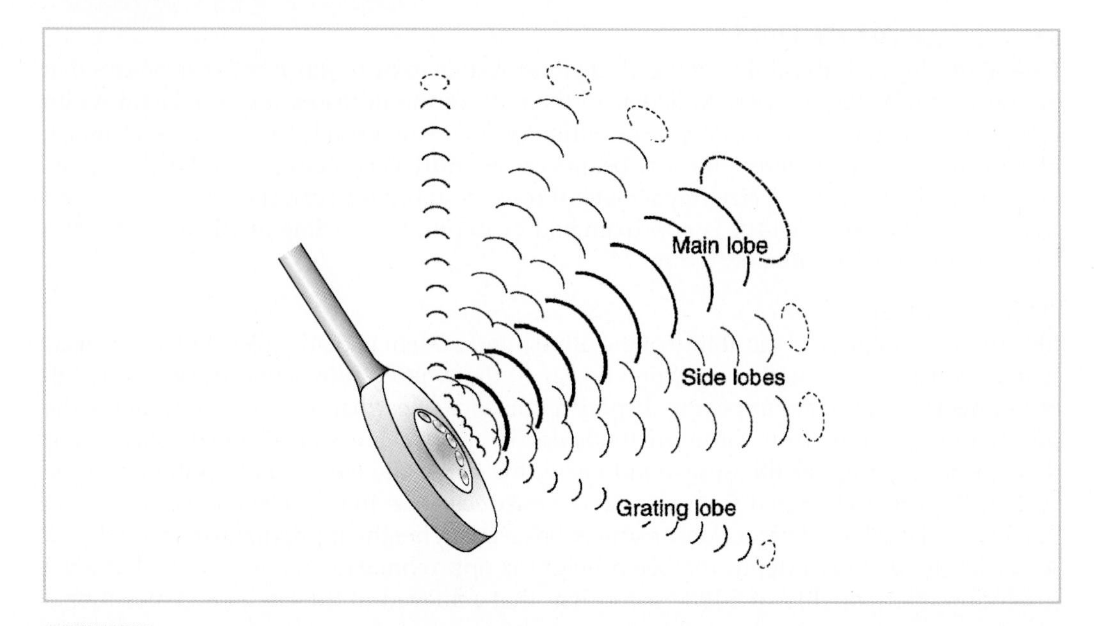

Figure 1.9. Side lobes. The sound energy emitted from ultrasound transducers has a typical pattern. Constructive interference of the individual wave fronts concentrates most of the energy on axis, in what is called the *main lobe*. However, constructive interference of individual wave fronts also causes lobes of energy to be directed off axis; these are known as *side lobes* and *grating lobes*. Reflections from these lobes reduce image quality and are a well-described source of imaging artifact.

SIDE LOBE ARTIFACTS

Both side and grating lobes contain less energy than the main beam and usually do not significantly affect the echocardiographic image. However, when these lobes of energy contact a highly reflective surface (catheter, prosthesis, calcium), sufficient energy can be reflected back to the transducer to create an artifact. The transducer believes these reflections have arisen from the main forwardly directed field and mistakenly displays them together with those from the main beam. To reduce such artifacts, the echocardiographer should minimize gain settings to decrease the likelihood of strong reflections from the weaker lobes. If they persist, to differentiate an artifact from a real structure, the field should be imaged from another window. An artifact is not likely to be reproduced in multiple planes.

SIGNAL RECEPTION AND PROCESSING

The conversion of reflected ultrasound signals into high-fidelity cardiac images is a complex process in which returning ultrasound pulses are received, electronically processed, and displayed. Understanding the basic principles of these steps is essential both to optimize image acquisition and avoid misdiagnosis caused by artifacts.

Cycling of Transducer Transmit and Receive Modes

The ultrasound transducer acts first as a transmitter and then as a receiver of sound signals. An oscillator signals the discharge of electric current to the piezoelectric crystal, thereby determining the rate of sound pulse transmission. After emitting a short burst of ultrasound, the transducer switches to receive mode to listen for the returning ultrasound reflections from the tissues.

Electrical Processing

AMPLIFICATION: GAIN CONTROLS

The echoes that return to the transducer are converted from sound energy to a radiofrequency electric signal by the piezoelectric crystal. A large portion of the sound energy is lost as the ultrasound wave travels, and the electric signal must be amplified before it can be further processed. This amplification is controlled by the **system gain** control. Furthermore, because signal attenuation is proportional to distance traveled, signals from distant structures can be 12 to 30 dB weaker than those from closer structures. **Time gain compensation** allows the echocardiographer to selectively amplify signals from structures of varying distances from the transducer. With this feature, signals from distant targets and weaker reflectors are boosted so that their amplitudes more closely match those from nearby structures.

COMPRESSION AND DISPLAY

The amplified and time gain–compensated electric signal must be processed before it can be displayed on a monitor. The radiofrequency signal has a large dynamic range of more than 100 dB, far too large for monitors to display. To reduce the dynamic range, two processes are commonly used. First, **reject** circuits filter out low-amplitude signals, which typically represent background noise or speckle. The remainder of the signal is then **compressed,** so that both low- and high-amplitude components can be displayed. **Digital scan conversion** then converts the electric signal into a standard video format for display.

PREPROCESSING AND POSTPROCESSING

The digital scan converter requires the analog electric signal to be digitized so it can be processed and then converted to an analog video format. This process offers two important opportunities for the echocardiographer to control the display of the imaging data. By adjusting the **preprocessing settings**, which affect the analog-to-digital conversion, and the **postprocessing settings**, which affect the conversion to analog video format, the echocardiographer can modify the appearance of the displayed image. These adjustments can be used, for example, to emphasize edge detection versus tissue texture or to improve the delineation of weaker reflectors. Again, the choice of these settings is dictated by the examination and the personal preferences of the echocardiographer.

DISPLAY FORMATS

The Golden Rule: Time Is Distance

Ultrasonic imaging is based on the amplitude and time delay of the reflected signals **(Figure 1.10)**. Because the velocity in tissue is relatively constant, only the distance of the structure from the transducer alters the time required for the ultrasound wave to travel to and from the reflected structure:

$$\text{Distance} = \text{velocity} \times \text{time} \quad [9]$$

As sound travels at a rate of 1,540 m/s through soft tissue, the round trip travel time for each centimeter of separation between transducer and reflector is calculated as:

$$\text{Travel time} = 13\ \mu\text{s/cm} \quad [10]$$

By timing the interval between transmission and return of the reflections, the echocardiography system can precisely calculate the location of a structure.

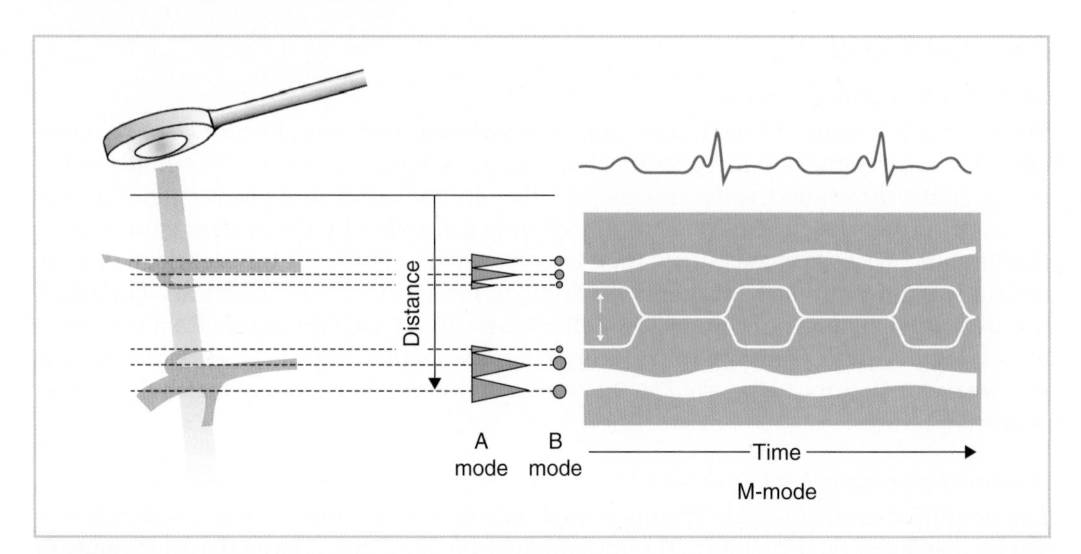

Figure 1.10. Display formats. The ultrasound beam is directed through the aortic valve leaflets. Amplitude mode (A-mode) display shows the resulting reflections as horizontal spikes. In the brightness mode (B-mode) display, the spikes are replaced with pixels of varying brightness. Motion mode (M-mode) shows sequential B-mode frames to capture cardiac motion. The "boxcar" pattern depicts normal opening and closing of the aortic valve leaflets.

Amplitude Mode

The original display format is a**mplitude mode** (A-mode), in which the amplitudes of the returning signals are represented as a series of horizontal spikes along the vertical axis of the display. The horizontal spikes correspond to the distance of the reflecting tissue and the strength of the returning echoes.

Brightness Mode

Current imaging is based on b**rightness mode** (B-mode) technology. Instead of horizontal spikes, the amplitudes of the returning echoes are represented as pixels of varying brightness along the vertical axis of the display. The brightness correlates with the strength of the returning signal.

Motion Mode

Motion mode (M-mode) adds temporal information to B-mode by displaying a series of collected B-mode images. M-mode echocardiography provides a one-dimensional, "ice pick" view through the heart and updates the B-mode images at a very high rate, allowing dynamic real-time imaging. *It is important to realize that before it emits the next pulse of energy, the transducer element must first receive the reflected energy of the previously emitted pulse.* The frequency at which the B-mode images are updated is the **frame rate and** is calculated as 1 sec/round trip travel time. The frame rate with M-mode imaging is very high (>2,000 frames/second), affording a superior display of dynamic motion in comparison with other techniques. However, M-mode imaging displays only axial motion and provides a limited view of cardiac anatomy. Because of its superior dynamics and axial resolution, M-mode is the best mode for examining the timing of cardiac events when displayed with the electrocardiogram.

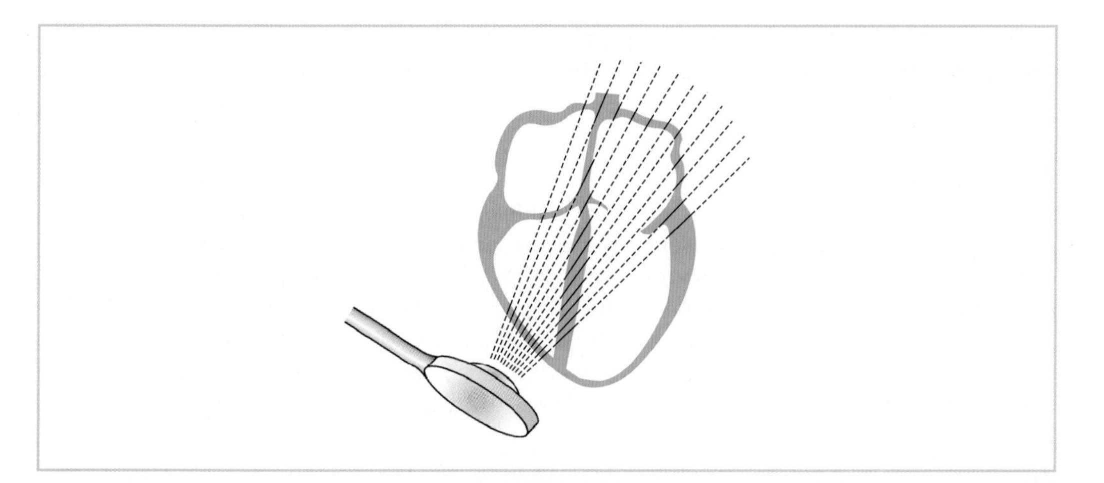

Figure 1.11. Scan lines. Illustration of the arced sector from a phased array two-dimensional echocardiogram. Each *dotted line* represents an individual B-mode (brightness mode) scan line. Any structure that interacts with a scan line will create reflections (*dark highlight*); however, structures that lie between the scan lines are not interrogated, and the echocardiography system averages the neighboring signals to fill in this defect. Accordingly, the closer the scan lines, the better the image quality. With a phased array scan, the gap between scan lines increases with the distance from the transducer.

Two-dimensional Echocardiography

Two-dimensional echocardiography is a modification of B-mode echocardiography and the mainstay of the echocardiographic examination. Instead of repeatedly firing ultrasound pulses in a single direction, the transducer in two-dimensional echocardiography sequentially directs the ultrasound pulses across a sector of the cardiac anatomy. In this way, two-dimensional imaging can display a tomographic section of the cardiac anatomy, and unlike M-mode, it can show shape and lateral motion **(Figure 1.11)**.

TWO-DIMENSIONAL SCAN SYSTEMS

Both electronic and mechanical systems have been developed to sweep the beam across an area of interest. Most commonly, the transducer consists of multiple crystals (or elements) aligned next to one another in a **linear array.** The individual sound waves from each crystal combine to provide a unified wave front that can be better focused and directed than that of a single crystal. Furthermore, with alterations in the timing of the electric activation of each crystal in the array, hence the term *phased array*, the beam can actually be steered without the transducer itself being moved. The advantages of an electronic system over a mechanical one, including an absence of moving parts and easy manipulation (steering, focusing, narrowing) of the ultrasound beam, have made it the dominant technology in echocardiography scanners. The two commonly used electronic scanning systems in medical ultrasound are the linear scanners and sector scanners.

Linear Scanners

The linear scanner uses a long transducer composed of several crystals. Groups of crystals are activated sequentially from one end of the transducer to the other. The firing of each group of crystals images the structures directly in front of them. With sequential firing of the groups of crystals, the anatomic features under the entire transducer are imaged.

However, the disadvantage of this approach is that the transducer face must be large enough to cover a broad anatomic area effectively. The linear array is commonly used in vascular and obstetric applications.

Sector Scanners

The phased array sector scanner is the most commonly used in echocardiography. This is an electronic system that by precisely timing the activation of the individual transducer elements is able to sweep the sound beam in an arc across a predetermined field. With activation of the transducer elements in different sequences, the ultrasound beam in the phased array system can be easily narrowed, steered, and focused **(Figure 1.8)**. The ability to direct a series of beams electronically over an arced sector also makes it possible to use the smaller transducer face required for TEE and transthoracic echocardiography.

CREATING THE TWO-DIMENSIONAL IMAGE

Imaging a Sector

To construct the two-dimensional image, the echocardiographic system records the B-mode data from the first pulse, redirects the next beam, records the returning signals, and so on until the entire sector has been scanned. Typically, the scanner images a sector of 30 to 90 degrees. The orientation of each B-mode line (also called the *scan line*) is recorded so that the information can be displayed in the correct position on the display screen. The two-dimensional scanner then repeats the entire process to update the image and capture motion. Each image created by a sector scan is a **frame.** Two-dimensional imaging typically requires 100 to 200 scan lines per frame, resulting in a **frame rate** of 30 to 60 frames/second. Because this rate is significantly slower than that of M-mode echocardiography, two-dimensional imaging is not as precise for demonstrating dynamic motion or the timing of cardiac events.

Image Quality and Dynamic Motion

Two-dimensional imaging is characterized by several factors that are operator controlled and have important (and often opposing) effects on image quality and dynamic motion. The proper settings vary depending on the particular examination at hand.

The **pulse repetition frequency** is the rate at which sound pulses are transmitted per second. The greater the pulse repetition frequency, the greater the number of scan lines that are emitted in a given period of time. The pulse repetition frequency is inversely related to the sector depth because a longer period of time is required for the ultrasound to travel increased distances.

The **frame rate** is the frequency at which the sector is rescanned. Each frame consists of one or two scans across the sector of interest. The information from two sweeps can be interlaced to improve image quality. A high frame rate improves the capture of movement. Typically, a frame rate greater than 30/s allows the dynamic representation of some relatively fine movements (e.g., intermediate positions of the aortic valve). The frame rate is critically dependent on the sector depth, which determines the time required for each scan line to be received, and sector width, which increases the number of scan lines to be processed. Consequently, increases in the sector size and depth come at the cost of a decreased frame rate.

The **scan line density,** calculated as the number of lines per degree of the sector, greatly affects the image quality. Line densities should be maintained at 1.5 to 2.2 lines per degree. Doubling the scan lines essentially doubles the lateral resolution. However, the cost is a decrease in the frame rate. The scan line density is calculated by dividing the number of scan lines per sweep by the angle of the sector. The greater the sector angle, the larger the area and the lower the line density. Because phased array transducers produce a fan-shaped sector, scan line density and hence lateral resolution is greater closer to the transducer and decreases in direct proportion to distance.

IMAGE QUALITY VERSUS DYNAMIC MOTION

It quickly becomes apparent that the echocardiographer must choose between the size of the imaging field and the frame rate. If the frame rate is high (100 frames/second), the number of scan lines per frame is reduced, resulting in a lower line density. Although the dynamics of the image may be excellent, the spatial image quality is decreased. We caution against the practice of assessing several structures in a single large view because it compromises both the dynamics and quality of the images. We recommend that the clinician focus each part of the examination on a given structure of interest and select the imaging plane that best delineates the structure in the near field. Motion can then be enhanced without costs in lateral resolution by decreasing the sector angle and depth. In situations in which the maximal frame rate is desired, M-mode should be considered. This results in a very dynamic image with a high level of axial resolution. For these reasons, M-mode echocardiography remains an important adjunct to both two-dimensional and color Doppler echocardiography.

SUMMARY

Two-dimensional echocardiography is based on the interaction of ultrasound and the patient. Between the generation of the ultrasound pulse and its subsequent reflection, reception, and display, a complex series of events takes place. Echocardiographers who ignore the physical realities of the imaging process will suffer two common causes of misdiagnosis: inadequate imaging and artifacts. However, expert echocardiographers, by applying an understanding of the principles involved and selecting the most appropriate views and machine settings, reliably optimize the imaging of a particular structure of interest. No patient or echocardiographic system is ideal. Rather, echocardiographers must compromise between conflicting imaging needs, such as between dynamic motion and the visual quality of an image, based on the primary diagnostic goal. We expand on the important relationship between the echocardiographer and the echocardiography machine in Chapter 21.

SUGGESTED READINGS

Geiser EA. Echocardiography: physics and instrumentation. In: Marcus ML, Skorton DJ, Schelbert AR, et al., eds. *Cardiac imaging*, 2nd ed. Philadelphia: WB Saunders, 1991.

Weyman A, ed. *Principles and practice of echocardiography*, 2nd ed. Philadelphia: Lea & Febiger, 1994:3–55.

QUESTIONS

1. All of the following statements regarding sound are true, except

a. Sound is a vibration in a physical medium.
b. Wavelength and frequency are inversely related.
c. The velocity of sound in soft tissue is relatively constant at 1,540 m/s.
d. Higher sound frequencies result in less absorption.

2. Which of the following statements regarding reflection of ultrasound is true?

a. Two-dimensional echocardiographic imaging consists of both specular and scattering reflections.
b. Scattered reflections come from larger, regular surfaces.
c. Specular reflections are greatest when the ultrasound beam and tissue interface is perpendicular to the beam.
d. Maximal reflection occurs at a tissue interface with an acoustic mismatch of zero.
e. Both **a** and **c.**

3. All of the following statements regarding reflection of the ultrasound beam are true, except

a. Reflection occurs at a tissue interface or area of acoustic mismatch.
b. Reflection is directly related to the absolute difference between the levels of acoustic impedance of two tissues.
c. The ultrasound beam is reflected at an angle equal and opposite to that of the incident beam.
d. Air is highly reflective because of its high acoustic impedance.

4. All of the following statements regarding attenuation are true, except

a. It is caused by friction.
b. It is caused by scattered reflection.
c. It is caused by dispersion.
d. Fluids rapidly absorb ultrasound energy.

5. All the following statements regarding wavelength and frequency are true, except

a. Resolution is improved with higher-frequency sound waves.
b. Resolution is improved with higher wavelengths.
c. Lower frequency sound waves are absorbed less than higher-frequency sound waves.
d. Higher-frequency sound waves create longer near fields.

6. All of the following statements regarding the ultrasound beam are true, except

a. It is more concentrated in the near field.
b. Width determines the axial resolution.
c. Width determines the lateral resolution.
d. Focusing increases far field divergence.

7. Resolution

a. Is improved with focusing.
b. Is better with high-frequency/low-wavelength sound.
c. Is better in the near field.
d. Consists of axial, lateral, and elevational components.
e. Is all of the above.

8. All of the following statements are true, except

a. Narrow ultrasound beams improve lateral resolution.

b. Higher frequencies increase the resolution and imaging of deeper structures.
c. Focusing improves resolution in the near field but creates a more divergent beam thereafter.
d. Beam width is related to the frequency of the sound wave.
e. Resolution is best in the near field.

9. All of the following statements regarding echocardiographic displays are true, except

a. A-mode imaging uses horizontal spikes along a vertical axis to represent tissue character and axial position.
b. M-mode imaging is characterized by high-resolution axial imaging and superdynamic display of cardiac motion.
c. M-mode imaging displays not only axial (vertical) motion but also lateral relations.
d. Two-dimensional imaging displays lateral and axial relations.
e. Two-dimensional imaging occurs at a much lower frame rate than M-mode imaging.

10. Which of the following statements is true with respect to scan systems?

a. An array consists of a single transducer element that is mechanically moved across the field of interest.
b. A linear array scan emits a narrow beam from a small transducer face, so that it is ideal for imaging through small apertures (echocardiographic windows).
c. A phased array scan sweeps the ultrasound beam over a fan-shaped sector.
d. Neither phased array nor linear array scans are subject to side or grating lobes.
e. Electronic activation of the multiple elements of a phased array scanner allows steering of the ultrasound beam, but not focusing.

Answers appear at the back of the book.

2 Two-Dimensional Examination*

Joseph P. Miller

The purpose of this chapter is to demystify echocardiographic image orientation and provide a stepwise approach to image acquisition. In the eyes of the novice, learning and applying transesophageal echocardiography (TEE) may seem like an insurmountable task. With the use of this stepwise approach, TEE will quickly become an integral part of your practice and a valuable aid for intraoperative decision making (1–6).

IMAGING PLANES AND ORIENTATION

Understanding the orientation of the imaging plane is crucial for both acquisition of the desired images and correct interpretation of the displayed cardiac anatomy. Although TEE is limited to the confines of the esophagus and stomach, the ability to alter the position and orientation of the ultrasound beam allows a broad view of the cardiac anatomy.

PROBE INSERTION

The TEE probe is passed into the esophagus in the same manner in which an orogastric tube is placed. The easiest way to insert the probe is to perform a jaw lift by grabbing the mandible with the left hand and inserting the probe with the right. The probe is inserted with constant gentle pressure in addition to a slight turning back and forth and from left to right to find the esophageal opening. If resistance is encountered, the cause most often is excessive extension of the head and neck. Advancement of the probe is stopped after the head of the probe has passed the larynx and cricopharyngeus muscle, where a distinct loss of resistance is felt. The imaging head will lie in the upper esophagus.

PROBE MANIPULATION

The position and orientation of the TEE probe can be altered by several types of manipulation **(Figure 2.1)**. By gripping the probe shaft near its entrance in the mouth, the probe can be **advanced** or **withdrawn.** The degree of insertion can be easily determined by the depth markings imprinted on the shaft. For cardiac imaging, the probe position ranges from the upper esophagus to the stomach. In the upper esophagus, the structure closest to the TEE probe is one of the great vessels. In the midesophagus (ME), the structure closest to the TEE probe is the left atrium, and in the transgastric (TG) position, the structure closest to the TEE probe is the left ventricle. Therefore, depending on the depth of insertion, the structure at the apex of the imaging sector will be one of the great vessels, the left atrium, or the left ventricle.

The orientation of the ultrasound beam can be further adjusted by manually **turning** the probe shaft to the left or right. The probe can be **anteflexed** or **retroflexed** by using the large knob on the probe handle. The small knob on the probe handle will **flex** the probe

*The opinions or assertions contained herein are the private views of the author(s) and are not to be construed as official or as reflecting the views of the Department of Defense.

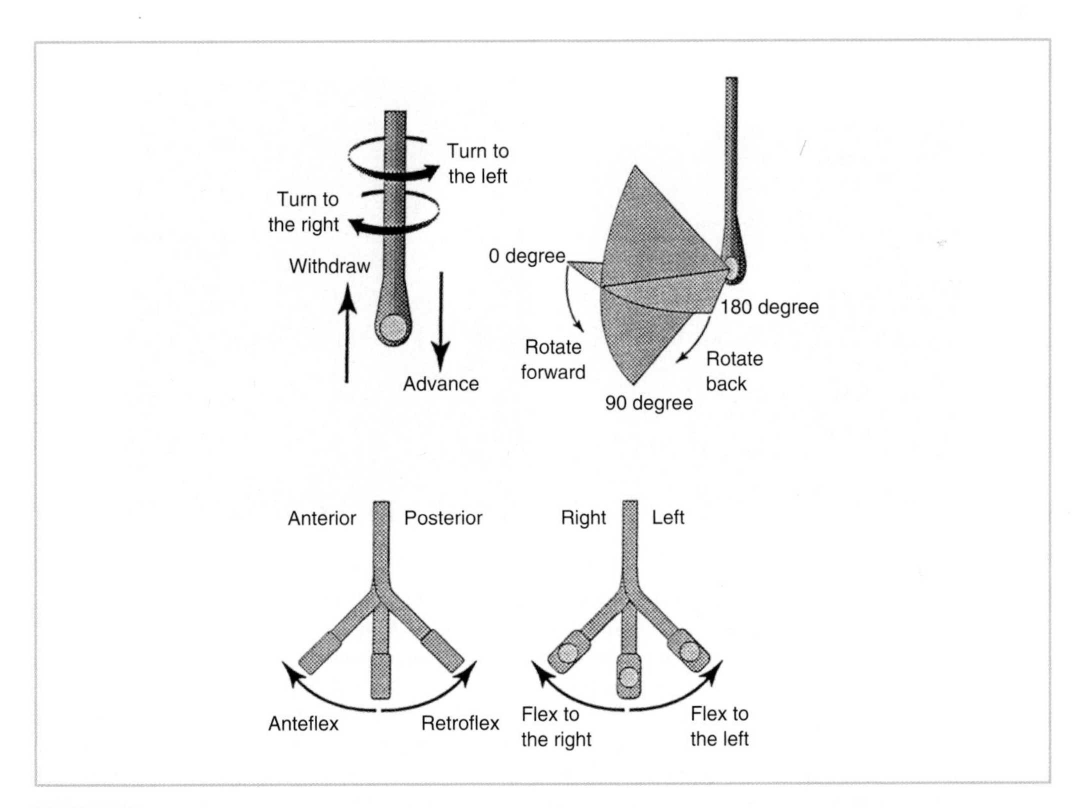

Figure 2.1. Terminology used to describe manipulation of the probe and transducer during image acquisition. (From Shanewise JS, Cheung AT, Aronson S, et al. ASE/SCA guidelines for performing a comprehensive intraoperative multiplane transesophageal echocardiographic examination: recommendations of the American Society of Echocardiography Council for Intraoperative Echocardiography and the Society of Cardiovascular Anesthesiologists Task Force for Certification in Perioperative Transesophageal Echocardiography. *Anesth Analg* 1999;89:870–884, with permission.)

leftward or rightward. These maneuvers allow precise user control over the direction of the ultrasound beam to visualize the structure of interest.

MULTIPLANE IMAGING ANGLE

The first clinically useful TEE probes were capable of producing a single or monoplane cross section of the heart. This imaging plane is generated perpendicular to the shaft of the probe and corresponds to the typical transverse views obtained with transthoracic echocardiography. The biplane probes of the next generation were able to produce two perpendicular views: the standard transverse cross sections and a longitudinal cross section. Currently, most of the probes in use in adult TEE are multiplane probes. Through an electronic switch on the probe handle, the operator selectively rotates the orientation of the imaging plane from 0 degree (transverse plane) through 180 degrees in 1-degree increments. This capability offers many advantages with respect to image acquisition but can also generate tremendous confusion for novice echocardiographers.

Experts rely on two key points to determine image orientation quickly. First, independent of the imaging plane, the ultrasound beam always originates from the esophagus or stomach and projects perpendicular to the probe. Consequently, on the monitor the apex

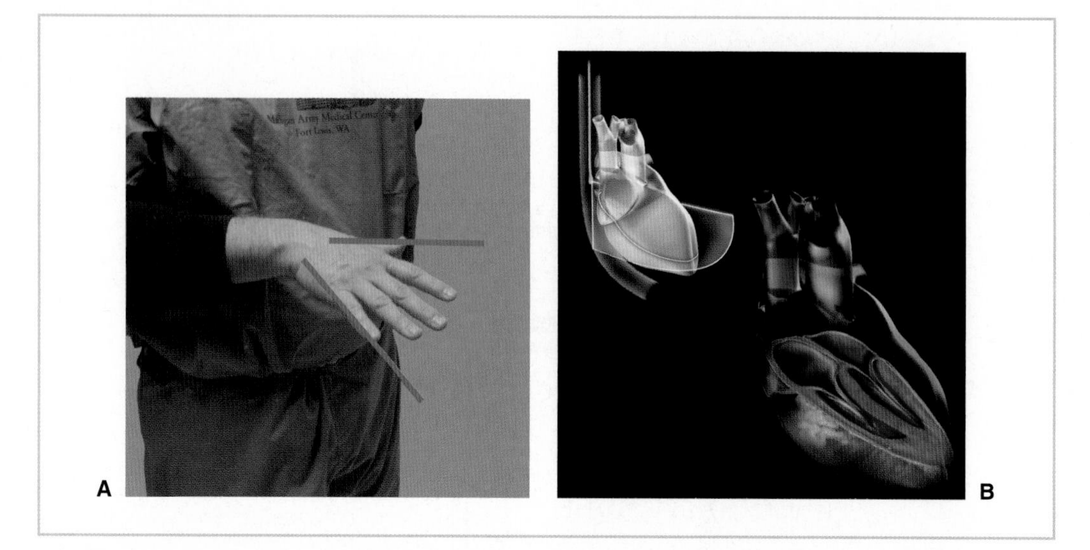

Figure 2.2. **A:** Orientation of your hand, as described in text, for an imaging plane of 0 degrees. The red and green lines correspond with the lines described in **figure 2.2B**. **B:** The top figure is a schematic representation of a transesophageal echocardiography (TEE) probe obtaining a midesophageal (ME) four-chamber view. The TEE probe lies in the esophagus posterior to the left atrium. The imaging plane is projected like a wedge anteriorly through the heart. The image is created by multiple scan lines traveling back and forth from the patient's left (green edge of imaging sector) to the patient's right (red edge). The resulting image is displayed on the monitor with the green edge of the sector displayed on the right side of the monitor and the red edge on the left. In the bottom image, the schematic is made transparent and the anatomy of the heart is displayed in the orientation seen in a ME four-chamber view.

of the sector displays structures that are closest to the TEE probe. As a general rule of thumb, structures seen near the apex of the image sector (i.e., closest to the TEE probe) will be posterior structures, and those close to the arc of the sector (i.e., more distant from the TEE probe) will be anterior structures.

Second, left and right orientation depends on the degree of rotation of the scan head. A simple way to orient yourself is to place your right hand at on your chest with your palm facing downward your extended thumb pointing leftward and anterior and your fingers rightward and anterior. This is the orientation of the imaging scan at 0 degrees and the scan lines begin at your fingers sweeping right to left towards your thumb. Consequently, your fingers point towards right heart structures that will be displayed on the left side on the monitor as you look at the screen **(Figure 2.2)**. Note that this right-to-left display orientation is similar to that of a chest x-ray.

Increases in the imaging plane angle proceed in a clockwise manner. For example, when the imaging plane is rotated to 90 degrees, the imaging orientation is mirrored by rotating your hand clockwise 90 degrees (fingers pointing downward) **(Figure 2.3)**.

Therefore, the scan now progresses from posterior to anterior structures (longitudinal plane).

The combination of probe manipulation and imaging plane angle provides a powerful tool for cardiac imaging **(Figure 2.4)**. For example, slight withdrawal of the probe and rotation

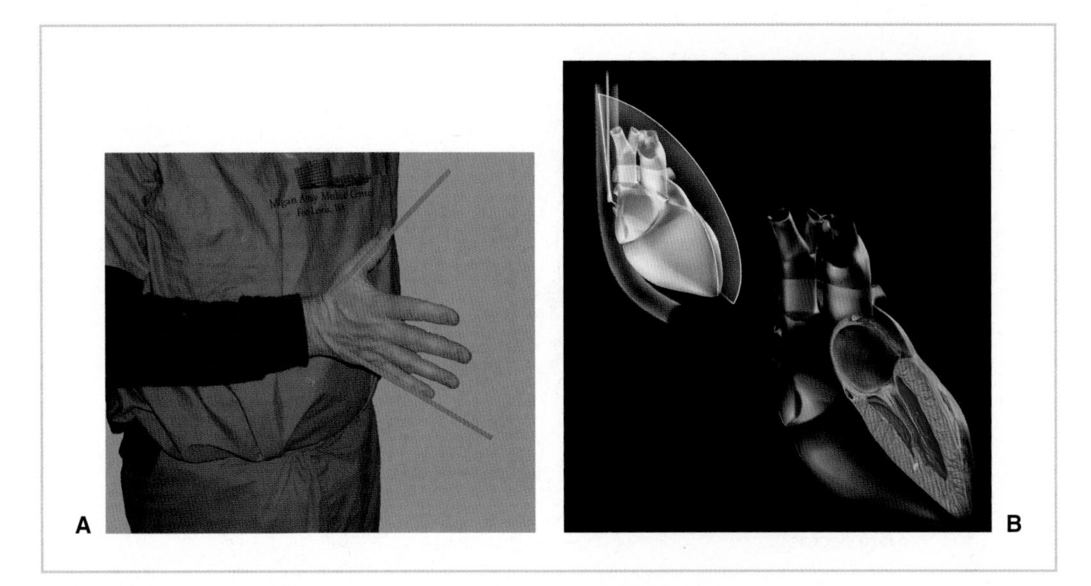

Figure 2.3. **A:** Orientation of your hand, as described in text, for an imaging plane of 90 degrees. The red and green lines correspond with the lines described in **figure 2.3B**. **B:** The top figure is a schematic representation of a transesophageal echocardiography (TEE) probe obtaining a midesophageal (ME) two-chamber view. The probe is in the same position as described in **Figure 2.2**. However, in this case the imaging sector is rotated so that the green sector edge has moved clockwise and is now cephalad, and the red sector edge is now caudad. As previously described, the green edge is displayed on the right side of the monitor's screen and the red edge on the left. In the bottom image, the schematic is made transparent and the anatomy of the heart is displayed in the orientation seen in a ME two-chamber view.

of the imaging plane to 40 degrees provides a short-axis view of the aortic valve **(Figure 2.5)**. In contrast, advancement of the probe into the stomach combined with anteroflexion with the imaging plane at 0 degrees provides a short-axis view of the left ventricle **(Figure 2.6)**.

GOALS OF THE EXAMINATION

TEE examinations, whether comprehensive or abbreviated, should display all pertinent structures in the heart. Each cardiac chamber and valve should be visualized in at least two orthogonal planes. All segments of the myocardium should also be visualized. This approach helps ensure the diagnosis of any significant abnormalities and minimizes the incorrect identification of artifacts.

Echocardiographers differ in their approach to a diagnostic TEE examination. Many prefer to start with those views that examine known pathology. Others believe the examination should first systematically examine for unknown pathology before the area of concern is evaluated. A common approach starts with TG views of the left ventricle because of the frequent abnormalities detected with these views. Each of these approaches has its advantages and disadvantages, and there is no one correct way. However, the goal of any approach must be a complete examination of all structures of the heart. A joint task force including members of the American Society of Echocardiography and the Society of Cardiovascular Anesthesiologists has published guidelines for performing a comprehensive intraoperative multiplane TEE examination (7). However, additional views are often required to assess a particular abnormality and no consensus has been

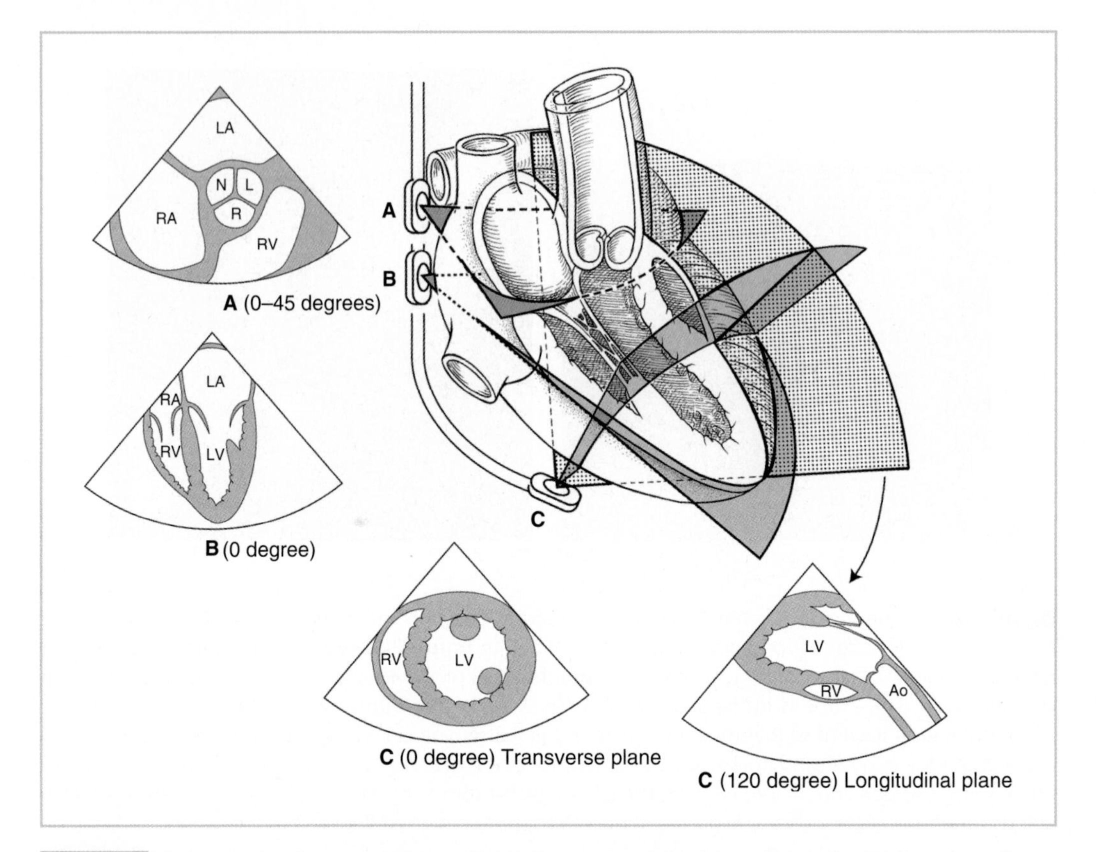

Figure 2.4. Through simple manipulations, the transesophageal echocardiography (TEE) probe offers a multifaceted picture of cardiac anatomy. Progressive advancement of the probe in the midesophagus provides a cross-sectional view of the aortic valve **(A)** followed by a long-axis view of the cardiac chambers **(B)** Further advancement and anterior flexion of the probe head **(C)** allows visualization of the left ventricle in the short axis. Rotation of the imaging plane expands the imaging capacity of TEE. In this example, the left ventricle and its outflow tract are brought into view by rotating the imaging plane to 120 degrees. LA, left atrium; RA, right atrium; N,non-coronary cusp; L, left-coronary cusp; R, right-coronary cusp; RV, right ventricle; LV, left ventricle; Ao, aorta.

reached regarding whether all 20 cross- sections described in the guidelines should be acquired in every surgical patient.

The examination is based on progressive esophageal advancement of the probe to evaluate cardiac anatomy and function followed by progressive withdrawal for the evaluation of the aorta. This approach minimizes manipulation of the TEE probe, thereby shortening the examination time. This author has not found the depth of probe insertion to be a reliable tool for identifying intracardiac anatomy. The preferred approach is to report the location of cardiac anatomy/pathology relative to known intracardiac structures and standard cross-sectional views. The progressive advancement/removal of the probe provides a systematic anatomic orientation (avoiding disorientation as to the displayed imaging plane) and allows for easy description of anatomy relative to other cardiac structures. Pathology in the aorta can be referred to the depth of probe insertion but this has more value in the long-term outpatient evaluation of lesions and, we believe, little value in the intraoperative examination.

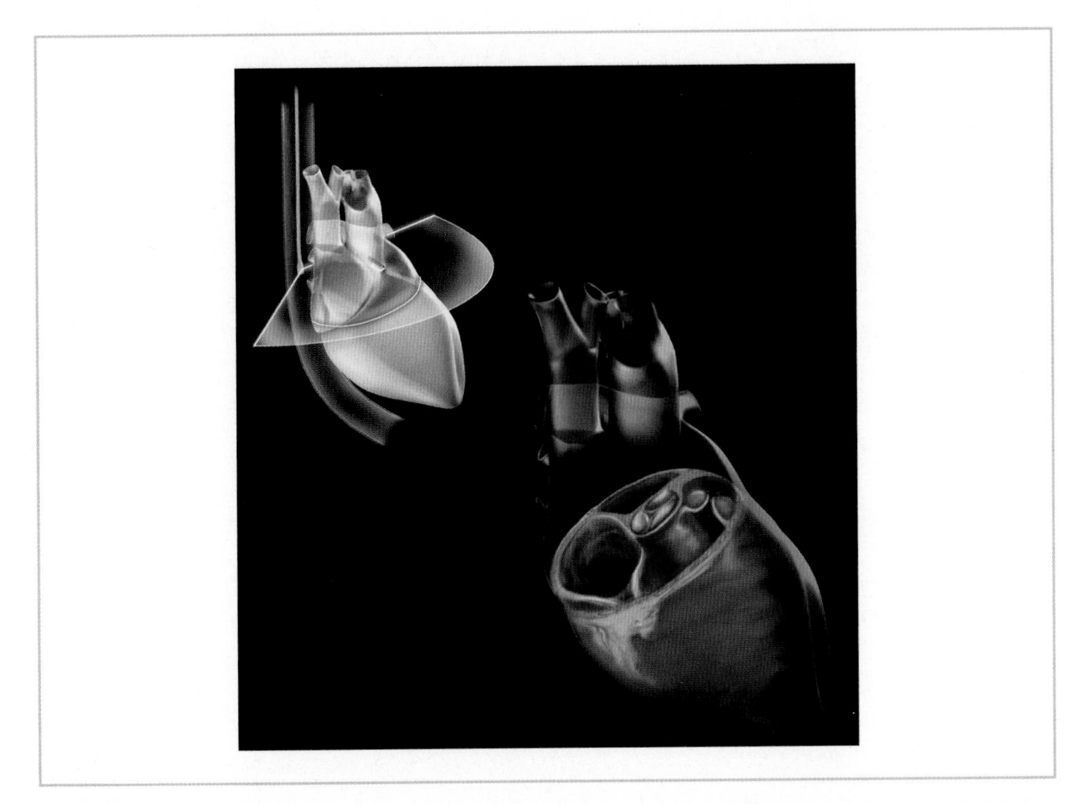

Figure 2.5. The top figure is a schematic representation of a transesophageal echocardiography (TEE) probe obtaining a midesophageal (ME) aortic valve short-axis view. The probe is in the esophagus is but slightly above the position in **Figures 2.2** and **2.3**. When the leaflets of the aortic valve are seen, the imaging plane is rotated from 0 degrees to approximately 40 degrees when the aortic valve is seen in a true cross section. The image on the monitor is generated from scan lines going back and forth from the green edge (right side of monitor) to the red edge (left side of monitor). In the bottom image the schematic is made transparent and the anatomy of the heart is displayed in the orientation seen in a ME aortic valve short-axis view.

The Comprehensive Examination

MIDESOPHAGEAL ASCENDING AORTIC SHORT-AXIS VIEW

From the initial position following passage into the esophagus instead of advancing to the aortic valve the probe is only advanced slightly until the proximal aorta is seen. The probe angle is then rotated until a true short axis is seen usually between 0 and 45 degrees. The main pulmonary artery is seen bifurcating and the right pulmonary artery will lie posterior and perpendicular to the proximal aorta **(Figure 2.7)**.

This view is useful for identifying pulmonary artery catheter placement as well as for visualizing thromboembolism in the pulmonary artery.

MIDESOPHAGEAL ASCENDING AORTIC LONG-AXIS VIEW

From the **short axis view,** the probe angle is rotated to visualize the proximal aorta in the long axis. This view may identify the proximal extent of a dissection, may allow for visualization of saphenous vein grafts and can also be used to interrogate the proximal suture line of an ascending aortic tube graft **(Figure 2.8)**.

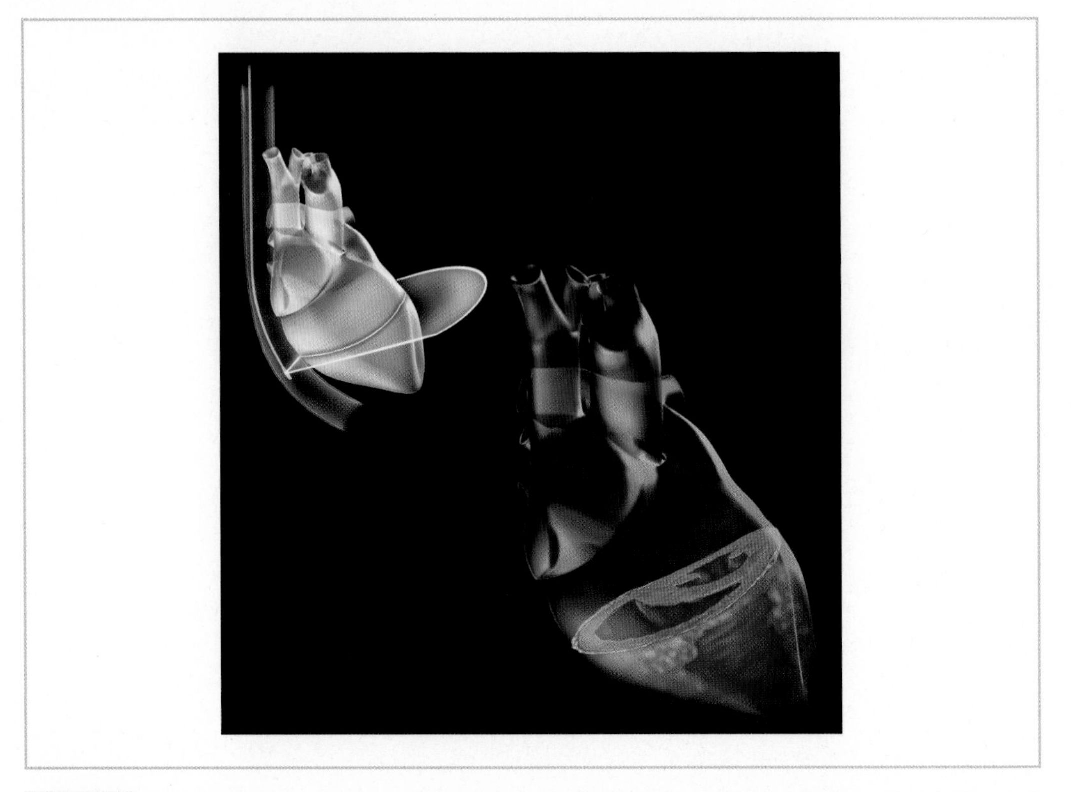

Figure 2.6. The top figure is a schematic representation of a transesophageal echocardiography (TEE) probe obtaining a transgastric (TG) mid short-axis view. The probe is advanced in to the stomach and anteroflexed until solid contact is made with the gastric wall. The imaging plane is projected from the probe at 0 degrees. The image on the monitor is generated from scan lines going back and forth from the green edge (right side of monitor) to the red edge (left side of monitor). In the bottom image, the schematic is made transparent and the anatomy of the heart is displayed in the orientation seen in a TG mid short-axis view.

MIDESOPHAGEAL AORTIC VALVE SHORT-AXIS VIEW

The probe is advanced until the leaflets of the aortic valve are seen. The imaging plane is then rotated to approximately 45 degrees to obtain the ME aortic valve short-axis view. The size of the aortic valve in comparison with the atrial chambers in addition to the mobility of the aortic leaflets and any leaflet calcification are carefully noted.

The primary diagnostic goals of this view are to define the general morphology of the aortic valve (e.g., bicuspid versus tricuspid) and to determine if aortic stenosis is present. The relative sizes of the aorta and the atria should be noted. The intra-atrial septum can be observed for openings consistent with an atrial septal defect or patent foramen ovale. In addition, look for continuous deviation of the septum away from an atrium with elevated pressures **(Figure 2.9)**.

MIDESOPHAGEAL RIGHT VENTRICULAR INFLOW–OUTFLOW

After completion of the ME short-axis view of the aortic valve, the next three views are obtained at the level of the aortic valve in the longitudinal plane. The first view is the ME right ventricular inflow–outflow view. Start at the ME aortic valve short axis and, without moving the probe, change the rotation of the imaging angle to approximately

Image Settings
- Angle: ~10 to 30 degrees
- Sector depth ~12 cm

Probe Adjustments
- Neutral

Primary Diagnostic Uses
- Aortic atherosclerosis
- Aortic dissection, dilation
- Pulmonary artery pathology (emboli, dilation, etc.)

Required Structures
- Aorta in cross section in transverse plane (0 degree)
- Pulmonary artery (main and proximal right)

Abbreviations
SVC: superior vena cava

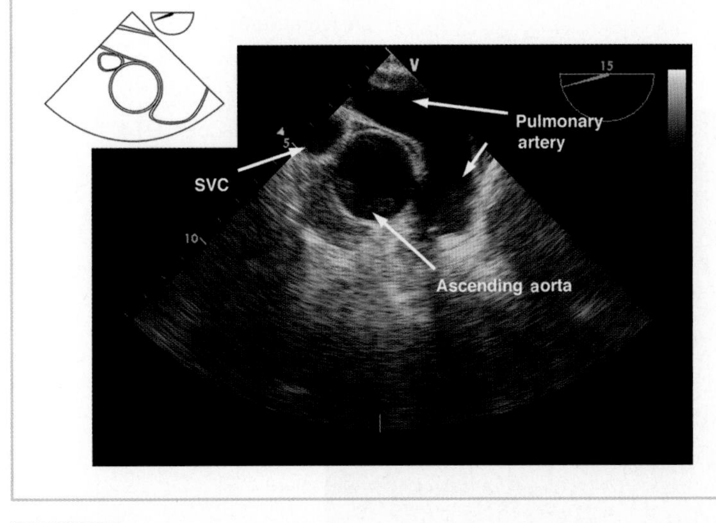

Figure 2.7. Mid-esophageal ascending aortic short-axis view.

Image Settings
- Angle: ~100 degree
- Sector depth: ~10 to 12 cm

Probe Adjustments
- Neutral

Primary Diagnostic Uses
- Aortic atherosclerosis
- Aortic dissection
- Ascending aortic dilation

Required Structures
- Ascending aorta in long axis
- Right pulmonary artery in cross section

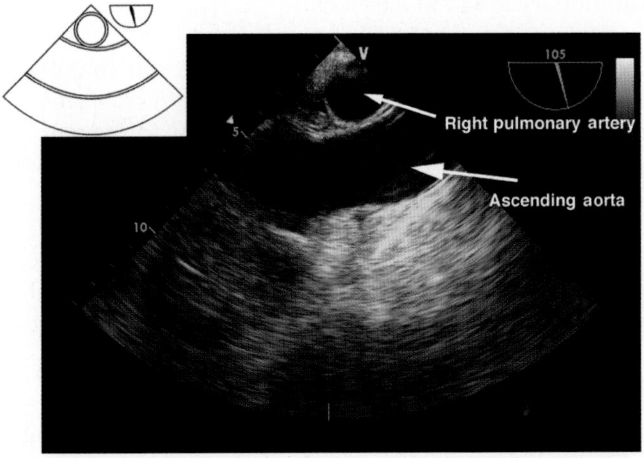

Figure 2.8. Mid-esophageal ascending aortic long-axis view.

Image Settings
- Angle: ~25 to 45 degrees
  Sector depth: ~10 to 12 cm

Probe Adjustments
- Neutral

Primary Diagnostic Uses
- Aortic stenosis
- Diagnosis of valve morphology

Required Structures
- Three valve leaflets[a]
- Commissures
- Coaptation point

[a]Except in congenitally abnormal valve

Abbreviations
RA: right atrium
LA: left atrium

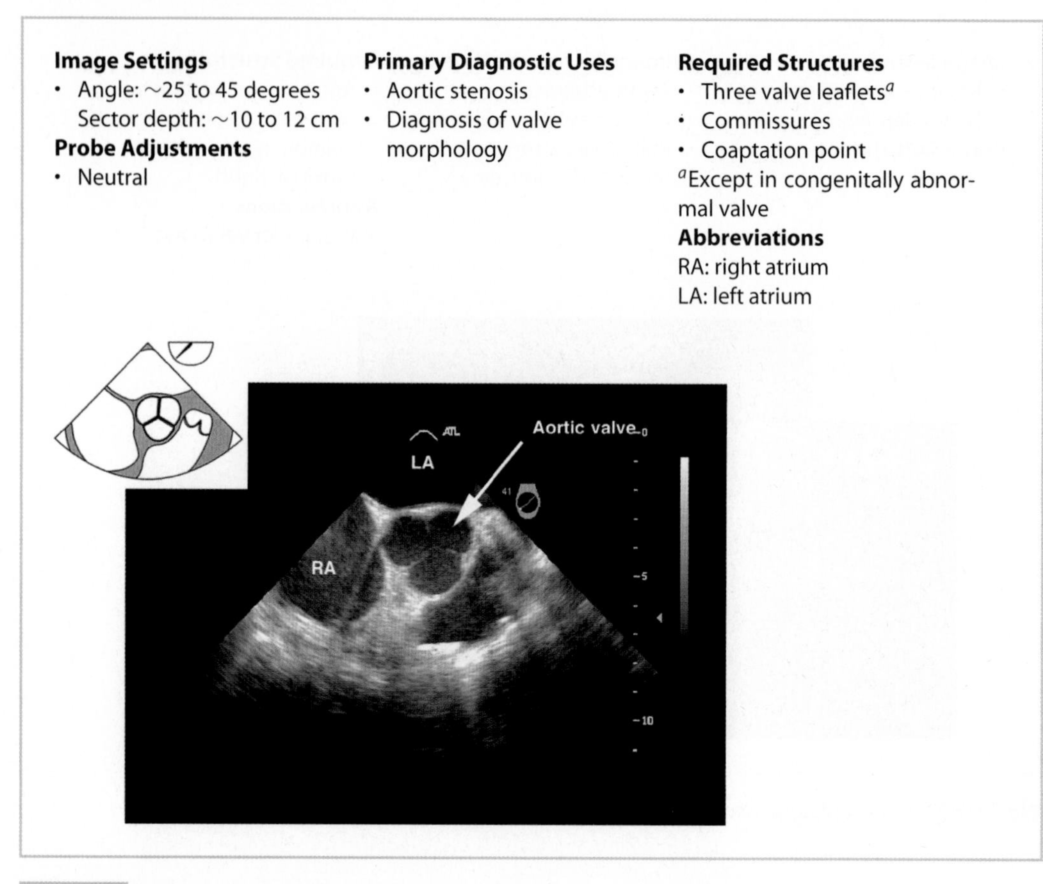

Figure 2.9. Midesophageal aortic valve short-axis view.

60 to 90 degrees. The desired imaging plane will visualize the tricuspid valve, right ventricular outflow tract, and proximal pulmonary artery. Note that the right atrium will be at 10 o'clock, the tricuspid valve at 9 o'clock, the right ventricular cavity at 6 o'clock, and the pulmonary valve and pulmonary artery at 3 o'clock.

The primary diagnostic goals of this view are to gauge the right ventricular chamber and pulmonary annulus size and to evaluate the pulmonic valve. *This view is often superior to the ME four-chamber view for Doppler interrogation of the tricuspid valve.* In adults with prior congenital heart surgery, evaluation of the right ventricular outflow tract and pulmonary valve may provide important diagnostic information.

This view may be helpful in confirming the location of a pulmonary artery catheter if a diagnostic waveform is not identified. The echodense linear pulmonary artery catheter will be seen in the proximal pulmonary artery if the catheter is in the correct location **(Figure 2.10)**.

MIDESOPHAGEAL AORTIC VALVE LONG-AXIS VIEW

The ME aortic valve long-axis view is obtained by further rotating the imaging angle to approximately 110 to 130 degrees. A slight turn of the probe toward the patient's right may be necessary to optimize this image. The view is complete when the left ventricular outflow tract, aortic valve, and proximal ascending aorta are displayed together. Additional

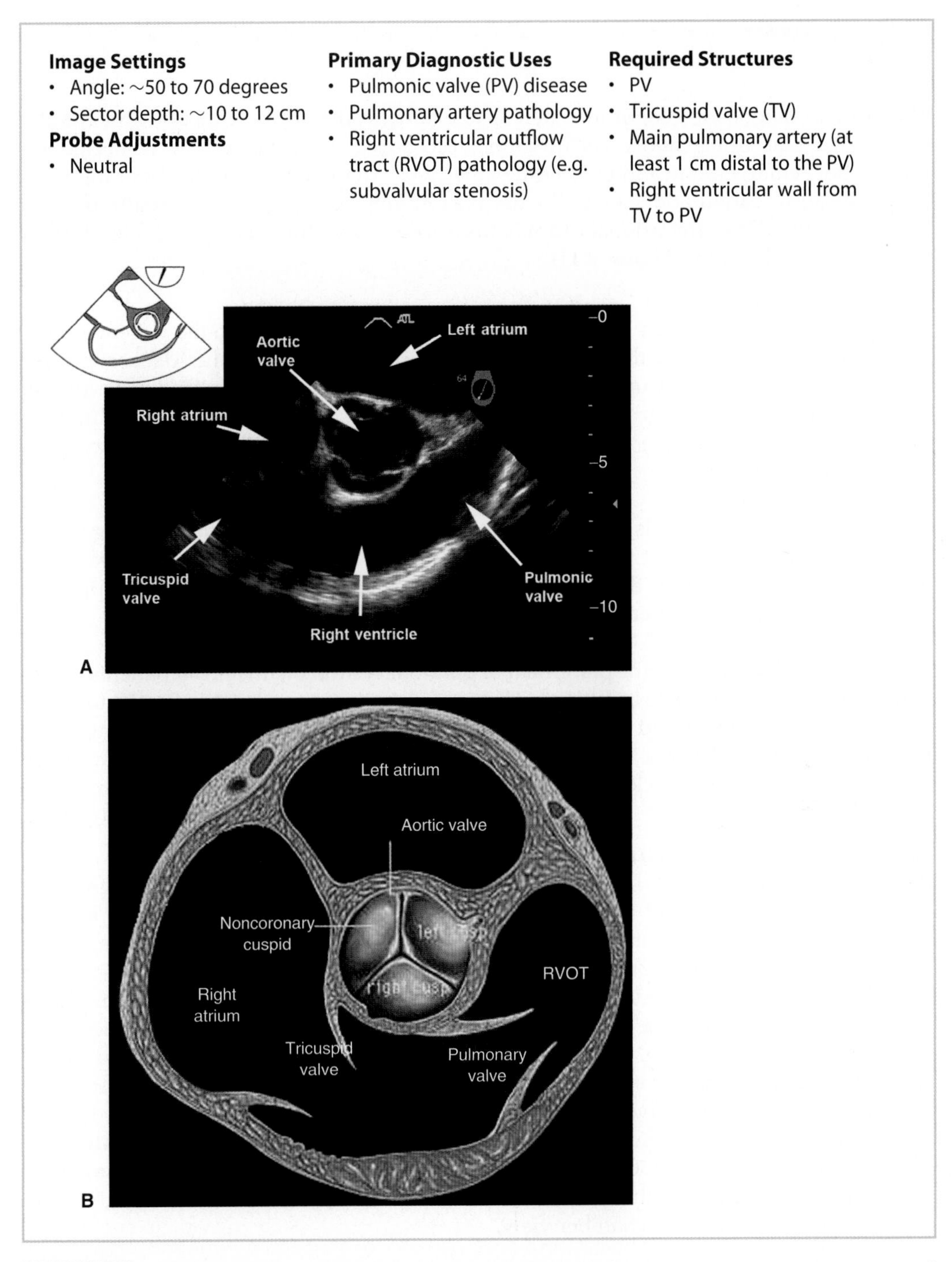

Image Settings
- Angle: ~50 to 70 degrees
- Sector depth: ~10 to 12 cm

Probe Adjustments
- Neutral

Primary Diagnostic Uses
- Pulmonic valve (PV) disease
- Pulmonary artery pathology
- Right ventricular outflow tract (RVOT) pathology (e.g. subvalvular stenosis)

Required Structures
- PV
- Tricuspid valve (TV)
- Main pulmonary artery (at least 1 cm distal to the PV)
- Right ventricular wall from TV to PV

Figure 2.10. A: Midesophageal (ME) right ventricular inflow-outflow. **B:** Anatomic representation of the ME right ventricular inflow-outflow view. The reader should compare this image to the adjacent echocardiographic image for a better understanding of cardiac anatomy. (B from Patrick J. Lynch; illustrator; C. Carl Jaffe; MD; cardiologist Yale University Center for Advanced Instructional Media Medical Illustrations by Patrick Lynch, generated for multimedia teaching projects by the Yale University School of Medicine, Center for Advanced Instructional Media, 1987–2000. Patrick J. Lynch, http://patricklynch.net Creative Commons Attribution 2.5 License 2006; no usage restrictions except please preserve our creative credits: Patrick J. Lynch, medical illustrator; C. Carl Jaffe, MD, cardiologist. http://creativecommons.org/licenses/by/2.5/)

structures to observe are the outflow tract itself, the sinus of Valsalva, and the sinotubular junction.

The primary diagnostic goal of this view is to evaluate aortic valve function and annular and sinotubular dimensions. The proximal ascending aorta should be inspected for calcification, enlargement, and protruding atheroma. An important limitation of this view is that the aortic cannulation site in the distal ascending aorta cannot be visualized. After completion of a two-dimensional examination, aortic valve function is evaluated further with color flow Doppler **(Figure 2.11)**.

MIDESOPHAGEAL BICAVAL VIEW

The ME bicaval view is then obtained by turning the probe further to the patient's right. This image is often best with 5 to 15 degrees less rotation than in the ME aortic valve long-axis view. The key structures in this view are the left and right atria, inferior and superior vena cavae, interatrial septum, and right atrial appendage. Minor adjustment to probe depth and multiplane angle will often bring the tricuspid valve or coronary sinus into view **(Figure 2.12)**.

The primary diagnostic goals of this view are to examine for atrial chamber enlargements and the presence of a patent foramen ovale or an atrial septal defect, and to detect intra-atrial air. If the integrity of the intra-atrial septum is questioned, color flow Doppler or bubble contrast should be performed.

This view may be helpful in the placement of pulmonary artery catheters in patients where entry into the right ventricle is difficult. The pulmonary artery catheter is floated to 20 cm and the balloon inflated and advanced. When the echodense inflated balloon enters the proximal superior vena cava it will be seen entering the right atrium. The catheter can be turned clockwise or counterclockwise to steer it towards the tricuspid valve at approximate 7 o'clock in the atrium rather then the inferior vena cava located at approximately 9 o'clock.

MIDESOPHAGEAL FOUR-CHAMBER VIEW

After completion of the ME bicaval view, the imaging angle is returned to 0 degree and the TEE probe is advanced to the mitral valve level. In the transverse plane, the ME four-chamber view is obtained **(Figure 2.13)**. This view allows visualization of all the chambers of the heart. The image rotation is approximately 0 to 10 degrees with some posterior flexion of the probe. Optimal position is achieved when the tricuspid annulus is at its maximal diameter. The key structures to observe are the left atrium, left ventricle, right atrium, right ventricle, the mitral and tricuspid valves, and the septal and lateral walls of the myocardium. If a portion of the left ventricular outflow tract and aortic valve is displayed (the so-called five-chamber view **[Figure 2.14]**), retroflexion of the probe and slight advancement or rotation of the imaging plane to 5 to 10 degrees should produce the ME four-chamber view. Remember that the aortic valve and left ventricular outflow tract are anterior structures, and these maneuvers will produce a true cross section of the more posteriorly located ME four-chamber view.

The ME four-chamber view is one of the most diagnostically valuable views in TEE. The diagnostic goals of this view include evaluation of chamber size and function, valvular function (both mitral and tricuspid), and regional motion of the septal and lateral walls of the left ventricle. An additional important use of this view is to look for intraventricular air following cardiopulmonary bypass. Air will appear as echodense small bubbles at the junction of the septum and apex. After two-dimensional interrogation of this view,

Image Settings
- Angle: ~115 to 130 degrees
- Sector depth: ~8 to 10 cm

Probe Adjustments
- Neutral

Primary Diagnostic Uses
- Aortic valve pathology
- Aortic pathology (ascending and root)
- Left ventricular outflow tract (LVOT) pathology

Required Structures
- LVOT (at least 1 cm proximal to the aortic valve)
- Aortic valve (visualized cusps approximately equal in size)
- Ascending aorta (at least 1 cm distal to the sinotubular junction)

Abbreviations
LA: left atrium
LV: left ventricle
LVOT: left ventricular outflow tract
RVOT: right ventricular outflow tract

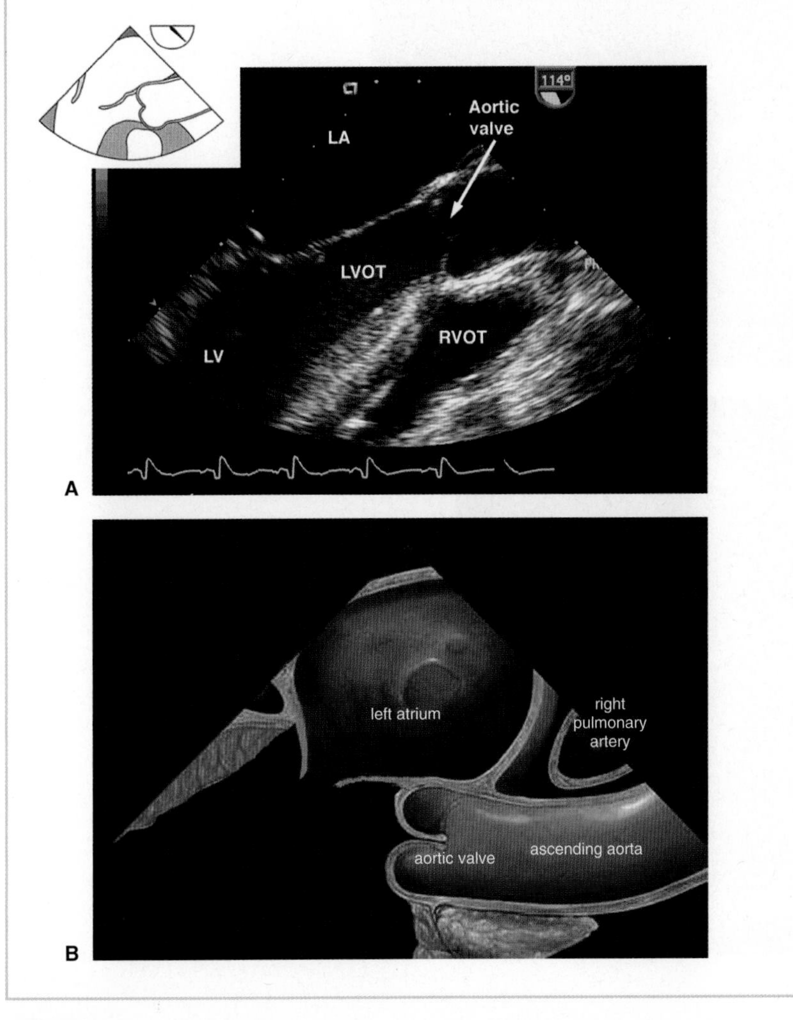

Figure 2.11. **A:** Midesophageal (ME) aortic valve long-axis view. **B:** Anatomic representation of the ME aortic valve long-axis view. (B from Patrick J. Lynch; illustrator; C. Carl Jaffe; MD; cardiologist Yale University Center for Advanced Instructional Media Medical Illustrations by Patrick Lynch, generated for multimedia teaching projects by the Yale University School of Medicine, Center for Advanced Instructional Media, 1987–2000. Patrick J. Lynch, http://patricklynch.net Creative Commons Attribution 2.5 License 2006; no usage restrictions except please preserve our creative credits: Patrick J. Lynch, medical illustrator; C. Carl Jaffe, MD, cardiologist. http://creativecommons.org/licenses/by/2.5/)

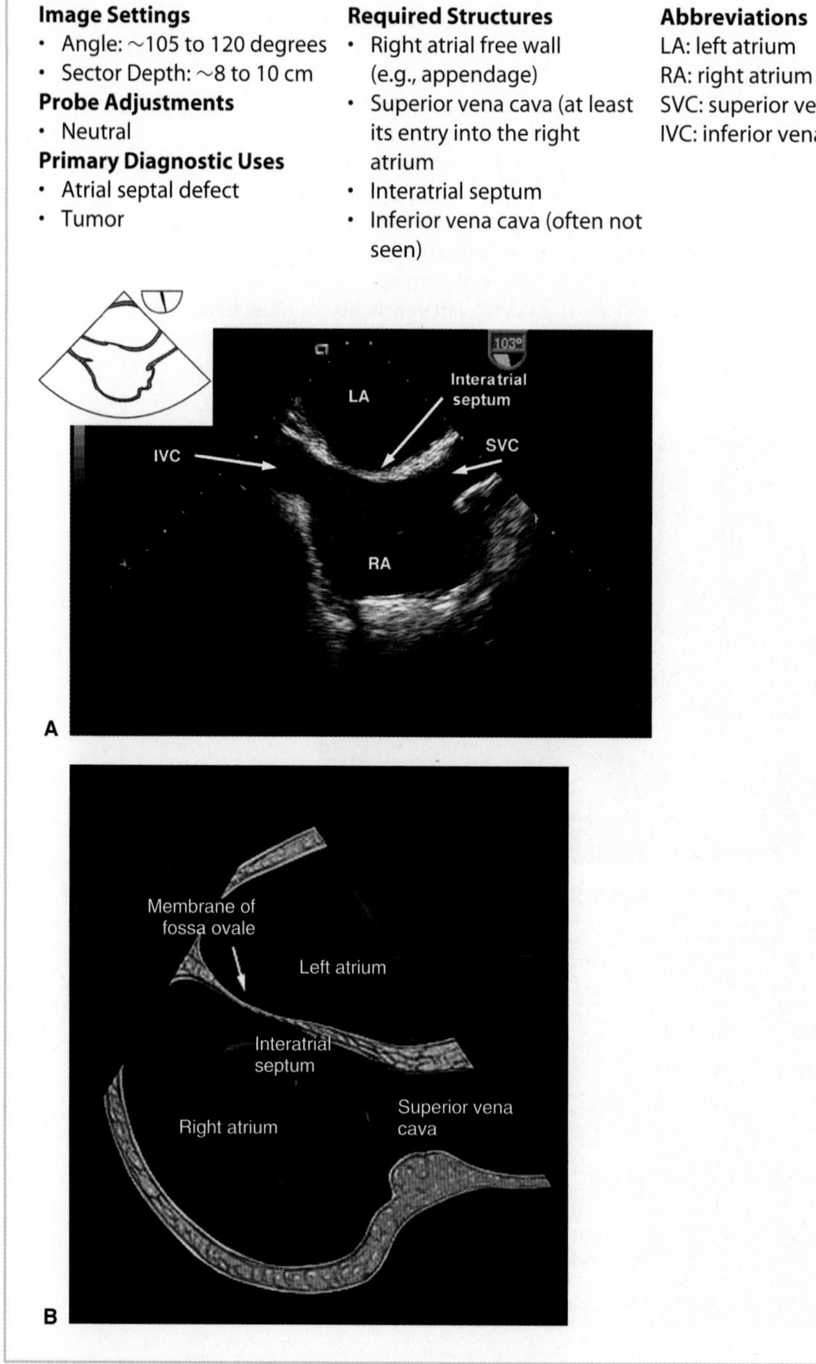

Image Settings
- Angle: ~105 to 120 degrees
- Sector Depth: ~8 to 10 cm

Probe Adjustments
- Neutral

Primary Diagnostic Uses
- Atrial septal defect
- Tumor

Required Structures
- Right atrial free wall (e.g., appendage)
- Superior vena cava (at least its entry into the right atrium
- Interatrial septum
- Inferior vena cava (often not seen)

Abbreviations

LA: left atrium
RA: right atrium
SVC: superior vena cava
IVC: inferior vena cava

Figure 2.12. **A:** Midesophageal bicaval view. **B:** Anatomic representation of the ME bicaval view. (B from Patrick J. Lynch; illustrator; C. Carl Jaffe; MD; cardiologist Yale University Center for Advanced Instructional Media Medical Illustrations by Patrick Lynch, generated for multimedia teaching projects by the Yale University School of Medicine, Center for Advanced Instructional Media, 1987–2000. Patrick J. Lynch, http://patricklynch.net Creative Commons Attribution 2.5 License 2006; no usage restrictions except please preserve our creative credits: Patrick J. Lynch, medical illustrator; C. Carl Jaffe, MD, cardiologist. http://creativecommons.org/licenses/by/2.5/)

Image Settings
- Angle: ~0 to 10 degrees
- Sector depth: ~12 to 14 cm

Probe Adjustments
- Neutral-retroflexed

Primary Diagnostic Uses
- Atrial septal defect
- Chamber enlargement/dysfunction
- Left ventricular regional wall motion (septal and lateral walls)
- Mitral disease
- Tricuspid disease
- Detection of intracardiac air

Required Structures
- Left atrium
- Left ventricle
- Right atrium
- Right ventricle
- Mitral valve
- Tricuspid valve (maximum annular dimension)

Abbreviations
LA: left atrium
LV: left ventricle
RA: right atrium
RV: right ventricle

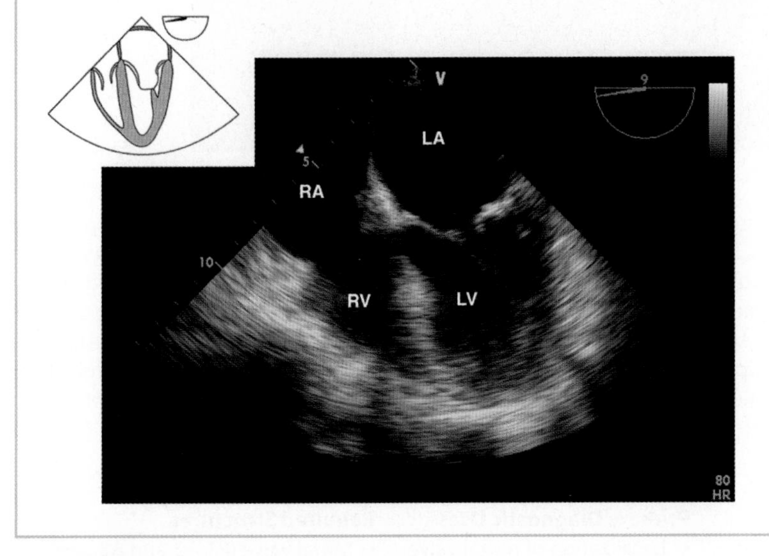

Figure 2.13. Midesophageal four-chamber view.

color flow Doppler should be placed on the mitral and tricuspid valves to detect valvular insufficiency and stenosis.

MIDESOPHAGEAL MITRAL COMMISSURAL VIEW

From the ME four-chamber view the imaging array is rotated to approximately 60 degrees to display the mitral valve in a characteristic P1-A2-P3 appearance. In this view, both the posteromedial and anterolateral papillary muscles will be visible with chordae seen going to the anterior and posterior leaflets. Small turns clockwise and counterclockwise as well as small amounts of ante- and retroflexion will optimize the image and provide a broader perspective of the mitral valve anatomy.

This view is especially helpful with localization of structural mitral valve pathology **(Figure 2.15)**.

MIDESOPHAGEAL TWO-CHAMBER VIEW

From the ME commissural view, rotate the imaging angle to approximately 60 to 90 degrees to obtain the ME two-chamber view. This view is identified by the appearance

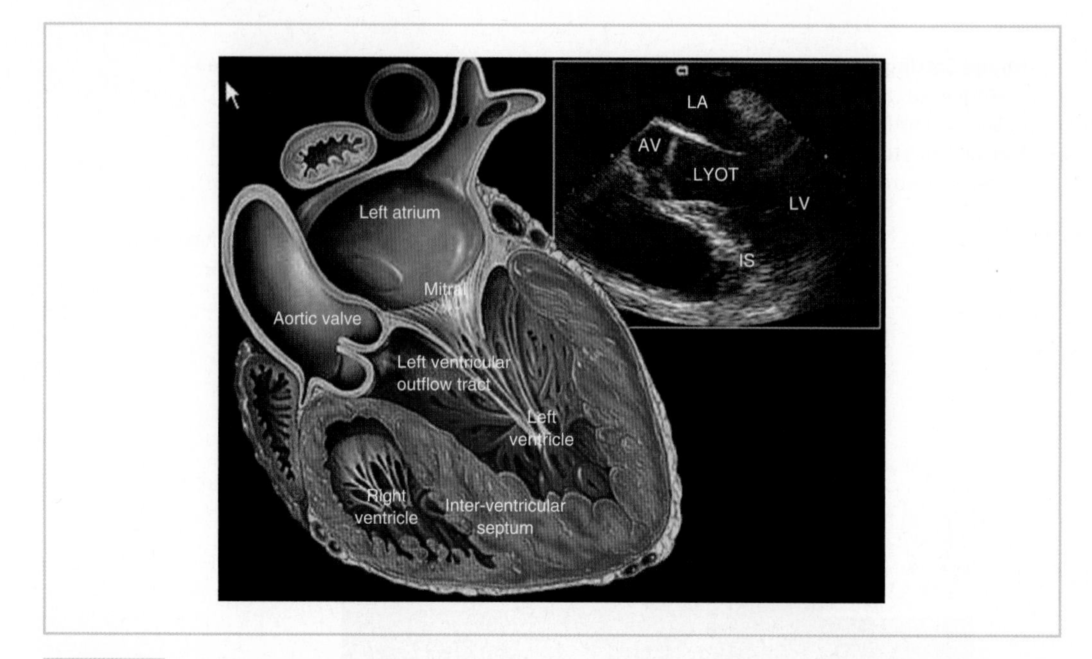

Figure 2.14. Anatomic representation of a midesophageal five-chamber view with the corresponding echocardiographic image. LA, left atrium; LV, left ventricle; RV, right ventricle; MV, mitral valve; AV, aortic valve; LVOT, left ventricular outflow tract. (From Patrick J. Lynch; illustrator; C. Carl Jaffe; MD; cardiologist Yale University Center for Advanced Instructional Media Medical Illustrations by Patrick Lynch, generated for multimedia teaching projects by the Yale University School of Medicine, Center for Advanced Instructional Media, 1987–2000. Patrick J. Lynch, http://patricklynch.net Creative Commons Attribution 2.5 License 2006; no usage restrictions except please preserve our creative credits: Patrick J. Lynch, medical illustrator; C. Carl Jaffe, MD, cardiologist. http://creativecommons.org/licenses/by/2.5/)

Image Settings
- Angle: ~60 to 75 degrees
- Sector depth: ~12 cm

Probe Adjustments
- Neutral

Primary Diagnostic Uses
- Localization of mitral valve pathology

Required Structures
- Mitral valve (P1, P3 and A2 scallops)
- Papillary muscles/chordae tendinae
- Left atrium
- Left ventricle

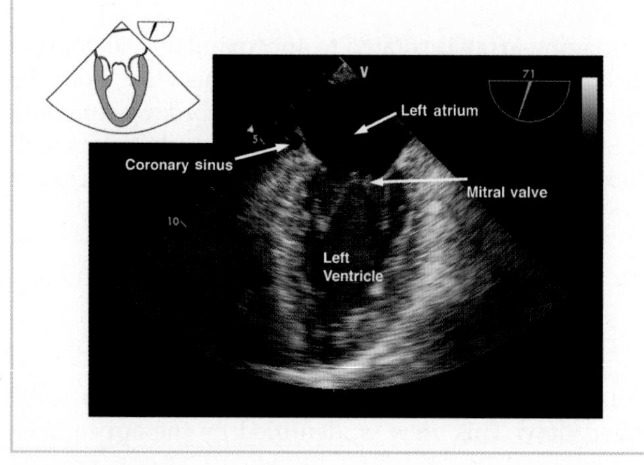

Figure 2.15. Midesophageal mitral commissural view.

of the left atrial appendage and the absence of right-sided heart structures, and it allows visualization of the anterior and inferior walls of the left ventricle. Occasionally, turning the probe shaft to the right will improve chamber alignment and this is the best TEE view for visualization of the true left ventricular apex. The apex is less mechanically active compared to the midcavity anterior and inferior segments which contract inward, like the narrowing of a V. If the apex rises with contraction, you are viewing a foreshortened left ventricle and not seeing the true apex, and the probe position should be adjusted. Ventricular thrombus or hypokinesis at the apex is often best appreciated in this view.

The primary goals of this view are to evaluate left ventricular function (especially the apex) and anterior and inferior regional wall motion. It can also be used to look for thrombus of the left ventricular apex and left atrial appendage. Another frequent use is to verify the correct position of a retrograde cardioplegia catheter in the coronary sinus. The catheter will be seen as an echodense structure visible in the coronary sinus located in the atrioventricular groove at approximately 9 o'clock in this cross section **(Figure 2.16)**.

MIDESOPHAGEAL LONG-AXIS VIEW

After evaluation of the ME two-chamber view, the probe is further rotated to approximately 120 degrees or when the left ventricular outflow tract is seen. Small amounts of rotation and flexion will allow for maximizing the diameter of the outflow tract. This view often appears similar to the ME aortic valve long axis; however, the ventricular inflow and outflow tracts are seen as well as a majority of the ventricular cavity.

Image Settings
- Angle: ~80 to 100 degrees
- Sector depth: ~12 to 14 cm

Probe Adjustments
- Neutral

Primary Diagnostic Uses
- Left atrial appendage mass or thrombus
- Left ventricular (LV) apex pathology
- LV systolic dysfunction
- LV regional wall motion (anterior & inferior walls)

Required Structures
- Left atrial appendage
- Mitral valve
- LV apex (maximum LV length)

Abbreviations
LA: left atrium
LV: left ventricle
MV: mitral valve

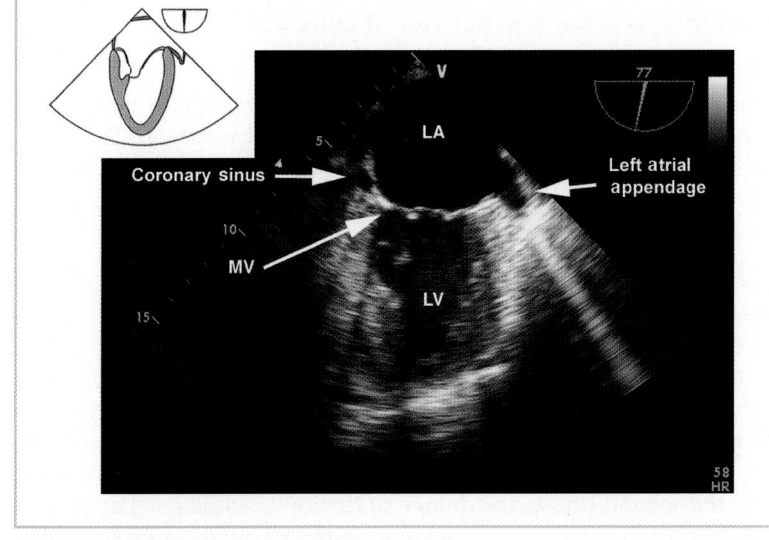

Figure 2.16. Midesophageal two-chamber view.

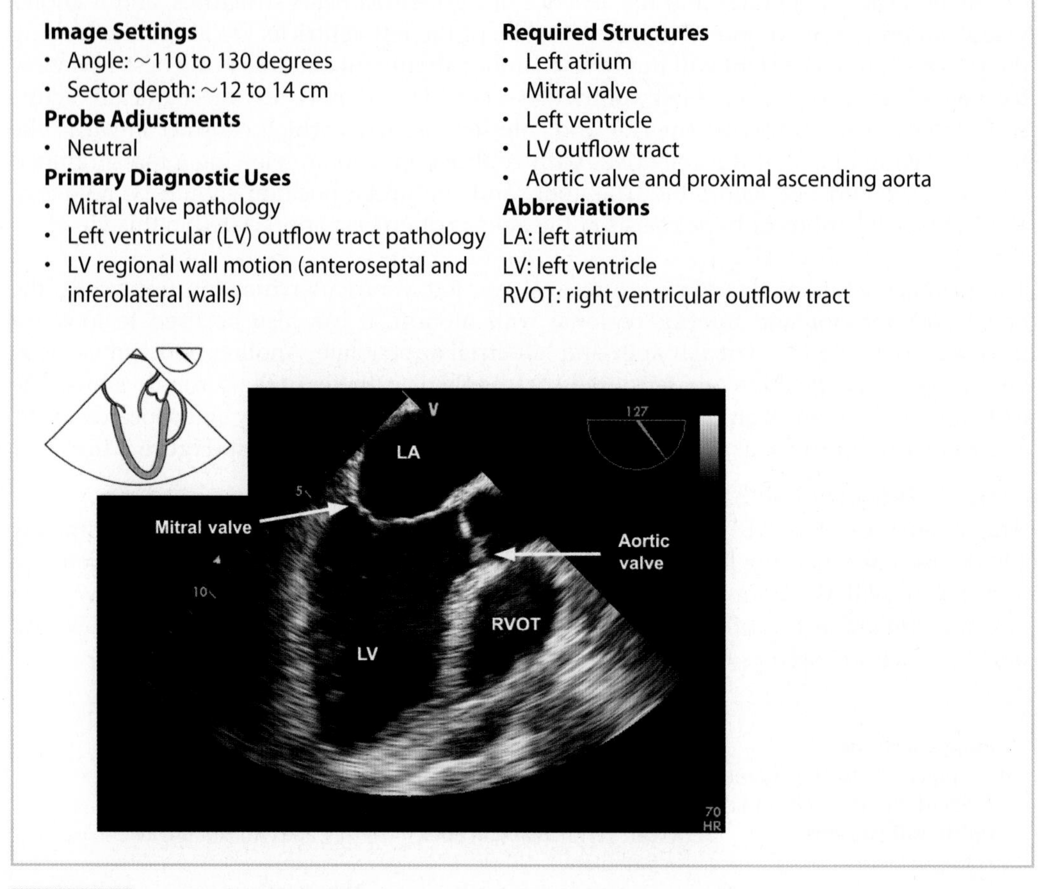

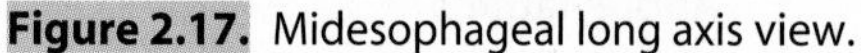
Figure 2.17. Midesophageal long axis view.

The mitral valve and left ventricular outflow tract can be evaluated in this view. Additionally, assesment of regional wall motion and global function of the anteroseptal and inferolateral walls of the ventricle is possible in this view **(Figure 2.17)**.

TRANSGASTRIC BASAL SHORT-AXIS VIEW

From the ME long axis the probe is rotated back to 0 degrees, advanced and anteflexed, and then withdrawn to obtain the TG basal short-axis view of the left ventricle. This view is often difficult to obtain. If the "fish mouth" view of the mitral valve is not obtained advancing to the TG mid short-axis then withdrawing the anteflexed probe may allow visualization of the TG basal short-axis **(Figure 2.18)**.

TRANSGASTRIC MIDPAPILLARY SHORT-AXIS VIEW

The probe is then advanced anteflexed and withdrawn until contact is made with the wall of the stomach and the **TG midpapillary short-axis** view is obtained. The key structures to visualize are the left ventricular walls and cavity in addition to the posteromedial and anterolateral papillary muscles. A true short-axis cross-section of the left ventricle is confirmed when the two papillary muscles are approximately of equal size. Fine-tuning this image may be challenging and is done in two phases. In the first phase, the depth of the probe is altered, and in the second phase, the degree of flexion is adjusted. The proper depth of the probe is obtained by focusing on the posteromedial papillary muscle, which

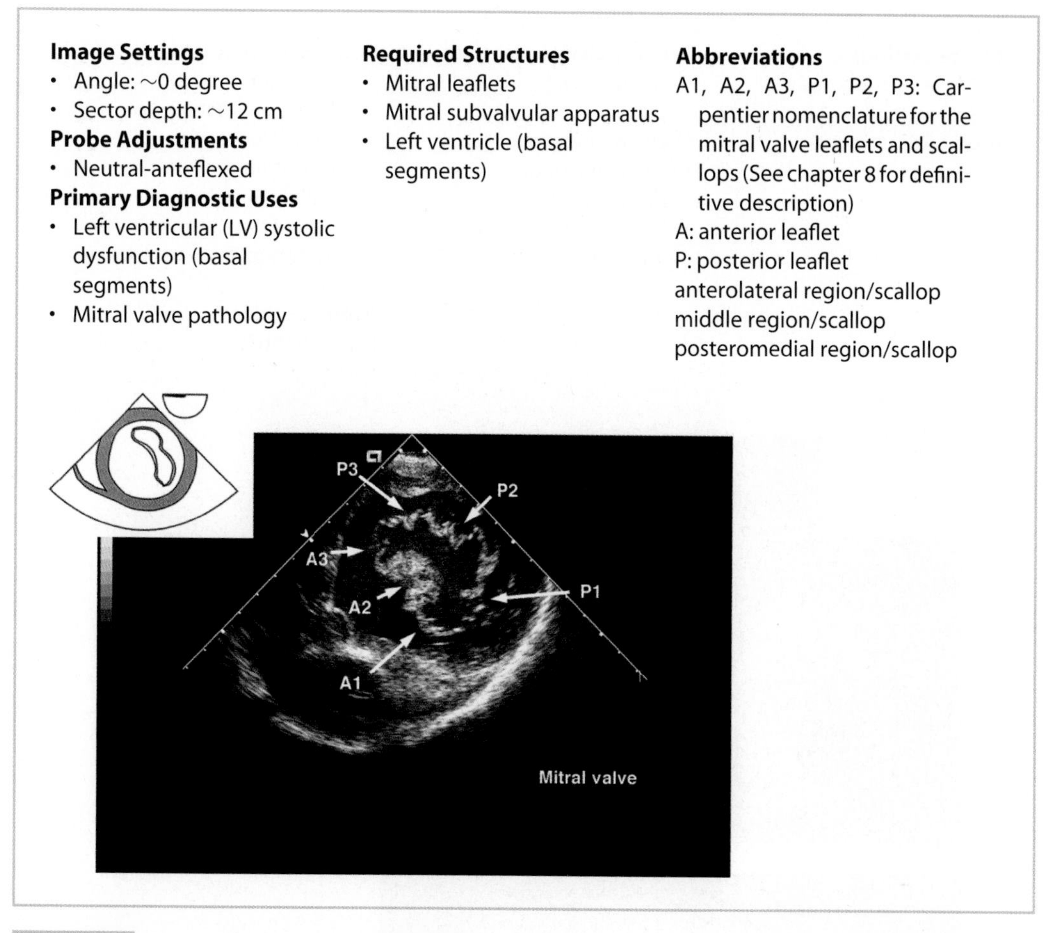

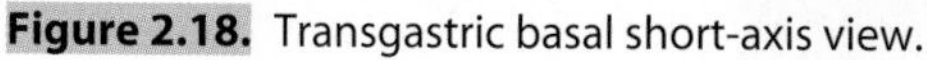
Figure 2.18. Transgastric basal short-axis view.

is the papillary muscle closest to the apex of the scan. If chordae tendineae are visible, the probe is too high and should be advanced. If no papillary muscle is visible, most often the probe is too low and should be withdrawn. Once the depth of the probe is appropriate, the flexion is adjusted to bring the anterolateral papillary muscle into the correct position. If any of the anterolateral chordae tendineae are visible, the probe is excessively anteflexed, and relaxation of the large wheel on the probe handle should bring the papillary muscle into the correct position.

The primary diagnostic goals of this view are assessment of left ventricular systolic function, left ventricular volume, and regional wall motion. Turning the probe rightward visualizes the right ventricle **(Figure 2.19)**.

TRANSGASTRIC TWO-CHAMBER VIEW

After completion of the TG mid–short-axis view, the imaging angle is rotated to approximately 90 degrees and the TG two-chamber view is obtained; this provides a long-axis view of the left ventricle, with the apex to the left of the display and the mitral valve to the right. The primary diagnostic goal of this view is analysis of regional wall motion. This is the preferred view for evaluation of the support structures of the mitral valve because they lie perpendicular to the ultrasound beam **(Figure 2.20)**.

Image Settings
- Angle: ~0 degrees
- Sector depth: ~12 cm

Probe Adjustments
- Anteflexed

Primary Diagnostic Uses
- Hemodynamic instability
- Left ventricular (LV) enlargement
- LV hypertrophy
- LV systolic dysfunction
- LV regional wall motion (mid segments)

Required Structures
- Left ventricle cavity
- LV walls (at least 50% of circumference with visible endocardium)
- Papillary muscles (approximately equal in size and distinct from ventricular wall)

Abbreviations
LV: left ventricle

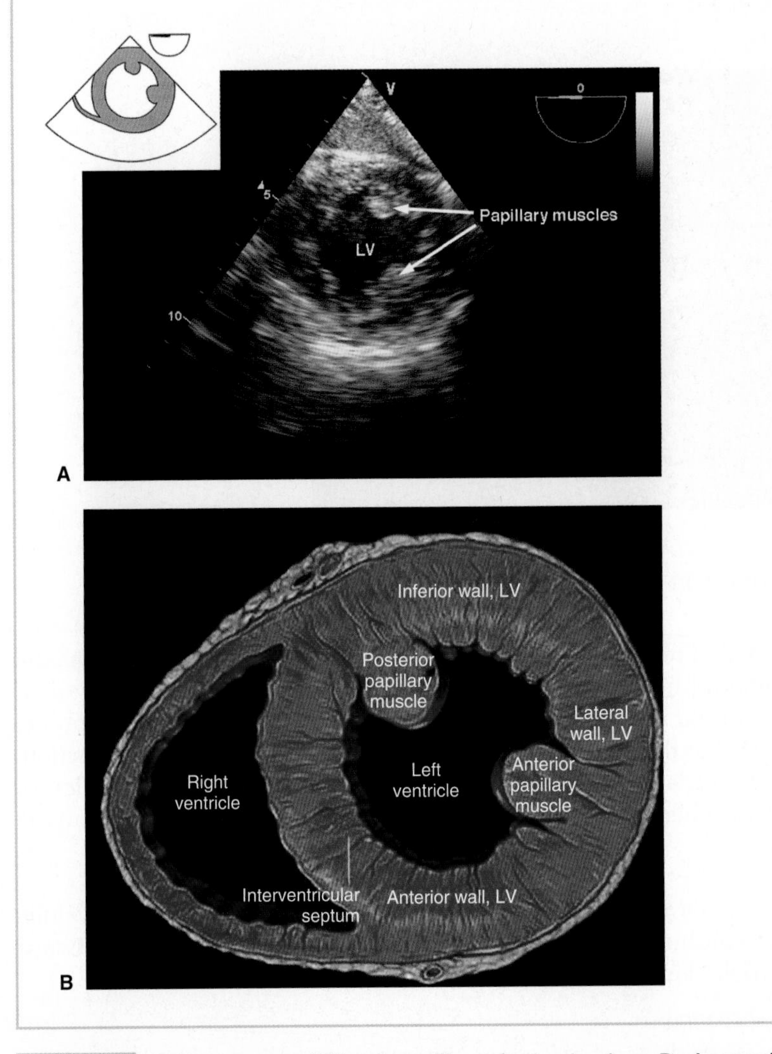

Figure 2.19. **A:** Transgastric (TG) midpapillary short-axis view. **B:** Anatomic representation of a TG mid short axis view. (B from Patrick J. Lynch; illustrator; C. Carl Jaffe; MD; cardiologist Yale University Center for Advanced Instructional Media Medical Illustrations by Patrick Lynch, generated for multimedia teaching projects by the Yale University School of Medicine, Center for Advanced Instructional Media, 1987–2000. Patrick J. Lynch, http://patricklynch.net Creative Commons Attribution 2.5 License 2006; no usage restrictions except please preserve our creative credits: Patrick J. Lynch, medical illustrator; C. Carl Jaffe, MD, cardiologist. http://creativecommons.org/licenses/by/2.5/)

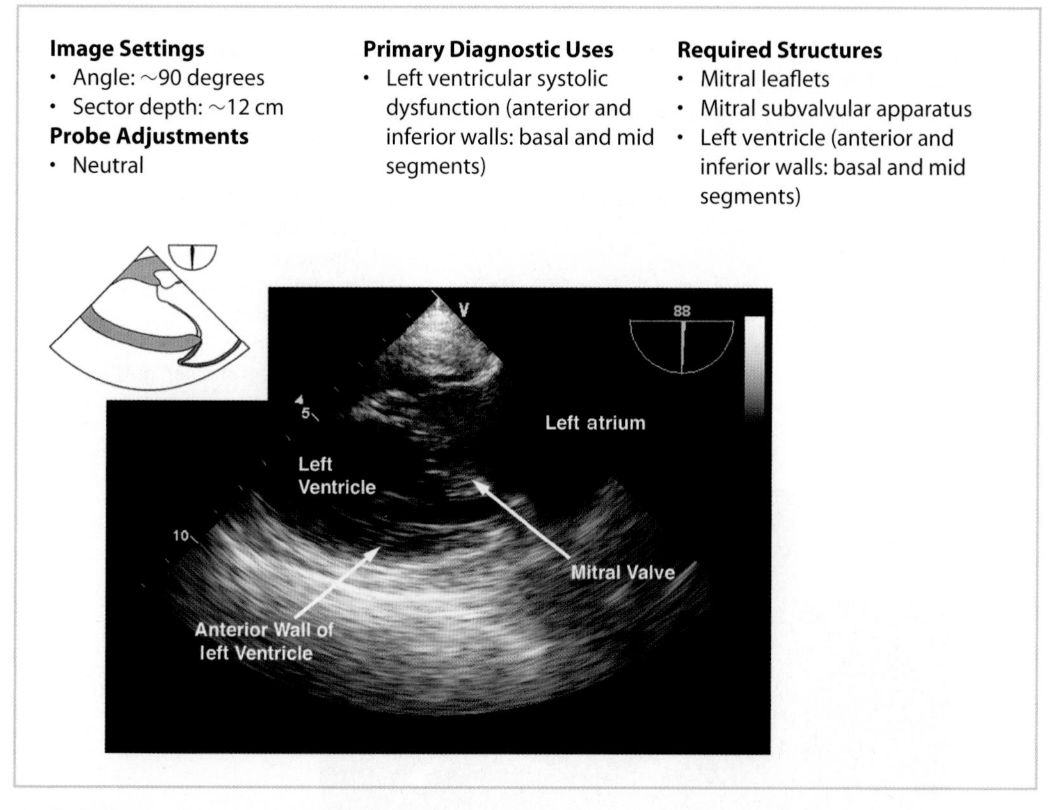

Figure 2.20. Transgastric two-chamber view.

TRANSGASTRIC LONG-AXIS VIEW

From the TG two-chamber view the probe is rotated to approximately 120 degrees. The left ventricular outflow tract and aortic valve should come into view at 4 o'clock. This view is especially helpful in the spectral Doppler interrogation of the aortic valve and left ventricular outflow tract **(Figure 2.21)**.

TRANSGASTRIC RIGHT VENTRICULAR INFLOW VIEW

From the TG long-axis the probe is turned toward the patient's right (clockwise) until the TG right ventricular inflow view is seen. This view is helpful in evaluating right ventricular wall thickening and tricuspid valve pathology **(Figure 2.22)**.

DEEP TRANSGASTRIC LONG-AXIS VIEW

The probe is then rotated back to 0 degrees, advanced toward the left ventricular apex then maximally anteflexed and slightly withdrawn to obtain the deep gastric long-axis view. Leftward flexion of the probe is often required. This view allows spectral Doppler interrogation of the outflow tract and aortic valves. Probe rotation may be necessary to optimize the Doppler interrogation angle **(Figure 2.23)**.

Aortic Examination

DESCENDING AORTA SHORT-AXIS VIEW

After completion of the evaluation of the ventricles, the probe is rotated to 0 degree and the probe shaft is turned to the patient's left and slightly withdrawn until a transverse

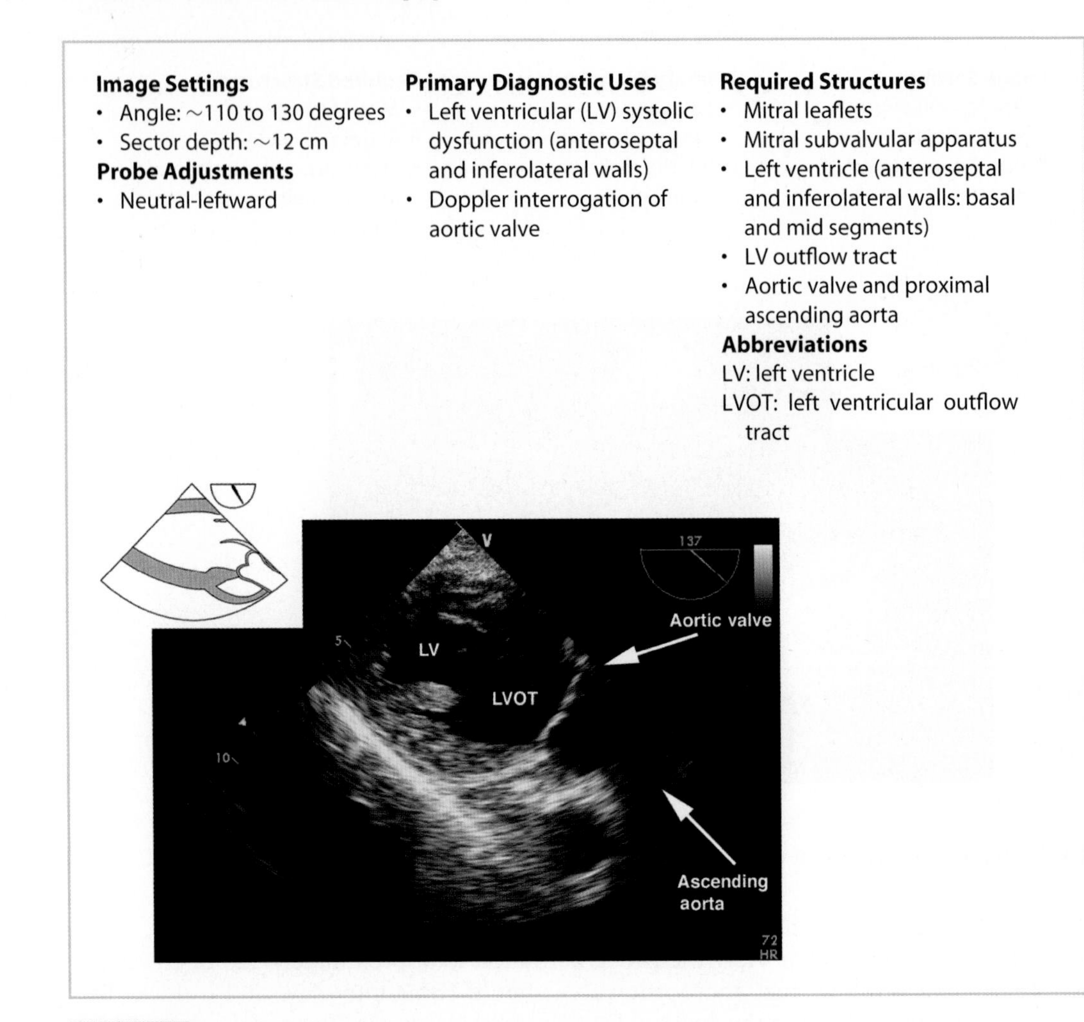

Figure 2.21. Transgastric long-axis view.

view of the descending aorta is obtained (the descending aorta short-axis view). Key factors in imaging the aorta are its small size and its proximity to the TEE probe head in the esophagus. Consequently, the following maneuvers are necessary to optimize aortic imaging. First, the image depth in reduced to enlarge the displayed aortic image. Second, the time gain compensation in the near field may have to be increased because it is often set at low levels during the cardiac examination. Finally, the frequency of the transducer can be increased to enhance resolution. In the author's experience, these changes in the settings have allowed the visualization of aortic atheromas that were not evident before the adjustments were made. The aorta is then examined along its course as the probe is slowly withdrawn. When the aorta begins to appear elongated, the probe has reached the level of the aortic arch **(Figure 2.24)**.

UPPER ESOPHAGEAL AORTIC ARCH LONG-AXIS VIEW

At the level of the arch the probe is turned rightward to visualize the distal ascending aorta and arch in long axis. This view is often useful in evaluating the distal ascending aorta, especially for the presence of calcification and/or atheroma at the cannulation site **(Figure 2.25)**.

Image Settings
- Angle: ~110 to 130 degrees
- Sector depth: ~12 cm

Probe Adjustments
- Neutral-rightward

Primary Diagnostic Uses
- Right ventricular (RV) systolic dysfunction
- Tricuspid valve pathology

Required Structures
- Right atrium
- Tricuspid valve
- Tricuspid subvalvular apparatus
- Right ventricle

Abbreviations
RA: right atrium
RV: right ventricle

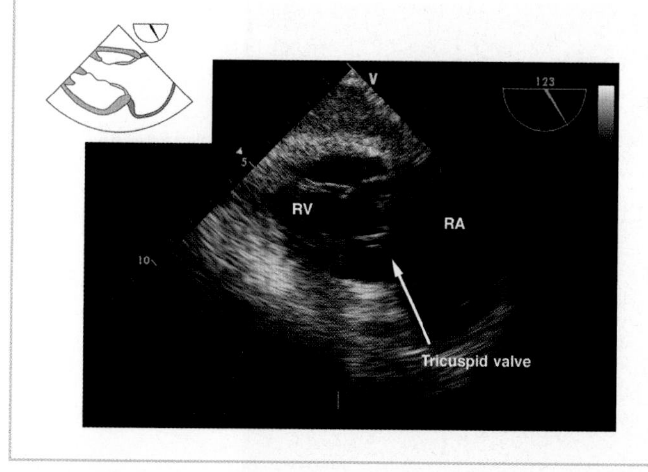

Figure 2.22. Transgastric right ventricular inflow view.

Image Settings
- Angle: ~0 degree
- Sector depth: ~16 cm

Probe Adjustments
- Anteflexed

Primary Diagnostic Uses
- Aortic valve pathology
- Left ventricular outflow tract (LVOT) pathology
- Doppler interrogation of aortic outflow

Required Structures
- Left ventricle
- Aortic valve
- Ascending aorta

Abbreviations
LV: left ventricle
LVOT: left ventricular outflow tract

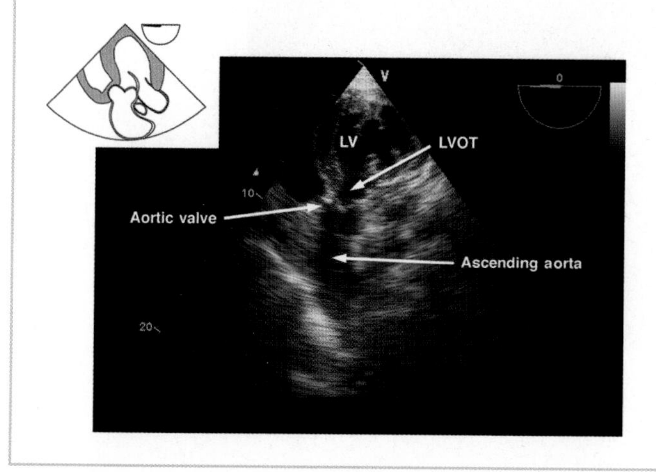

Figure 2.23. Deep transgastric long-axis view.

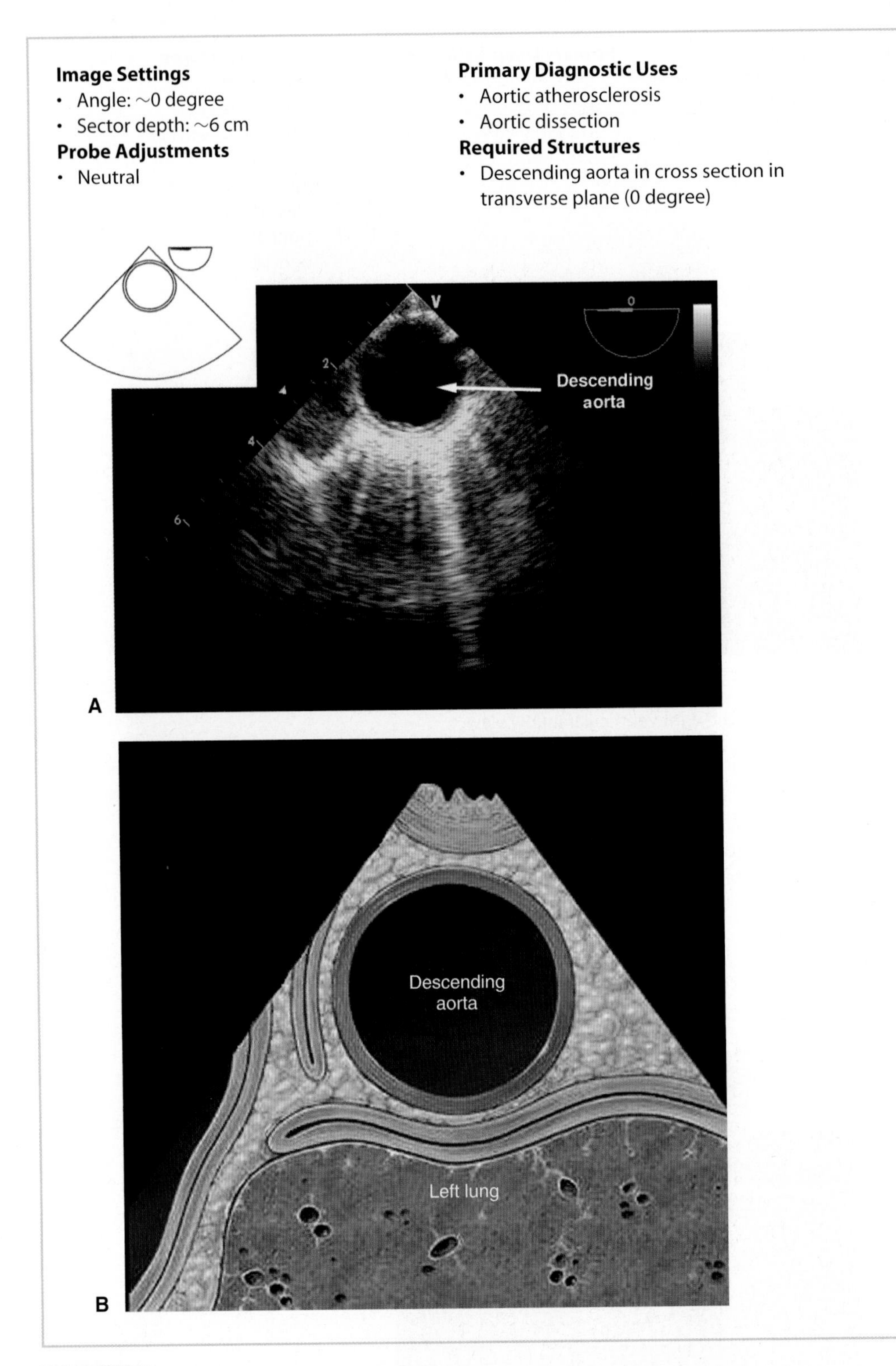

Figure 2.24. Descending aorta short-axis view.

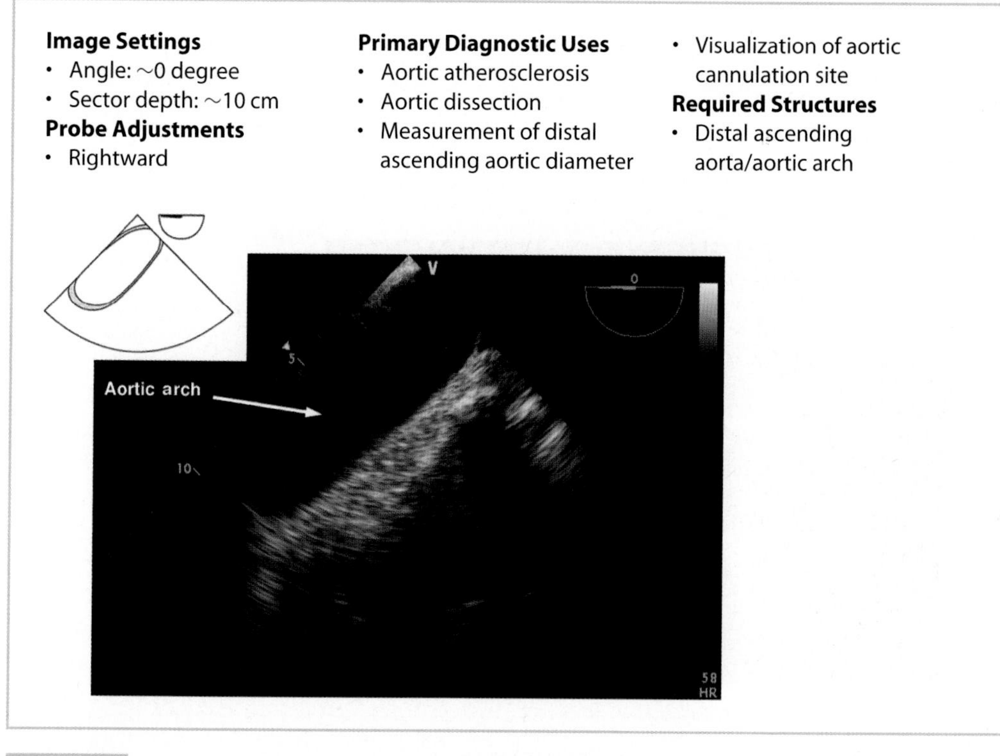

Figure 2.25. Upper esophageal aortic arch long axis view.

UPPER ESOPHAGEAL AORTIC ARCH SHORT-AXIS VIEW

The imaging angle is then turned to 90 degrees to obtain the upper esophageal aortic arch short-axis view. Small left and right turns of the probe shaft will allow you to interrogate the arch for calcification, enlargement, and foreign bodies. You may see the origins of the great vessels at approximately 3 o'clock in the short axis of the aortic arch. The innominate vein and the origin of the left subclavian artery are visualized in this view. The pulmonary artery lies parallel to the imaging beam affording excellent Doppler interrogation **(Figure 2.26)**.

DESCENDING AORTA LONG-AXIS VIEW

After completion of the aortic arch views, the probe is slowly advanced to obtain the longitudinal view of the descending aorta (the descending aorta long-axis view). As the probe is advanced, small left and right turns of the probe permit better interrogation of the aortic walls **(Figure 2.27)**.

AN ABBREVIATED EXAMINATION

The operating room is often a busy, hectic environment. Anesthesiologists are constantly multitasking and often responsible for not only the management of the anesthetic but the simultaneous performance and interpretation of the echocardiogram. A comprehensive examination may not be practical or indicated in this environment especially during circumstances of hemodynamic instability. In such cases an abbreviated or focused examination is more appropriate. An example sequence is found in **Figure 2.28**. This examination can be completed in 3 to 5 minutes and focuses on pathologic conditions that require immediate therapy. All chambers and valves (except pulmonic) are viewed

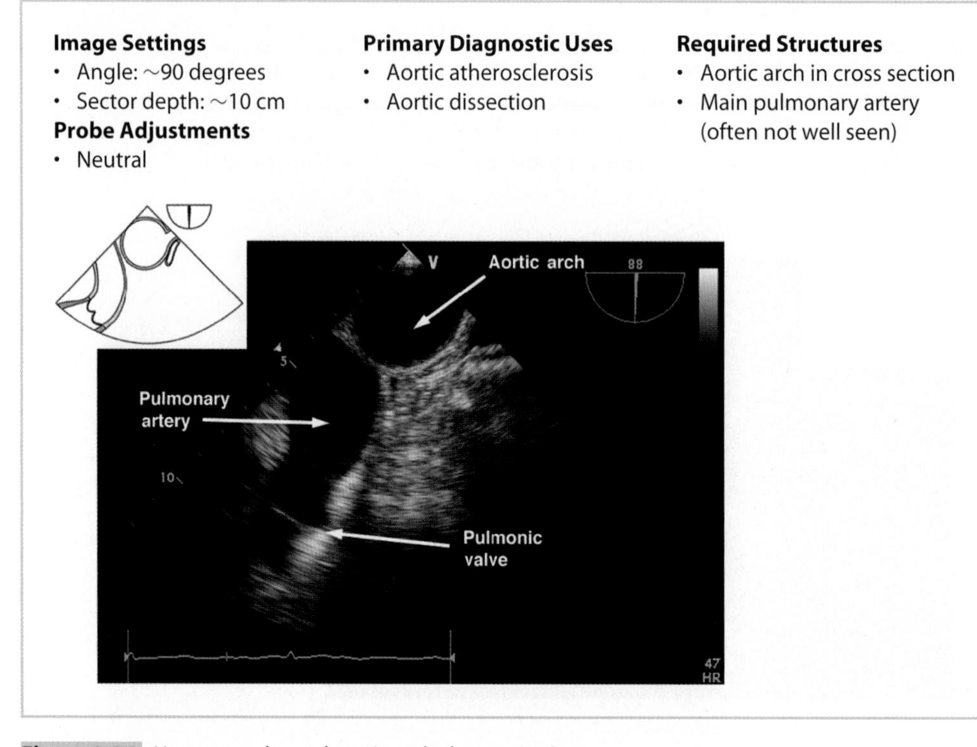

Figure 2.26. Upper esophageal aortic arch short-axis view.

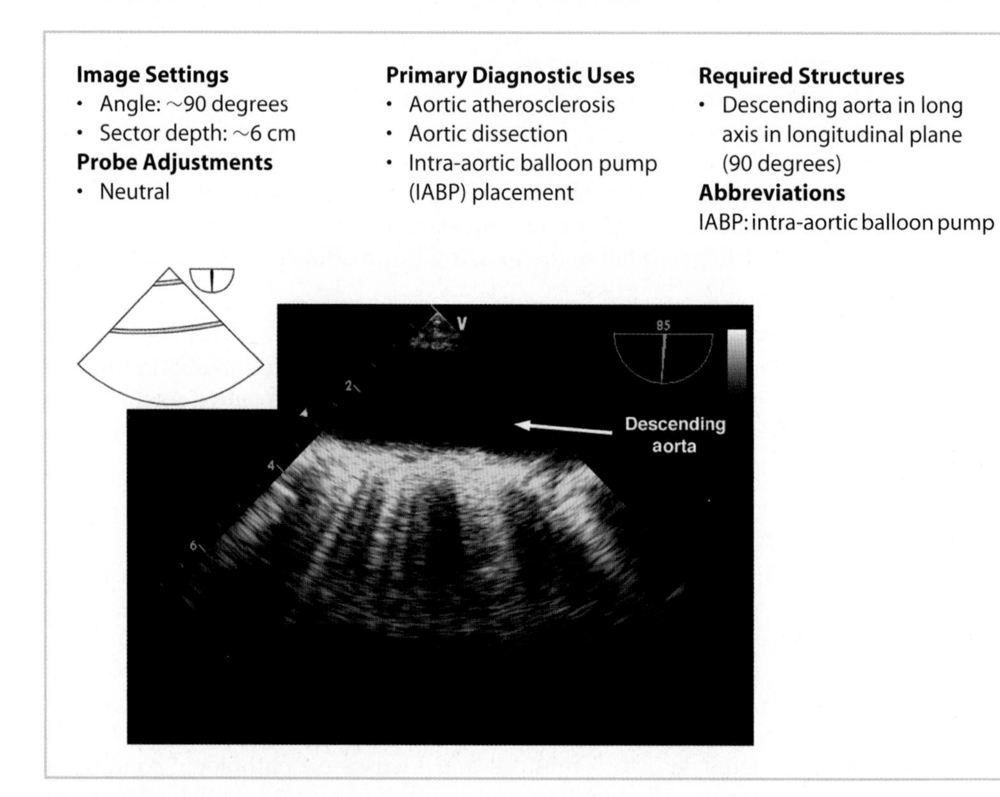

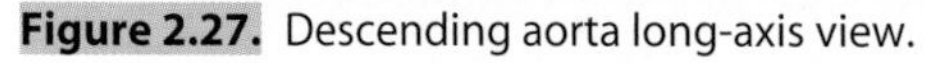
Figure 2.27. Descending aorta long-axis view.

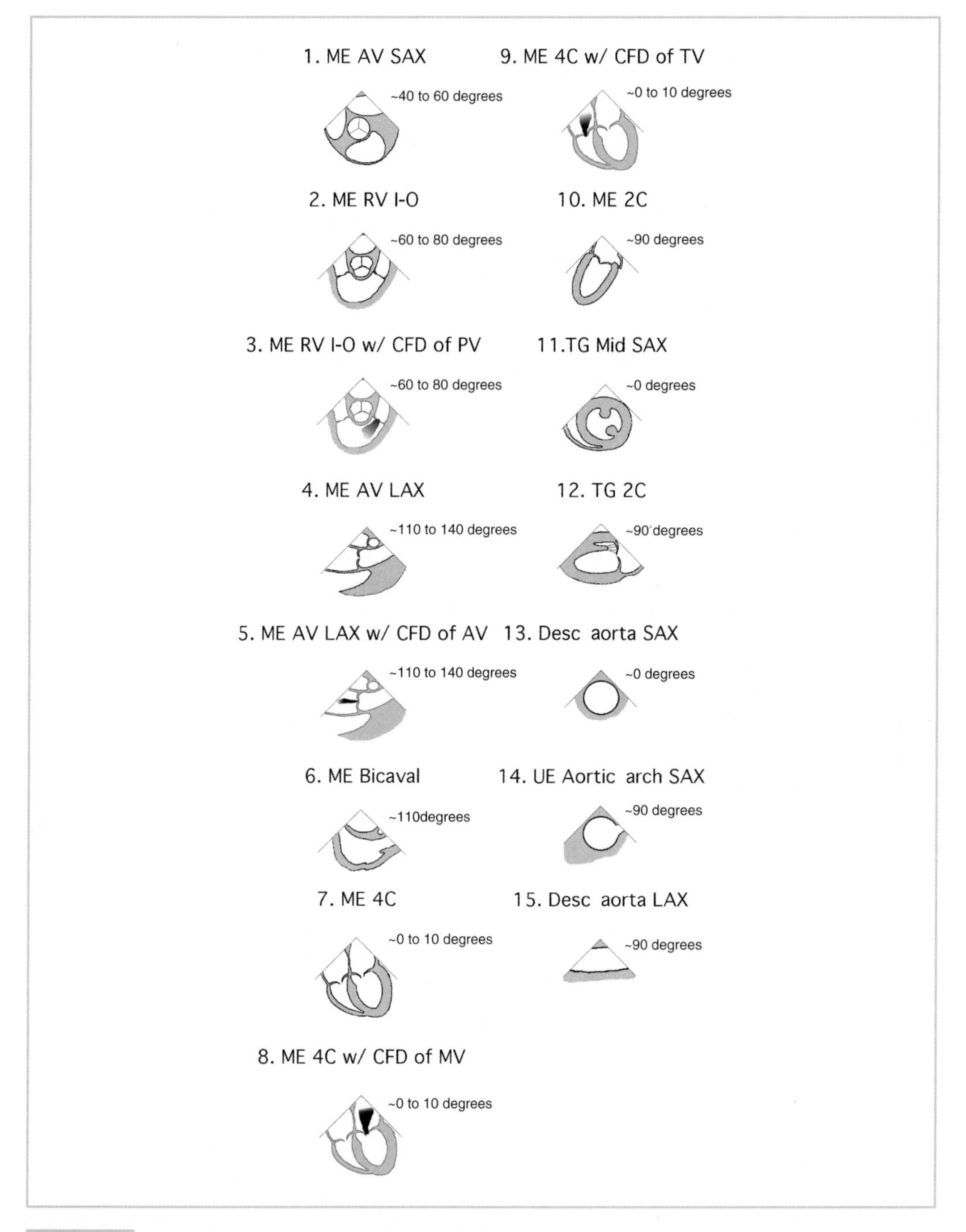

Figure 2.28. The author's recommended basic transesophageal echocardiography cardiac examination. ME, midesophageal; AV, aortic valve; CFD, color Doppler flow; TV, tricuspid valve; RV, right ventricular; I-O, inflow-outflow; PV, pulmonary valve; TG, transgastric; SAX, short-axis; LAX, long-axis; Desc, descending; 2C, two-chamber; 4C, four-chamber. (Modified from Miller JP, Lambert SA, Shapiro WA, et al. The adequacy of basic intraoperative transesophageal echocardiography performed by experienced anesthesiologists. *Anesth Analg* 2001;92:1103–1110, with permission.)

in at least two planes. On the basis of the findings, specific pathology and be further evaluated using additional two dimensional and Doppler techniques. In the intraoperative and critical care settings the abbreviated exam plays an important role.

SUMMARY

Mastering the two-dimensional echocardiographic examination requires an understanding of the imaging planes and practical experience. No two patients' anatomy is identical, and the images obtained in clinical practice vary from the textbook examples. Some TEE views cannot be obtained in certain patients. A common setback is disorientation with the displayed images. *To recover your anatomic orientation, it is often best to return the imaging plane to 0 degree because many structures are more easily identified from the transverse plane.* Next, identify the structure at the apex of the scan. This structure will be one of the great vessels (most often the aorta), the left atrium, or the left ventricle. Next, advance or withdraw the probe until you can identify a major structure in the view (e.g., aortic valve). Finally, with the known structures in view, rotate the imaging plane. In this way, an unknown structure can be identified by its association with the neighboring anatomy.

This chapter has described a stepwise approach to ensure an efficient yet systematic examination of the pertinent anatomy. Whether performing an abbreviated or comprehensive examination a definable and reproducible sequence should be followed. The habit of jumping around leads to the all too common error of omitting views and missing clinically important and unrecognized abnormalities.

REFERENCES

1 Sheikh KH, De Bruijn NP, Rankin JS, et al. The utility of transesophageal echocardiography and Doppler color flow imaging in patients undergoing cardiac valve surgery. *J Am Coll Cardiol* 1990;15:363–372.
2 Sheikh KH, Bengtson JR, Rankin JS, et al. Intraoperative transesophageal Doppler color flow imaging used to guide patient selection and operative treatment of ischemic mitral regurgitation. *Circulation* 1991;84:594–604.
3 Stevenson JG. Adherence to physician training guidelines for pediatric transesophageal echocardiography affects the outcome of patients undergoing repair of congenital cardiac defects. *J Am Soc Echocardiogr* 1999; 12:165–172.
4 Ungerleider RM, Kisslo JA, Greeley WJ, et al. Intraoperative echocardiography during congenital heart operations: experience from 1,000 cases. *Ann Thorac Surg* 1995;60(Suppl 3):S539–S542.
5 Savage RM, Lytle BW, Aronson S, et al. Intraoperative echocardiography is indicated in high-risk coronary artery bypass grafting. *Ann Thorac Surg* 1997;64:368–374.
6 American Society of Anesthesiologists. Practice guidelines for perioperative transesophageal echocardiography. A report by the American Society of Anesthesiologists and the Society of Cardiovascular Anesthesiologists Task Force on Transesophageal Echocardiography. *Anesthesiology* 1996;84:986–1006.
7 Shanewise JS, Cheung AT, Aronson S, et al. ASE/SCA guidelines for performing a comprehensive intraoperative multiplane transesophageal echocardiographic examination: recommendations of the American Society of Echocardiography Council for Intraoperative Echocardiography and the Society of Cardiovascular Anesthesiologists Task Force for Certification in Perioperative Transesophageal Echocardiography. *Anesth Analg* 1999;89:870–884.
8 Miller JP, Lambert SA, Shapiro WA, et al. The adequacy of basic intraoperative transesophageal echocardiography performed by experienced anesthesiologists. *Anesth Analg* 2001;92:1103–1110.

QUESTIONS

1. The large knob on the TEE hand piece controls
  a. Anteflexion/retroflexion.
  b. Left/right flexion.
  c. Image rotation.
  d. Image depth.

2. The small knob on the TEE hand piece controls
  a. Anteflexion/retroflexion.
  b. Left/right flexion.
  c. Image rotation.
  d. Image depth.

3. When a standard orientation is used, at 0 degree, the image seen on the right side of the display is
  a. On the patient's left.
  b. On the patient's right.
  c. Cephalad.
  d. Caudad.

4. When a standard orientation is used, at 90 degrees, the image seen on the right side of the display is
  a. On the patient's left.
  b. On the patient's right.
  c. Cephalad.
  d. Caudad.

5. The primary diagnostic purpose of the ME aortic valve short-axis view is to
  a. Identify aortic valve stenosis.
  b. Identify aortic valve insufficiency.
  c. Measure the sinotubular junction.
  d. Identify both **a** and **b.**

6. The view that best visualizes the left ventricular apex is the
  a. ME two-chamber view.
  b. TG two-chamber view.
  c. TG mid–short-axis view.
  d. ME four-chamber view.

7. The view that is not commonly useful in assessing LV systolic function is the
  a. ME four-chamber view.
  b. ME two-chamber view.
  c. TG mid–short-axis view.
  d. ME bicaval view.

8. Increasing the near field time gain compensation is especially important in an interrogation of the
  a. Left atrium.
  b. Right atrium.
  c. Left ventricle.
  d. Aorta.

9. The origins of the great vessels (e.g., carotid, subclavian) can be seen in the

a. ME four-chamber view.
b. Descending aorta short-axis view.
c. Descending aorta long-axis view.
d. Upper esophageal aortic arch short-axis view.

10. The left atrial appendage is best seen in the

a. ME bicaval view.
b. ME two-chamber view.
c. TG mid–short-axis view.
d. TG two-chamber view.

Answers appear at the back of the book.

3 Left Ventricular Systolic Performance and Pathology

Susan Garwood

Of all the indications for echocardiography, the evaluation of left ventricular (LV) systolic function is perhaps the most common; in part because it is the best understood parameter of cardiac function but also because it has consistently been shown to be a predictor of morbidity and mortality. Left ventricular systolic performance is usually assessed in practically every echocardiogram, even if it is not the primary focus of the exam. The American Society of Echocardiography (ASE) recommends that every complete echocardiographic examination should include the evaluation of LV chamber size and function and emphasizes the importance of these measurements for clinical decision making (1).

WHAT IS LEFT VENTRICULAR SYSTOLIC FUNCTION?

LV systolic function describes the contractility of the LV. Contractility of the myocardial fibers of the heart is described by the Frank-Starling relationship whereby increases in preload (left ventricular end diastolic pressure [LVEDP]) result in increased contractility. Therefore, contractility or systolic function is load dependent and strictly speaking, should be assessed over a range of preload and afterload. This is not usually clinically feasible and true load-independent assessments of LV systolic function are difficult using echocardiography. Consequently, the preload status at the time of the examination is frequently reported along with the systolic function as the LV chamber dimension either as a diameter, area, or volume. LV thickness or mass is also usually reported with systolic function and LV chamber size to complement the overall estimate of LV systolic performance.

Quantitative Measures of Left Ventricular Systolic Performance

LV systolic performance may be assessed qualitatively or quantitatively with echocardiography. There are a number of parameters which describe LV systolic function, the most commonly used being ejection fraction. Ejection fraction is expressed mathematically as a fraction of a diastolic dimension minus the corresponding systolic dimension divided by the original diastolic dimension, where this dimension can be a linear measurement, an area, or a volume. For example:

$$\{(LVEDV - LVESV)/LVEDV\} \times 100\%$$

where LVEDV is LV end diastolic volume and LVESV is LV end systolic volume. A normal ejection fraction is equal to or greater than 55% for both men and women.

An echocardiographer may become quite efficient and accurate at visually estimating left ventricular ejection fraction (LVEF). However, accuracy and reproducibility are dependent upon the individual interpreter's skill and interobserver measurements may vary considerably. Consequently, calibrated measurements are preferred, and the ASE recommends that even experienced echocardiographers regularly cross- check qualitative evaluations against calibrated measurements (1).

QUANTITATIVE EVALUATION OF LEFT VENTRICULAR SYSTOLIC FUNCTION–LINEAR MEASUREMENTS

Linear measurements (whether made from motion mode [M-mode] or two-dimensional [2-D] images) have the lowest interobserver variability as compared to area or volume measurements, render quite accurate estimates of systolic function in healthy subjects, but are probably the least representative of overall LV systolic function in cardiac diseases that produce regional abnormalities of the myocardium. Linear measurements are preferably made from M-mode tracings, because the higher pulse rate compared to 2-D provides better temporal resolution.

Endocardial fractional shortening

Endocardial fractional shortening (%): $= \{(\text{LVIDd} - \text{LVIDs})/\text{LVIDd}\} \times 100$

Normal values: men 25% to 43%, women 27% to 45% (1).

The measurements required for this quantitative estimate of systolic function are LV internal diameter at end diastole (LVIDd also called *end diastolic diameter LVEDD*) and LV internal diameter at end systole (LVIDs also called *end systolic diameter LVESD*). These are measured from endocardial border to endocardial border (known as *leading edge to leading edge*) (2) from an M-mode tracing of a transgastric short axis (TG SAX) view taken just above the papillary muscles (Figure 3.1).

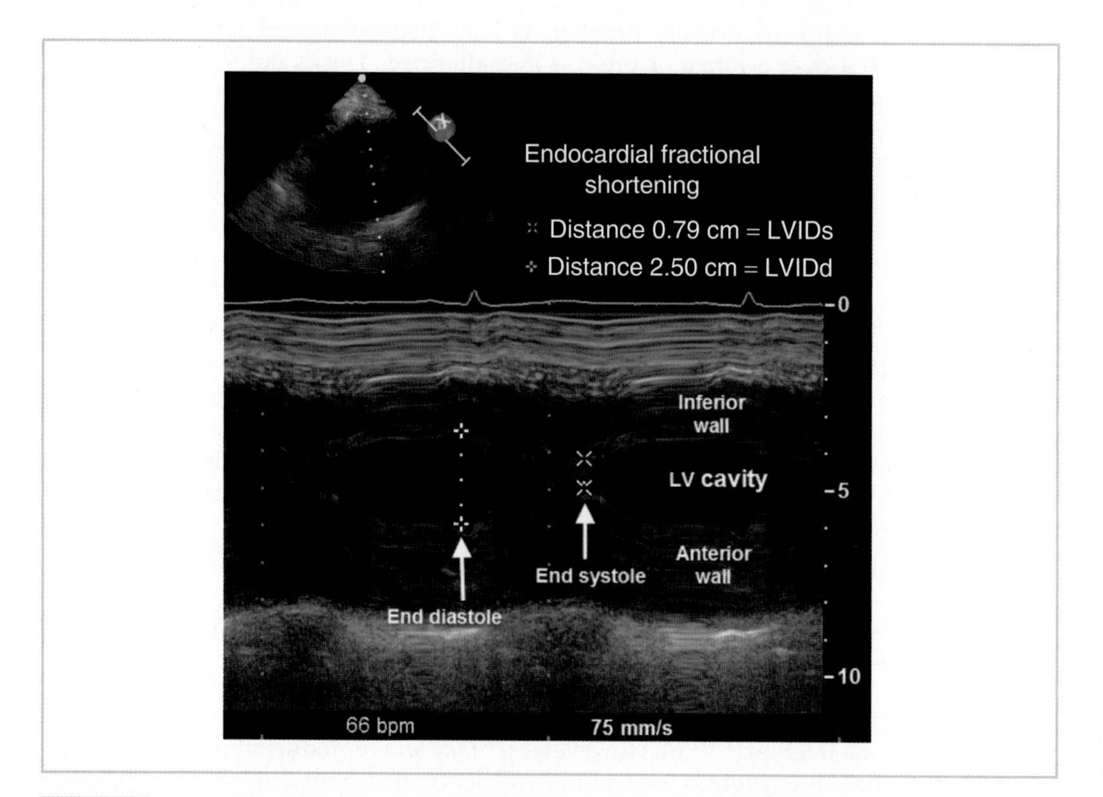

Figure 3.1. Transgastric mid short-axis view demonstrating M-mode measurements of ventricular cavity dimensions in systole and diastole using the leading edge to leading edge technique. LVIDd, left ventricular internal diameter at end diastole; LVIDs, left ventricular internal diameter at end systole; LV, left ventricular.

Although fractional shortening gives a rapid and simple estimate of LV systolic function, it is not a representative measurement in asymmetric ventricles such as those with regional wall abnormalities or aneurismal deformation (1).

Left Ventricular Wall Thickness

Normal values: men 0.6 to 1.0 cm, women 0.6 to 0.9 cm (1).

Measurements of LV wall thickness are made using the TG mid SAX view. Usually both septal wall thickness at end diastole (SWTd) and posterior wall thickness at end diastole (PWTd) are reported. Septal wall thickness is measured from the right septal surface to the left septal surface, whereas posterior wall thickness is measured from epicardial surface to endocardial surface (being careful not to include pericardial tissue), using leading edge methodology for M-mode (2) and trailing edge to leading edge for 2-D (1).

Relative wall thickness

Relative wall thickness (RWT) mm: $= (2 \times \text{PWTd})/\text{LVIDd}$

or $(\text{PWTd} + \text{SWTd})/\text{LVIDd}$.

Normal values: men 0.24 to 0.42 cm, women 0.22 to 0.42 cm (1).

RWT is often used in patients with LV hypertrophy. In transesophageal echocardiography (TEE), the measurements are usually made in a TG SAX (just above the papillary muscles) and may be calculated from either of the two formulae given earlier. RWT is expressed as a decimal and used to describe LV hypertrophy and remodeling. An RWT equal to or greater than 0.42 denotes concentric hypertrophy (wall thickness is increased in the presence of a normal internal diameter) and an RWT less than 0.42 denotes eccentric hypertrophy (dilated internal ventricular dimension). The distinction between the two forms of hypertrophy is of prognostic interest, as concentric hypertrophy is associated with a higher incidence of cardiovascular events than eccentric hypertrophy.

QUANTITATIVE EVALUATION OF LEFT VENTRICULAR SYSTOLIC FUNCTION–PLANIMETRIC MEASUREMENTS

Area measurements offer improvements in accuracy over linear dimensions, as more of the LV is represented in the measurement.

Fractional area change

Fractional area change (FAC) (%): $= \{(\text{LVAd} - \text{LVAs})/\text{LVAd}\} \times 100$

Normal values: men 56% to 62%, women 59% to 65% (3).

The area of the LV cavity is measured at end systole (LVAs) and at end diastole (LVAd) and used to calculate FAC. Most commonly these measurements are made from the TG mid SAX view of the LV, but when this view is suboptimal long axis views can be substituted. The endocardium is manually traced around the LV cavity ignoring the papillary muscles.

Alternatively, automated border detection obviates the need to manually trace cavity area and provides real time, beat-to-beat measures of LVAd, LVAs, and FAC (Figure 3.2). The acoustic properties of tissue and blood are discriminated because they create significantly different backscatter and thereby signal strength, allowing for automated detection of the endocardial border. A software package computes and displays the area of the LV (blood pool) cavity, superimposes it upon a 2-D display of the ventricle and calculates the FAC

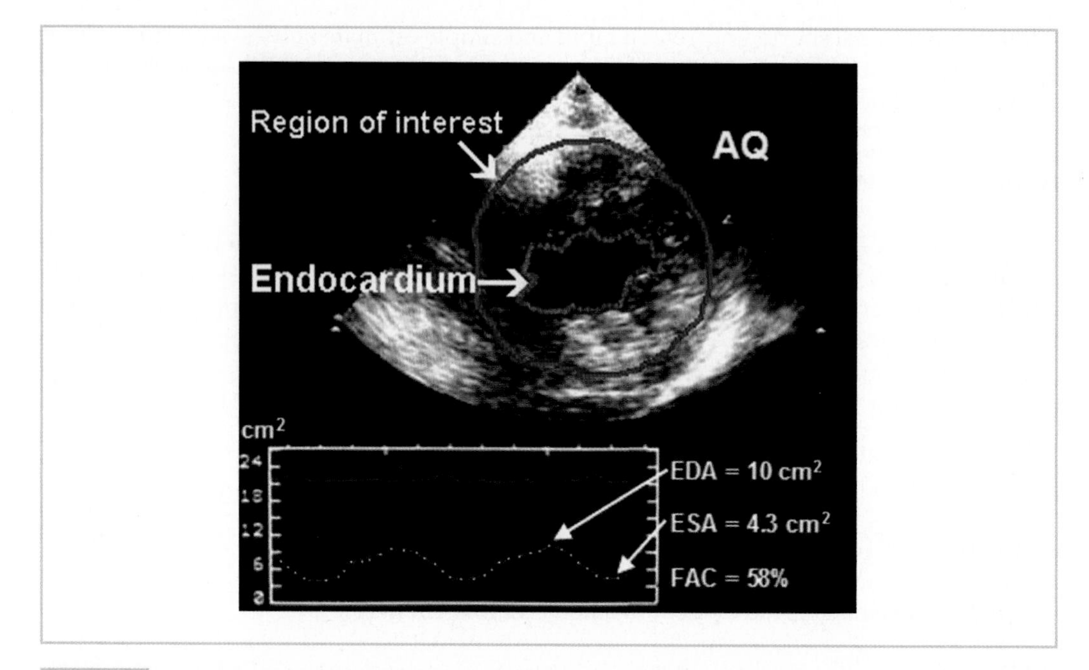

Figure 3.2. Transgastric mid short-axis view demonstrating automated border detection measurement (*red line*) of fractional area of change (lower panel). EDA, end diastolic area; ESA, end systolic area; FAC, fractional area of change.

on a beat-to-beat basis in the TG mid SAX view. The echocardiographer adjusts the time compensated gain, lateral gain, and overall gain settings to ensure that the displayed automated border tracks the endocardium throughout the cardiac cycle. For example, attenuation (or drop out) caused by the relative parallel orientation of myocardial fibers in the septal and lateral walls to the ultrasound beam in the SAX view decreases backscatter and therefore signal strength. Accordingly, adjustments to the lateral gain compensation are used to enhance receiver gain in these areas and allow for better tracking of the borders by the software.

QUANTITATIVE EVALUATION OF LEFT VENTRICULAR SYSTOLIC FUNCTION–LEFT VENTRICULAR VOLUMES

LV volumes measured at end systole and end diastole are used to calculate ejection fraction. However, LV systolic volumes in and of themselves have prognostic value. Values greater than 70 mL are associated with increased risk for morbidity and mortality.

Left ventricular volume, volumetric equations using linear measurements

There are a number of formulae in use which derive a 3-D LV volume from linear measurements. These are based on geometric models, which approximate the shape of a *symmetric* LV.

The Cubed formula

Cubed formula: LV Volume (mL) $= (\text{LVID}_{\text{minor}})^3$.

This formula assumes that the LV is approximated by a prolate ellipse, which has a SAX (minor axis, $\text{LVID}_{\text{minor}}$) equal to one half of the long axis (or major axis $\text{LVID}_{\text{major}}$) (Figure 3.3). Measurement of the minor axis can be performed in the midesophageal (ME)

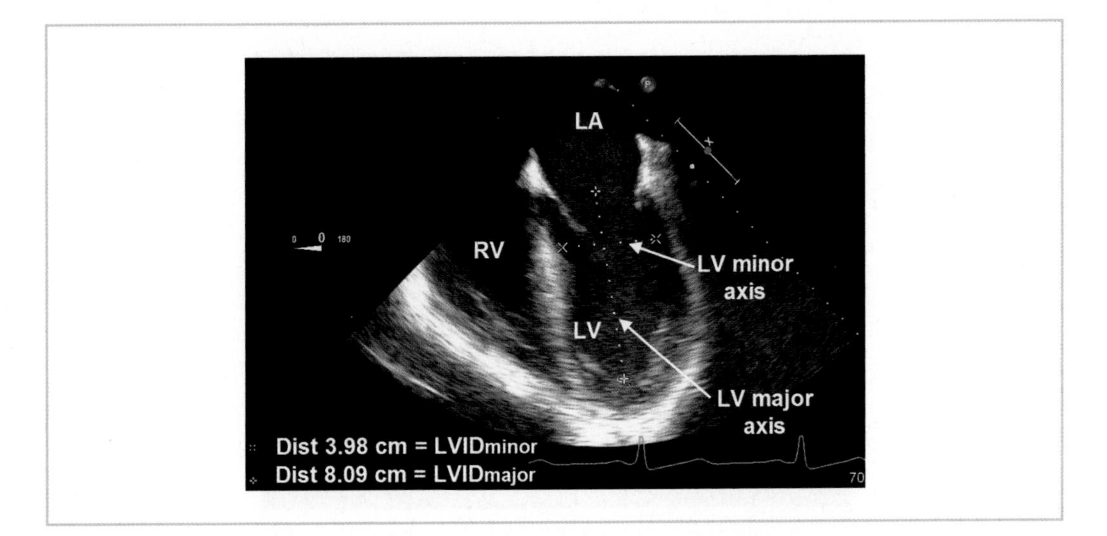

Figure 3.3. Midesophageal four chamber demonstrating left ventricle (LV) as a prolate ellipse, which has a short axis (left ventricular internal diameter minor axis [$LVID_{minor}$]) equal to one half of the long axis (or major axis $LVID_{major}$). The minor axis is used for the cubed formula. LA, left atrium; RV, right ventricle; LVID, left ventricle internal diameter.

two- or four- chamber or the TG two-chamber view and are taken at the mitral chordae level (1). Although the cube formula is the simplest formula, it compounds measurement errors because of the cube function and overestimates the volume of dilated ventricles. This occurs because the LV dilates primarily along the SAX, becoming more spherical in shape.

Volumetric equations using planimetric measurements

Again, these formulae are derived from geometric models which approximate a symmetrically shaped LV.

1. *Single plane ellipsoid*

$$\text{Single plane ellipsoid method: LV volume (mL)} = 8 \times (LVA_{LAX})^2/3\pi LVID_{major}$$

   The LV volume is calculated assuming an ellipsoid shape (Figure 3.4). The long axis diameter ($LVID_{major}$) and corresponding LV cavity area (LVA_{LAX}) obtained from a single long axis view (ME four or two chamber, or TG two chamber) are required for this formula. The basal border of the LV cavity area is best delineated by a straight line connecting the mitral valve (MV) insertions at the lateral and septal borders of the annulus (1).
2. *Biplane ellipsoid*

$$\text{Biplane ellipsoid method: LV volume (mL)} = (\pi\ LVID_{major}/6) \times (4\ LVA_{SAX}/\pi\ LVID_{minor}) \times (4\ LVA_{LAX}/\pi\ LVID_{major})$$

   This model incorporates the LV major axis diameter $LVID_{major}$ (acquired from a ME two- or four-chamber view or TG two-chamber which are view, all long axis views) and the LV cavity area from the same image (LVA_{LAX}); plus the LV minor axis diameter ($LVID_{minor}$) acquired from the TG SAX of the LV view just above the papillary muscles; plus the corresponding LV cavity area from the same image (LVA_{SAX}).

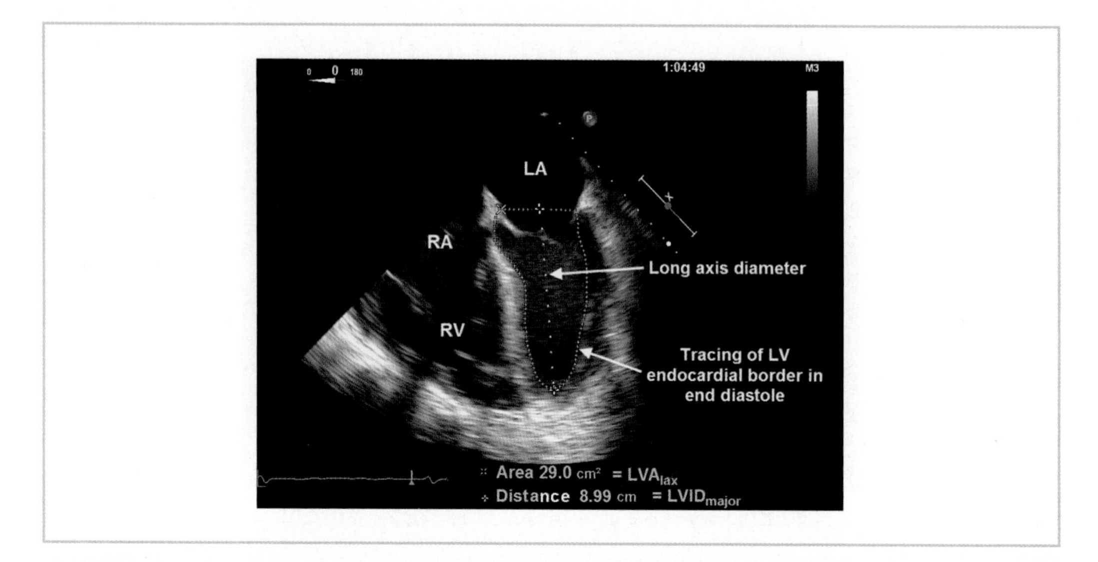

Figure 3.4. Midesophageal two chamber demonstrating the measurements required for single plane ellipsoid formula; a long axis diameter ($LVID_{major}$) and the left ventricle (LV) area from the same long axis view (LVA_{LAX}). LA, left atrium; RA, right atrium; RV, right ventricle.

3. *Hemisphere-cylinder or bullet formula*

Hemisphere-cylinder (or bullet formula): LV volume (mL) = $5/6 \times LVA_{SAX} \times LVID_{major}$

This model approximates the LV to the shape of a bullet (Figure 3.5). Volume is calculated from a long axis diameter ($LVID_{major}$) and the LV cavity area from the TG mid SAX view (LVA_{SAX}). This formula is also known as the *area length formula*.

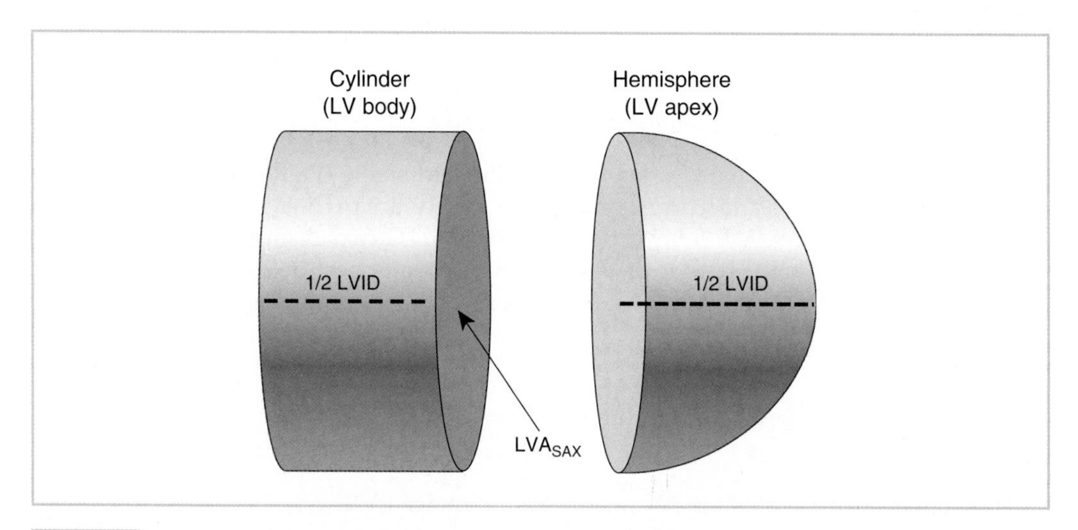

Figure 3.5. Demonstrates how the geometry of a cylinder plus a hemisphere approximates the left ventricle (LV) as a bullet. The length of the cylinder and the radius of the hemisphere are both equal to one half left ventricular internal diameter major axis ($LVID_{major}$). *LVA_{SAX}*, left ventricle area from the short axis view.

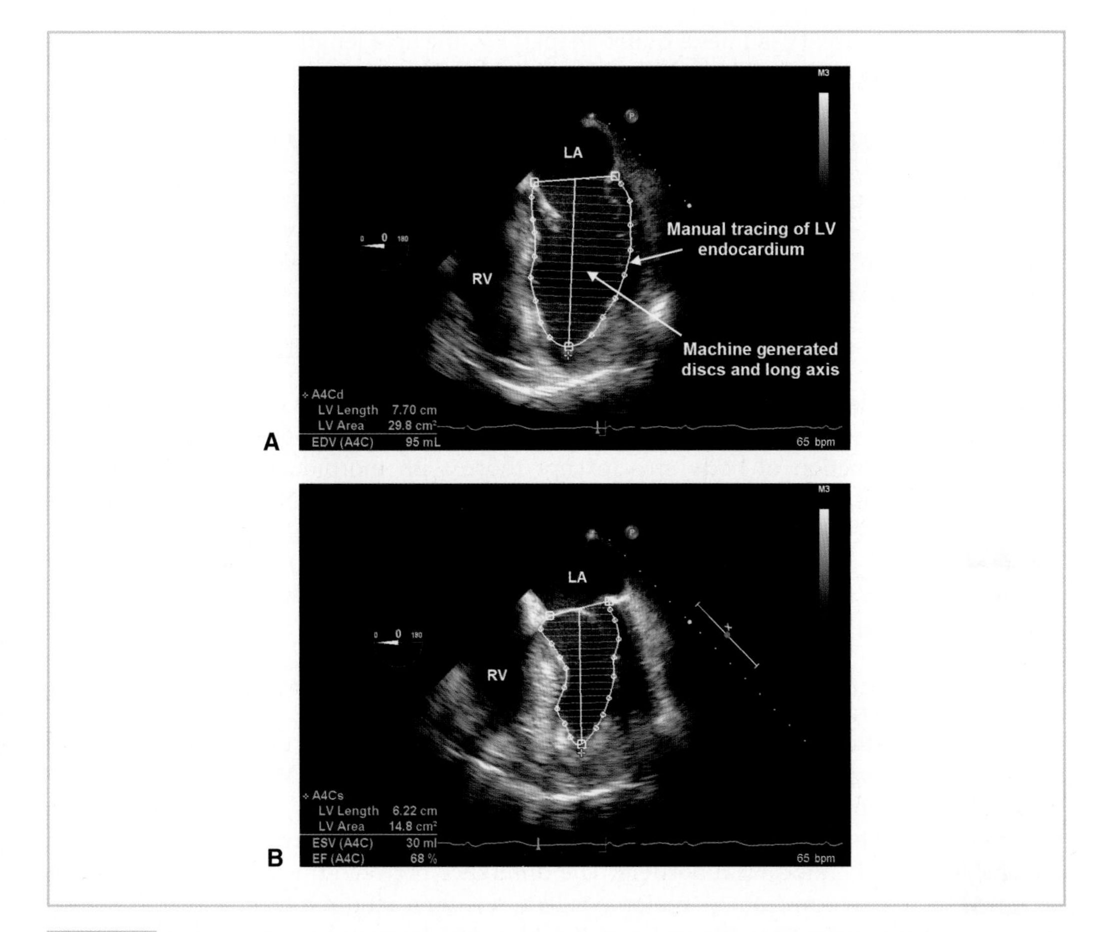

Figure 3.6. Midesophageal (ME) four-chamber views demonstrating the left ventricle (LV) measurements required for the method of disks (modified Simpson's rule) to estimate LVEF. **A:** ME four-chamber view at end diastole; the endocardium is manually traced and the software calculates the $LVID_{major}$ and divides the LV cavity into 20 discs. **B:** ME four-chamber view at end systole; the same measurements are made as in part A. These measurements also required in the ME two-chamber view. LA, left atrium; RV, right ventricle; EDV, end diastolic volume; ESV, end systolic volume; EF, ejection fraction.

4. *Method of disks (modified Simpson's rule)*

Modified Simpson's rule: LV Volume (mL) =

$$(\pi/4)\Sigma_{(n=1-20)}\ (\text{LVIDn}_{\text{minor(ME 2 chamber)}} \times \text{LVIDn}_{\text{minor(ME 4 chamber)}}) \times \text{LVID}_{\text{major}}/20$$

In this method, the LV is described as a series of 20 disks from the base to the apex of the LV, like a stack of coins of decreasing size. The views required for this calculation are ME 4- (Figure 3.6) and two-chamber views. The computer software package calculates the volume of each disk as area × height and the volumes are summated to give a total LV volume. Foreshortening of the LV will result in underestimation of volume (1). *Because biplane planimetry (area acquired using both the ME four- and two-chamber views) corrects for shape distortion and minimizes mathematical assumptions, the method of disks is the recommended technique for volumetric measurements of the LV, particularly in those patients with regional wall motion abnormalities or an aneurysm* (1). In cases where the endocardial border of the apex is not well seen, the area length method becomes the method of choice (1). Because it assumes a bullet-shaped LV, the area length method compensates for the inability to detect the apical endocardial borders.

QUANTITATIVE EVALUATION OF LEFT VENTRICULAR SYSTOLIC FUNCTION–LEFT VENTRICULAR MASS; LINEAR MEASUREMENTS

All LV mass calculations are based on the subtraction of the volume of the LV cavity from the volume encompassed by the LV epicardium. This leaves LV myocardial volume, which is then multiplied by the density of myocardial tissue to calculate LV mass. The ASE recommends the following formula:

$$\text{LV mass (g)}=0.8 \times [1.04 \times \{(\text{LVID}_{\text{major}} + \text{PWT} + \text{SWT})^3 - (\text{LVID}_{\text{major}})^3\}] + 0.6\text{ g}$$

Increased LV mass is a stronger predictor than low EF for all cause mortality and cardiac event rates in both hypertensive and normotensive populations. Because LV mass increases as a function of body size (except those with morbid obesity), LV mass is preferably expressed as a function of body surface area (BSA) (1). Normal values for LV mass are given as 67 to 162 g for women and 88 to 224 g for men. Indexed to BSA this becomes 43 to 95 g/m^2 for women and 49 to 115 g/m^2 for men (1) (Table 3.1). LV mass may be combined with RWT to categorize patients into various classes of hypertrophy (1) (see following section on 'Left Ventricular Hypertrophy').

QUANTITATIVE EVALUATION OF LEFT VENTRICULAR SYSTOLIC FUNCTION–LEFT VENTRICULAR MASS, PLANIMETRIC MEASUREMENTS

In the determination of LV mass using planimetric measurements, either the area length method or the truncated ellipsoid method are recommended (1,4). Most current echocardiography machines include the software to calculate LV mass by one or both of these two methods. The LV is acquired in the TG mid SAX view. An area tracing is made of the epicardial and endocardial borders. The difference between the two areas is the area occupied by the myocardium. A major axis length is then acquired from a long axis view and the software calculates the mass of the LV according to the formulae used by the vendor (1,4), Figure 3.7.

QUANTITATIVE EVALUATION OF LEFT VENTRICULAR SYSTOLIC FUNCTION–RATE OF VENTRICULAR PRESSURE RISE

The rate of rise in ventricular pressure (dP/dT) has been demonstrated to be well correlated with systolic function. The greater the contractile force exerted, the greater the rise in ventricular pressure. Previously this could only be measured invasively with LV catheterization; however continuous wave Doppler (CWD) determination of the velocity of a mitral regurgitant (MR) jet allows calculation of instantaneous pressure gradients between the left ventricle and the left atrium. Left atrial pressure variations in early systole can be considered to be negligible; therefore, the rising segment of the MR velocity curve should essentially reflect LV pressure increase only. If the rate of rise in ventricular pressure is reduced because of poor LV function, the rate of increase of the MR jet velocity will also be low.

To perform a dP/dT measurement (Figure 3.8), the MR jet is interrogated with CWD. The cursor is placed on the MR velocity profile at 1/ms and then at 3/ms and the time interval between the two points is determined (5). Using the simplified Bernoulli equation, the pressure differential is $[4(3)^2] - [4(1)^2]$ or 32 mm Hg. dP/dT is therefore 32 mm Hg divided by the time interval in seconds. Normal values exceed 1,000 mm Hg/s.

Table 3.1 Normal values for echocardiographic left ventricular systolic parameters published by the American Society of Echocardiography (ASE) compared to magnetic resonance imaging data from the Framingham Heart Study

Parameter	[a]ASE (echocardiography) range	[b]Framingham Heart Study (MRI) Mean (95% upper limit)
	Left ventricular wall thickness	
Posterior wall thickness (mm)	♂ 6–10 ♀ 6–9	♂ 9.9 (11.2) ♂ 8.7 (9.8)
Septal wall thickness (mm)	♂ 6–10 ♀ 6–9	♂ 10.1 (11.7) ♀ 8.9 (10.1)
	Left ventricular volumes	
LV end systolic volume (mL)	♂ 22–58 ♀ 19–49	♂ 36.3 (65.0) ♀ 25.1 (40.9)
LV end systolic volume/BSA (mL/m²)	♂ 12–30 ♀ 12–30	♂ 18.1 (30.8) ♀ 14.8 (24.0)
	Left ventricular mass	
LV mass (g)	♂ 88–244 ♀ 67–162	♂ 115.1 (201.4) ♀ 103.0 (134.0)
LV mass/BSA (g/m²)	♂ 49–115 ♀ 43–95	♂ 77.9 (95.0) ♀ 60.8 (74.7)
LV mass/height (g/m)	♂ 52–126 ♀ 41–99	♂ 88.6 (114.0) ♀ 63.6 (81.9)
LV mass/height$^{2.7}$ (g/m$^{2.7}$)	♂ 20–48 ♀ 18—44	

[a]Lang RM, Bierig M, Devereux RB, et al. Chamber Quantification Writing Group. American Society of Echocardiography's Guidelines and Standards Committee. European Association of Echocardiography. Recommendations for chamber quantification: a report from the American Society of Echocardiography's Guidelines and Standards Committee and the Chamber Quantification Writing Group, developed in conjunction with the European Association of Echocardiography, a branch of the European Society of Cardiology. *J AmSoc Echocardiogr* 2005;18(12):1440–1463.
[b]Salton CJ, Chuang ML, O'Donnell CJ, et al. Gender differences and normal left ventricular anatomy in an adult population free of hypertension. A cardiovascular magnetic resonance study of the Framingham Heart Study Offspring cohort. *J Am Coll Cardiol* 2002;39(6):1055–1060.
LV, left ventricular; ♂, men; ♀, women; BSA, body surface area.

NEWER ECHOCARDIOGRAPHIC MODALITIES FOR ASSESSING LEFT VENTRICULAR SYSTOLIC FUNCTION

Three-dimensional echocardiography

The event of three-dimensional echocardiography (3DE) has revolutionized the acquisition and understanding of echocardiographic data. Currently there are two methods of acquiring 3DE images. One technique utilizes a set of 2-D images acquired simultaneously, which are then used to reconstruct the 3-D image. This method requires an "offline" reconstruction. The second technique employs a matrix array transducer, which scans a pyramidal shaped sector and displays the image in real time.

The advantage of 3DE for measuring LV volumes and masses is that the LV can be acquired and displayed in its true shape avoiding the need for mathematical modeling. This means that regional function can be included in the overall estimates, producing

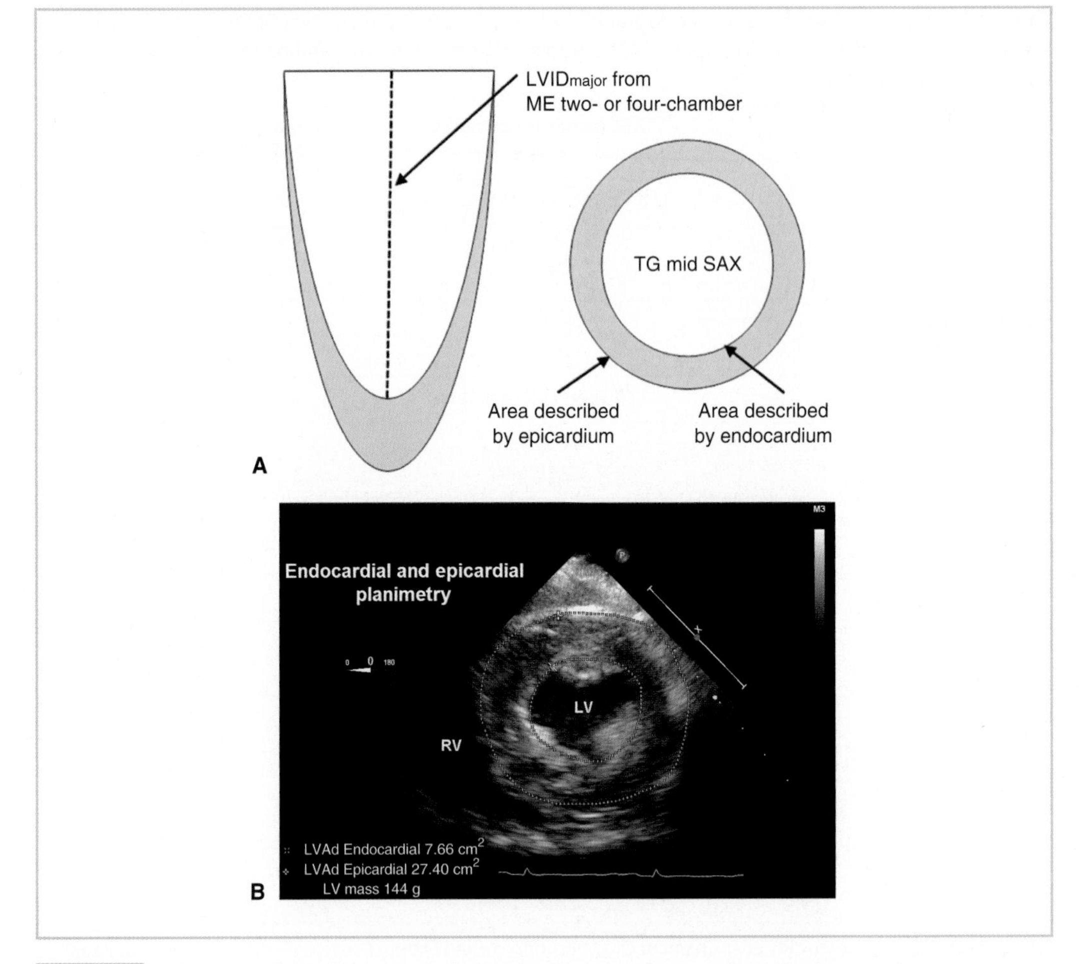

Figure 3.7. Left ventricular (LV) mass calculation. **A:** Diagram representing the views and measurements required for planimetric LV mass calculation. **B:** The endocardium and epicardium are traced in the transgastric mid short axis view and the software calculates LV mass using left ventricular internal diameter major axis ($LVID_{major}$) (from a long axis view as in part **A**) and density of myocardial tissue. LVAd, area of left ventricular cavity measured at end systole.

a more accurate measurement. Furthermore, inaccuracies do not occur because of plane positioning errors and foreshortening. 3DE is highly correlated with the gold standard of imaging (magnetic resonance imaging [MRI]), producing a better agreement with lower inter and intraobserver variation than 2DE (6). Visual display of 3-D systolic performance varies from vendor to vendor. The LV may be displayed as raw images, a wire framework, or a reconstructed volumetric figure (Figure 3.9).

Limitations of 3DE currently include time to reconstruction and the need for a regular cardiac rhythm. Even "real time" imaging requires the acquisition of several cardiac cycles, so unlike 2DE, beat-to-beat changes cannot be followed continuously during surgery. With respect to epicardial 3DE, the matrix probe is currently quite bulky and difficult to place in the mediastinal cavity for long axis imaging. Furthermore, placing the probe directly on the heart may cause some compression of the LV, mimicking regional wall abnormalities

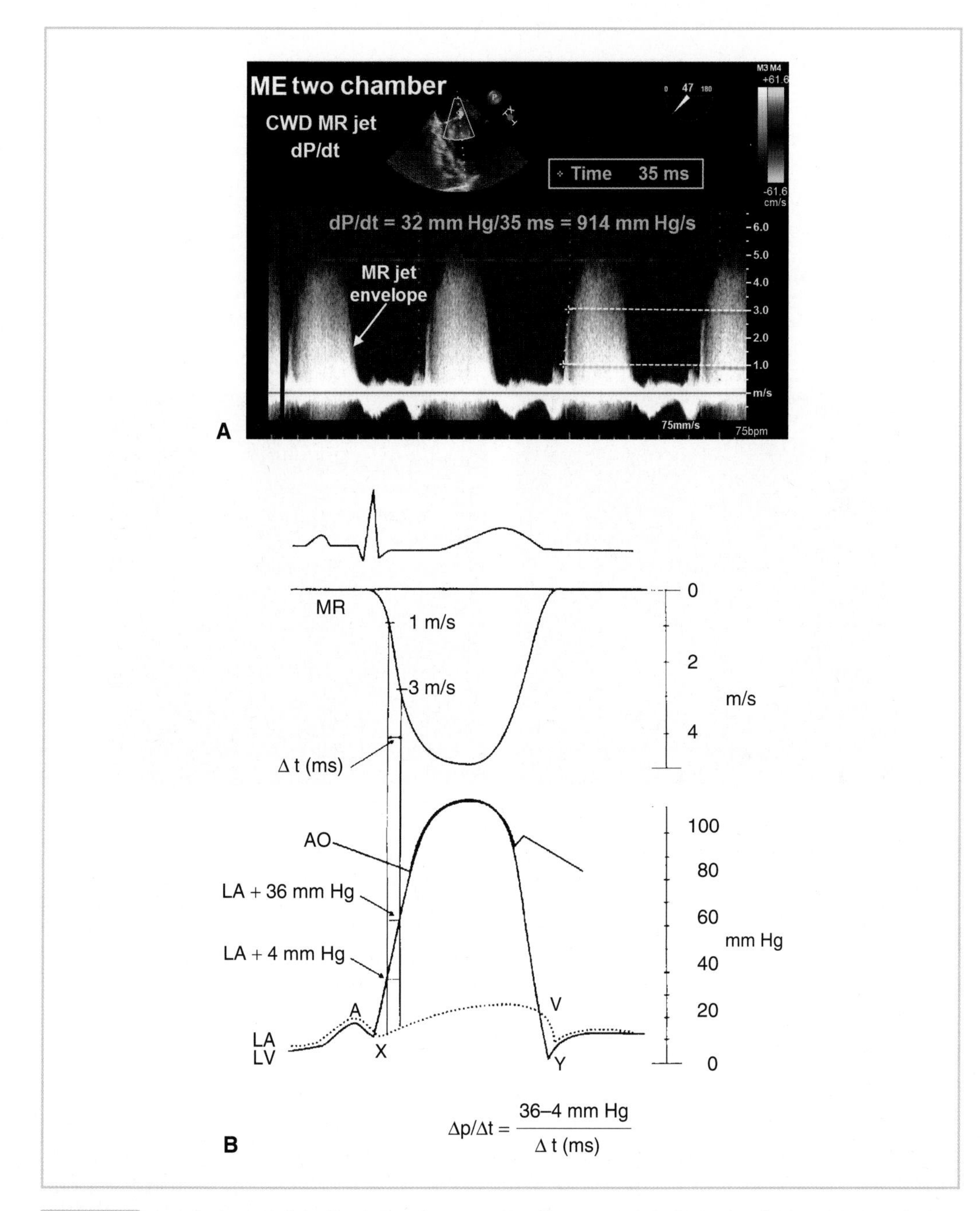

Figure 3.8. **A:** Calculation of dP/dT. Place caliper on mitral regurgitant (MR) jet envelope at 1 m/s and again at 3 m/s to measure the time for the instantaneous pressure gradient between the left ventricle (LV) and left atrium (LA) to rise from 4 mm Hg to 36 mm Hg. **B:** Upper panel; electrocardiography (ECG). Middle panel; Doppler trace of MR jet (acquired from transthoracic approach). Lower panel; equivalent pressure recordings at catheterization. CWD, continuous wave Doppler. (Part B from Pai RG, Bansal RC, Shah PM. Doppler-derived rate of left ventricular pressure rise. Its correlation with the postoperative left ventricular function in mitral regurgitation. *Circulation* 1990;82:514–520.)

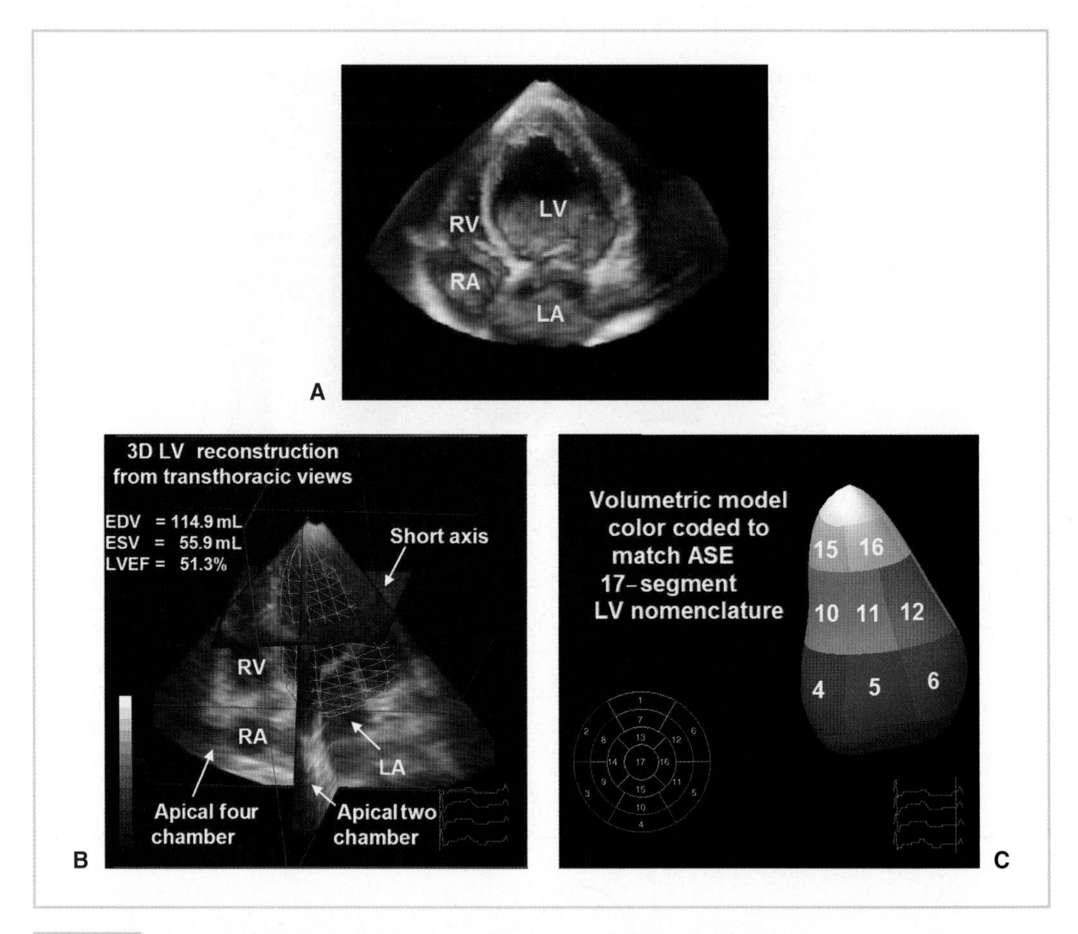

Figure 3.9. Three-dimensional (3DE) echocardiography. **A:** Apical four-chamber view (transthoracic approach) of a dilated left ventricle (LV) as raw 3-D images. **B:** 3-D representation of a left ventricle as a wire framework. **C:** 3-D representation of a left ventricle reconstructed volumetric model depicting the 17 segments used in regional wall motion analysis. RV, right ventricle; RA, right atrium; LA, left atrium; EDV, end diastolic volume; ESV, end systolic volume; LVEF, left ventricular ejection fraction; RV, right ventricle; RA, right atrium; LA, left atrium; ASE, American Society of Echocardiography. (Courtesy of Philips.)

and rendering volumetric calculations inaccurate. 3DE TEE probes are currently under development.

Tissue Doppler imaging

The high temporal resolution of Doppler imaging is specifically suited to the accurate measurement of velocities at precise locations in the heart. When Doppler is used in its original application to measure blood flow, high-pass filters are employed to screen out the low velocities from the myocardium, valvular structures and vessel walls. In contrast, tissue Doppler imaging (TDI or tissue Doppler echocardiography, TDE) measures the velocity of myocardial tissue using low-pass filters to screen out higher velocities generated by blood flow. Unlike blood flow Doppler signals that are typified by high velocity and low amplitude, myocardial motion is characterized by low velocity and high amplitude. Tissue motion creates Doppler shifts that are approximately 40 dB higher than Doppler signals from blood flow and their velocities rarely exceed 20 cm/s. To record low wall motion velocity, gain amplification is reduced and high-pass filters are bypassed.

During image acquisition, it is important to optimize temporal resolution by selecting as narrow an image sector as possible, which increases frame rate (>150/s is recommended, Figure 3.10). Equally important is to select the appropriate velocity scale. These parameters should be optimized at the time of imaging, as it is not possible to modify the frame rate and the velocity scale during postprocessing image analysis.

In TDI, a small pulsed wave sampling volume measures the velocities of the myocardium as it moves toward and away from the transducer. The sample volume is placed in the middle of a segment of the heart and velocities within that area are measured. A velocity against time plot is displayed, using the convention that tissue moving towards

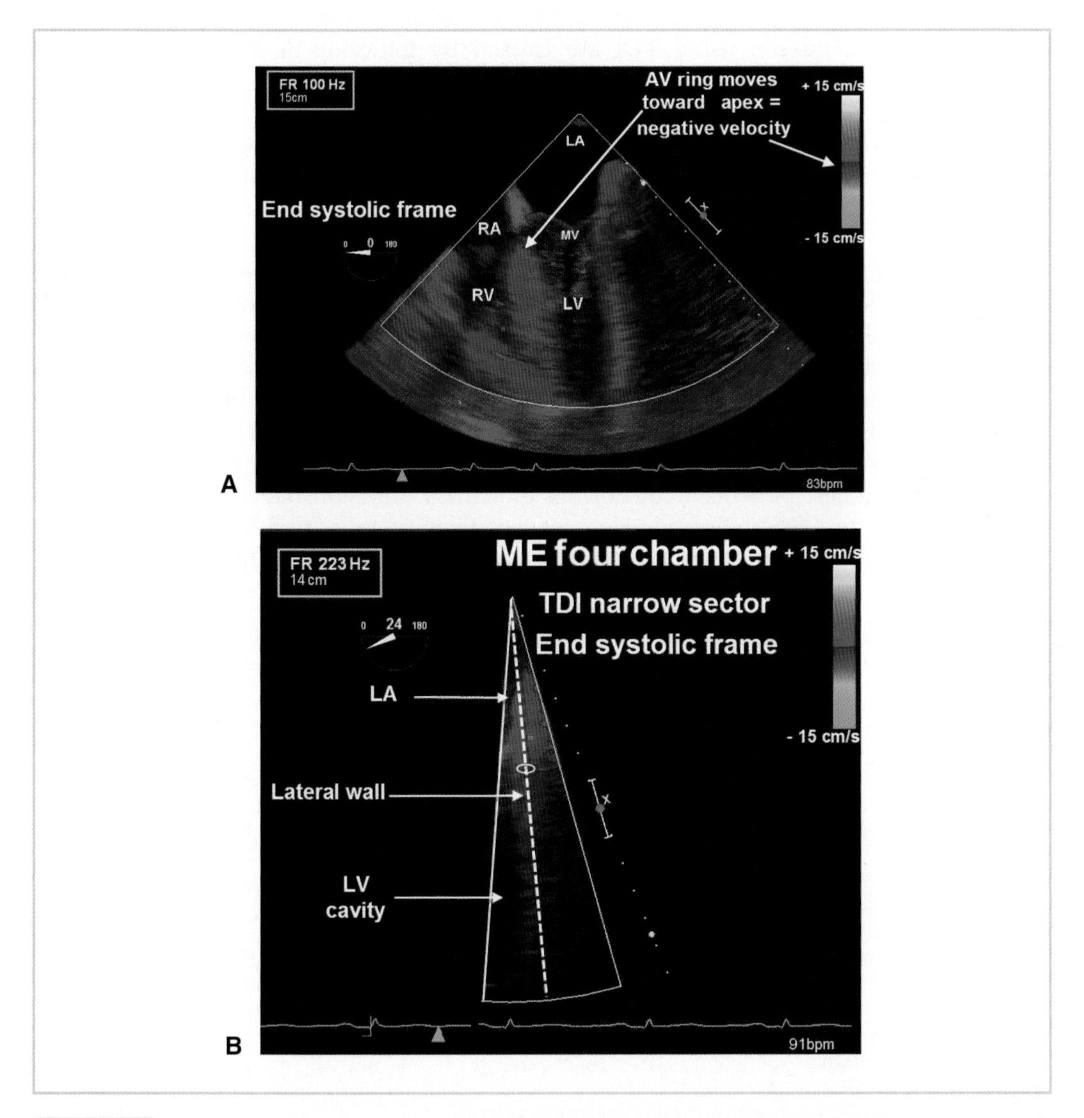

Figure 3.10. Tissue Doppler imaging (TDI). **A:** TDI of a midesophageal (ME) four-chamber view acquired as a full sector view; frame rate is 100 Hz. **B:** The same image is acquired but the sector is narrowed down to improve frame rates. Note that frame rates have increased from 100 Hz to 223 Hz. LA, left atrium; RA, right atrium; MV, mitral valve; RV, right ventricle; LV, left ventricle.

the transducer is positive. For example, during interrogation of the basal segment of the septum in the ME four-chamber view, as the heart contracts and thickens during systole the atrioventricular ring moves toward the apex and thereby will move away from the transducer producing a negative deflection.

Because this is a Doppler technique, TDI will underestimate the myocardial velocities if the angle of interrogation is not parallel to motion (7). Although most ultrasound platforms allow for correction of the Doppler equation for the angle of incidence, this is not recommended (7). Rather, it is recommended that for an ME view, the wall to be interrogated is placed in the center of the imaging sector to better align the angle of interrogation (Figure 3.10).

Other errors encountered using TDI are caused by tethering as velocity imaging is confounded by velocities from adjacent segments. For example, in a ME four-chamber view, an akinetic segment at the basal part of the septum should by definition have a longitudinal systolic velocity of zero. However, if the midventricular segment of the septal wall moves normally the tethering effect will cause the akinetic basal segment to move longitudinally.

In general, longitudinal measurements are made of the basal and midventricular segments, obtained from the ME two- and four-chamber views. A gradient of systolic velocities exists from the base of the heart to the apex. Peak systolic longitudinal velocities at the MV annulus (Sa) are greater compared to those at the midventricular segments (Sm). Sm velocities are more representative of overall systolic function. Annular velocities are difficult to acquire in patients with mitral annular calcification or with a prosthetic valve or annuloplasty ring. Myocardial velocities are age and gender dependent (Table 3.2). From transthoracic studies, patients with normal global LV function have systolic velocities greater than 7.5 cm/s (8) whereas velocities less than or equal to 5.5 cm/s indicate LV failure (9). Systolic velocities less than 3 cm/s are associated with a significant increased

Table 3.2 Factors affecting tissue Doppler imaging velocity measurements

Parameter	Tissue Doppler velocities (cm/s)			
Age differences in cardiac patients	<65 years Average Sa = 6.7 ± 1.8[a]		>65 years Average Sa = 5.7 ± 1.7[a]	
Gender differences in healthy subjects with mild hypertension	Male Sa lateral wall = 10.2(9.6–11.0)[b]		Female Sa lateral wall = 8.9(8.4–9.5)[b]	
Point of interrogation i.e., longitudinal velocity gradient (Healthy subjects)	Septum Sa = 5.7 ± 1.6[a] Sm = 4.3 ± 1.1[a] Apex = 3.1 ± 1.0[a]	Lateral Sa = 8.7 ± 2.4[a] Sm = 7.9 ± 2.4[a] Apex = 7.1 ± 2.4[a]	Posterior Sa = 6.4 ± 1.1[a] Sm = 5.4 ± 1.2[a] Apex = 4.2 ± 1.4[a]	Anterior Sa = 7.7 ± 2.0[a] Sm = 6.3 ± 2.2[a] Apex = 4.8 ± 2.5[a]

[a]Mean ± standard deviation.
[b]Mean (95% confidence intervals).
Sa, mitral annular systolic velocity; Sm, midventricular systolic velocity.
From Bountioukos M, Schinkel AF, Bax JJ, et al. Pulsed-wave tissue Doppler quantification of systolic and diastolic function of viable and nonviable myocardium in patients with ischemic cardiomyopathy. *Am Heart J* 2004;148(6):1079–1084 and Lim JG, et al. *Am Heart J* 2005;150(5):934–940; Kowalski M, Kukulski T, Jamal F, et al. Can natural strain and strain rate quantify regional myocardial deformation? A study in healthy subjects. *Ultrasound Med Bio.* 2001;27(8):1087–1097.

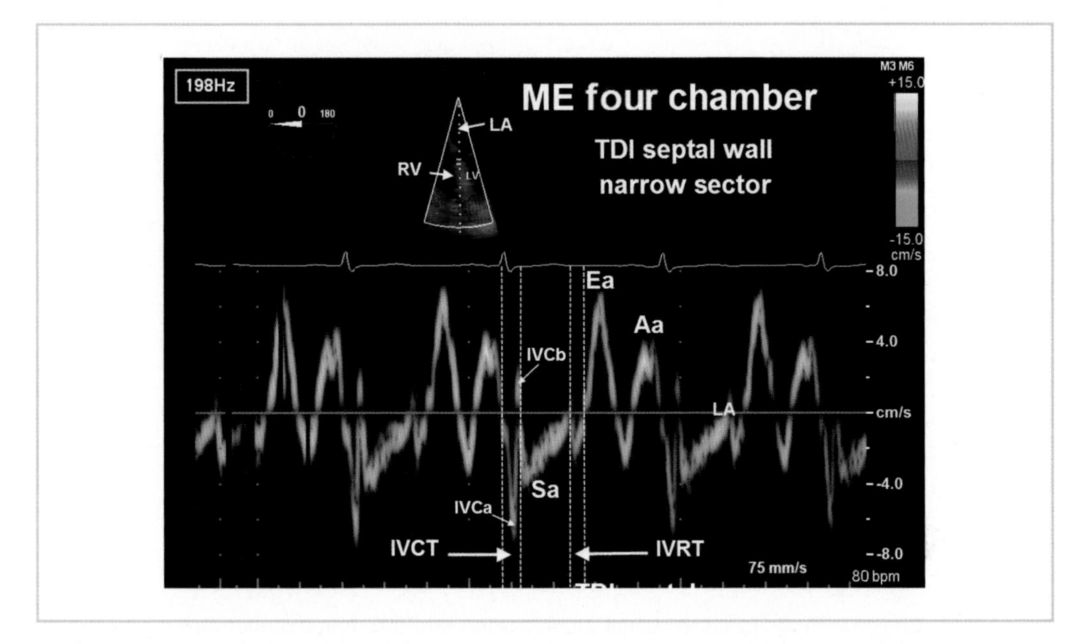

Figure 3.11. Typical left ventricle mitral annulus tissue Doppler imaging (TDI). LA, left atrium; RV, right ventricle; LV, left ventricle; Ea, early diastolic peak tissue velocity; Aa, atrial contraction (late diastolic) tissue velocity; IVC, isovolumic contraction; Sa mitral annular systolic tissue velocity; IVCT, isovolumic contraction time; IVRT, isovolumic relaxation time.

risk of cardiac death within 2 years (10). (Note that values are positive because transthoracic measurements are acquired from the apex of the heart.)

The typical systolic TDI profile (Figure 3.11) has two parts with a biphasic wave during isovolumic contraction (IVCa and IVCb) and a monophasic wave during systolic ejection. IVCa corresponds to the timing of the MV closure, and represents early myocardial activation at the base of the heart; occurring 20 to 30 ms earlier in the anteroseptal than the posterior free wall (11). The movement of the myocardium at the annulus is inward and toward the apex. The second wave IVCb is in the opposite direction caused by subsequent contraction of the apex making the base bulge up and outward just before ejection. The systolic wave is directed inward and toward the apex and represents contraction of the LV during ejection.

Color tissue Doppler

In the same way that conventional Doppler can be color coded to provide a color map of blood flow patterns, tissue Doppler can be color coded to display myocardial velocities; red depicting positive velocities and blue for negative velocities. The display is of real-time 2-D gray-scale images overlain by color-coded myocardial velocities (Figure 3.10).

Placing markers at various points along a ventricular wall produces a graphic representation of velocity against time called *curved M-mode* (Figure 3.12). This form of color TDI combines spatial resolution with high temporal resolution and can be displayed in real time. *Color tissue Doppler measures mean velocities and therefore has lower values for a given segment than tissue Doppler which measures peak instantaneous velocities.* The advantage of color tissue Doppler over tissue Doppler is the ability to utilize spatial information and therefore assess regional and global LV function. The advantage of color tissue Doppler

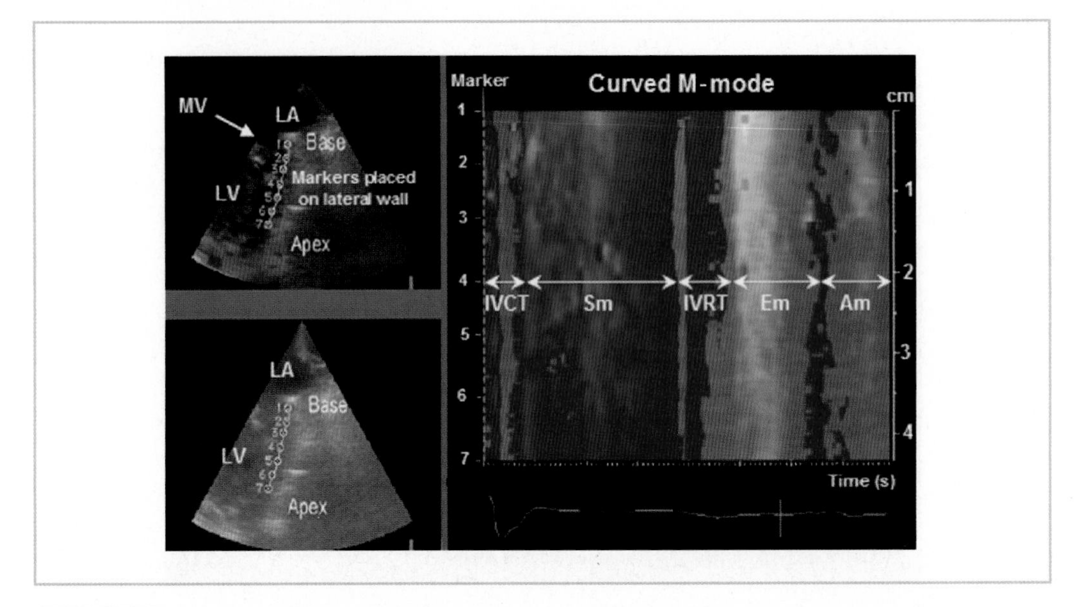

Figure 3.12. Curved M-mode. Left lower panel: 2-D midesophageal (ME) four chamber showing placement of markers on lateral wall of left ventricle (LV). Left upper panel: tissue Doppler imaging ME four chamber showing placement of markers on lateral wall of LV. Right panel: Curved M-mode, displaying mean tissue velocities of the marked positions (y axis) against time (x axis). MV, mitral valve; LA, left atrium; IVCT, Isovolumic contraction time; Sm, systolic systolic tissue velocity; IVRT, isovolumic relaxation time; Em, early diastolic tissue velocity; Am, late diastolic tissue velocity. (From Maclaren G, Kluger R, Prior D, et al. Tissue Doppler, strain, and strain rate echocardiography: principles and potential perioperative applications. *J Cardiothorac Vasc Anesth* 2006;20(4):583–593.)

over 2-D echocardiography is that the endocardial borders do not need to be clearly identified; drop out in walls which lie parallel to the path of the ultrasound beam is no longer a limitation in assessing LV function.

Strain and strain rate

Strain (ϵ) and strain rate (SR) are an extrapolation of TDI technology. Strain measures segmental myocardial deformation (or shape change) whereas SR measures the rate of this change. Deformation is the result of the complex interaction of intrinsic contractile force and extrinsic loading conditions applied to a tissue with variable elastic properties (Table 3.3). Therefore, changes in preload and afterload, and changes in myocardial stiffness, are important determinants of myocardial deformation. Therefore it follows that *ϵ and SR are not direct measures of contractility.*

Table 3.3 Normal strain and strain rate patterns

	Wall	Average value in normal subjects
Longitudinal strain (%)	Lateral, posterior, anterior	18 ± 5
	Septal	22 ± 5
Longitudinal strain rate (/s)	Anterior, septal	1.5 ± 0.4
	Lateral, posterior	1.2 ± 0.3

Adapted from Kowalski M, Kukulski T, Jamal F, et al. Can natural strain and strain rate quantify regional myocardial deformation? A study in healthy subjects. *Ultrasound Med Biol* 2001;27(8):1087–1097.

The use of ϵ and SR imaging overcomes the limitations inherent in using tissue Doppler velocity profiles because tissue Doppler myocardial velocities may be influenced by either global heart motion (translation and rotation) or by segmental motion induced by contraction of adjacent myocardial segments (tethering). By convention, an increase in myocardial length is denoted by a positive value, whereas a decrease in myocardial length is denoted by a negative value. In the ME long axis views, as the ventricle contracts, the longitudinal length becomes smaller and ϵ and SR values will be negative. Conversely, during diastole the ventricle elongates and ϵ and SR will have positive values. However, note that during systole in a SAX view of the LV, the myocardium thickens, so that the measured myocardial length (thickness) increases and ϵ and SR will have positive systolic values; with negative values during diastole as the myocardium thins out.

Modern echocardiographic machines color code strain such that positive strain is displayed as blue and negative strain is encoded red (Figure 3.13). *Note that this is the opposite of TDI color coding*. Akinetic myocardial tissue does not change dimension (no strain) and is displayed in green. Because ϵ and SR are localized measures of myocardial deformation and they do not suffer from the disadvantage of being influenced by tethering as in TDI; ϵ and SR perform better at differentiating between infracted and noninfracted myocardium. In a study of off-pump coronary revascularization, ischemia during transient occlusion of

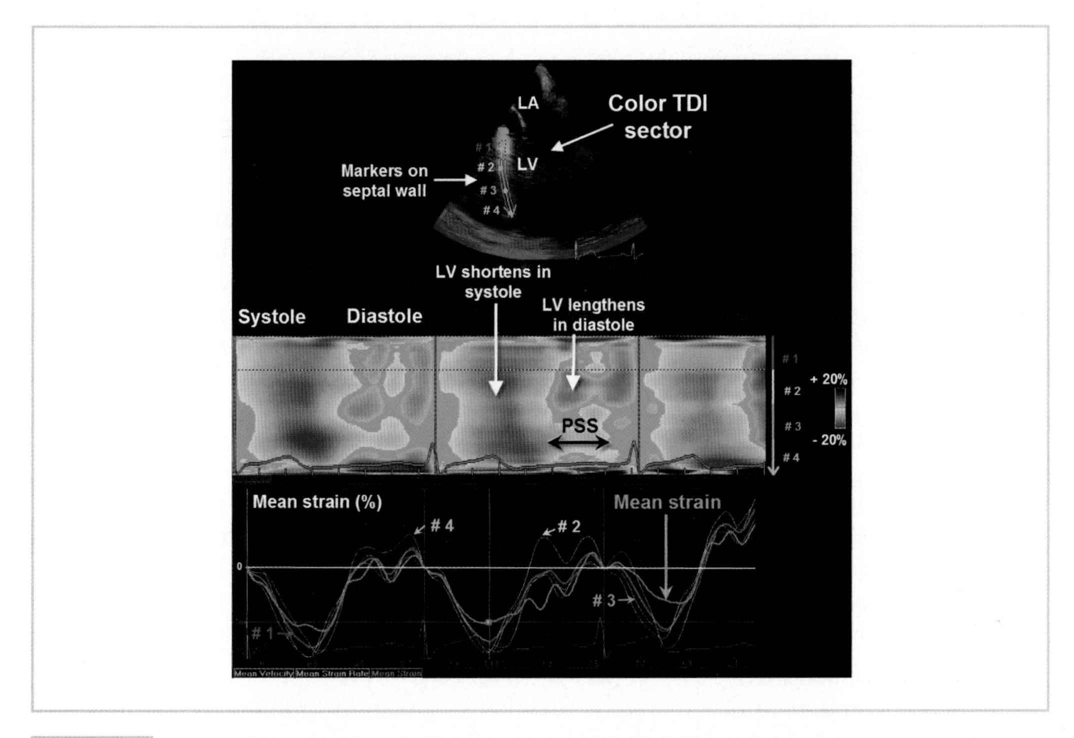

Figure 3.13. Strain. Upper panel: midesophageal (ME) four-chamber color tissue Doppler imaging (TDI) with markers placed on the septal wall. Middle panel: Color-coded strain imaging (deformation) of the left ventricle (LV) displayed for each marker (y axis) against time (x axis); blue denotes positive strain (lengthening in diastole) and red denotes negative strain (shortening in systole); green denotes zero strain (no change in length). Note that in the apical regions (# 3, 4) the myocardium contracts during diastole (postsystolic shortening). Lower panel: individual strain values for each marker, plus mean strain. LA, left atrium; PSS, post systolic shortening.

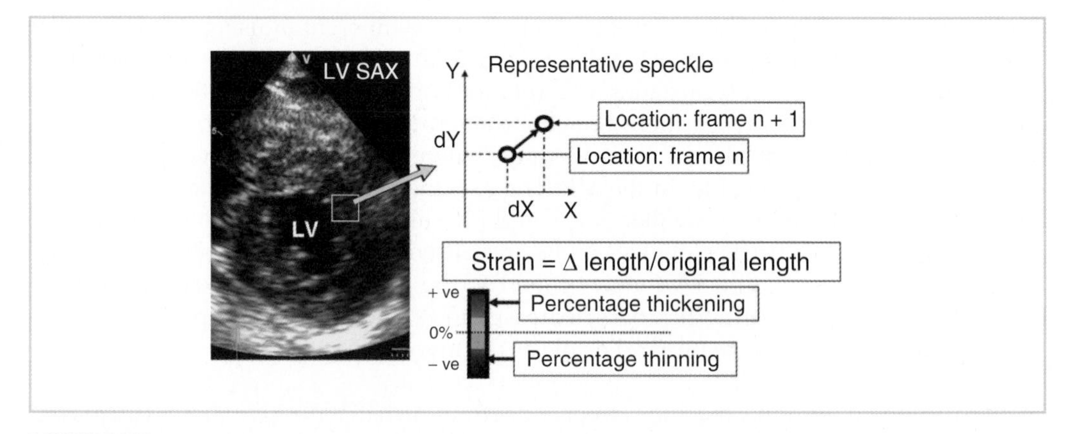

Figure 3.14. Tissue (speckle) tracking. Localized region of the myocardium is marked by box; speckles are identified in frame (n) and tracked over time to frame (n + 1); velocity vector is calculated and used to derive strain. LV, left ventricle; SAX, short axis. (From Suffoletto MS, Dohi K, Cannesson M, et al. Novel speckle-tracking radial strain from routine black-and-white echocardiographic images to quantify dyssynchrony and predict response to cardiac resynchronization therapy. *Circulation* 2006;113(7):960–968.)

the left anterior descending coronary artery was detected by a reduction in ϵ in the mid anterior wall segment and not detected by TDI velocities or hemodynamic monitoring (12).

Speckle tracking (tissue tracking)

A novel modality termed *speckle tracking* (or *tissue tracking*) utilizes routine gray-scale 2-D echocardiography images to calculate myocardial strain (13) (Figure 3.14). Stable patterns of unique acoustic markers (speckles) are identified in localized regions of the myocardium and tracked over time, measuring velocity and direction of movement. The image-processing software automatically subdivides a user-defined region of interest into blocks of approximately 20 to 40 pixels containing these stable patterns of speckles. Subsequent frames are then analyzed automatically by searching for the new location of each of the blocks. The location shift of these acoustic markers from frame to frame (which represents tissue movement) provides the spatial and temporal data used to calculate velocity vectors. Temporal alterations in these stable speckle patterns are identified as moving further apart or closer together, and a series of regional strain vectors are calculated as change in length/initial length. SR can also be calculated from speckle tracking.

Because this modality does not rely on Doppler velocity measurements, ϵ and SR calculated from speckle tracking is independent of the angle of interrogation. In comparison to ϵ and SR derived from TDI, which can only be measured in specific walls because of the angle dependency, speckle tracking ϵ and SR can be measured in any wall that can be visualized by 2-D echocardiography. This technique requires high frame rates and image quality.

Left ventricular synchrony

An important component of LV systolic function is synchronization of ventricular contraction. As LV systolic function begins to fail, segments of the myocardium contract dyssynchronously, typically with the posterior and lateral walls displaying delayed contraction. Dyssynchrony is caused by disease of the conducting system itself (electrical dyssynchrony, classically left bundle branch block) or mechanical dyssynchrony, caused by scarring from previous infarction which interrupts the electrical impulse within the LV. The presence of LV dyssynchrony leads to inefficient LV contraction which shifts the blood volume within the LV rather than contributing to effective ejection, resulting in a

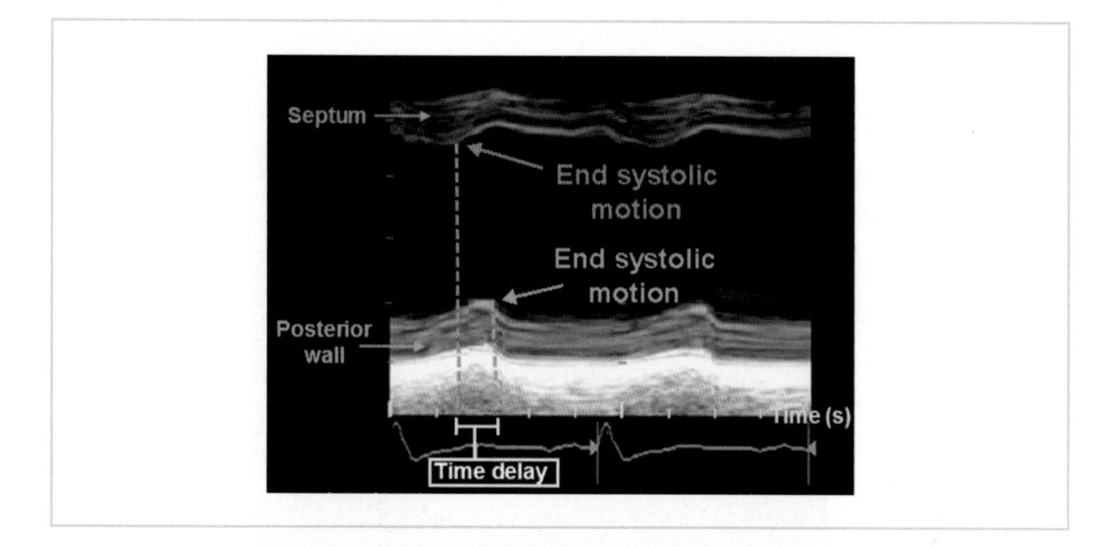

Figure 3.15. Left ventricular synchrony. Transthoracic M-mode of transgastic short axis showing septal wall and posterior wall. Identify maximal contraction of each wall and calculate time difference.

lower stroke volume. LV dyssynchrony is recognized as an important predictor of poor outcome and patients with New York Heart Association class III and IV heart failure have been shown to improve with cardiac resynchronization therapy (CRT) (14).

To better identify patients with LV dyssynchrony and predict those who will respond favorably to CRT, a number of echocardiographic approaches are in use. M-mode echocardiography has been used to measure the mechanical delay between the septum and the posterior wall (septal to posterior wall motion delay) where a delay of greater than 130 ms between systolic motion of the septum and posterior wall indicates severe LV dyssynchrony, Figure 3.15.

TDI is the preferred screening tool for dyssynchrony and to stratify patients before CRT and during follow-up. Using this method, a septal to lateral wall delay of greater than 65 ms predicts responders to CRT (14) (Figure 3.16). However, as noted in the preceding text, segmental TDI velocities do not indicate whether a segment is actively contracting or moving passively because of the tethering effect. This may explain the fact that up to 20% of patients do not respond to CRT when screened in this manner. This may be overcome by analyzing the velocity profile throughout the complete cardiac cycle during a stress test where viable segments of myocardium will display an increase in systolic velocity whereas infracted and scarred areas will not. In addition, TDI can be used to detect postsystolic shortening which represents myocardial contraction after closure of the aortic valve (AoV) during the isovolumic relaxation time (IVRT) period. This form of dyssynchrony has deleterious effects on ventricular filling and subsequent ejection (Figure 3.13).

VENTRICULAR PATHOLOGY

Cardiomyopathies

Cardiomyopathy is a common diagnosis and encompasses a diverse range of cardiac disease states (Figure 3.17). A recent reclassification (15) divides cardiomyopathies into primary cardiomyopathies (disease confined to the heart, which may be genetic,

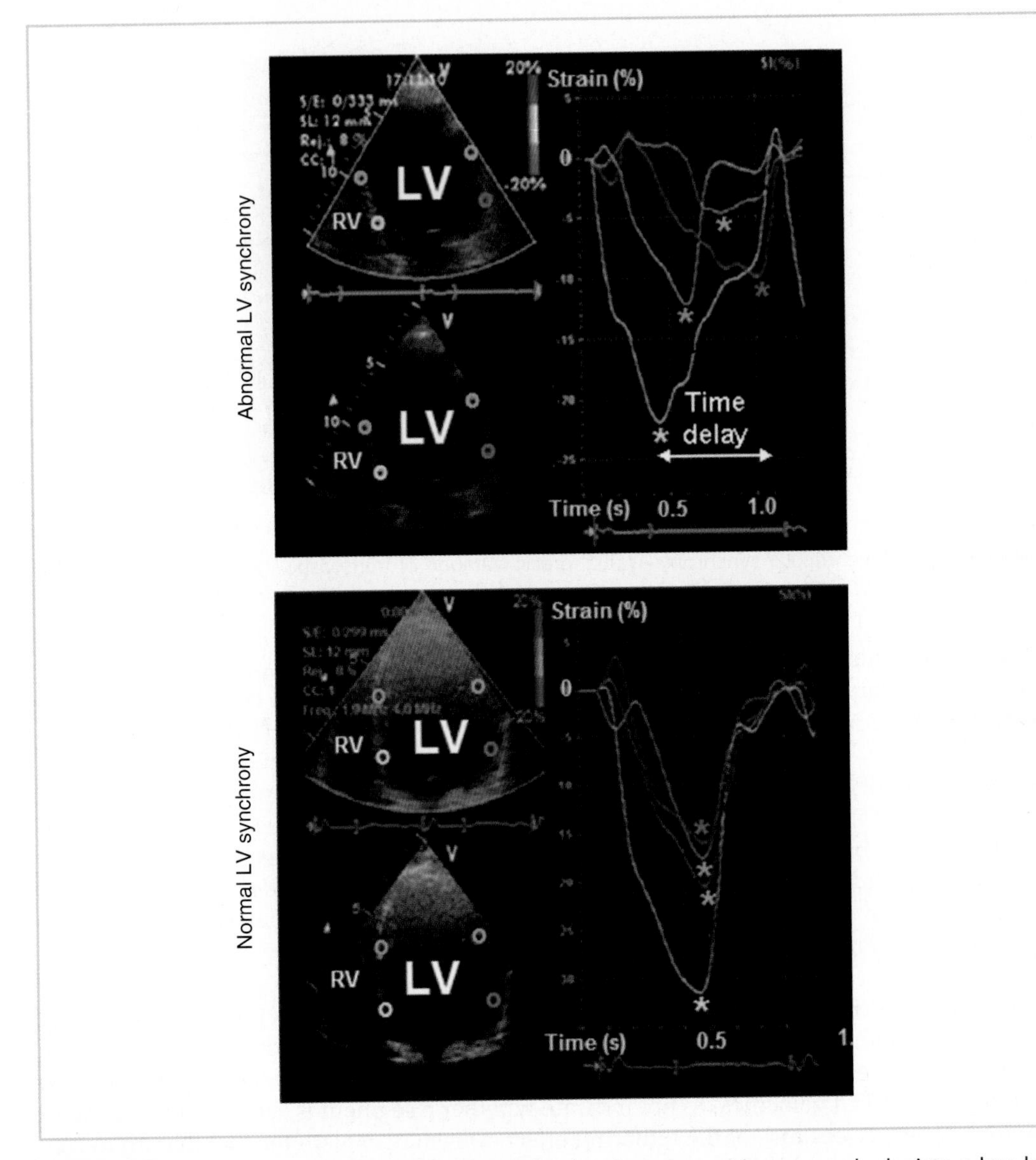

Figure 3.16. Left ventricular synchrony. Left hand side of upper and lower panels depicts a low left ventricular ejection fraction (dilated cardiomyopathy); markers are placed on the septal and lateral walls. Right hand side of upper and lower panels depicts individual strain waveforms for each marker. The upper panel shows a delay between septal and lateral wall deformation (abnormal LV synchrony); this patient is therefore a candidate for cardiac resynchronization therapy. RV, right ventricle; LV, left ventricle. (Mele D, Pasanisi G, Capasso F, et al. Left intraventricular myocardial deformation dyssynchrony identifies responders to cardiac resynchronization therapy in patients with heart failure. *Eur Heart J.* 2006;27(9):1070–1078.)

nongenetic, or acquired) and secondary cardiomyopathies (disease involves the heart as part of a generalized process which also affects other organs).

PRIMARY GENETIC CARDIOMYOPATHIES

1. ***Hypertrophic cardiomyopathy (HCM).*** HCM forms a heterogeneous group of genetic cardiac diseases characterized by a hypertrophied, nondilated LV which is not secondary

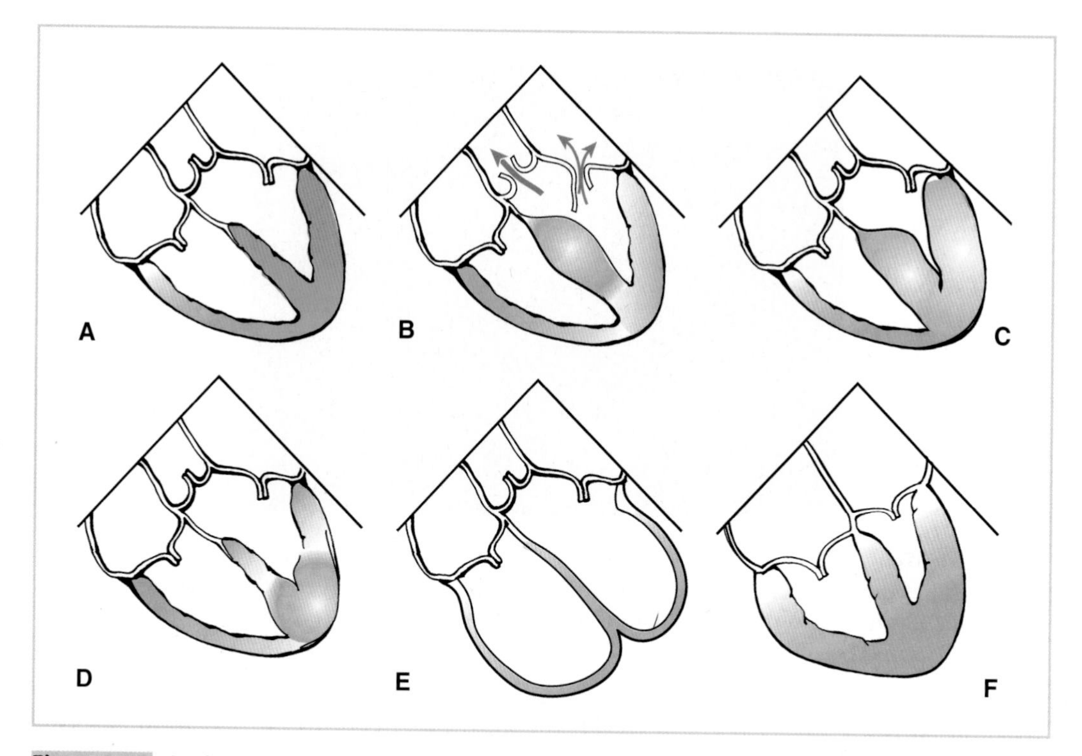

Figure 3.17. Cardiomyopathy variants. **A:** Normal. **B:** Septal hypertrophic cardiomyopathy (HCM). Note left ventricular outflow obstruction (LVOT) causing increased LVOT gradient, systolic anterior motion of the mitral valve, and mitral regurgitation. **C:** Concentric HCM. The posterobasal wall is frequently spared. **D:** Apical HCM. **E:** Dilated cardiomyopathy; dilation may be confined to the left ventricle or biventricular with or without atrial involvement. **F:** Restrictive cardiomyopathy. Note thick ventricles with small intraventricular cavities and biatrial enlargement.

to other disease processes such as hypertension or aortic stenosis. Clinical diagnosis is made by the 2-D echocardiography finding of LV wall thickening with a small LV cavity in a patient without other causes for LV hypertrophy. Many HCM patients have the propensity to develop dynamic obstruction of the left ventricular outflow tract (LVOT) either under resting or provoked conditions. This LVOT obstruction is produced by systolic anterior motion (SAM) of the MV in which the anterior mitral leaflet (AML) coapts with the bulging septum. Several theories have been proposed to explain of SAM, such as the LVOT dynamic obstruction creates a Venturi effect causing coaptation of the AML with the septum; abnormally oriented papillary muscles secondary to LV remodeling; an abnormal AML which is elongated with an increased surface area facilitating coaptation with the septum. Echocardiographic findings of SAM in HCM include AML septal contact during systole, posterolaterally directed midsystolic MR associated with SAM which can persist into diastole, a turbulent color flow Doppler pattern in the LVOT, a late systolic peaking velocity profile on continuous wave interrogation of the LVOT, and systolic "notching" on the M-mode tracing of AoV (premature closure of the AoV).

HCM is caused by a number of mutations but is invariably expressed as an autosomal dominant inheritance and there are several phenotypic expressions that are recognized with the hypertrophy being concentric (Figure 3.18), limited to the septum or to the apex of the LV. HCM limited to the septum, which may be either diffuse hypertrophy

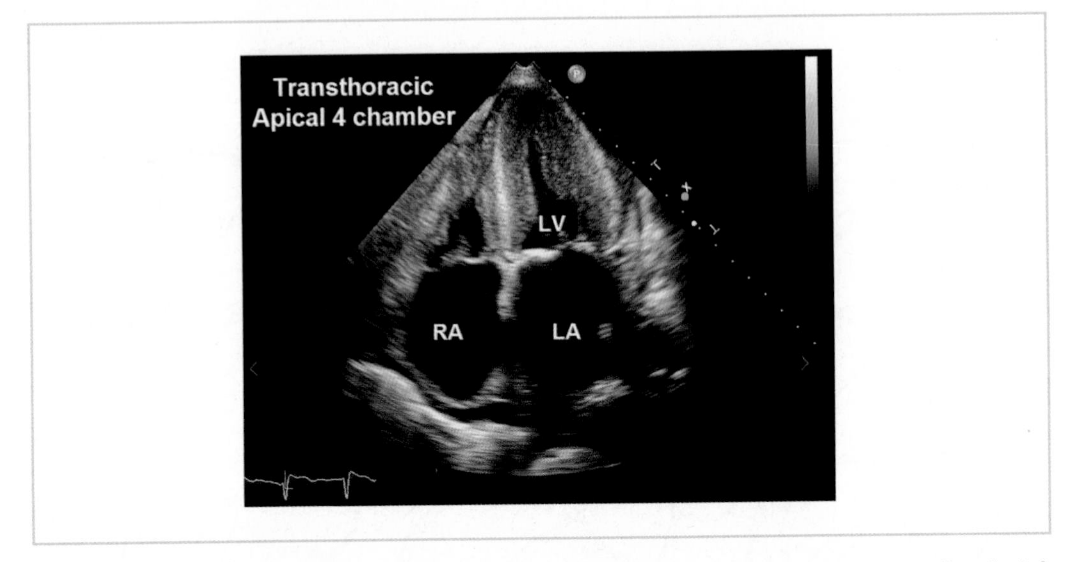

Figure 3.18. Hypertrophic cardiomyopathy. Note hypertrophy of the right ventricle (RV) as well as the left ventricle (LV). RA, right atrium; LA, left atrium. (Courtesy of Philips.)

throughout the septum or only in the basal or mid-wall regions, has also been known as *asymmetric septal hypertrophy* (ASH) or idiopathic hypertrophic subaortic stenosis (IHSS). Asymmetry is expressed by a septal wall to free wall (posterior wall) thickness ratio greater than 1.4. Although systolic function is usually preserved in HCM until late in the disease, LV dyssynchrony is common in all forms.

2. ***Noncompaction of the left ventricle (Figure 3.19).*** Noncompaction of the LV is a congenital cardiomyopathy, which involves predominantly the apex of the LV with

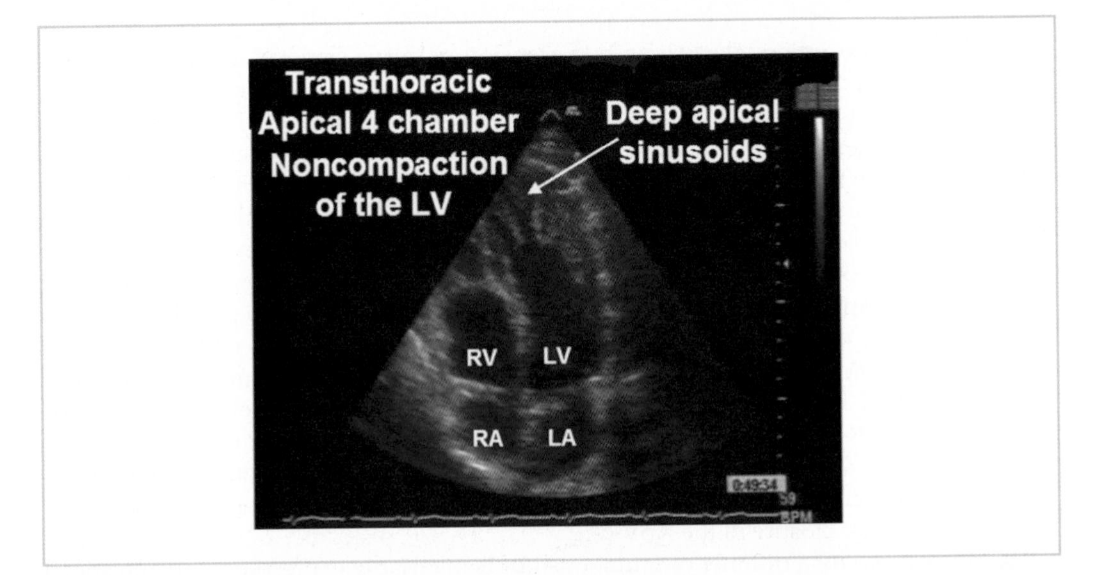

Figure 3.19. Noncompaction of the left ventricle (LV) showing deep apical sinuses and enlarged trabeculae. RV, right ventricle; RA, right atrium; LA, left atrium. (Murphy RT, Thaman R, Blanes JG, et al. Natural history and familial characteristics of isolated left ventricular non-compaction. *Eur Heart J.* 2005;26(2):187–192.)

deep sinusoids between enlarged trabeculae caused by arrested embryogenesis of the LV. A cross-section of the apex of the LV thereby resembles the structure of a natural sponge. Noncompaction of the LV may be an isolated finding or may be associated with other congenital heart anomalies such as complex cyanotic congenital heart disease. Noncompaction of the LV results in systolic dysfunction and heart failure although arrhythmias and sudden death are also frequent clinical presentations. Thrombi may form within the sinusoids and being in continuity with the LV cavity may produce embolic events.

PRIMARY MIXED (GENETIC AND NONGENETIC) CARDIOMYOPATHIES

1. ***Dilated cardiomyopathy (DCM) (Figure 3.20).*** DCM is a common cardiomyopathy with an estimated prevalence of 1:2,500; it is the third most common cause of heart failure and the most frequent reason for patients being listed for heart transplantation.

   It is characterized by LV enlargement in the presence of normal wall thickness with an increased cardiac mass. The LV becomes more globular as dilation occurs preferentially along the SAX and the sphericity index (long axis/SAX) is reduced from the normal (>1.5) and approaches 1. All measures of systolic function are abnormally low and LV dyssynchrony is invariably present.

   Frequent associated findings are mitral annular dilation, reduced excursion of the mitral leaflets and abnormally oriented papillary muscles resulting in functional MR, dilated right ventricle (RV), biatrial enlargement, apical thrombus, and diastolic dysfunction. DCM is associated with arrhythmias, thromboembolic events, and increased cardiac-related death.

   Approximately one third of the patients with DCM are found to be familial, most frequently autosomal dominant. The DCM phenotype may also occur secondary to infectious agents (particularly viruses), toxins (alcohol, chemotherapeutic agents, heavy metals), autoimmune diseases, collagen vascular disorders, pheochromocytoma, neuromuscular, mitochondrial, metabolic, endocrine disorders, and nutritional deficiencies.

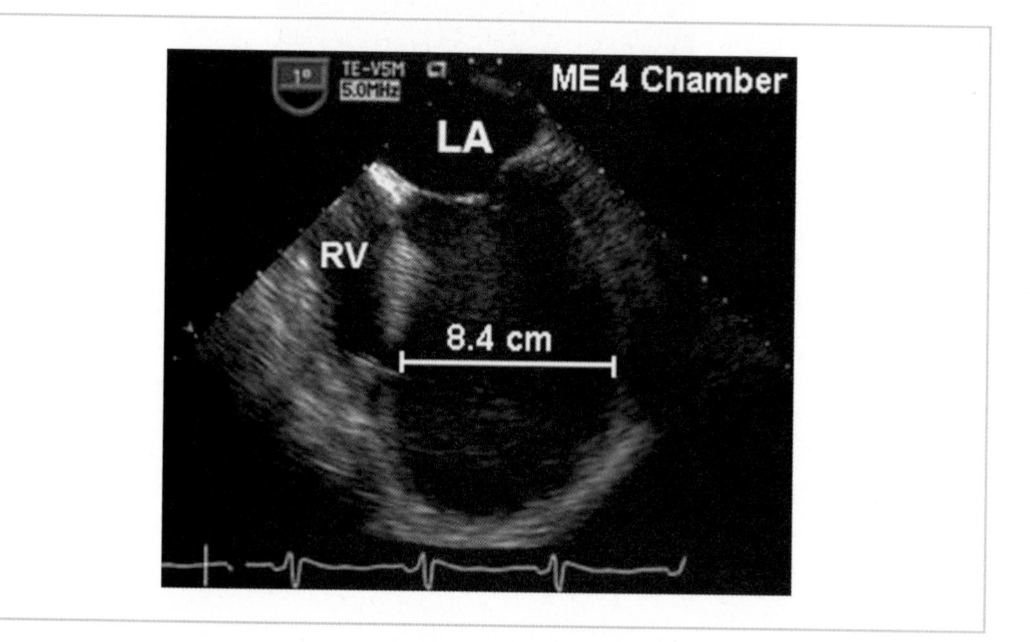

Figure 3.20. Dilated cardiomyopathy. ME, midesophageal; LA, left atrium; RV, right ventricle.

2. ***Primary restrictive cardiomyopathy.*** Primary restrictive cardiomyopathy is characterized by a normal or decreased volume of both ventricles associated with biatrial enlargement, normal wall thickness and normal valves, impaired (restrictive) diastology, and normal or near normal systolic function. Both familial and sporadic forms have been described.

ACQUIRED PRIMARY CARDIOMYOPATHIES

1. ***Myocarditis.*** Myocarditis may be an acute or chronic inflammatory process caused by infective agents, drugs, toxins, and a number of other less common agents and typically results in DCM and arrhythmias.
2. ***Tako-Tsubo (apical ballooning) cardiomyopathy.*** Tako-Tsubo cardiomyopathy (Figure 3.21) takes its name from the Japanese word for a traditional octopus trap, which resembles a vase with a narrow neck and a ballooned out base. This is a rapidly developing cardiomyopathy, typified by extensive myocardial stunning in the mid and apical segments of the LV. The apical half of the LV becomes akinetic or dyskinetic ballooning out during systole mimicking extensive infarction, whereas the basal segments are hypercontractile. It is apparently associated with extreme stress and high levels of circulating sympathetic hormones and has a higher incidence in females than males. Treatment of the underlying cause of stress and control of the sympathomimetic imbalance usually results in rapid and full recovery.

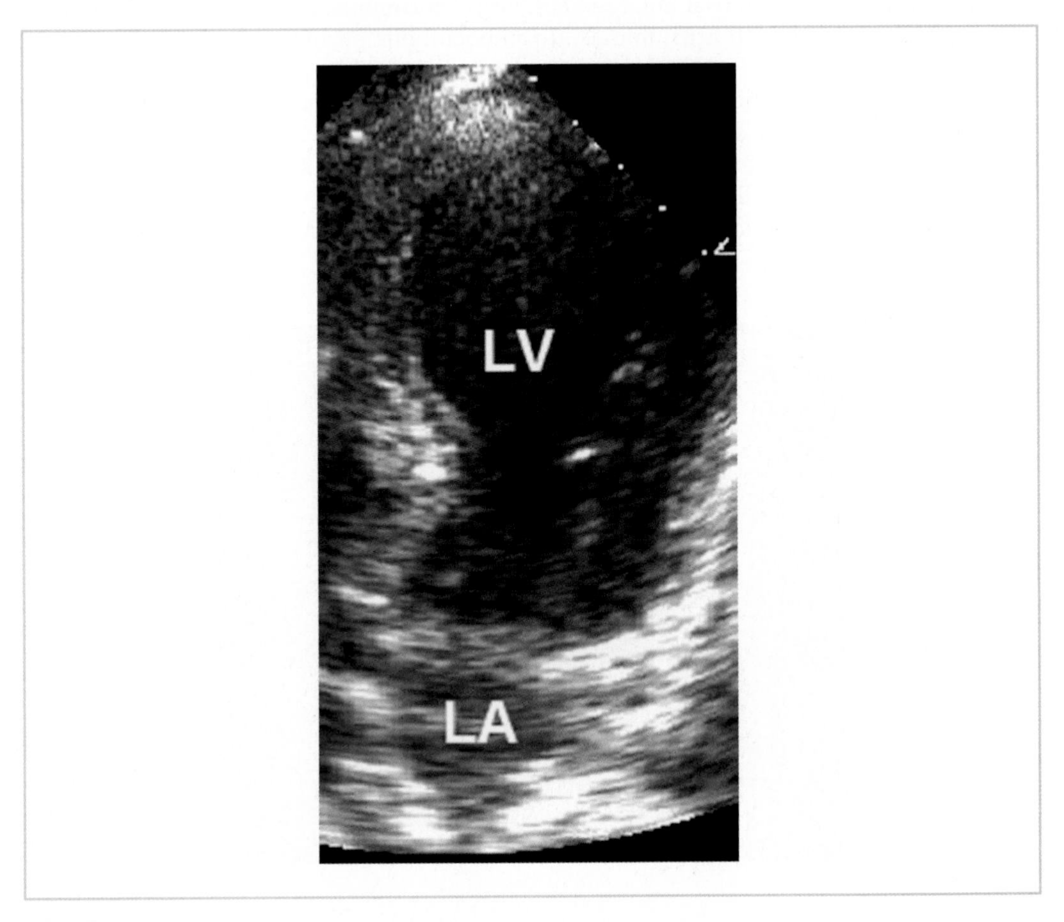

Figure 3.21. Tako-Tsubo cardiomyopathy. LV, left ventricle; LA, left atrium.

3. ***Peripartum cardiomyopathy.*** Peripartum cardiomyopathy is fortunately a rare cause of severe DCM appearing at any time between the third trimester of pregnancy up to 5 months postpartum. Prognosis is variable with approximately half the number of the women affected progressing onto persistent heart failure whereas the remainder recover to normal function.

SECONDARY CARDIOMYOPATHIES

The list of causes of secondary cardiomyopathies is extensive and includes infiltrative diseases, storage diseases, toxic exposure, inflammatory processes, genetic, and autoimmune diseases. Presentation may be typified by signs and symptoms of either a hypertrophied or DCM depending upon the disease process.

Note that other myocardial pathologic processes and ventricular dysfunction such as that which occurs with valvular heart disease, congenital heart disease, ischemic heart disease, and hypertension are not included in this classification (15). Therefore the LV hypertrophy that occurs with hypertension is discussed in the subsequent text in the section on 'Left Ventricular Hypertrophy'.

THE ROLE OF ECHOCARDIOGRAPHY IN CARDIOMYOPATHIES

Although echocardiographic findings in patients with symptomatic cardiomyopathy tend to be characteristic of the specific phenotype, some of the more important roles for echocardiography in cardiomyopathies are as follows:

1. ***Screening for cardiomyopathy in family members of affected subjects in cardiomyopathies of genetic or familial origin.*** Most genetic cardiomyopathies do not display signs or symptoms until early adulthood. Most of the traditional echocardiography parameters of systolic and diastolic function do not distinguish between patients with cardiomyopathy and healthycontrols until symptoms develop. The more recent modalities of TDI, ϵ, and SR have proved useful in distinguishing between healthy subjects, asymptomatic genetic carriers, and full-blown phenotypic expression in HCM (16).
2. ***Distinguishing between HCM and LV hypertrophy secondary to systemic hypertension or LV hypertrophy in athletes.*** The distinction between these entities may be difficult on grounds of history and examination. Again traditional echocardiographic markers are not able to distinguish readily between HCM and athlete's heart or HCM and LV hypertrophy secondary to systemic hypertension. Newer echocardiographic modalities based on TDI may help differentiate between HCM and athletes heart (17).
3. ***Distinguishing between restrictive cardiomyopathy and constrictive pericarditis (CP).*** The clinical distinction between restrictive cardiomyopathy (RCM, typified by amyloid infiltration of the heart) and CP is often very challenging because of the similar clinical presentation and hemodynamic findings. Conventional M-mode and 2-D images may aid in the diagnosis by demonstrating a significantly thickened pericardium in CP or a pattern of sparkling, granular LV in amyloid (RCM) (Figure 3.22). Doppler blood flow patterns have proved helpful in differentiating the two entities and the respiratory variation in transvalvular velocity blood flow is the most frequently used diagnostic parameter (Table 3.4). In CP, the total cardiac volume is defined by the pericardium. During spontaneous inspiration, blood flows to the right atrium increasing right-sided volumes, necessitating a reciprocal drop in left-sided volumes as the septum moves toward the left ventricle (may be seen as septal flattening). These changes are reflected in the E wave (early diastolic filling) across both the tricuspid valve (TV) and the MV. During inspiration, the tricuspid E wave increases whereas the mitral E wave decreases. During expiration, tricuspid E wave decreases whereas mitral E wave increases. These

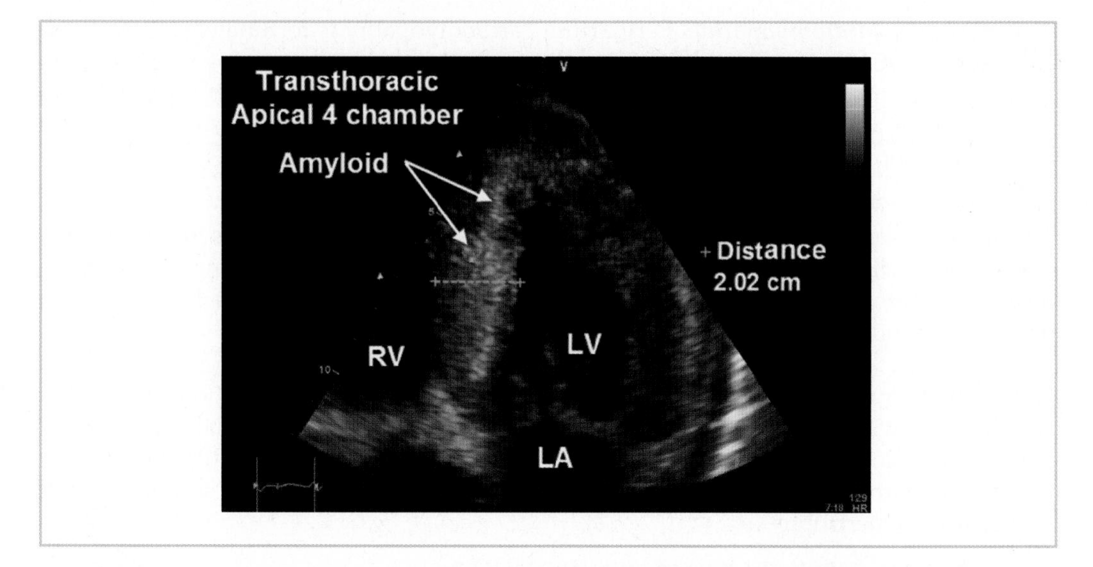

Figure 3.22. Amyloid restrictive cardiomyopathy. RV, right ventricle; LV, left ventricle; LA, left atrium.

changes are most noticeable on the beat after the start of inspiration or expiration. If the pulse wave Doppler (PWD) sweep speed is set to 150 mm/s, a characteristic undulating increase and decrease of the height of the E wave can be seen to coincide with the respiratory pattern. Note that in ventilated patients, the changes will be reciprocal because positive inspiratory pressure reduces blood flow to the right side, thereby causing a decreased tricuspid E wave and an increased mitral E wave. Respiratory variation also occurs in healthy subjects but the percentage difference in mitral E waves between inspiration and expiration is usually less than 5%. *A difference of greater than 25% in mitral E waves between inspiration and expiration is highly suggestive of CP*. However, respiratory variation is not invariably present in CP and also occurs in patients with chronic obstructive airway disease, where the variation is somewhere in the range of 10% to 15% (18). TDI has proved useful in the differential diagnosis of RCM and CP. An early diastolic mitral annular velocity (Ea) cutoff value greater than 8 cm/s has a 95% sensitivity and 96% specificity for differentiating CP from RCM (19).

Left Ventricular Hypertrophy

LV hypertrophy is a compensatory adaptation of the ventricle to stress. *Concentric hypertrophy* is a thickening of the ventricular wall as a consequence of parallel replication of sarcomeres without significant chamber enlargement; it occurs secondary to chronic pressure overload of the ventricle, as in systemic hypertension and aortic stenosis. The increased impedance to ejection causes marked rises in ventricular wall stress. Concentric hypertrophy is a compensatory response that reduces wall stress (the law of Laplace) and enables the ventricle to develop the exaggerated intracavitary pressures necessary to contract effectively against the increased afterload. Other physiologic alterations of the ventricle that occur in concentric hypertrophy include a prolongation of isovolumetric relaxation, a reduction in compliance that leads to diastolic dysfunction, and eventual worsening of cardiac function as compensatory limits are reached. Echocardiographic analysis of concentric hypertrophy involves a determination of LV thickness and LV mass which have both been described in the preceding text (Figure 3.23).

Table 3.4 Two-dimensional and Doppler characteristics of constrictive pericarditis and restrictive cardiomyopathy

	Constrictive pericarditis	**Restrictive cardiomyopathy**[a]
	Two-dimensional echocardiography or M-mode	
Thickened pericardium	+++	±
Biatrial enlargement	±	+++
LV chamber size	±	Small
Wall thickness	±	↑↑
Myocardium	Normal	Sparkling, granular
Systolic function	Intact	Reduced
Septal movement	Septal "bounce" = rapid anterior movement during early diastole; clinically = pericardial knock. Ventricular interdependence: septum moves towards LV during inspiration	No ventricular interdependence
IVC and hepatic veins	Enlarged	Enlarged
Mitral regurgitation	±	Usually present
Tricuspid regurgitation	±	Usually present
	Doppler findings	
E/A ratio	May be normal or <1	>2.2
MV inflow deceleration time (ms)	Low normal	Shortened (<150)
Mitral E wave changes during respiration	>25% reduction in inspiration and increase in expiration[b] (reciprocal changes seen in tricuspid E wave)	Normal (~5%)
IVRT during inspiration	↑↑	No variation
Pulmonary vein flow (left-sided filling pattern)	Inspiration S approximately = D, expiration produces ↑ D waves	S<D, S/D ratio <0.5 deep and wide a wave; no respiratory variation
Hepatic vein flow (right sided filling pattern)	W wave form (prominent a wave, prominent y descent), with respiratory variations (↓ diastolic flow during expiration)	Blunted systolic flow, deep atrial reversal, may be reversal during systole (2° to significant TR).

[a]Findings in for example late cardiac amyloidosis.
[b]In spontaneously breathing patient. Pattern would be reversed in positive pressure ventilation.
LV, left ventricle; IVC, inferior venacava; E, early diastolic filling; A, late diastolic filling; MV, mitral valve; IVRT, isovolumic relaxation time; TV, tricuspid valve; W wave form, reversal of flow in late systole and late diastole; TR, tricuspid regurgitation.

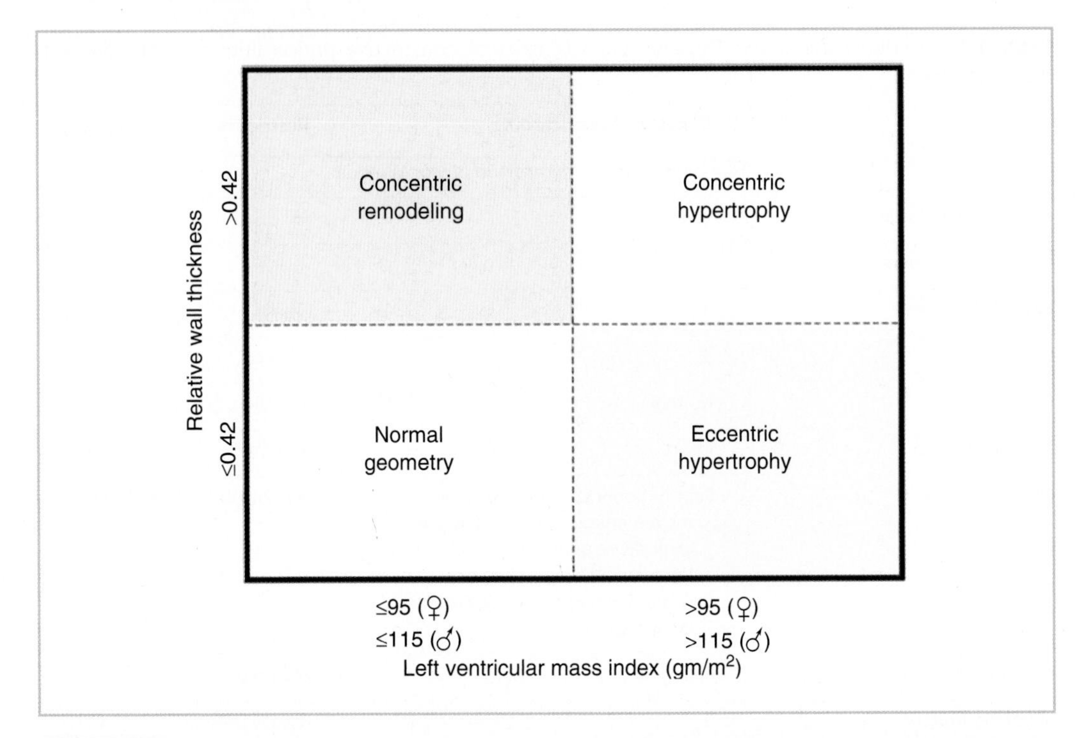

Figure 3.23. Left ventricular mass may be combined with relative wall thickness to categorize patients into various classes of left ventricle (LV) hypertrophy. TG, transgastric; SAX, short axis; RV, right ventricle; LV, left ventricle. (From Lang RM, Bierig M, Devereux RB, et al. Chamber Quantification Writing Group. American Society of Echocardiography's Guidelines and Standards Committee. European Association of Echocardiography. Recommendations for chamber quantification: a report from the American Society of Echocardiography's Guidelines and Standards Committee and the Chamber Quantification Writing Group, developed in conjunction with the European Association of Echocardiography, a branch of the European Society of Cardiology. *J Am Soc Echocardiogr* 2005;18(12):1440–1463.)

Eccentric hypertrophy is an enlargement or dilation of the LV chamber as a consequence of serial replication of sarcomeres and occurs secondary to chronic volume overload of the ventricle; aortic regurgitation is the classic example.

Left Ventricular True Aneurysm

Most LV aneurysms are located at the apex and are predominantly a consequence of anterior myocardial infarctions. Within 90 days of an anterior myocardial infarction, LV aneurysms develop in 22% of patients (20). No new true aneurysms develop more than 3 months after myocardial infarction. Early aneurysm formation, within the first 5 days of myocardial infarction, is associated with increased mortality.

TWO-DIMENSIONAL CHARACTERISTICS

A ventricular aneurysm is characterized as a dilated dyskinetic area with myocardial thinning. A narrow band of myocardium lines a "true" aneurysm and distinguishes it from a pseudoaneurysm (discussed later). As demonstrated in Figure 3.24, a smooth, gradual transition is seen between the aneurysm and normal myocardium, with a gradual, obtuse tapering of the myocardium into a dilated, thinned area that has a wide neck or opening. The ratio of the size of the aneurysmal opening from the ventricle to the maximal aneurysmal diameter ranges between 0.9 and 1.0 (21).

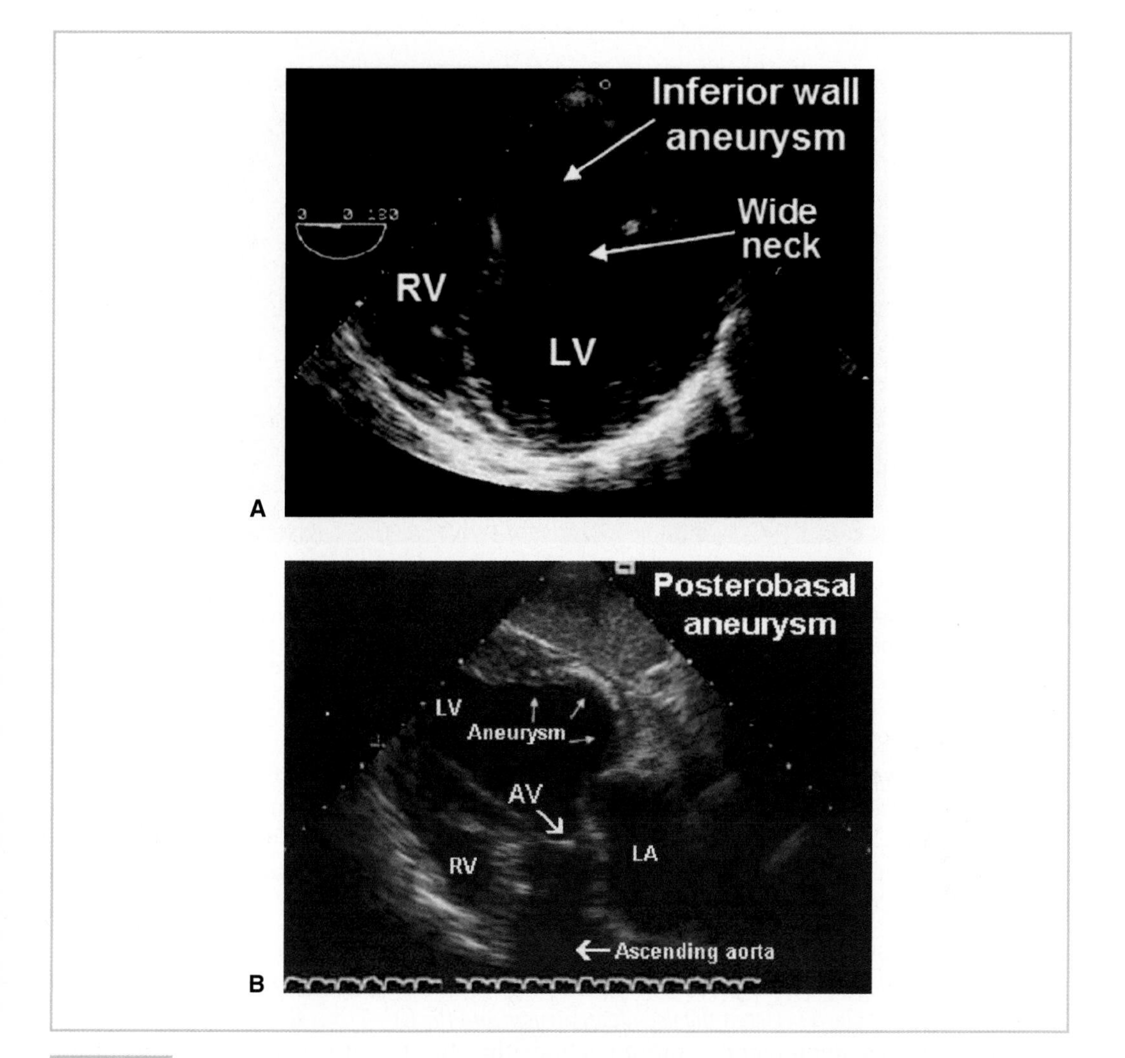

Figure 3.24. Left ventricular aneurysm. **A:** Transgastric mid short axis view of inferior wall true aneurysm. Note wide neck. **B:** TG long axis view of posterobasal aneurysm. Note wide neck and gradual transition from normal myocardium to the aneurysm. RV, right ventricle; LV, left ventricle; AoV, aortic valve; LA, left atrium.

ASSOCIATED FINDINGS

Intraoperative TEE is useful to detect thrombus formation within the aneurysm. Thrombus appears as an area of increased echogenicity that can be clearly delineated from the endocardium and is a frequent finding as a consequence of stasis of blood within the dilated aneurysm.

Left Ventricular Pseudoaneurysm

The ability to distinguish a true aneurysm from a pseudoaneurysm is critical because pseudoaneurysms have a high incidence of spontaneous rupture and therefore require surgical correction (21). A pseudoaneurysm represents a chronic ventricular rupture contained by pericardium. Therefore, a pseudoaneurysm is a saccular structure that communicates directly with the pericardial space.

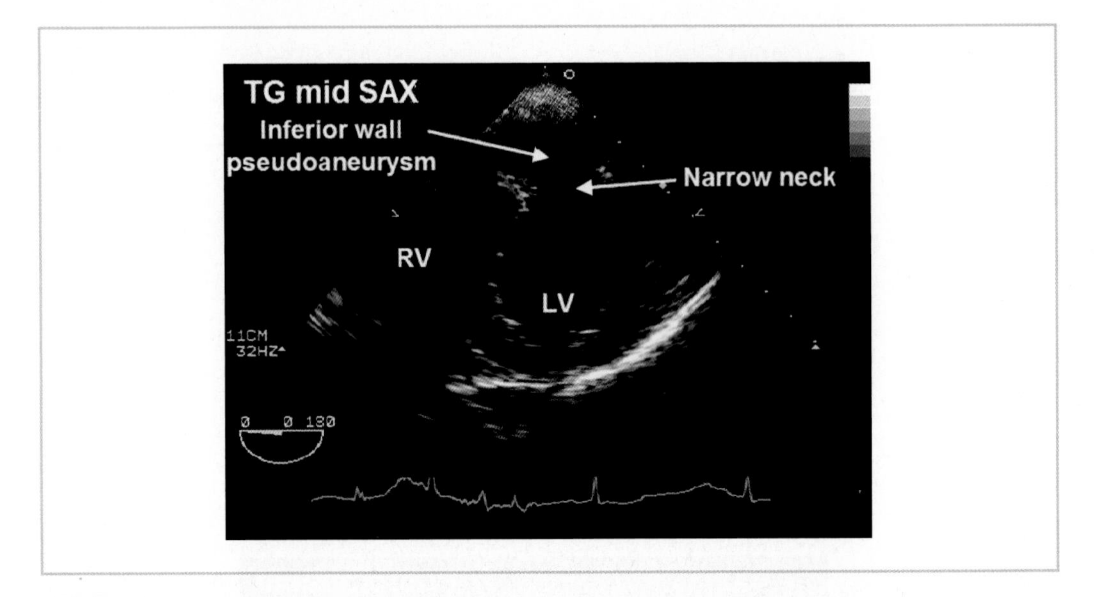

Figure 3.25. Left ventricular pseudoaneurysm. Note narrow neck which is less than one half of the parallel internal diameter of the pseudoaneurysm. TG, transgastric; SAX, short axis; RV, right ventricle; LV, left ventricle.

TWO-DIMENSIONAL CHARACTERISTICS

A pseudoaneurysm is characterized by a narrow orifice (neck) arising from the ventricular chamber; the ratio of the size of the orifice to the maximal aneurysmal diameter is less than 0.5 (Figure 3.25). The size of the small neck rarely exceeds half the maximal parallel internal diameter of the aneurysmal sac (22). The LV cavity size decreases in systole while the false aneurysm gradually expands.

QUANTITATIVE DOPPLER CHARACTERISTICS

Doppler echocardiography has proved useful in diagnostically difficult cases and demonstrates bidirectional flow of blood between the pseudoaneurysm and the LV. Color flow Doppler echocardiography usually demonstrates mosaic jets exiting the LV in systole and entering the pseudoaneurysm cavity. In diastole, this mosaic pattern occurs within the LV, confirming the turbulent ebb and flow of blood to and from the pseudoaneurysm. One may also see a profound variation in maximal Doppler flow velocity throughout the respiratory cycle, with inspiration causing a significant increase in the maximal flow velocity (22).

ASSOCIATED FINDINGS

Spontaneous echo contrast and thrombus within the pseudoaneurysm cavity are frequent findings.

CONCLUSION

LV systolic function is the most common assessment made during intraoperative echocardiography and a number of parameters are available for measuring it. These vary in complexity from measurements made on 2-D gray-scale imaging through 3-D representation and on to some of the newer modalities based on TDI. Although subjective and qualitative assessment of LV systolic function have been shown to correlate well with quantitative measurements and with clinical outcome, the ASE advises that even the most experienced clinician calibrates the findings against actual measurements on a regular basis.

Quantitative measurements of LV systolic function such as wall thickness and FAC can be easily acquired by novice practitioners, producing meaningful data for use in daily practice. Current echocardiography software also assists in the rapid acquisition of some of the more complicated but more accurate parameters such as LV mass and volume. Although the newer technologies based on TDI are rapidly becoming standard of care in echocardiography laboratories, their robustness has yet to be confirmed in the operating room setting.

REFERENCES

1 Lang RM, Bierig M, Devereux RB, et al. Chamber Quantification Writing Group. American Society of Echocardiography's Guidelines and Standards Committee. European Association of Echocardiography. Recommendations for chamber quantification: a report from the American Society of Echocardiography's Guidelines and Standards Committee and the Chamber Quantification Writing Group, developed in conjunction with the European Association of Echocardiography, a branch of the European Society of Cardiology. *J Am Soc Echocardiogr* 2005;18(12):1440–1463.

2 Sahn DJ, DeMaria A, Kisslo J, et al. American Society of Echocardiography. Recommendations regarding quantitation in M-mode echocardiography: results of a survey of echocardiographic measurements. *Circulation* 1978;58(6): 1072–1083.

3 Skarvan K, Lambert A, Filipovic M, et al. Reference values for left ventricular function in subjects under general anaesthesia and controlled ventilation assessed by two-dimensional transoesophageal echocardiography. *Eur J Anaesthesiol* 2001;18(11):713–722.

4 Schiller NB, Shah PM, Crawford M, et al. Recommendations for quantitation of the left ventricle by two-dimensional echocardiography: The American Society of Echocardiography committee on standards, subcommittee on quantitation of two-dimensional echocardiograms. *J Am Soc Echocardiogr* 1989;2: 358–367.

5 Chung N, Nishimura RA, Holmes DR Jr, et al. Measurement of left ventricular dP/dT by simultaneous Doppler echocardiography and cardiac catheterization. *J Am Soc Echocardiogr* 1992;5(2):147–152.

6 Gopal AS, Keller AM, Rigling R Jr, et al. Left ventricular volume and endocardial surface area by three-dimensional echocardiography: comparison with two-dimensional echocardiography and nuclear magnetic resonance imaging in normal subjects. *J Am Coll Cardiol* 1993;22(1):258–270.

7 Quinones MA, Otto CM, Stoddard M, et al. Doppler Quantification Task Force of the Nomenclature and Standards Committee of the American Society of Echocardiography. Recommendations for quantification of Doppler echocardiography: a report from the Doppler Quantification Task Force of the Nomenclature and Standards Committee of the American Society of Echocardiography. *J Am Soc Echocardiogr* 2002;15(2):167–184.

8 Alam M, Wardell J, Andersson E, et al. Effects of first myocardial infarction on left ventricular systolic and diastolic function with the use of mitral annular velocity determined by pulsed wave Doppler tissue imaging. *J Am Soc Echocardiogr* 2000;13(5):343–352.

9 Vinereanu D, Lim PO, Frenneaux MP, et al. Reduced myocardial velocities of left ventricular long-axis contraction identify both systolic and diastolic heart failure-a comparison with brain natriuretic peptide. *Eur J Heart Fail* 2005;7(4):512–519.

10 Wang M, Yip GW, Wang AY, et al. Peak early diastolic mitral annulus velocity by tissue Doppler imaging adds independent and incremental prognostic value. *J Am Coll Cardiol* 2003;41(5):820–826.

11 Garcia MJ, Rodriguez L, Ares M, et al. Myocardial wall velocity assessment by pulsed Doppler tissue imaging: characteristic findings in normal subjects. *Am Heart J* 1996;132(3):648–656.

12 Skulstad H, Andersen K, Edvardsen T, et al. Detection of ischemia and new insight into left ventricular physiology by strain Doppler and tissue velocity imaging: assessment during coronary bypass operation of the beating heart. *J Am Soc Echocardiogr* 2004;17(12):1225–1233.

13 Ingul CB, Torp H, Aase SA, et al. Automated analysis of strain rate and strain: feasibility and clinical implications. *J Am Soc Echocardiogr* 2005;18(5):411–418.

14 Bax JJ, Bleeker GB, Marwick TH, et al. Left ventricular dyssynchrony predicts response and prognosis after cardiac resynchronization therapy. *J Am Coll Cardiol* 2004;44(9):1834–1840.

15 Maron BJ, Towbin JA, Thiene G, et al. American Heart Association. Council on Clinical Cardiology, Heart Failure and Transplantation Committee. Quality of Care and Outcomes Research and Functional Genomics and Translational Biology Interdisciplinary Working Groups. Council on Epidemiology Prevention. Contemporary definitions and classification of the cardiomyopathies: an American Heart Association

Scientific Statement from the Council on Clinical Cardiology, Heart Failure and Transplantation Committee; Quality of Care and Outcomes Research and Functional Genomics and Translational Biology Interdisciplinary Working Groups; and Council on Epidemiology and Prevention. *Circulation* 2006;113(14):1807–1816.

16 De Backer J, Matthys D, Gillbert TC, et al. The use of tissue Doppler imaging for the assessment of changes in myocardial structure and function in inherited cardiomyopathies. *Eur J Echocardiogr* 2005;6:245–250.

17 Palka P, Lange A, Fleming AD, et al. Differences in myocardial velocity gradient measured throughout the cardiac cycle in patients with hypertrophic cardiomyopathy, athletes and patients with left ventricular hypertrophy due to hypertension. *J Am Coll Cardiol* 1997;30(3):760–768.

18 Hatle LK, Appleton CP, Popp RL. Differentiation of constrictive pericarditis and restrictive cardiomyopathy by Doppler echocardiography. *Circulation* 1989;79(2):357–370.

19 Ha JW, Ommen SR, Tajik AJ, et al. Differentiation of constrictive pericarditis from restrictive cardiomyopathy using mitral annular velocity by tissue Doppler echocardiography. *Am J Cardiol* 2004;94(3):316–319.

20 Visser CA, Kan G, Meltzer RS, et al. Incidence, timing and prognostic value of left ventricular aneurysm formation after myocardial infarction: a prospective, serial echocardiographic study of 158 patients. *Am J Cardiol* 1986;57:729–732.

21 Brown SL, Gropler RJ, Harris KM. Distinguishing left ventricular aneurysm from pseudoaneurysm. A review of the literature. *Chest* 1997;111:1403–1409.

22 Roelandt JRTC, Sutherland GR, Yoshida K, et al. Improved diagnosis and characterization of left ventricular pseudoaneurysm by Doppler color flow imaging. *J Am Coll Cardiol* 1988;12:807–811.

QUESTIONS

1. Which of the following measurements is/are normal?

a. End systolic volume greater than 70 mL
b. Left ventricular mass = 150 g in a 65-year-old male
c. Posterior wall thickness = 13 mm
d. Relative wall thickness = 0.32 cm

2. A patient has the following left ventricular (LV) measurements taken from an M-mode tracing:

Left ventricular internal diameter (LVID) in diastole, 5.2 cm
LVID in systole, 3.1 cm

a. Calculate the fractional shortening.
b. Is the LV function normal based on this measurement?

3. Which parameters measured by transesophageal echocardiography (TEE) correlate with systolic ventricular performance?

a. End systolic volume
b. Ejection fraction
c. Fractional shortening
d. Fractional area change (FAC)
e. All of the above

4. Left ventricular volumes in a patient with an inferior aneurysm are best measured by

a. Area length formula
b. Cubic formula
c. Method of disks

5. If you cannot image the endocardial border of the left ventricular apex of a patient, which formula should you use to calculate LV volume?

a. Area length formula
b. Cubic formula
c. Method of disks

6. All of the following are echocardiographic manifestations of an LV pseudoaneurysm except

a. A wide neck opening
b. A decreasing LV cavity size in systole while the pseudoaneurysm expands
c. Spontaneous echo contrast within the pseudoaneurysm cavity
d. Demonstration by color Doppler of bidirectional flow into the pseudoaneurysm

7. All of the following statements regarding dilated cardiomyopathy are true except

a. The ventricular end diastolic volume is increased.
b. Severe contractile dysfunction is present.
c. Only the left atrium (LA) and LV are enlarged.
d. Functional mitral regurgitation (MR) may be present.

8. In dilated cardiomyopathy

a. The mitral leaflets are typically normal.
b. Abnormal displacement of the papillary muscles can cause significant MR.
c. Annular dilation can cause incomplete coaptation of the mitral valve leaflets.
d. The mitral leaflet excursion may be decreased.
e. All of the above.

9. All of the following statements about asymmetric hypertrophic cardiomyopathy (HCM) are true except
a. It is an autosomal dominant disorder.
b. Outflow obstruction occurs during systole.
c. There may be premature closing of the aortic valve.
d. The basal posterior LV wall is equally hypertrophied.

10. Which of the following statements has been proposed as an explanation of mitral valve pathology in asymmetric HCM?
a. Anterior motion of the mitral valve contributes to the left ventricular outflow tract (LVOT) obstruction.
b. A "Venturi" effect may occur through the narrowed LVOT, thereby drawing the anterior leaflet toward the septum.
c. An altered orientation of the papillary muscles leads to systolic anterior motion of the mitral valve.
d. The anterior leaflet may be enlarged in asymmetric septal hypertrophy.
e. All of the above.

11. Constrictive pericarditis can be best distinguished from restrictive pericarditis by which of the following:
a. Ejection fraction
b. Clinical presentation
c. Transmitral flow patterns during respiration
d. Two-dimensional echocardiography

12. The following statements are true regarding HCM except
a. Only the asymmetric form of HCM (also known as *asymmetric septal hypertrophy* or *idiopathic hypertrophic subaortic stenosis*) has dynamic outflow obstruction.
b. Left ventricular dyssynchrony is common.
c. Tissue Doppler imaging is better than traditional echocardiography for distinguishing between HCM and LV hypertrophy secondary to hypertension or athlete's heart.
d. There is more than one genotype responsible for HCM.

13. Which of the following echo modalities are derived from tissue Doppler imaging?
a. Systolic tissue velocity
b. Strain
c. Strain rate
d. Tissue tracking (speckle tracking)
e. Curved M-mode

14. In a midesophageal four-chamber view, the tissue Doppler imaging systolic wave measured at the mitral annulus (septal wall) is positive or negative?

15. In a midesophageal four-chamber view, strain during systole measured at the mitral annulus (septal wall) is positive or negative?

Answers appear at the back of the book.

4 Diagnosis of Myocardial Ischemia

Martin J. London

Perioperative transesophageal echocardiography (TEE) is a valuable monitor for detecting myocardial ischemia, capable of rapidly and decisively guiding anti-ischemic therapy. Currently, the qualitative recognition of regional wall motion abnormalities (RWMAs) is the basis of the clinical use of TEE for ischemia detection. Although newer technologies may allow easier, more precise, and quantitative analysis, the basic physiologic principles underlying RWMAs are not likely to change in the near future.

CLINICAL RELEVANCE OF TRANSESOPHAGEAL ECHOCARDIOGRAPHY IN DIAGNOSING MYOCARDIAL ISCHEMIA

TEE may improve the outcome in certain high-risk subsets of patients (1). However, the magnitude of this effect, relative to the greater expense and training required for TEE than for other commonly used methods of perioperative monitoring (e.g., electrocardiography [ECG], pulmonary artery catheterization [PAC]), remains controversial. Early clinical studies of TEE, particularly during vascular surgery, were somewhat overly optimistic about its value because it was mistakenly thought that new intraoperative RWMAs identified *all patients sustaining perioperative myocardial ischemia*. However, cardiology research subsequently documented more complex manifestations of myocardial ischemia, particularly myocardial stunning and hibernation, that complicate the *immediate assessment* of myocardial viability (2,3) (Table 4.1). More recent studies report a much lower predictive value for new intraoperative RWMAs because they relate to postoperative myocardial ischemia, and enthusiasm for "routine" TEE monitoring in noncardiac surgery *for the sole purpose of detecting ischemia* has waned (4,5).

In contrast, the use of TEE for ischemia detection and other applications during coronary artery bypass graft (CABG) surgery continues to increase (6). Given that epidemiologic studies convincingly demonstrate long-term survival advantages of CABG relative to medical therapy or percutaneous coronary interventions (i.e., percutaneous transluminal coronary angioplasty), particularly in patients with a depressed ejection fraction, it is likely that clinical interest in monitoring patients at high risk for ischemia with TEE will continue to grow (7). Also, the use of off-pump coronary artery bypass graft (OPCABG) has increased dramatically. In OPCAB, TEE is useful in evaluating the early efficacy of revascularization and, perhaps of greater importance, assessing the impact of surgical complications (e.g., inadequate anastomosis, inability to tolerate temporary occlusion of a distal vessel, hemodynamic consequences of cardiac displacement by stabilizers) (8,9).

The intraoperative echocardiographer must have a firm grounding in the physiologic, technical, and clinical aspects of ultrasonographic imaging because it relates to acute and chronic myocardial ischemia and infarction. Although ischemia and infarction lie at the ends of a continuous physiologic spectrum, obvious physiologic differences and morphologic changes specific to myocardial infarction (e.g., chronic wall thinning, calcification, septal rupture) may substantially affect clinical decision making with TEE. These changes tend to reduce the sensitivity and specificity of TEE, although recognition of the chronic irreversible consequences of infarction can have important implications for hemodynamic

Table 4.1 Characteristics of currently postulated forms of myocardial ischemia

	Conventional ischemia	Stunned myocardium	Hibernating myocardium	Preconditioned myocardium
Regional function	Reduced, usually in proportion to reduction in CBF	Reduced	Reduced	Possibly reduced during preconditioning stimulus, protected with repeated stimulus
Coronary blood flow	Severe reduction for akinesia, dyskinesia	Partial to full restoration after relief of ischemia	Moderate reduction to normal at rest, reduced with stress	Dependent on clinical situation, reduced during OPCAB
Energy metabolism	Reduced during low CBF	Normal to moderate reduction	Reduced in relation to contractile decrease	Reduced during preconditioning stimulus
Duration	Minutes to hours	Hours to weeks	Days to months	Minutes to hours after stimulus
Outcome	Infarction if severe enough	Full to partial recovery	Full recovery with revascularization	Decreased postischemic infarct or ischemic damage
Perioperative implications	Most "treatable" form	Common following CPB	May show immediate improvement after CPB	Sometimes used during OPCAB, volatile anesthesia preconditioning effects

CBF, cerebral blood flow; OPCAB, off-pump coronary artery bypass; CPB, cardiopulmonary bypass.
Modified from Opie LH. The multifarious spectrum of ischemic left ventricular dysfunction: relevance of new ischemic syndromes. *J Mol Cell Cardiol* 1996;28:2403–2414, with permission.

management. Also, the detection of thrombus in an infarcted segment or aneurysm can prevent devastating cerebrovascular consequences.

The American Society of Anesthesiologists/Society of Cardiovascular Anesthesiologists practice guidelines for the use of perioperative TEE accorded TEE only a category II indication (i.e., supported by weaker evidence than category I, possibly useful in improving clinical outcomes but appropriate indications less certain) for use in patients at increased risk for ischemia and infarction (10). It was given an even lower rating (category III: little current scientific or expert support) for evaluating myocardial perfusion, coronary artery anatomy, or graft patency. Given the logistic difficulties of performing clinical research on the impact of monitoring technology on patient outcomes, it is unlikely that the indications will be upgraded in subsequent revisions of these somewhat dated guidelines. However, significant clinical research based on newer technology continues to show promise for a wider application of TEE in ischemia monitoring.

PHYSIOLOGIC BASIS FOR THE DETECTION OF ISCHEMIA

Experimental animal and human clinical studies document the extraordinary sensitivity of ultrasonographic technology in detecting the rapid reduction in regional myocardial function associated with an acute reduction in myocardial blood flow in the perfusion territory of an affected coronary artery. These changes usually occur within a significantly shorter time than either ST-segment changes on the ECG or increased filling pressures noted by PAC, allowing earlier diagnosis. Although the ECG is also sensitive for ischemia detection, a number of physiologic factors lower its specificity (e.g., bundle branch block, pacing, Q waves or nonspecific ST-segment changes), so that *at least during the intraoperative period,* TEE is useful in a wider range of patients (11).

The most sensitive change associated with ischemia is a reduction or cessation of systolic wall thickening, which normally increases by 50% of the end-diastolic value (12) (Figure 4.1). With a complete cessation of coronary flow, systolic *wall thinning* may occur, leading to outward bulging of the affected wall (Figure 4.2). However, because the function of the heart is to eject blood *through a reduction in chamber size* by inward motion of the endocardial surface during systole, a reduction in *endocardial excursion* is a more obvious sign, especially when referenced to movement of the normal walls. It is also well established that in unaffected, nonischemic regions, exaggerated inward movement (termed *compensatory hyperkinesis*) develops, offsetting the adverse effects of regional dysfunction on cardiac stroke volume. This is the principal reason why changes in systemic hemodynamics with ischemia are a late (and particularly ominous) sign and usually occur only with very severe regional (particularly dyskinetic) or global ischemia.

When wall motion is scored, it should be appreciated that our eyes (and brain) can integrate several factors, particularly the translation and rotation movements of the heart in the chest, in "real time" to arrive at the "semiquantitative" classification of wall motion agreed on by echocardiographers (13) (Tables 4.2 and 4.3; Figure 4.3). These same factors greatly complicate computer analysis. Currently, despite the promotion of automated boundary detection techniques and their refinements (i.e., color kinesis), which are based on the detection of very low-level echo signals ("tissue backscatter"), the visual analysis of wall motion is the only viable option for use in clinical practice (14).

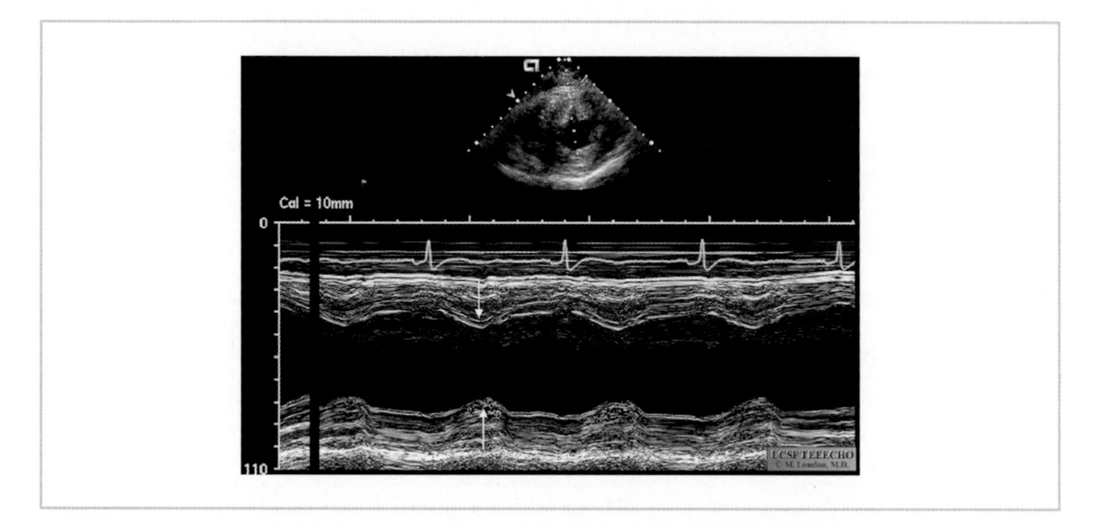

Figure 4.1. Normal wall M-mode (motion mode). Normal inward endocardial excursion and wall thickening are illustrated on an M-mode image through the inferior (**top**) and anterior (**bottom**) walls in the transgastric short-axis view (**top inset**). Systole starts at the onset of the QRS complex and ends near the end of the T wave (*arrows*). M-mode imaging through transesophageal echocardiography can on occasion provide helpful information regarding the timing of wall motion, particularly when coupled with the electrocardiogram.

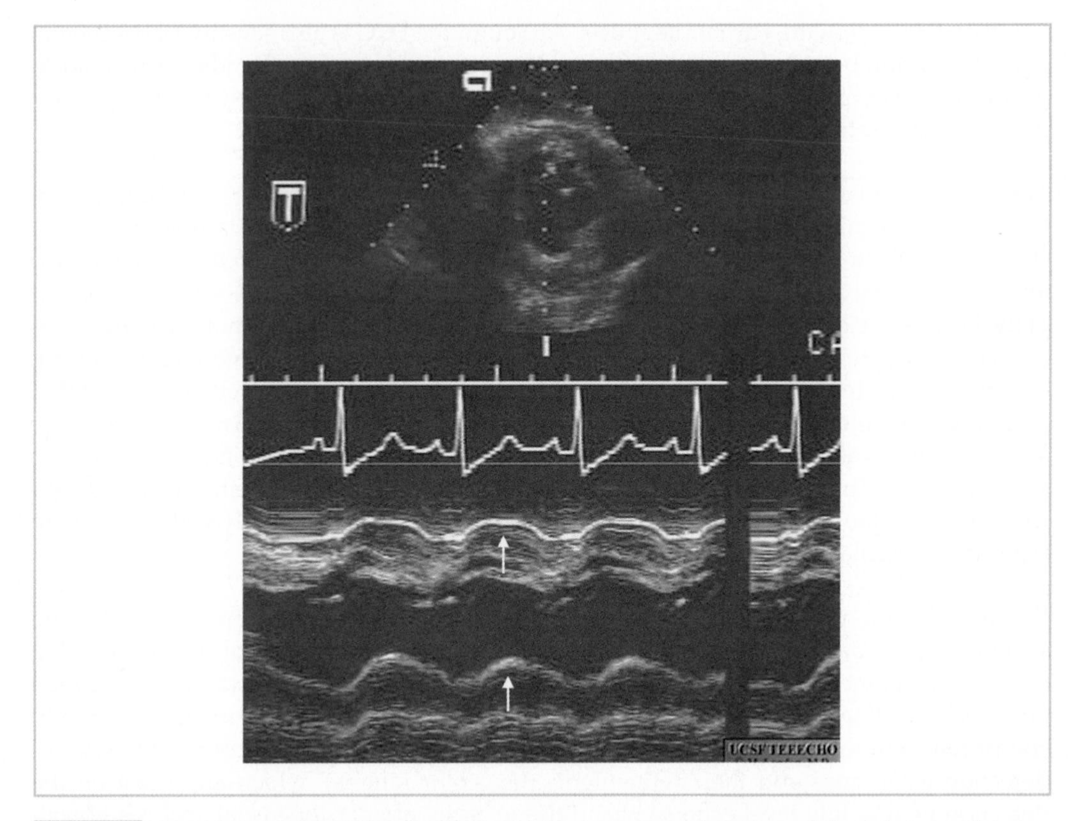

Figure 4.2. M-mode (motion mode) dyskinesis. Dyskinetic outward motion of the inferior wall (*upper arrow*) in a patient with a chronic inferior wall infarction (note the increased density of the myocardium on both the M-mode and two-dimensional images). Orientations are identical to those in Figure 4.1.

Table 4.2 Endocardial excursion versus wall thickening

Endocardial excursion	Wall thickening
Advantages	
Relies on a more readily defined interface (endocardium)	Independent of a center of reference
More readily measured around the entire circumference of the ventricle	Unaffected by translation or rotation
	Unaffected by shape changes
Disadvantages	
Centroid (center of mass)–dependent	Difficult to measure around the entire circumference of the ventricle because of poor epicardial definition
Affected by translation and rotation of the left ventricle in the chest	Tends to be "all or none" phenomenon
	More difficult to correlate with other imaging modalities (i.e., radionuclide or contrast ventriculograms)

From Mann DL, Gillam LD, Weyman AE. Cross-sectional echocardiographic assessment of regional left ventricular performance and myocardial perfusion. *Prog Cardiovasc Dis* 1986;29:1, with permission.

Table 4.3 Scoring of segmental wall motion abnormalities

Grade	Endocardial excursion (%)	Wall thickening (%)
Normal	>30	30–50
Hypokinesis		
Mild	10–30	30–50
Severe	<10	<30
Akinesis	0	<10
Dyskinesis	Outward bulging	Absent or systolic thinning
Hyperkinesis	>"Normal"	>"Normal"

It is important to appreciate that in most experimental studies, changes in endocardial excursion substantially overestimate the area of hypoperfused ischemic myocardium, whereas wall thickening more closely approximates it (15). The leading explanation for this overestimation is "tethering" of the abnormal myocardium to adjacent muscle segments, with complex mechanical effects (16). The clinician should always remember that endocardial excursion substantially overestimates the degree of ischemia. It is also critical to appreciate that other physiologic and morphologic conditions can "mimic" ischemia by causing abnormal endocardial

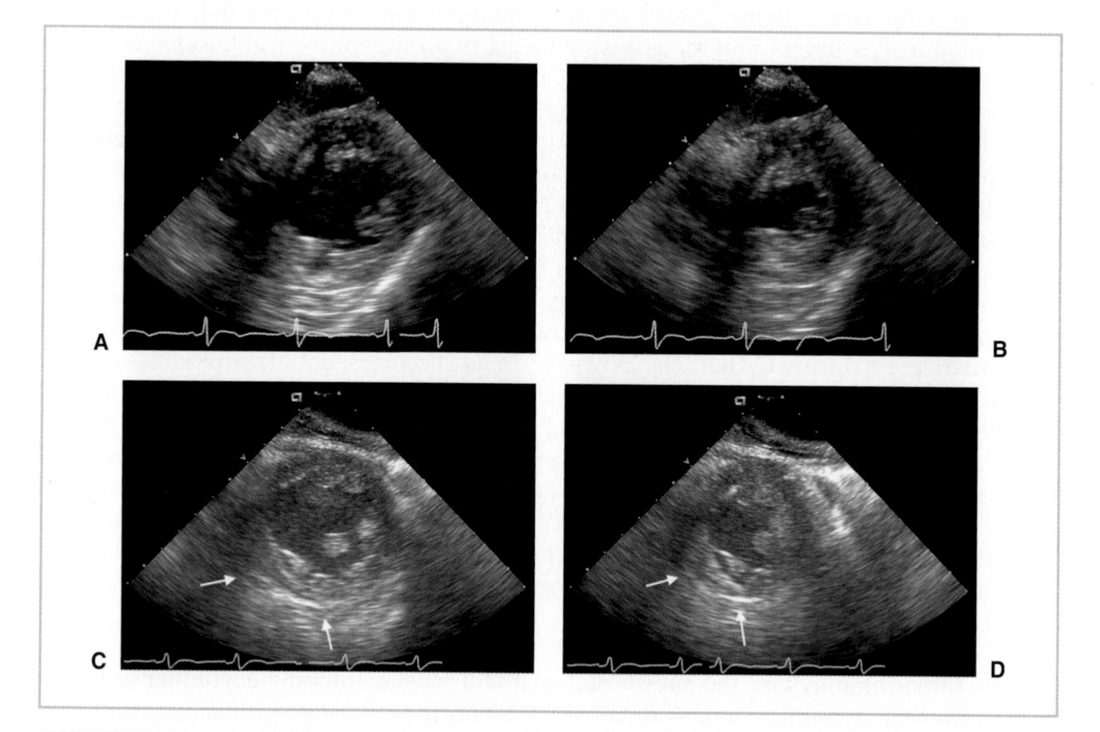

Figure 4.3. Anteroseptal akinesis following cardiopulmonary bypass. The upper frames show normal endocardial excursion and wall thickening from end-diastole **(A)** to end-systole **(B)** in the transgastric short-axis view in a patient undergoing coronary artery bypass grafting. The lower frames show akinesis of the mid-anterior and anteroseptal segments (*arrows*) on weaning from coronary bypass. **C:** End-diastole. **D:** End-systole.

excursion (discussed later). However, in these situations, *systolic wall thickening should be normal*. Finally, it is important to recognize that the magnitude of endocardial excursion and wall thickening can vary between different regions of the heart and between different "normal" individuals (17). Therefore, using the patient's baseline status as a control is necessary.

Precise numeric relations between coronary blood flow and regional function are controversial. The subendocardium, with its higher metabolic requirements and greater susceptibility to the adverse effects of elevated intracavitary filling pressures, is more sensitive to flow reduction and shows earlier change in thickening (12). In the nonsurgical setting, myocardial infarction is usually related to coronary obstruction at the epicardial level and, depending on the site of obstruction and the status of the collateral circulation, results in transmural or subendocardial ischemia. An often quoted cardiology study suggests that regional function may cease with only a 20% reduction in transmural flow (18). This observation forms the basis for the considerable interest of cardiologists in assessing myocardial viability because an RWMA in the resting state indicates little regarding potential improvement (i.e., return to normal wall motion) after medical or surgical intervention. Myocardial viability is most commonly assessed with measures of metabolism (positron emission tomography), intact microvascular circulation (thallium imaging, perfusion contrast echocardiography), and, of particular interest to the cardiac anesthesiologist, mechanical contractile reserve (dobutamine stress testing). Each of these methods yields slightly different (and complementary) information (19).

Increasing emphasis is being placed on dobutamine stress testing for risk stratification before noncardiac surgery and for assessing the early postoperative wall motion response to CABG. With low doses of dobutamine, normal myocardium becomes hyperkinetic and coronary blood flow increases (20). The development of hypokinesis or akinesis in a previously normal segment with dobutamine indicates myocardial ischemia. A chronic transmural infarction will not increase wall thickening in response to either low or high doses of dobutamine. Improvement of function in a kinetic segment with low-dose dobutamine indicates the presence of *viable myocardium with contractile reserve*, called *stunned myocardium*. A *biphasic response*, in which improvement occurs at a low dose followed by deterioration at a higher dose, is characteristic of *hibernating myocardium*. One study suggests a potential role for intraoperative dobutamine stress testing before revascularization during CABG (21). However, in most centers, dobutamine stress echo or other tests of viability are routinely performed during the preoperative workup for CABG. The development of short-term myocardial stunning during cardiopulmonary bypass (CPB) can complicate the early interpretation of viability. *Although early studies suggested that the development of new RWMAs on termination of CPB was an indication for graft revision, a more widespread appreciation of the complexities of myocardial stunning suggests that only when the surgeon suspects technical problems (e.g., intramyocardial vessel, difficulty in locating proper vessel, need for endarterectomy of the vessel, intimal flaps) should a new RWMA prompt a potentially morbid return to CPB.*

Despite these complexities, the anesthesiologist will most commonly encounter ischemia related to more dynamic changes in coronary blood flow during surgical manipulation (i.e., with retraction of the heart during OPCAB) or to hemodynamic abnormalities caused by surgery (e.g., profound hypotension, tachycardia, marked increase in afterload). In these situations, new RWMAs are more likely to be coupled to acute changes in coronary blood flow caused by the altered hemodynamics and are therefore usually more amenable to immediate treatment.

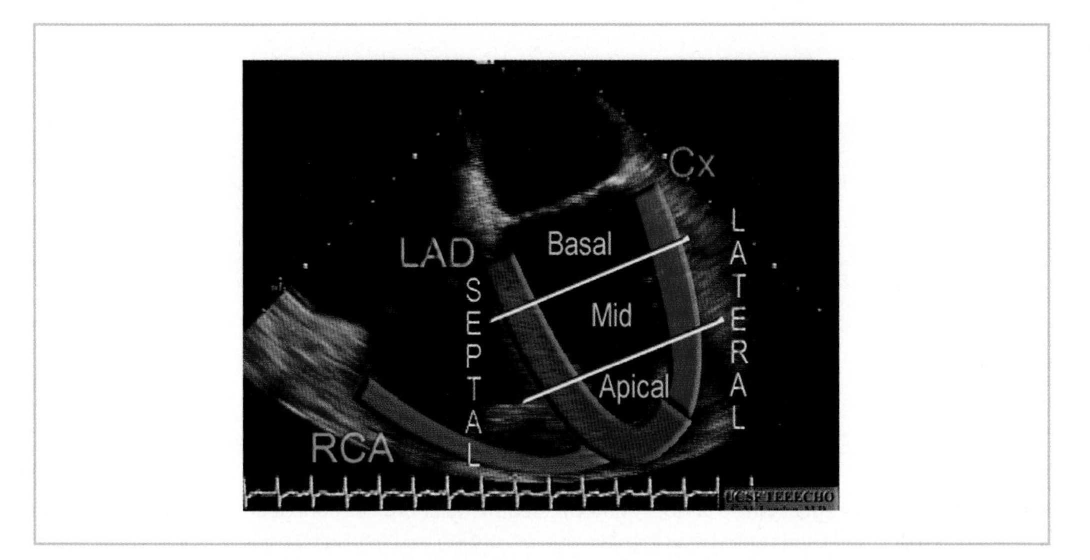

Figure 4.4. Midesophageal four-chamber anatomic segments and perfusion. Segmental anatomy of the left ventricle in the midesophageal four-chamber view according to the American Society of Echocardiography classification system. Also depicted are the approximate perfusion zones of the left anterior descending (LAD), circumflex (Cx), and right coronary (RCA) arteries.

ECHOCARDIOGRAPHIC DETECTION OF ISCHEMIA

Anatomic Localization of Ischemia: The 17-Segment System

The precise anatomic localization of left ventricular (LV) RWMAs is essential to guide clinical decision making, particularly in localizing the likely diseased coronary artery, and to gauge the impact of therapy. It is also important for accurate documentation in the medical record and for communication with surgeons and cardiologists. The 17-segment model adopted by the American Heart Association is universally accepted in this country (22) (Figures 4.4–4.7). This system is based on division of the LV into apical, mid, and basal zones. The basal and mid zones each contain six segments, the apical zone with its smaller area has only four and the apex is the final segment. To assess all 17 segments completely requires interrogation of five imaging planes: the midesophageal (ME) four-chamber, two-chamber, and long-axis views, and the transgastric (TG) mid and basal views.

In the author's experience, the basal TG view can be problematic to obtain, and interpreting wall motion in this region so close to the fibrous atrioventricular (AV) skeleton of the heart can be challenging. Therefore, some clinicians omit this view, substituting the three longitudinal ME views to assess the basal segments. Although this method allows visualization of at least a portion of each of the six basal segments, it is technically *incomplete* because the entire radius of each segment is not visualized. However, if these segments appear normal in the longitudinal orientation, it is likely that the remaining portion will be. It is important to remember that to obtain a "true" ME four-chamber view, one must rotate the multiplane transducer approximately 10 degrees to "remove" the anteriorly located LV outflow tract, which allows visualization of the basal septal segment.

Although assessing all 17 segments can be laborious for the busy clinician, it is important for the effective communication of findings.

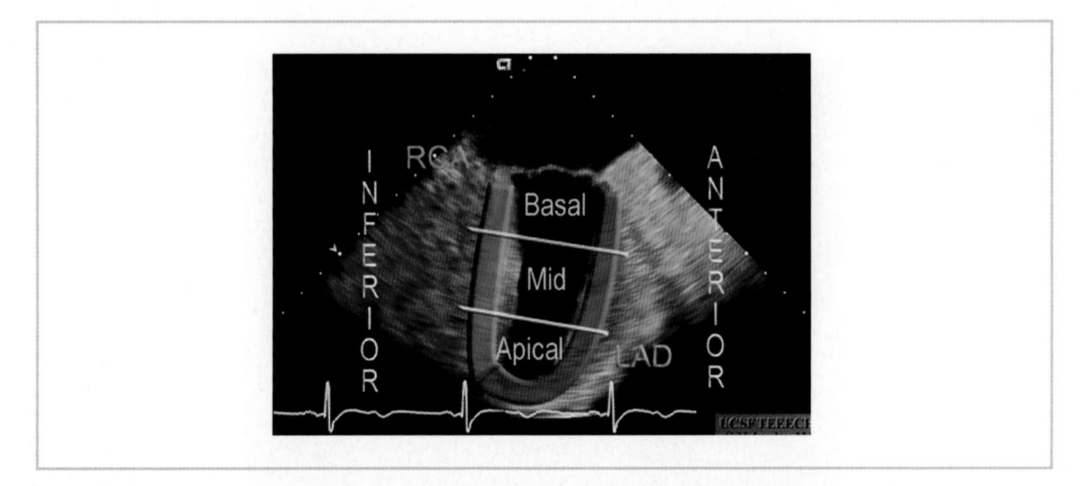

Figure 4.5. Midesophageal two-chamber anatomic segments and perfusion. Segmental anatomy of the left ventricle in the midesophageal two-chamber view according to the American Society of Echocardiography classification system. Also depicted are the approximate perfusion zones of the left anterior descending (LAD) and right coronary (RCA) arteries.

CLINICAL CAVEAT: IMAGING THE APICAL SEGMENTS

Recognition by the clinician that new apical RWMAs are commonly encountered in patients undergoing CABG and that complications of infarction, particularly aneurysm and thrombus formation, are commonly encountered in this region mandates careful attention to the apex during the baseline echocardiographic examination.

It is difficult to obtain a transverse apical image, although it is facilitated by retroflexion at the level of the TG short-axis view (Figure 4.8). Therefore, assessment of the apex is nearly exclusively performed with the ME longitudinal orientations. However, TEE

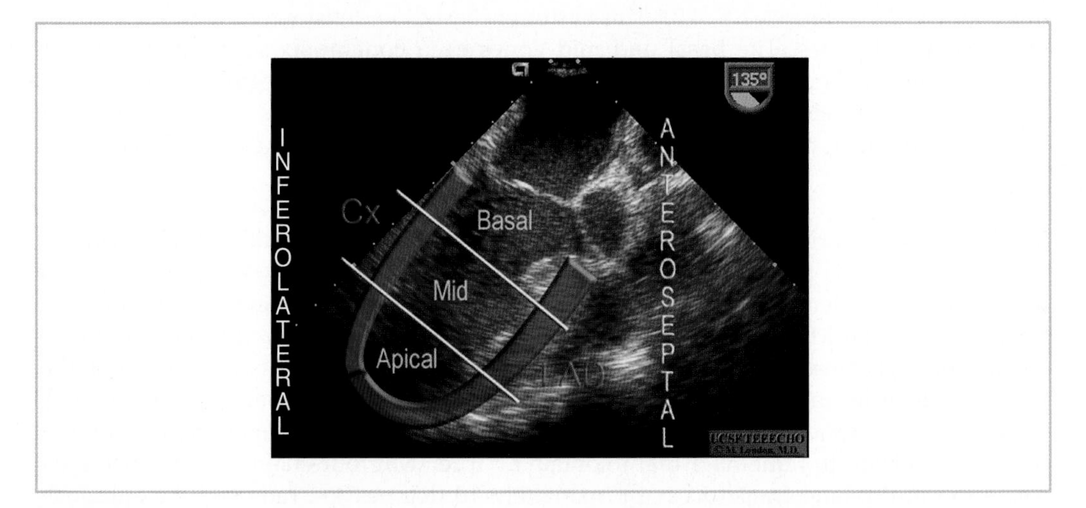

Figure 4.6. Midesophageal long-axis anatomic segments and perfusion. Segmental anatomy of the left ventricle in the midesophageal long-axis view according to the American Society of Echocardiography classification system. Also depicted are the approximate perfusion zones of the major left anterior descending (LAD) and circumflex (Cx) arteries.

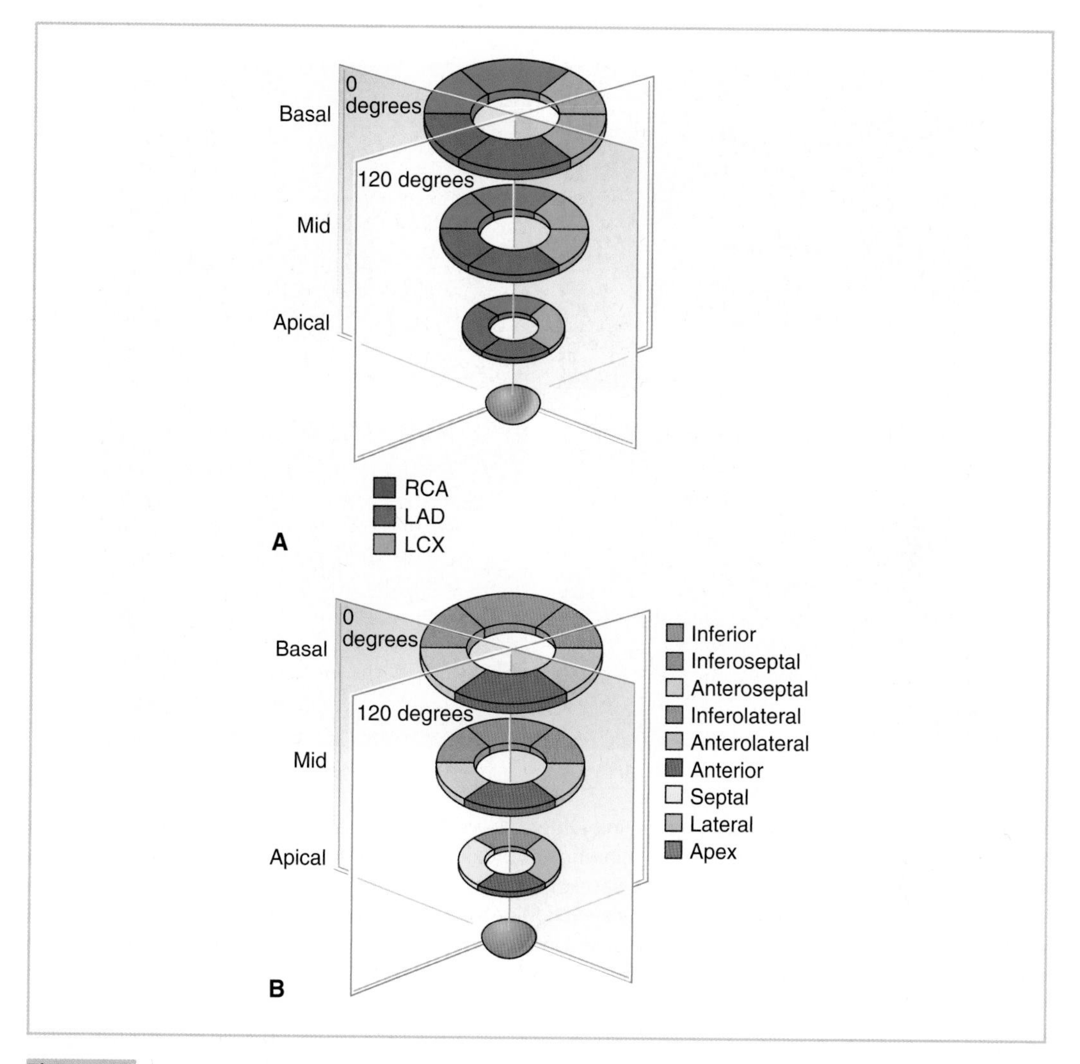

Figure 4.7. **A:** Coronary artery distribution as demonstrated in the transgastric short axis views. RCA, right coronary artery; LAD, left anterior descending artery; LCX left circumflex artery. **B:** Seventeen-segment left ventricular nomenclature. (Adapted from Cerqueira MD, Weissman NJ, Dilsizian V, et al. Standardized myocardial segmentation and nomenclature for tomographic imaging of the heart. *Circulation* 2002;105:539.)

has documented limitations for assessing the "true apex," and it is well known that TEE long-axis images can be "foreshortened," with the echo beam exiting the ventricle somewhere above the true apex (23). The ability of transthoracic echocardiography (TTE) to image the apex more reliably given the ability of the echocardiographer to move the transducer freely on the chest wall is one of the few advantages of TTE over TEE. Despite these limitations, TEE imaging of the apex can be accomplished in nearly all patients with focused effort by an experienced echocardiographer. Given that the apex is in the "far field" of the image, it is important to optimize gain/time gain compensation settings in this region. To optimize visualization of the apex, place the focal zone over the apex, select as low a frequency as is consistent with optimal resolution (usually no higher than 6 MHz), and if the ultrasonographic system allows, use the "zoom" feature. The TG long-axis

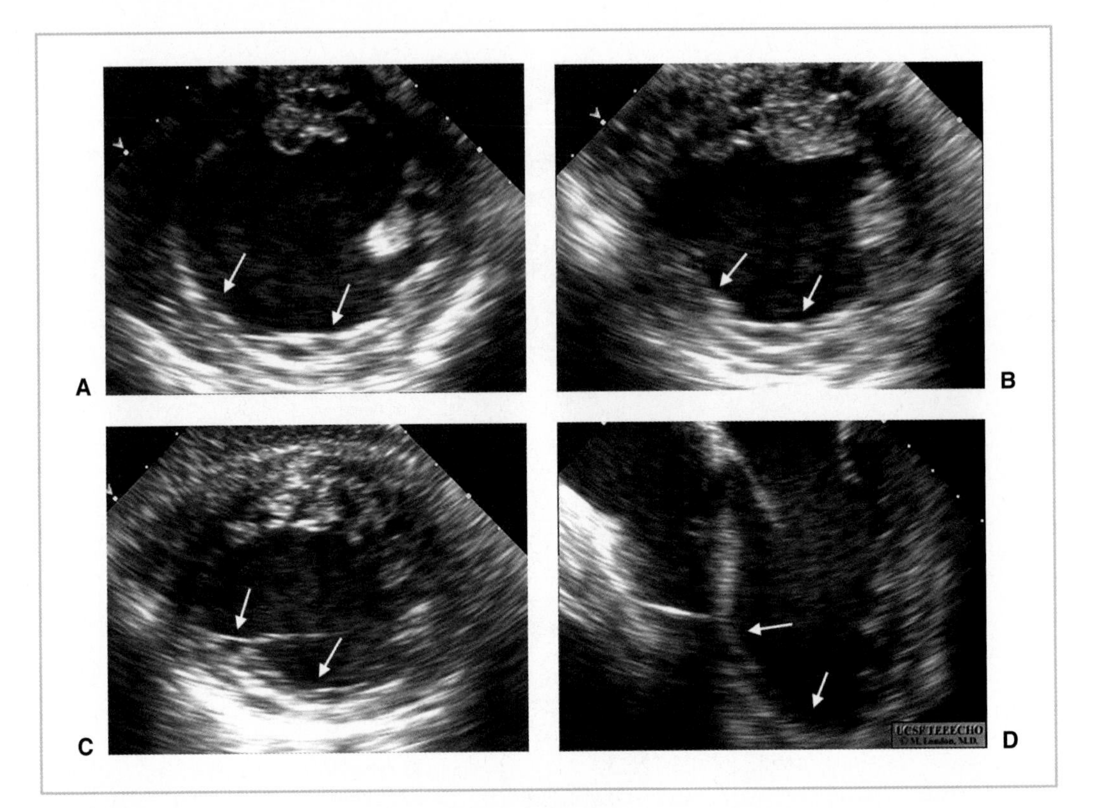

Figure 4.8. Chronic anteroseptal infarction in multiple views. A large area of infarction in the anteroseptal region is characterized by chronic wall thinning (approximately outlined by *arrows*), and akinesis is visualized in multiple imaging planes. **A:** Basal transgastric short-axis view. **B:** Midtransgastric short-axis view. **C:** Apical transgastric short-axis view. **D:** Midesophageal four-chamber view. A "hinge point" characteristic of the junction between normal and infarcted myocardium is evident at the *top arrow* in the frame. Calcification of the anteromedial papillary muscle is also evident.

view can be of particular value in further assessing anterior and inferior wall motion in a complementary fashion to the TG short-axis view, particularly when imaging from the ME planes is poor. However, apical imaging is not possible from this view.

CORONARY ARTERY PERFUSION ZONES

The 17-segment system was adopted by the American Society of Echocardiography in part because the coronary artery perfusion territories are relatively constant in the various segments (Figures 4.4–4.7). One of the reasons for the popularity of the TG short-axis view (besides that it is the easiest one in which to assess intracavitary area/volume continuously) is that it is the only view in which *a portion of the territories of all three main coronary arteries perfusing the LV can be visualized*. In Figure 4.7, the four-chamber view, right coronary perfusion of the right ventricular (RV) free wall, but not of the LV, can be assessed. Therefore, with a significant reduction in flow in one of the three main coronary arteries, one will *usually* see a new RWMA. However, if ischemia is caused by stenosis in a vessel distal to this region (i.e., perfusing the apical segments), wall motion will remain normal in the TG short-axis view, and the clinician must remain "vigilant" and use other views.

Variation in the normal coronary anatomy further complicates simple mapping of the coronary artery distributions by anatomic segments. The most important factor is the origin of the posterior descending artery from the right coronary artery in a *right-dominant system* versus its origin from the circumflex coronary artery in the less common left-dominant system. The size of the perfusion zone can vary by individual, and overlap between territories is usual, most commonly in the inferolateral segments and the inferoapical and lateral apical segments. The left anterior descending coronary artery usually perfuses these apical segments, although the posterior descending (inferoapical segment) or circumflex (lateral apical segment) coronary artery may also be present.

WALL MOTION SCORE INDEX

Once wall motion has been scored in each of the 17 LV segments, a global wall motion score can easily be calculated by assigning an integer score to each category of wall motion (increasing the number with increasing severity of wall motion) (13). The sum for all the segments is divided by the total number of segments visualized (with the realization that all segments may not be adequately imaged) to obtain a wall motion score index. This approach has been validated by cardiology studies comparing echo wall motion analysis with other imaging modalities, particularly thallium perfusion methods. However, given that akinesis can occur with flow reductions affecting only 25% of wall thickness, the correlation of a wall motion index with myocardial viability, particularly in acute myocardial infarction, can be variable. It is rarely if ever used by anesthesiologists, and there is no literature basis for its value in the perioperative period.

Ischemic Mitral Regurgitation

Mitral regurgitation (MR) is commonly associated with acute, severe ischemia and provides valuable information regarding its severity and, more importantly, the efficacy of therapy as it resolves. In a previously normal mitral valve, the regurgitation is central in origin and is associated with marked elevation of the pulmonary artery pressures. A variety of theories about etiologic factors have been proposed, including acute ventricular dilation leading to incomplete leaflet coaptation, ischemic dysfunction of one or both papillary muscles, and hypokinesia of the ventricular segment underlying an otherwise normally functioning papillary muscle (24). Newer studies based on three-dimensional modeling have noted acute annular enlargement with displacement of the papillary muscle tips, resulting in what is termed *loitering* (i.e., a slow response of the mitral valve leaflets to coapt properly in early systole) (25). It may occur with severe global subendocardial ischemia. *In the author's experience, MR occurs almost universally in sudden, severe intraoperative ischemia.* Therefore, rapid color flow interrogation of the mitral valve should be a "second nature" maneuver for the clinician who suspects that ischemia may be present.

With myocardial infarction, additional factors contributing to MR include LV cavity and annular dilation, aneurysmal or pseudoaneurysmal changes, particularly of the basal segments, and in the most severe and life-threatening situation, papillary muscle rupture. Rupture most commonly involves the posteromedial muscle in the setting of either a right or circumflex infarction because the posteromedial papillary muscle is perfused by a single coronary artery, whereas the anteromedial papillary muscle has a dual arterial supply.

Recognizing the Complications of Myocardial Infarction

It is important to recognize the chronic manifestations and complications of myocardial infarction for the following reasons:

1. Often, the myocardial infarction will preclude monitoring for ischemia in the affected segments.

Table 4.4 Complications of acute myocardial infarction

Complications
Acute phase
LV systolic dysfunction
Rupture
Free wall rupture
Ventricular septal defect
Papillary muscle rupture
Subepicardial aneurysm
Mitral regurgitation
LV dilatation
Papillary muscle dysfunction
Papillary muscle rupture
LV thrombus
Pericardial effusion/tamponade
RV infarct
LV outflow tract obstruction
Chronic phase
Infarct expansion
Ventricular aneurysm
True aneurysm
Pseudoaneurysm
LV thrombus

LV, left ventricular; RV, right ventricular.
Adapted from Oh JK, Seward JB, Tajik AJ. *The echo manual*, 2nd ed. Philadelphia: Lippincott Williams & Wilkins, 1999:77.

2. Certain complications, if unrecognized, can have serious or fatal consequences (e.g., mural thrombus causing a cerebrovascular accident, ruptured pseudoaneurysm causing pericardial tamponade) (Table 4.4 and Figure 4.9).

An end-diastolic wall thickness of 0.6 cm or less has been shown to exclude the potential for recovery of function with myocardial revascularization (26). Recognition of a chronically

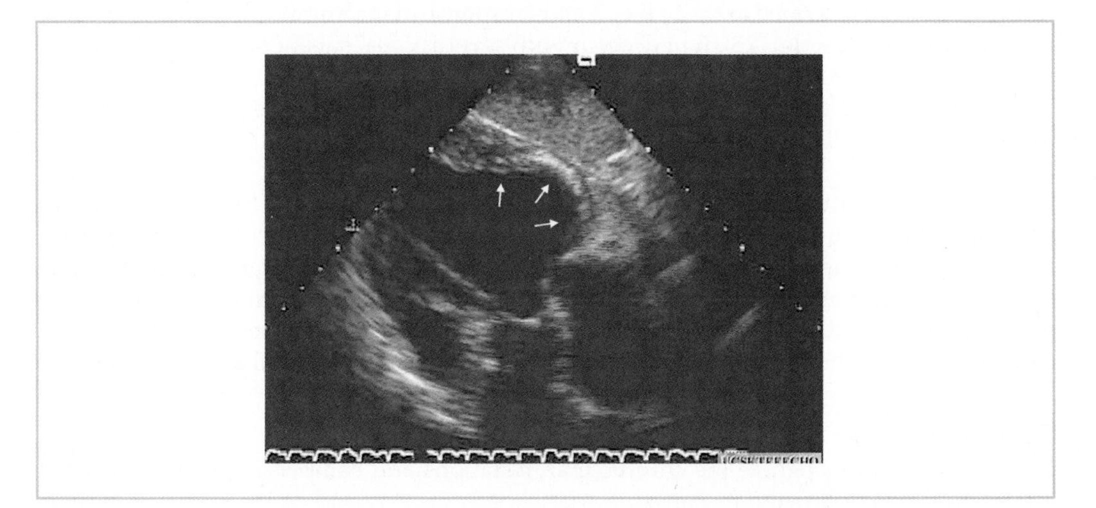

Figure 4.9. Inferobasal aneurysm. Aneurysm (boundaries noted by *arrows*) of the inferobasal segment imaged in the transgastric long-axis view. Note the increased density of the myocardium, consistent with fibrosis.

infarcted, fibrotic, or, in the later phases, calcified segment is important to distinguish these findings from acute ischemia. However, the dyskinesis seen in these longstanding conditions does not have the ominous potential that results from acute dyskinesis (with wall thinning) in a previously normal segment, although it is obvious that the latter situation is more likely to be amenable to therapy.

Mural thrombi may pose a particular challenge because they are often difficult to appreciate on routine echocardiographic examination. The sessile, laminated thrombus that commonly occurs with a large anterior infarction may blend in with the wall. Apical thrombi are more likely to be recognized because they may present as unique shapes in the apex, occasionally as pedunculated masses. Recognition of thrombi is important because the use of an LV vent during CABG or valve surgery can dislodge thrombus, with potentially fatal consequences.

Clinical Caveats: Detection of Ischemia

DIGITAL CAPTURE OF CINE LOOPS

To monitor for RWMAs, the clinician must accurately distinguish between systole and diastole. Although this seems trivial, in fact it can be quite challenging, particularly if the patient has abnormal resting function or morphology (particularly LV hypertrophy) or if the ventricle is paced (as often occurs after separation from bypass) and loading conditions are markedly abnormal. Application of a three-lead ECG cable from the ultrasonography machine to the patient is standard operating procedure in the echocardiography laboratory and should also be used routinely in the operating room, particularly if images are acquired digitally and displayed as "cine loops." When the capture button is pushed, digital image capture is triggered as the R wave signals the onset of systole. In the absence of an ECG R-wave trigger, a capture of 1 second or more is acquired. Although this is more than adequate to capture several complete cardiac cycles, a lack of precise timing (i.e., onset of systole) at the start of image capture makes it difficult to play clips acquired at different time periods in a quad or split screen format *in a synchronized manner*. This makes careful comparison of loops considerably more difficult.

IMAGING PITFALLS

A variety of technical and patient-specific factors may complicate the detection of ischemia. The most common technical factor is endocardial "dropout," common in segments parallel to the ultrasound beam. In this situation, use of an echo "contrast agent" will in most instances precisely delineate the endocardial border. However, given the expense of these agents and storage issues, their use in the operative setting is uncommon. Foreshortening of the apex is also commonly encountered and can prevent accurate imaging of the apex. In the author's experience, with careful probe manipulation, the apex can be adequately imaged. An oblique orientation of the probe in the TG short-axis view can lead to misinterpretation of septal motion as a consequence of incorporation of a portion of the LV outflow tract into the image. This is usually easily recognized because the ventricle chamber will not be circular but oblique in shape.

ABNORMAL LOADING CONDITIONS

Common patient-specific factors include abnormal loading conditions, which at either end of the volume or pressure spectrum complicate the interpretation of RWMAs (27). With hypervolemia or an elevated afterload secondary to severe hypertension, wall motion can appear severely hypokinetic. This is usually easily recognized, especially in that all walls are affected equally and wall motion promptly returns to normal with a reduction in pressure or volume. Hypovolemia is more problematic because it accentuates any regional disparity in endocardial excursion and can cause "pseudo" dyskinetic motion in an already akinetic segment. Usually, this occurs only with gross hypovolemia. However, in a long case with major fluid shifts, clinicians may "lose" their frame of reference as to what constitutes normovolemia. Therefore, a baseline image acquired shortly after the induction of anesthesia (with care taken to note any obvious loading changes during induction) is helpful when displayed alongside the later images.

OTHER CAUSES OF ABNORMAL WALL MOTION

Patients with severe LV hypertrophy are more difficult to image, and appreciating changes in wall motion is challenging. The intracavitary area may be reduced, so that the appreciation of changes in endocardial excursion becomes more difficult. In the worst-case scenario, hypertrophic cardiomyopathy, the ground glass appearance of the myocardium, greatly complicates the assessment of wall motion. Pacing of the ventricle, particularly ventricular pacing with endocardial wires during open chest cardiac procedures, can be problematic. Earlier studies suggested that septal wall motion abnormalities were particularly common in the post-CPB setting, either caused by the release of pericardial restraint or accentuated by pacing. However, in the author's clinical practice, major septal abnormalities resulting from these factors sufficiently significant to be confused with ischemia are rare.

Right Ventricular Ischemia and Infarction

The RV is a complex and important part of the heart that is often overlooked by the busy intraoperative echocardiographer. Although major abnormalities of RV function and ischemia are infrequently encountered in routine adult surgical practice, when they occur, they can be very difficult to treat. Given the anterior location of the RV in the chest and its thin walls, it is more susceptible than the LV to incomplete myocardial preservation, particularly with radiant warming during CPB. When severe RV failure occurs, as evidenced by the absence of a response to inotropic and vasodilator support, a very invasive pulmonary artery balloon pump or RV assist device may be required.

The right coronary artery perfuses most of the RV, although the conus branch of the left anterior descending artery may supply a small portion of the RV free wall (28). Patients with severe chronic obstructive pulmonary disease and coronary artery disease are particularly susceptible to RV ischemia/failure during CABG. Tricuspid regurgitation commonly accompanies RV ischemia and is severe during RV failure. The preferred imaging plane for the detection of RV ischemia is usually the ME four-chamber view, although portions of the RV can be imaged in other views, including TG planes. Gross RV dilation is common and in the absence of a major elevation of pulmonary artery pressure is usually diagnostic of RV ischemia.

CLINICAL APPLICATIONS

Use of Preoperative Data to Guide Monitoring

The clinician can tailor TEE monitoring to the particular patient by a careful consideration of the results of preoperative diagnostic testing. Obviously, careful assessment of a preoperative echocardiographic study will allow the most direct comparison of any change in the patient's state, particularly new or worsened RWMAs, worsened ventricular function, and MR. Results of a preoperative dobutamine stress test can be particularly helpful in identifying which segments are at greatest jeopardy for becoming ischemic and warrant the closest monitoring (29).

Recommendations for Monitoring

Several intraoperative factors will influence the monitoring plan for a specific patient. Patient-, clinician-, and procedure-specific variables must be considered. The availability of imaging planes based on the location of surgery, the particular patient's body habitus, and other mechanical factors clearly affect the ability to assess wall motion in all 17 segments. The level of difficulty of the surgery and the time available (or lack thereof) for the clinician to focus on the TEE images are also major factors. Given the variable impact of TEE on patient outcome during different types of surgery, the most basic recommendation is to attempt to perform as complete an examination of all segments, valvular function, and contractility as is possible under the clinical circumstances immediately after induction of anesthesia. Cardiac surgical procedures in which CPB is used usually involve additional examinations just before CPB is applied and immediately after weaning. The clinician's choice of a monitoring plane that is continuously displayed between comprehensive examinations is variable; many clinicians prefer the TG mid short-axis view, which allows a rapid estimation of cavitary area and wall motion, whereas others prefer the ME long-axis view, particularly the four- or five-chamber view, which allows continuous assessment of mitral valve structure and apical wall motion.

Primary Coronary Artery Bypass Grafting (with Cardiopulmonary Bypass)

As noted earlier, a careful assessment of wall motion is advised at several points during the procedure, although the speed at which many private surgeons operate may on occasion mandate an abbreviated examination that should focus on the individual patient's "high-risk" anatomy. Transient ischemia during CABG has numerous causes, the detection of which is greatly facilitated by the use of TEE (Table 4.5).

Redo Coronary Artery Bypass Grafting

Patients undergoing redo CABG are at high risk for the development of ischemia in the prebypass period, particularly during the manipulation of existing grafts, which can be easily damaged during dissection and are likely to contain atheromatous debris that can readily form emboli, resulting in catastrophic ischemia. Hemodynamic perturbations, particularly hypotension and tachycardia, may precipitate ischemia in the setting of multiple occluded grafts.

Table 4.5 Causes of acute ischemia during coronary artery bypass grafting

Causes
Pre-CPB ischemia
Hemodynamic abnormalities (tachycardia, hypotension most common)
Sudden ventricular fibrillation
Ischemia during cannulation (hypotension most common)
Dislodgement of atheromatous debris from previous graft (redo CABG)
Post-CPB ischemia
Low cardiac output states
Graft problems (intimal flap, total occlusion from thrombus, inadvertent graft into vein, graft too short or kinked during closure of chest)
Air embolus from pooled air in cardiac apex or from pulmonary veins (most commonly right coronary distribution)
Sudden ventricular fibrillation

CPB, cardiopulmonary bypass; CABG, coronary artery bypass graft.

Off-Pump Coronary Artery Bypass

The use of OPCAB is increasing rapidly, adding new challenges to anesthetic management. TEE imaging is compromised when surgical packing is placed posteriorly and the heart is lifted to facilitate surgical exposure of the arteries (9). The best images are usually obtained during the left anterior descending artery anastomosis because only minor displacement is required. However, during circumflex and right coronary artery dissection, imaging is poor and TG planes are usually not possible. Monitoring with ME four- or two-chamber views often reveals very distorted LV anatomy but is usually the only option during this period. Fortunately, newer stabilization devices allow the elimination of posteriorly placed surgical packing and improve TEE visualization.

Because the stabilizer apparatus "tethers" the adjacent myocardium during the procedure, wall motion is usually grossly abnormal, so that analysis of regional wall motion is not reliable for detecting ischemia. Preconditioning for each of the vessels is controversial, and not all surgeons use it. For those who do use preconditioning, assessing the wall motion response (in the absence of the stabilizer) can be helpful. It is not uncommon to see new wall motion abnormalities that last for a short period of time after completion of the anastomosis, presumably caused by myocardial stunning (8). However, these should resolve relatively quickly, and if they do not, either reinspecting the anastomosis or using on-graft Doppler imaging to verify graft patency should be considered.

Transmyocardial Laser Revascularization

In this new (and controversial) procedure, a laser is used to burn approximately 1-mm transmural channels (approximately one channel per square centimeter) through myocardium not amenable to routine revascularization (30). The mechanism of angina relief is controversial, although some form of angioneogenesis is the leading explanation. These patients are at high risk for the development of ischemia and may have impaired ventricular function as a result of previous infarction. A complete examination of the LV segments is mandatory to monitor for ischemia. In this procedure, the echocardiographer has the important and unique responsibility of notifying the surgeon when the laser has penetrated the full thickness of the myocardium. This is easily recognized by the sudden appearance of numerous bubbles within the LV cavity (Figure 4.10). The task is important because a burn that is too deep or too long can damage the mitral valve chordae or other valvular components. Therefore, careful examination of the mitral and aortic valves by two-dimensional and color Doppler imaging before and after a series of laser treatments is mandatory.

Valve Surgery

Ischemia can develop during valve surgery secondary to either concurrent coronary artery disease or embolism. The latter is most commonly caused by air that often originates from the pulmonary veins or cardiac apex (31). Because the anteriorly located ostia of the right coronary artery is at a 90-degree angle to the aortic root, air exiting the ventricle in large quantities can cause clinically significant ischemia in this distribution. Prompt recognition of coronary air embolism is important because it can be easily treated by "blowing the air through" and using high doses of phenylephrine or returning to CPB. Ischemia can also be caused by subendocardial hypoperfusion during low cardiac output states following a technically difficult valve repair/replacement requiring a very long pump run or a failed repair.

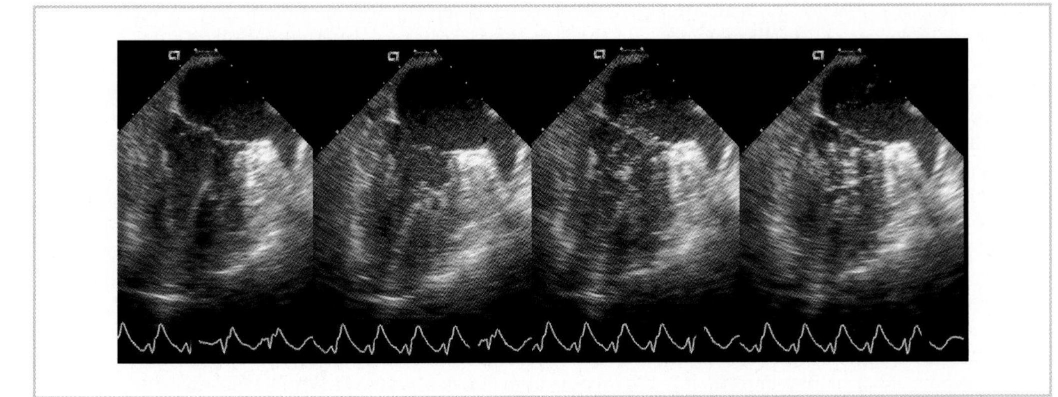

Figure 4.10. Sequential image frames from a transmyocardial laser revascularization procedure illustrating penetration of the laser beam into the left ventricle, evidenced by microbubbles at the point of entrance in the basal portion of the anterior wall (midesophageal two-chamber view). Note the temporary current of injury on the electrocardiogram.

SUMMARY

The detection of myocardial ischemia is an important priority for the practicing clinician, especially as our population ages and the incidence of coronary artery disease increases. A clinically based framework for the anatomic, physiologic, technical, and procedure-specific factors involved in ischemia has been presented here. These are only the basics, and with the increasing sophistication of echocardiographic technology (particularly applications of integrated backscatter technology and tissue Doppler imaging), the methods will undergo further refinement. It is likely that newer technology will facilitate capture of the earliest presentations of ischemia, a scenario that ultimately should enhance patient outcome.

REFERENCES

1 Savage RM, Lytle BW, Aronson S, et al. Intraoperative echocardiography is indicated in high-risk coronary artery bypass grafting. *Ann Thorac Surg* 1997;64:368–373; discussion 373–374.

2 Kloner RA, Jennings RB. Consequences of brief ischemia: stunning, preconditioning, and their clinical implications: part 1. *Circulation* 2001;104:2981–2989.

3 Kloner RA, Jennings RB. Consequences of brief ischemia: stunning, preconditioning, and their clinical implications: part 2. *Circulation* 2001;104:3158–3167.

4 London MJ, Tubau JF, Wong MG, et al. S.P.I. Research Group. The natural history of segmental wall motion abnormalities in patients undergoing noncardiac surgery. *Anesthesiology* 1990;73:644–655.

5 Dodds TM, Burns AK, DeRoo DB, et al. Effects of anesthetic technique on myocardial wall motion abnormalities during abdominal aortic surgery. *J Cardiothorac Vasc Anesth* 1997;11:129–136.

6 Morewood GH, Gallagher ME, Gaughan JP, et al. Current practice patterns for adult perioperative transesophageal echocardiography in the United States. *Anesthesiology* 2001;95:1507–1512.

7 Eagle KA, Guyton RA, Davidoff R, et al. ACC/AHA guidelines for coronary artery bypass graft surgery: executive summary and recommendations: a report of the American College of Cardiology/American Heart Association Task Force on Practice Guidelines (committee to revise the 1991 guidelines for coronary artery bypass graft surgery). *Circulation* 1999;100:1464–1480.

8 Malkowski MJ, Kramer CM, Parvizi ST, et al. Transient ischemia does not limit subsequent ischemic regional dysfunction in humans: a transesophageal echocardiographic study during minimally invasive coronary artery bypass surgery. *J Am Coll Cardiol* 1998;31:1035–1039.

9 Mathison M, Edgerton JR, Horswell JL, et al. Analysis of hemodynamic changes during beating heart surgical procedures. *Ann Thorac Surg* 2000;70:1355–1360.

10 *Anesthesiology.* Practice guidelines for perioperative transesophageal echocardiography. A report by the American Society of Anesthesiologists and the Society of Cardiovascular Anesthesiologists Task Force on Transesophageal Echocardiography 1996;84:986–1006
11 London MJ, Kaplan JA. Advances in electrocardiographic monitoring. In: Kaplan JA, Reich DL, Konstadt SN, eds. *Cardiac anesthesia,* 4th ed. Philadelphia: WB Saunders, 1999:359–400.
12 Gallagher KP, Kumada T, Koziol JA, et al. Significance of regional wall thickening abnormalities relative to transmural myocardial perfusion in anesthetized dogs. *Circulation* 1980;62:1266–1274.
13 Schiller NB, Shah PM, Crawford M, et al. Recommendations for quantitation of the left ventricle by two-dimensional echocardiography. American Society of Echocardiography Committee on Standards, Subcommittee on Quantitation of Two-Dimensional Echocardiograms. *J Am Soc Echocardiogr* 1989;2:358–367.
14 Koch R, Lang RM, Garcia MJ, et al. Objective evaluation of regional left ventricular wall motion during dobutamine stress echocardiographic studies using segmental analysis of color kinesis images. *J Am Coll Cardiol* 1999;34:409–419.
15 Buda AJ, Zotz RJ, Pace DP, et al. Comparison of two-dimensional echocardiographic wall motion and wall thickening abnormalities in relation to the myocardium at risk. *Am Heart J* 1986;111:587–592.
16 Homans DC, Asinger R, Elsperger KJ, et al. Regional function and perfusion at the lateral border of ischemic myocardium. *Circulation* 1985;71:1038–1047.
17 Pandian NG, Skorton DJ, Collins SM, et al. Heterogeneity of left ventricular segmental wall thickening and excursion in two-dimensional echocardiograms of normal human subjects. *Am J Cardiol* 1983;51:1667–1673.
18 Lieberman AN, Weiss JL, Jugdutt BI, et al. Two-dimensional echocardiography and infarct size: relationship of regional wall motion and thickening to the extent of myocardial infarction in the dog. *Circulation* 1981;63:739–746.
19 Oh JK, Seward JB, Tajik AJ. Stress echocardiography. *The echo manual,* 2nd ed. Philadelphia: Lippincott Williams & Wilkins, 1999:91–101.
20 Lualdi JC, Douglas PS. Echocardiography for the assessment of myocardial viability. *J Am Soc Echocardiogr* 1997;10:772–780.
21 Aronson S, Dupont F, Savage R, et al. Changes in regional myocardial function after coronary artery bypass graft surgery are predicted by intraoperative low-dose dobutamine echocardiography. *Anesthesiology* 2000;93:685–692.
22 Cerqueira MD, Weissman NJ, Dilsizian V, et al. Standardized myocardial segmentation and nomenclature for tomographic imaging of the heart. *Circulation* 2002;105:539–542.
23 Smith MD, MacPhail B, Harrison MR, et al. Value and limitations of transesophageal echocardiography in determination of left ventricular volumes and ejection fraction. *J Am Coll Cardiol* 1992;19:1213–1222.
24 Kono T, Sabbah HN, Rosman H, et al. Mechanism of functional mitral regurgitation during acute myocardial ischemia. *J Am Coll Cardiol* 1992;19:1101–1105.
25 Glasson JR, Komeda M, Daughters GT, et al. Early systolic mitral leaflet "loitering" during acute ischemic mitral regurgitation. *J Thorac Cardiovasc Surg* 1998;116:193–205.
26 Cwajg JM, Cwajg E, Nagueh SF, et al. End-diastolic wall thickness as a predictor of recovery of function in myocardial hibernation: relation to rest-redistribution Tl-201 tomography and dobutamine stress echocardiography. *J Am Coll Cardiol* 2000;35:1152–1161.
27 Seeberger MD, Cahalan MK, Rouine-Rapp K, et al. Acute hypovolemia may cause segmental wall motion abnormalities in the absence of myocardial ischemia. *Anesth Analg* 1997;85:1252–1257.
28 Bowers TR, O'Neill WW, Grines C, et al. Effect of reperfusion on biventricular function and survival after right ventricular infarction. *N Engl J Med* 1998;338:933–940.
29 Boersma E, Poldermans D, Bax JJ, et al. Predictors of cardiac events after major vascular surgery: role of clinical characteristics, dobutamine echocardiography, and beta-blocker therapy. *JAMA* 2001;285:1865–1873.
30 Lee LY, O'Hara MF, Finnin EB, et al. Transmyocardial laser revascularization with excimer laser: clinical results at 1 year. *Ann Thorac Surg* 2000;70:498–503.
31 Orihashi K, Matsuura Y, Sueda T, et al. Pooled air in open heart operations examined by transesophageal echocardiography. *Ann Thorac Surg* 1996;61:1377–1180.

QUESTIONS

1. **Transesophageal echocardiography (TEE) is useful in off-pump coronary artery bypass (OPCAB) for**
   a. Evaluating the adequacy of the coronary anastomosis.
   b. Evaluating the ability of the patient to tolerate vessel occlusion.
   c. Evaluating the hemodynamic consequences of cardiac displacement.
   d. All of the above.

2. **The most sensitive TEE indicator of myocardial ischemia is**
   a. A reduction of systolic wall thickening
   b. The presence of systolic wall thinning
   c. A reduction in endocardial excursion
   d. The presence of compensatory hyperkinesis

3. **Which of the following statements is false regarding dobutamine stress echo testing?**
   a. Low doses will cause normal myocardium to become hyperkinetic.
   b. New-onset hypokinesis indicates myocardial ischemia.
   c. A biphasic response with improvement at low doses and deterioration at higher doses of dobutamine is termed *stunned myocardium*.
   d. A chronic transmural infarction will show no response to low-dose dobutamine.

4. **All of the following statements are true regarding digital cine loops except**
   a. Electrocardiography (ECG) monitoring from the echocardiographic machine should be standard practice.
   b. The cine loop captures off the P wave.
   c. In the absence of an ECG tracing, a capture of 1 second or more is acquired.
   d. Ventricular systole is more difficult to determine with paced rhythms.

5. **The 17-segment model for assessing wall motion adopted by the American Society of Echocardiography/Society of Cardiovascular Anesthesiologists requires evaluation of all the following views except**
   a. Midesophageal (ME) four-chamber
   b. ME two-chamber
   c. ME long-axis
   d. Transgastric (TG) basal short-axis
   e. TG mid short-axis

6. **All of the following "tricks" are helpful in attempting to visualize the left ventricular (LV) apex except**
   a. Retroflexion at the level of the TG short-axis view
   b. Optimizing far field gain and time gain compensation settings
   c. Moving the focal zone over the apex
   d. Maximally increasing the frequency of the transducer in the ME four-chamber view

7. **The TG mid short-axis view is commonly used for monitoring during coronary artery bypass graft (CABG) surgery because**
   a. Changes in intracavitary volume are easily determined.
   b. Territories of all three main coronary arteries perfusing the LV are visualized.
   c. The papillary muscles serve as a useful reference point to ensure that the same territory is being evaluated.
   d. All of the above.

8. All of the following are common imaging pitfalls in attempting to diagnose myocardial ischemia with TEE except

a. Endocardial dropout
b. Images of poor quality
c. Oblique orientation of the TG mid short-axis view
d. Foreshortening of the apex

9. The following may be associated with wall motion abnormalities:

a. Hypervolemia
b. Hypovolemia
c. Hypertrophic cardiomyopathy
d. Ventricular pacing
e. All of the above

10. Chronic ischemic mitral regurgitation (MR) is postulated to occur through all the following mechanisms except

a. Ventricular dilation with incomplete leaflet coaptation
b. Papillary muscle rupture
c. Ischemic dysfunction of one or both papillary muscles
d. Hypokinesis of the ventricular segment underlying a normal papillary muscle

Answers appear at the back of the book.

Essentials of Doppler Echocardiography

5 Doppler Technology and Technique

Albert C. Perrino, Jr.

The high-resolution display of cardiac structures in motion obtained with two-dimensional echocardiography is remarkable. Yet despite the ability to reveal the most intricate anatomic detail, two-dimensional imaging is unable to visualize blood flow. Blood flow in cardiac chambers and the great vessels is simply presented in black on the two-dimensional display. Because the movement of blood is the *raison d'étre* of the cardiovascular system, this limitation presents a serious challenge to the diagnostic capability of echocardiography. Doppler ultrasonography overcomes this limitation in the assessment of blood flow. Its color flow display affords the echocardiographer dramatic views of blood flow. Additionally, spectral Doppler provides the tools to quantify the magnitude and direction of flow. Because Doppler evaluation is quantitative, it provides a means of grading the severity of disease in many cases in which two-dimensional echocardiography merely demonstrates the presence of an abnormality. As such, mastery of Doppler examinations is a critical element in the training of a perioperative echocardiographer.

DOPPLER FREQUENCY SHIFT

Doppler examinations are based on principles fundamentally different from those underlying two-dimensional imaging. As is addressed in the sections that follow, these differences necessitate altered approaches and techniques when Doppler examinations are performed. Many times, the required view and imaging frequencies are contrary to those selected for two-dimensional imaging of the same anatomic region. To obtain an optimal assessment of both the form and function of the desired cardiac structure, it is essential to remain cognizant of the underlying physical principles of the two approaches and how they differ.

The Doppler Effect

As explained in Chapter 1, two-dimensional imaging is based on the intensity and time delay of reflected ultrasound. *To determine the velocity of blood flow, Doppler systems examine the change in frequency of the ultrasound reflected from red blood cells.* Our ability to use the movement of red blood cells to gauge blood flow velocity dates back to the experiments of the Austrian physicist Christian Doppler. Trumpeters on a high-speed locomotive played a tone at a specific pitch so that the effects of motion on sound frequency could be examined. A second group of musicians stationed on a loading dock played the same tone as the train passed by. As Doppler had predicted, the two tones were audibly different. The change in pitch, known as the *Doppler effect,* occurs because the motion of an object causes the sound wave to be compressed in the direction of the motion and expanded in the direction opposite to the motion.

Signal Frequency and Blood Flow

Red blood cells reflect ultrasound as they travel through the blood stream. By directing an ultrasound signal at flowing blood and listening for the change in frequency produced by

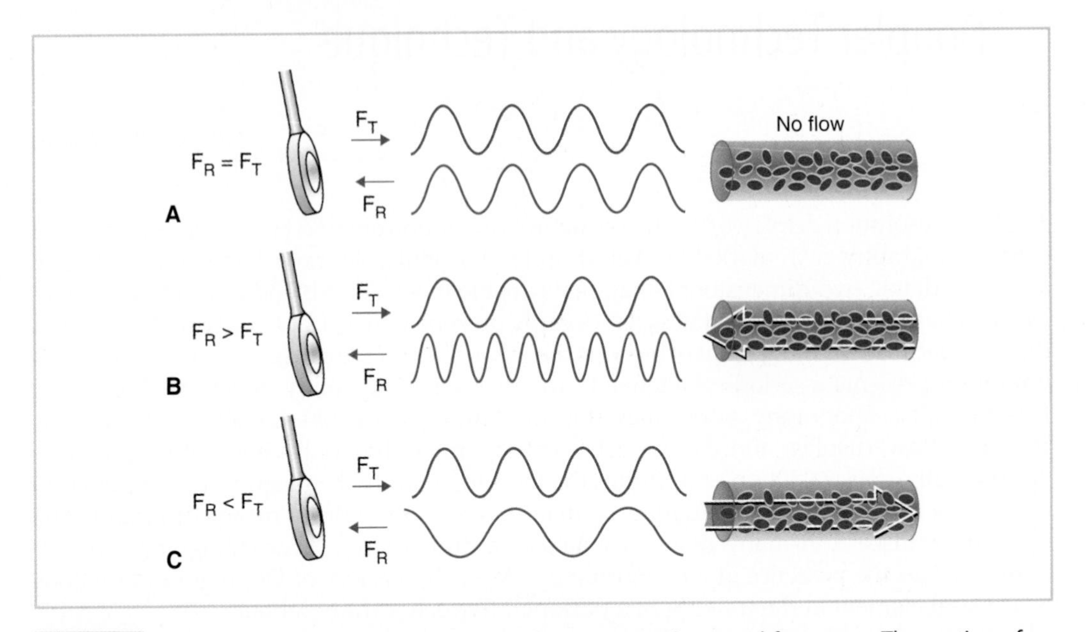

Figure 5.1. Detecting blood flow: effects of red cell motion on ultrasound frequency. The motion of an object alters the frequency of a reflected ultrasound signal. **A:** The reflected echoes from a stationary target are of the same frequency as the transmitted signal. **B:** Objects such as red blood cells moving toward the transducer compress the sound signal, and the reflected frequency is increased. **C:** When red cells travel away for the transducer, the frequency of the reflected echoes is decreased. These modulations in the frequency of the reflected ultrasound are used to detect blood flow. F_T, transmitted signal frequency; F_R, reflected signal frequency.

the red cell reflections, Doppler echocardiography can assess the direction and speed of blood flow.

Figure 5.1 illustrates the principle of the Doppler effect for cardiac applications. When ultrasound is transmitted to blood, it is scattered by the multitude of red blood cells, and a small portion of this scattering is reflected back toward the transducer. The strength of the echoes returning to the transducer is related to the number of particles reflecting the ultrasound. If the hematocrit is increased, more interfaces are available for reflection and the ultrasound signal is stronger. However, this effect is self-limited because at a hematocrit exceeding 30%, the reflected signal strength is weakened by destructive interference. Modern echocardiography systems are designed to detect Doppler signals over a wide range of hematocrit values.

If the red cells are stationary, the signal is reflected at the same frequency as the transmitted signal. Because no Doppler frequency shift occurs, the situation is similar to that of two-dimensional echocardiography. When blood flows toward the ultrasound transducer, the reflected signal is compressed by the motion of the red cells, and its frequency is higher than that of the transmitted signal. Conversely, when blood flows away from the ultrasound transducer, the frequency of the reflected signal received by the transducer is lower than that of the transmitted signal. The technical term for the alterations in the frequency of the ultrasound signals caused by the Doppler effect is *modulation*. Through analysis of the modulated signal, both the direction and speed of the red blood cells can be determined.

DOPPLER ANALYSIS

The Doppler Equation: Linking the Frequency Shift to Velocity

The *Doppler equation* describes the relationship between the alteration in ultrasound frequency and blood flow velocity (Figure 5.2):

$$\Delta f = v \times \cos\theta \times 2f_t/c$$

where Δf is the difference between transmitted frequency (f_t) and received frequency, v is blood velocity, c is the speed of sound in blood (1,540 m/s), and θ is the angle of incidence between the ultrasound beam and blood flow.

Conceptually, the equation can be simplified based on the observation that the change in ultrasound frequency is directly related to just two variables: blood velocity and $\cos\theta$. The remaining factors in the equation, the speed of sound in blood (c) and the transmitted frequency (f_t), are constants. The Doppler signal is shifted only by the component of the blood velocity that is in the direction of the beam path (i.e., $v\cos\theta$). For example, when the direction of the ultrasound beam is parallel to the blood flow, the observed Δf fully reflects total blood velocity ($\cos\theta = 1$). With nonparallel orientation of the ultrasound beam to blood flow, Δf is reduced by the factor $\cos\theta$. As illustrated in Figure 5.3, when the beam angle divergence is small, the effects on Δf are limited. However, *with angles greater than 30 degrees, the value of* $\cos\theta$ *decreases rapidly*. When the direction of the beam is perpendicular to the blood flow (90 degrees, $\cos 90 = 0$), the movement of blood is no longer appreciated by the Doppler system ($\Delta f = 0$).

Implications of Beam Orientation

The effect of the beam angle on Doppler measurements has important clinical implications. In clinical practice, the ultrasound system measures the frequency shift to calculate

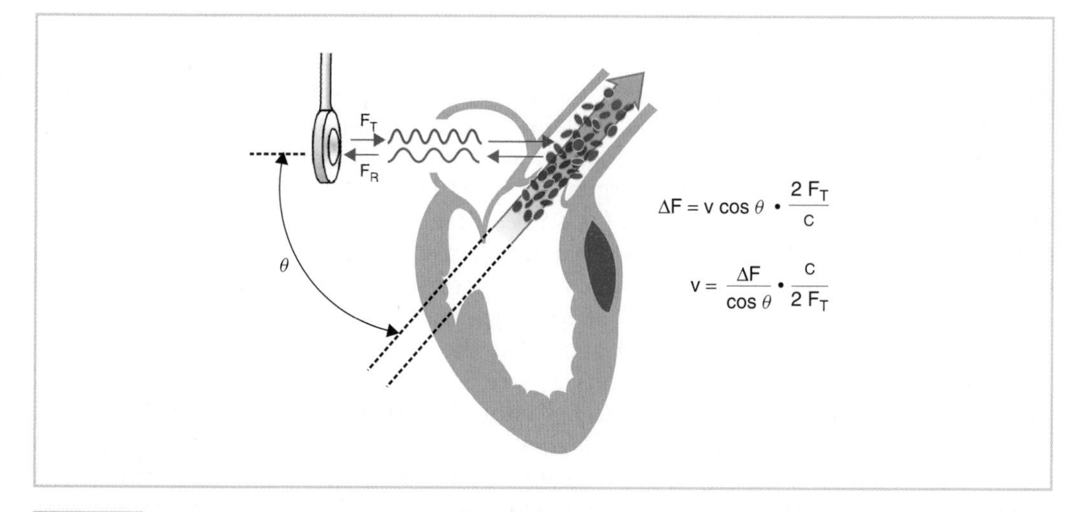

Figure 5.2. Calculating blood flow velocity: the Doppler equation. The Doppler equation calculates blood flow velocity based on two variables: the Doppler frequency shift (ΔF) and the cosine of the angle of incidence between the ultrasound beam and the blood flow. The Doppler frequency shift is measured by the echocardiographic system, but $\cos\theta$ is unknown, and manual entry by the echocardiographer is required for its estimation. v, blood flow velocity; F_T, transmitted signal frequency; F_R, reflected signal frequency; ΔF, difference between F_R and F_T; c, speed of sound in tissue; θ, angle of incidence between the orientation of the ultrasound beam and that of the blood flow.

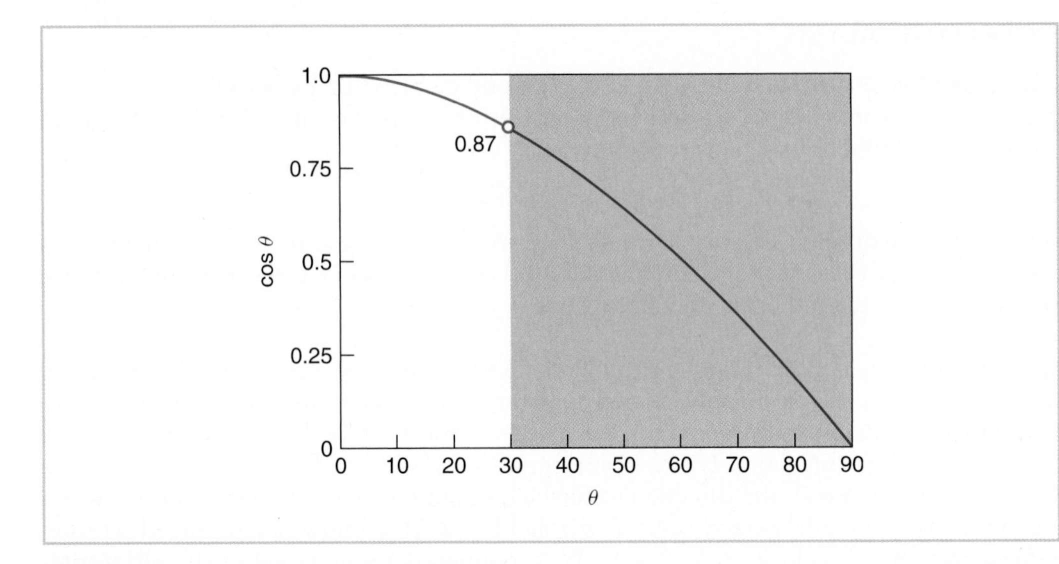

Figure 5.3. Cosine relationship. Most devices default to a simplified Doppler equation in which cos θ is ignored, with the assumption that the Doppler beam is nearly parallel to the blood flow so that the cos θ factor is negligible. However, at angles between beam and blood flow greater than 30 degrees, a precipitous drop in the cosine curve results in a substantial underestimation of blood flow velocity. θ, angle of incidence between the orientation of the ultrasound beam and that of the blood flow.

velocity. By rearranging the Doppler equation, the calculated blood velocity is derived as follows:

$$v = \Delta f/\cos\theta \times c/2f_t$$

The angle of incidence between the beam and the blood flow is not easily determined. Although a two-dimensional image of the blood vessel allows the echocardiographer to estimate the angle in the x- and y-planes, the orientation in the z-plane remains indeterminate. Assessment of the interrogation angle is further complicated by eccentrically directed blood flow, as in mitral regurgitation. Most Doppler systems default to a value of cos θ of 1, with the assumption that the echocardiographer has directed the ultrasound beam to be nearly parallel with the blood flow of interest. This approach has the advantages of stronger Doppler signals and a lower rate of errors as a consequence of the plateau shape of the cosine curve at angles of low incidence. Therefore, in clinical practice, the transducer should be positioned such that the beam and blood flow are nearly parallel for accurate velocity calculations. Figure 5.3 illustrates the basis for the clinical practice of requiring the beam angle to be within 30 degrees of the direction of blood flow, so that the rate of angle-related errors remains less than 15%. The assumption that the orientation of the ultrasound beam is parallel to the blood flow leads to a common error in Doppler velocity calculations. *Because of the shape of the cosine curve, when the incident angle between the beam and the blood flow is greater than 30 degrees, the blood flow is markedly underestimated* (Figure 5.4). However, even the 30-degree standard may not be acceptable in certain conditions. For example, when very high velocities are interrogated, as in aortic stenosis, even a 15% underestimation will correspond to a large difference in velocity and may result in an underestimation of the severity of aortic stenosis.

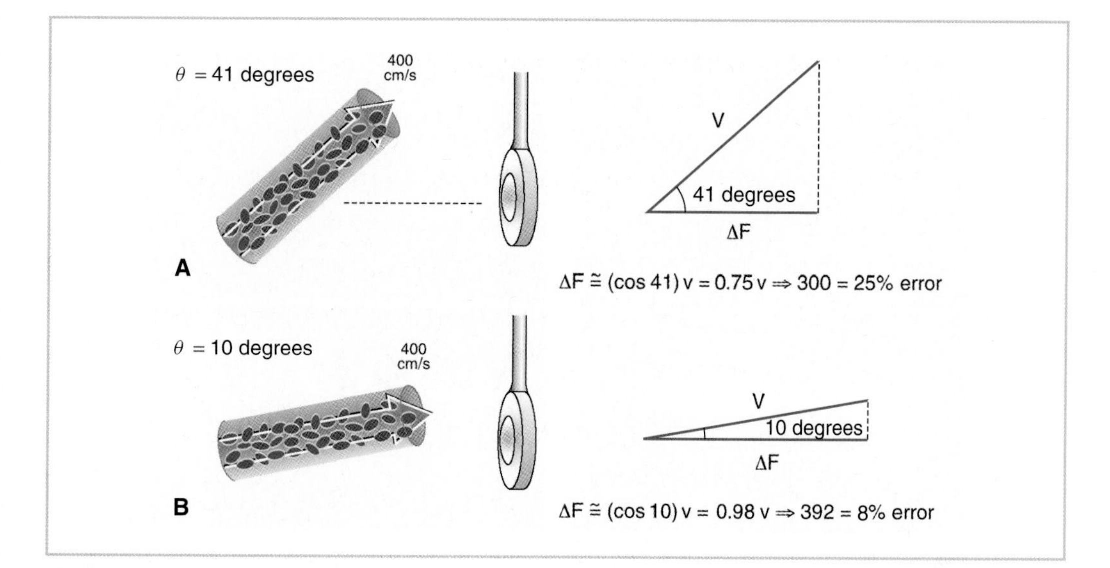

Figure 5.4. Underestimation of blood flow velocity with nonparallel beam orientation. **A:** With an angle of 41 degrees, the vector component of blood flow velocity in the direction of the ultrasound beam is only 75% of the total. Therefore, a velocity estimation based on ΔF alone will lead to a clinically unacceptable underestimation of the true blood flow velocity of 25%. **B:** With an angle of 10 degrees, the vector component of blood flow velocity in the direction of the ultrasound beam is 92%, and the practice of ignoring the cos θ leads to a clinically acceptable 8% underestimation of velocity. ΔF, difference between F_R and F_T; v, blood flow velocity; θ, angle of incidence between the orientation of the ultrasound beam and that of the blood flow.

Clinical Caveats in Transesophageal Echocardiographic Doppler Examinations

1. Positioning the transesophageal echocardiography (TEE) probe so that the orientation of the Doppler beam is parallel to the blood flow is often a significant challenge. Unlike the position of a transthoracic probe, which can be moved freely about the chest wall to achieve proper orientation, the position of the TEE probe is limited to the confines of the esophagus and stomach.
2. The standard views used for two-dimensional imaging are often inadequate for Doppler assessments. Optimal two-dimensional images are obtained by directing the beam perpendicular to the structure of interest to obtain strong, mirrorlike reflections. Paradoxically, Doppler measurements are best obtained when the beam is parallel to the blood flow to avoid underestimates of blood flow velocity. The view that provides the best two-dimensional image of a structure typically provides only limited flow information and can result in a failure to detect abnormal flow. Figure 5.5 illustrates the application of this principle in examining the aortic valve.

Isolating the Doppler Frequency Shift

For the Doppler system to determine the frequency shift caused by red blood cells, it must first distinguish red cell–modulated echoes from all the other non–frequency-shifted echoes created by reflections from tissue (Figure 5.6). This *demodulation process* is often accomplished by comparing the returning echoes with internal reference signals that are in phase and 90 degrees out of phase with the transmitted signal, a process known as *quadrature demodulation*. Once the Doppler signal has been isolated, its frequency content

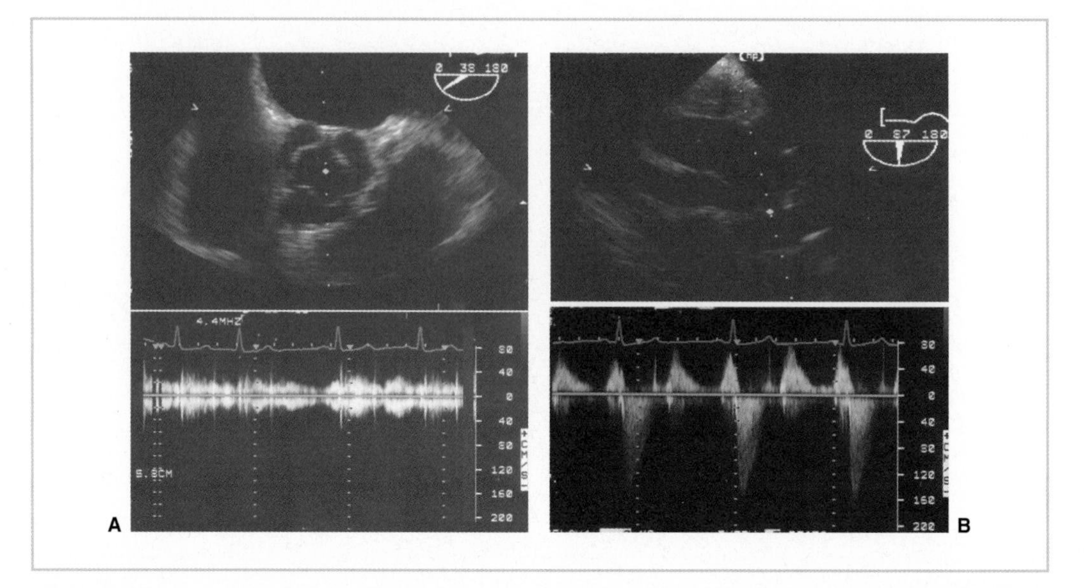

Figure 5.5. Comparison of views selected for two-dimensional imaging versus Doppler flow measurement. **A:** Two-dimensional echocardiography from the midesophageal aortic valve short-axis view (**top**) provides high-fidelity images of the valve leaflets and their excursion. Because the direction of blood flow is orthogonal to the ultrasound beam in this view, the continuous wave Doppler measurement of blood flow velocity (**bottom**) will substantially underestimate blood flow velocity. **B:** After repositioning of the probe to obtain the transgastric long-axis view (**top**), the direction of the ultrasound beam is parallel to the left ventricular outflow tract and ascending aorta, providing excellent continuous wave measurements of blood flow velocity (**bottom**).

can then be determined by means of the *fast Fourier transform* technique. This approach transforms the demodulated Doppler signal into its individual frequency components. The process is analogous to identifying the individual harmonics that comprise a musical chord. At each time point, the analysis provides the range of frequencies (i.e., velocities) detected and their magnitude (i.e., the number of red cells moving at this speed).

PRESENTATION OF DOPPLER DATA

Audible Broadcast

Blood flow in the heart and great vessels creates a Doppler frequency shift in the kiloHertz range, with a high-velocity aortic stenotic jet generating a Doppler frequency shift in the order of 20 kHz. Because these frequencies are within the audible range, most echocardiography machines provide a sound system that amplifies and broadcasts the signal to the operator. *By listening to the loudness and pitch of the broadcast Doppler frequencies, the echocardiographer can precisely position the Doppler beam to interrogate the desired flow signal.* Typically, the ideal location is identified when the signal reaches its highest frequency and greatest loudness. Soft, low-decibel signals indicate that the Doppler beam is misdirected and is only glancing a small part of the blood flow. In addition, the texture and pitch of the Doppler signal are useful in diagnosis. For example, when transvalvular flow across the aortic valve is examined, a coarse, high-pitched signal is diagnostic of a high-velocity, turbulent jet caused by aortic stenosis and contrasts markedly with the smooth-sounding, low-pitched signals generated by the laminar flow in a normal aortic valve. The ability to use the audible Doppler signal to guide beam positioning is a favored technique of

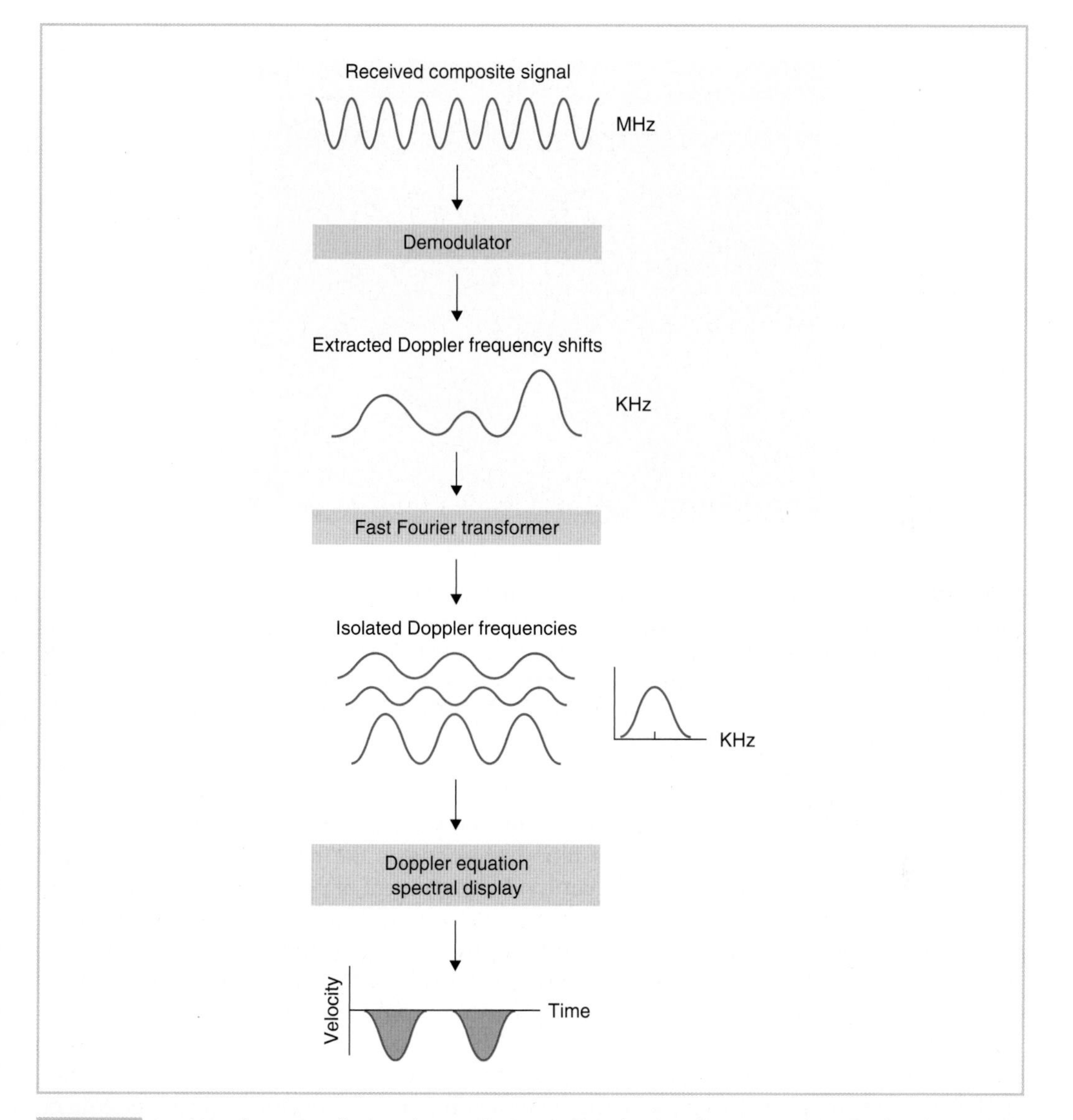

Figure 5.6. Looking for a needle in a haystack. Extracting the low-frequency, low-amplitude Doppler signal for the received composite signal is a technical challenge requiring several procedures, including demodulation and fast Fourier transform. Once isolated, the Doppler frequencies can be analyzed and displayed.

experienced echocardiographers, and development of this skill remains a goal for all trainees.

Spectral Display

Presenting Doppler data as a time-velocity plot is known as a *spectral display* (Figure 5.7). At each point in time, the spectrum of velocities detected by the Fourier transformation are displayed. For blood flow measurements, the low velocity signals emanating from myocardial motion are filtered and not displayed (the use of these "tissue Doppler" signals is presented in Chapters 3 and 7). Frequencies with greater amplitude (loudness)

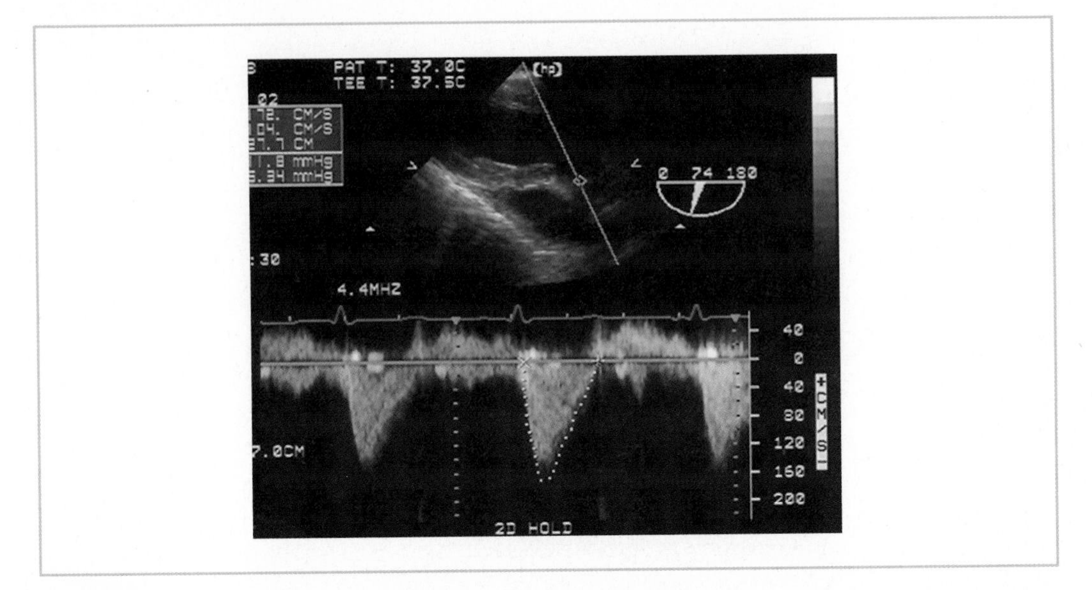

Figure 5.7. Doppler spectral display. Blood flow through the left ventricular outflow tract and aorta is captured by using continuous wave Doppler directed from the transgastric long-axis view. This time-velocity display shows the Doppler-calculated velocities on the x-axis, with flow toward the transducer as positive deflections and flow away from the transducer as negative deflections. Planimetry of the velocity waveform has been performed by the operator, and the machine's analysis package calculates the velocity-time integral and the mean and peak flow velocities.

are marked with brighter pixels. The excellent temporal resolution of the spectral display allows beat-to-beat assessment of blood flow and is the basis for the quantitative calculations of cardiovascular hemodynamics. Measurement of peak velocity, acceleration ($\Delta v/\Delta t$), and the time-velocity integral (represented by the area under the velocity-time plot from a single cardiac cycle) are examples of the many important measurements that are easily obtained from the spectral display (see Chapter 6 for a detailed examination of the use of these measurements in clinical echocardiography).

Despite the ease with which velocity measurements are made from the spectral display, vigilance is required on the part of the echocardiographer. The measurements will be accurate only when the underlying principles of good Doppler technique have been followed. First, the Doppler beam must be properly positioned to interrogate the targeted blood flow. For example, small alterations in beam position determine whether the displayed spectral velocities represent a targeted high-frequency jet of mitral stenosis or the lower blood flow velocities found along its perimeter. Second, the direction of the Doppler beam must be parallel to the path of the targeted blood flow. Errors in diagnosis are often related to failure to meet these essential requirements.

Poor ultrasound technique can often be detected by an examination of the spectral display. High-quality signals result in a pattern commonly referred to as a *clean envelope*, denoted by a sharply demarcated border, bright pixels, and clear peaks. When these features are lacking, the echocardiographer should be reluctant to accept the data from the spectral display and improve the Doppler signal through alterations in probe position or imaging view (Figure 5.8). Inexplicably, seemingly minor alterations can resolve difficulties in

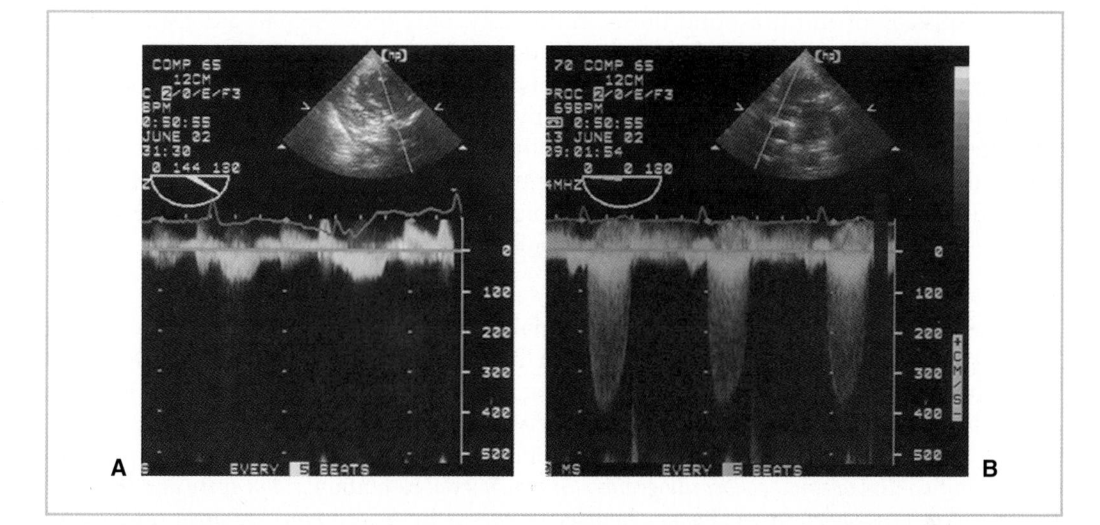

Figure 5.8. Hunting for the jet core. **A:** Despite high-quality two-dimensional imaging of the transgastric long-axis view, Doppler interrogation of the transvalvular flow fails to detect the high-velocity flow of aortic stenosis. The wispy signal waveform provides no clear definition of peak velocities. **B:** After adjustment of the probe position to obtain the deep transgastric long-axis view, the resulting Doppler interrogation detects a 400-cm/s high-velocity jet, revealing aortic stenosis. Note the potential for misdiagnosis if the echocardiographer bases the diagnosis on the initial signal obtained in **A**.

obtaining a flow signal. In this regard, there is no substitute for perseverance and experience.

DOPPLER TECHNIQUES

Two Doppler techniques, *pulsed wave* and *continuous wave*, are commonly used to evaluate blood flow. A thorough understanding of the advantages and disadvantages of each technique is critical in selecting the one most appropriate for the clinical setting at hand.

In clinical practice, pulsed wave and continuous wave Doppler are frequently used in conjunction with two-dimensional imaging. The two-dimensional image is used to identify the area of interest and guide the echocardiographer in precisely localizing the sampling volume in a pulsed wave study or in directing the beam in a continuous wave study.

Pulsed Wave Doppler

The pulsed wave transducer uses a single crystal as both the emitter and the receiver of ultrasound waves. Like the pulsed echo system described for two-dimensional imaging, the pulsed wave Doppler system transmits a short burst of ultrasound toward the target and then switches to receive mode to interpret the returning echoes. Because the speed of sound (c) in tissue is constant, the time delay for a signal to reach its target and return to the transducer depends solely on the distance (d) to the target:

$$\text{Timedelay} = 2d/c$$

Consequently, reflected signals from locations more distant from the transducer return after a greater time interval. The electronic circuitry of the pulsed wave transducer interprets returning echoes only after a predetermined time period has elapsed because the transmission of an ultrasound pulse. In this way, only those signals associated with a specific depth or location are selected for evaluation, a process known as *time gating*. It is important to remember that the transducer transmits a three-dimensional beam. Therefore, the small portion of reflected sound accepted by the time-gating process corresponds to a volume of blood at a specific location, called the *sample volume*. The pulse length, which equals the product of the wavelength and the number of cycles contained in each sound pulse, determines the length of the sample volume. The width and height of the sample volume are related to the transducer size, signal frequency, and beam focus.

CLINICAL CAVEATS FOR PULSED WAVE DOPPLER

Because red cells scatter the ultrasound signal, the reflected Doppler signal returning to the transducer represents only a fraction of the transmitted signal. Therefore, the returning signal is much weaker than the strong specular reflections from tissue interfaces. Accordingly, the clinician faces a tradeoff between good range resolution (i.e., a small sample length) and an accurate determination of velocity. *In contrast to the preferred settings in two-dimensional echocardiography, in which axial resolution is a priority and the pulse length is kept very short, large Doppler sample volumes (length >10 mm) are preferred by most echocardiographers to improve the accuracy of the velocity measurement because they provide more wavelength for demodulation.* A more powerful Doppler signal is produced because the signal-to-noise ratio is increased.

In summary, pulsed wave Doppler allows the echocardiographer to select both the location and dimensions of the sample volume to determine blood flow velocity at a discrete location. The ability to select a sample volume from which to record blood velocities was a major advancement in the diagnostic capability of echocardiography.

PULSED WAVE DOPPLER SYSTEM PROCESSING

The pulsed Doppler system uses a repeating pattern of ultrasound transmission and reception. After producing a short burst of ultrasound, it waits for a period of time, proportional to the selected distance, to receive the signal from the sample volume. The transducer then sends another burst of ultrasound, waits and receives, and so on. The rate at which the device repeatedly generates sound bursts is known as the *pulse repetition frequency* (*PRF*). The longer the pulsed wave system waits for the returning echoes, the lower the PRF. Because the speed of sound through tissue is a constant, the PRF is directly related to the depth of the sample volume. The PRF is analogous to the frame rate of a movie camera. Like the multiple frames on a roll of movie film, each ultrasound pulse interacts with the blood flow for a brief period of time, and just as a series of movie frames display motion, a series of pulsed cycles are consecutively analyzed to determine the blood flow. The demodulation process examines the returning echoes from a series of pulses to determine the Doppler frequency shift and calculate blood flow velocity.

LIMITATIONS OF PULSED WAVE DOPPLER

Because the Doppler data are collected intermittently, the maximal frequency and blood flow velocity that can be accurately measured by pulsed wave Doppler are limited. The maximal frequency, which equals one half the PRF, is known as the *Nyquist limit*. Figure 5.9 illustrates the principle of the Nyquist limit with the example of an orbiting comet. A similar effect is seen in movie animation, in which a rapidly spinning wheel appears to spin backward because of the slow frame rate. At Doppler shifts above the Nyquist limit, analysis of the returning signal becomes ambiguous, so that the velocity is indeterminate. This ambiguous signal for frequencies above the Nyquist limit, known as *aliasing*, appears on the spectral display as a signal on the other side of the baseline, often referred to as

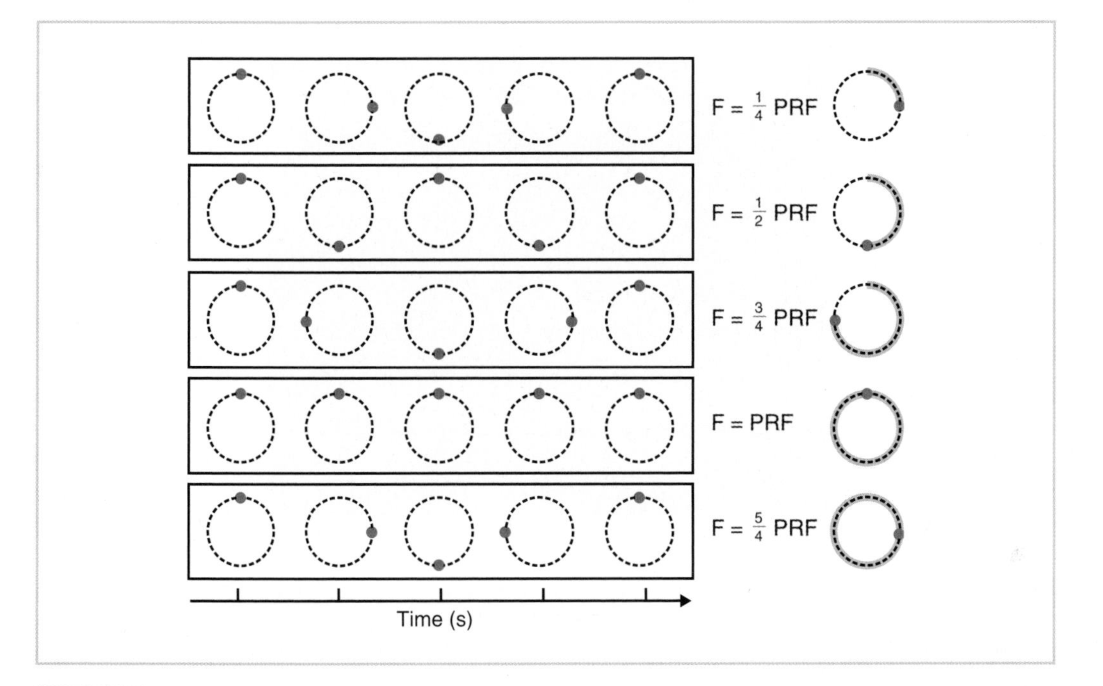

Figure 5.9. Nyquist illusions. The Nyquist limit of one half the pulse repetition frequency (PRF) applies to any system based on intermittent observation. In this illustration, the position of the orbiting comet at each observation point is displayed. The orbiting velocity of the comet is progressively increased from the top to the bottom rows. At the low orbiting velocity of one fourth PRF, the serial observations properly portray the comet as moving in a clockwise direction. As the speed of the comet is increased so that its orbiting velocity is three fourths the PRF, it appears to be traveling counterclockwise. It appears to be moving not at all when its orbiting velocity equals the PRF. At five fourths the PRF, it appears to be orbiting at the same speed as when it was traveling at the much slower speed of one fourth the PRF.

wraparound (Figure 5.10). The intermittent sampling of the pulsed system can resolve only frequencies that are less than half the pulse repetition rate.

MAXIMIZING PULSED WAVE VELOCITY MEASUREMENTS

The echocardiographer has several techniques available to maximize the velocity performance of a pulsed wave system:

1. The first clinical principle is to select the view that places the transducer closest to the sample volume. Lessening the target distance increases the PRF, thereby increasing the velocity that can be assessed.
2. The second clinical principle is to select a low transmitted frequency. The lower transmitted frequency has two major advantages:
   a. The modulated echo (f_r) will be of a lower frequency for any given blood velocity because $f_r = f_t + \Delta f$. Therefore, increased velocities can be measured without the aliasing that would be caused by a Doppler signal with a higher transmitted frequency.
   b. Lower frequencies provide a stronger signal because they are less attenuated by tissue. This is important because Doppler signals are much weaker than those used for imaging. Figure 5.11 illustrates the importance of target distance and transmitted frequency to the velocity performance of a Doppler system.

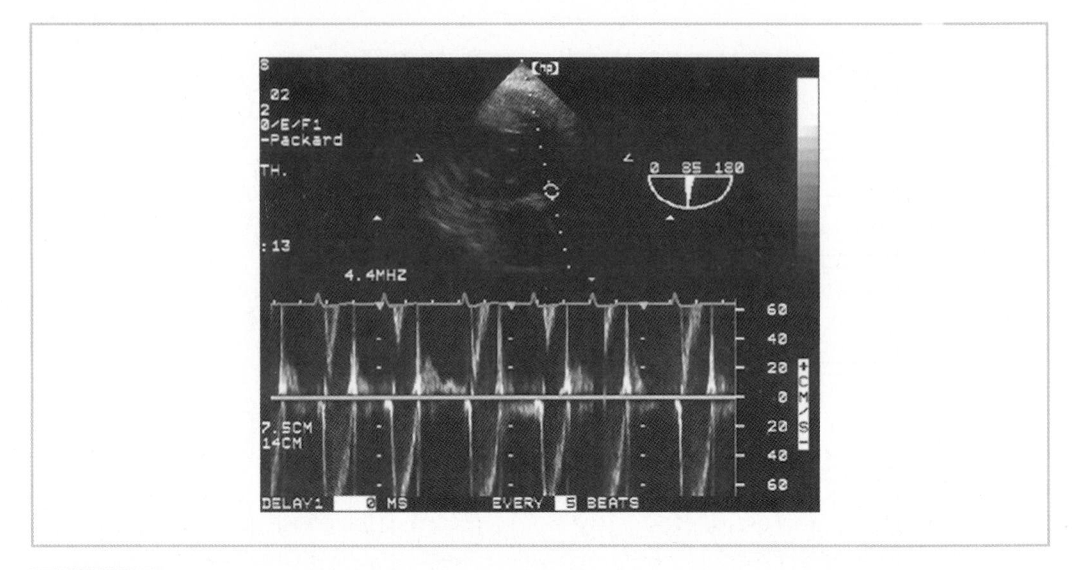

Figure 5.10. Alias artifact. Alias artifact appears once velocities exceed the Nyquist limit. In this example, the pulsed wave Doppler sample volume is located in the left ventricular outflow tract, and when the peak velocities of the spectral signal exceed 70 cm/s, aliasing occurs and they appear on the opposite side of the baseline, a condition known as *wraparound*.

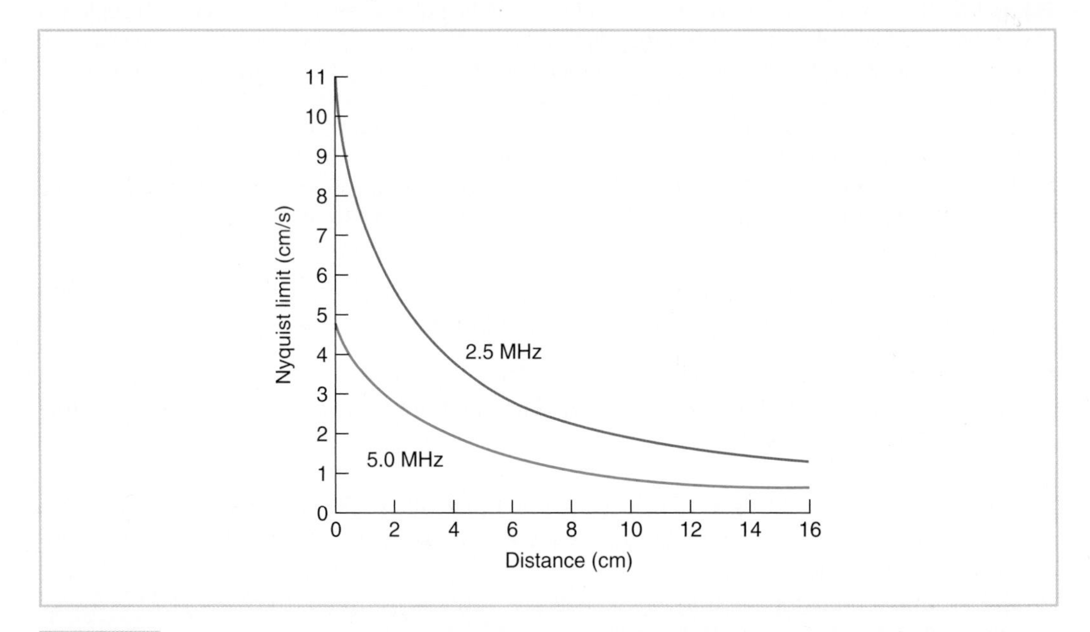

Figure 5.11. Effect of distance and frequency on the Nyquist limit. Two important variables under the echocardiographer's control that can be used to minimize the potential for aliasing in Doppler signals are target distance and transmitted frequency. As the transducer is moved closer to the target or the transmitted frequency is lowered, the pulsed wave Nyquist limit rises substantially, allowing higher-velocity signals to be measured accurately.

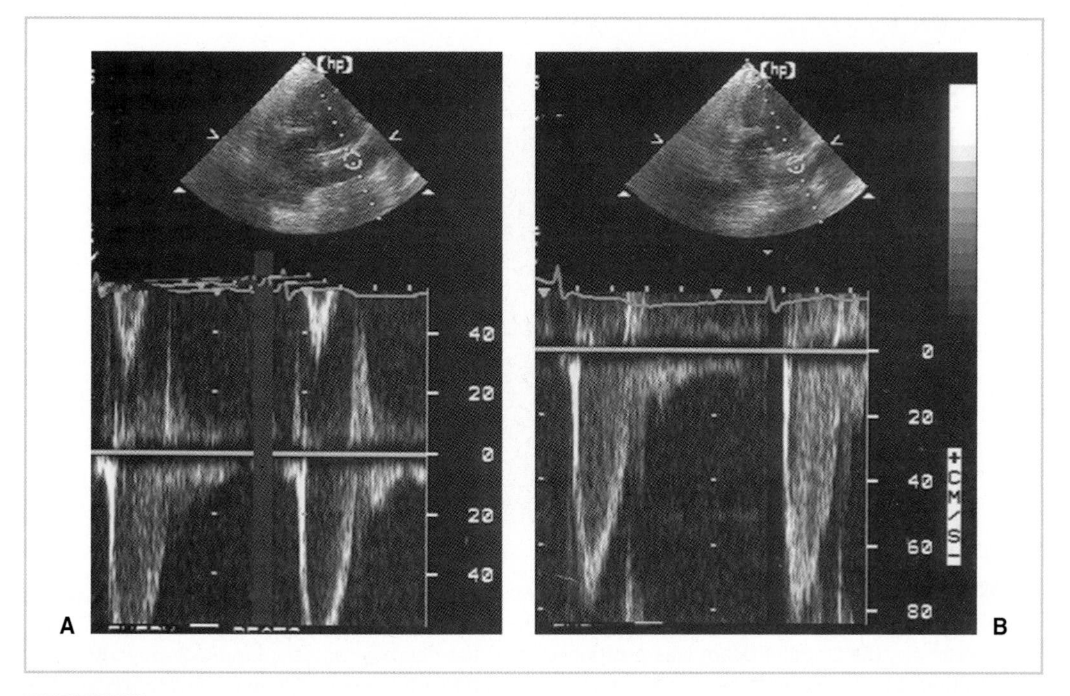

Figure 5.12. Effect of baseline setting on pulsed wave Doppler aliasing. **A:** With the velocity baseline set in the midportion of the display, the signal aliases at 50 cm/s. **B:** The baseline has been adjusted to the upper portion of the display, which increases the Nyquist limit to more than 80 cm/s for flow away from the transducer and captures the spectral signal without aliasing.

3. The third clinical principle is to set the baseline of the spectral display to provide the greatest range of velocities in the direction of interest. Figure 5.12 illustrates the practical implications of baseline adjustment.

Echocardiography technology has also tried to address the velocity limitation of pulsed wave Doppler systems with the development of *high-frequency pulsed Doppler*. This approach sacrifices some of the spatial resolution of the pulsed wave system in exchange for the ability to measure significantly faster flows. The principle of high-frequency pulsed Doppler is to emit a second or third pulse signal before the first signal has returned. In this way, the PRF is doubled or tripled, and it becomes possible to calculate a greater maximal velocity. However, with high-frequency pulsed Doppler, the operator cannot be sure that the reflected echoes have come from the intended target rather than from other targets located more proximally.

Despite technologic advancements, the Nyquist limit remains a major impediment to the measurement of high-velocity blood flows, such as those across stenotic valves and in congenital cardiac lesions, with pulsed wave Doppler. This limitation has led to an alternative approach for the Doppler assessment of high-velocity blood flows, which is continuous wave Doppler.

Continuous Wave Doppler

The continuous wave Doppler technique avoids the maximal velocity limitation of pulsed wave systems. The transducer of a continuous wave system is composed of two crystals, one

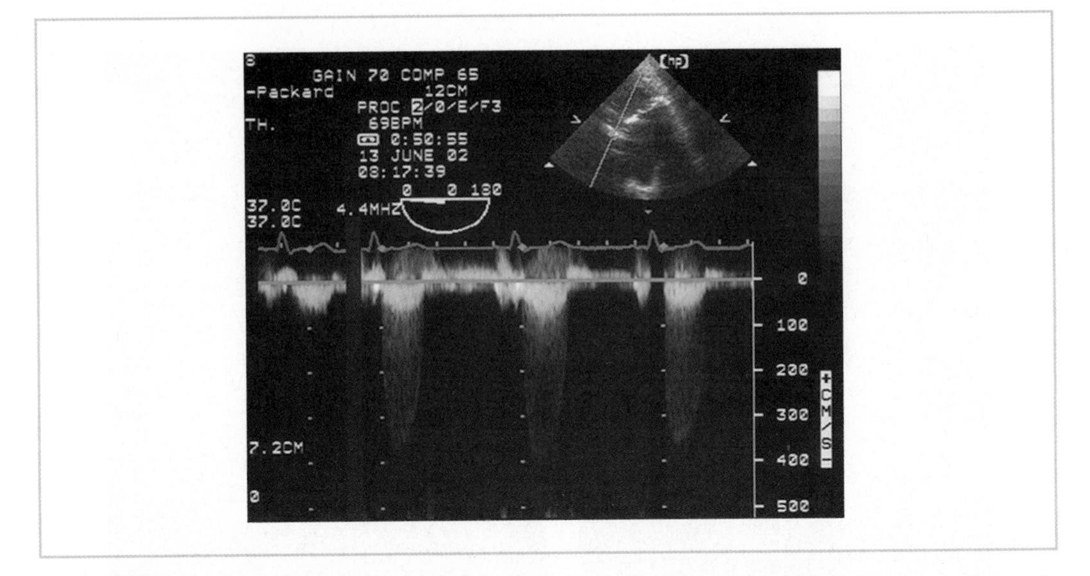

Figure 5.13. Continuous wave spectral signal. Whereas pulsed wave Doppler obtains targeted sample volume recordings, the continuous wave system detects blood flow along the entire beam path. **Top:** In this example, the Doppler beam was positioned from the deep transgastric long-axis view. **Bottom:** The resulting spectral signal shows two distinct peaks, a pattern often referred to as a *double envelope*. The major peak at 400 cm/s is the high-velocity jet caused by aortic stenosis recorded from that portion of the beam in the aorta. The minor peak of 100 cm/s represents the blood velocity in the left ventricular outflow tract.

continuously transmitting and the other continuously receiving the reflected ultrasound signal. With continuous reception of the Doppler signal, the Nyquist limit is not applicable, and blood flows with very high velocities can be recorded accurately. A continuous wave transducer can measure velocities in excess of 7 m/s and is therefore useful in measuring the high-velocity flows associated with stenotic valvular disease. Other differences between the pulsed wave and continuous wave techniques are important. Because the continuous wave signal is not time-gated like the pulsed wave technique, the continuous wave mode receives reflected signals from blood flow throughout its beam path. Unlike the clean envelope achieved with pulsed wave Doppler, the spectral display of continuous wave Doppler is typically shaded with the multitude of velocities recorded along the beam path (Figure 5.13). Consequently, the use of continuous wave Doppler is limited primarily to detecting the highest velocities along the beam path, represented by the edge of the spectral envelope.

Color Flow Mapping

Color flow mapping provides a dramatic display of both blood flow and cardiac anatomy. To achieve these remarkable images, the technique combines two-dimensional ultrasonic imaging and pulsed wave Doppler methods. The pulsed wave Doppler used for color flow mapping differs from that previously discussed in two important ways. First, instead of recording from a single, operator-selected sample volume, color flow mapping performs multiple pulsed wave sample determinations of velocity along the depth of each scan line. Multiple sample volume recordings are obtained along each scan line as the beam is swept through the sector. This approach provides flow data matched with the structural data obtained by two-dimensional imaging. The second difference is that the Doppler velocity data from each sample volume is color-coded and superimposed on top of the gray scale two-dimensional image. *In the most widely accepted color code, red indicates flow toward the transducer and blue indicates flow away from the transducer.* In addition to flow direction, flow velocity alters the color map. Increasing flow velocities are displayed by various hues; high-velocity flow toward the transducer is displayed as yellow, and high-velocity flow away from the transducer is displayed as cyan. Flow with directional variance, as in areas of turbulence, is displayed as green.

The ability to provide a real-time, integrated display of flow and structural information makes color flow Doppler useful for assessing valvular function, aortic dissection, and congenital heart abnormalities. However, several important caveats to its use in the clinical setting must be noted. Because it relies on pulsed wave Doppler measurements, color flow mapping is susceptible to alias artifacts. In fact, *color flow will alias at a lower velocity than a conventional pulsed wave device because part of the signal must be used for image generation, and this effectively decreases the PRF*. Aliasing in the color flow map is illustrated in Figure 5.14. At the extreme of accurate velocity measurement (e.g., bright yellow for flow toward the transducer), progressively increasing flow rates appear cyan, then dark blue, and then dark red. In a high-velocity jet, several cycles of color alias can occur, which appear as a tiger stripe pattern in hues of red and blue. Because of the complex acquisition of multiple Doppler samples and the sharing of acquisition time with the imaging processor, the velocities displayed by the color flow mapper lack the fidelity of a conventional pulsed wave device. Color flow mapping cannot measure blood flow velocity nor track alterations in velocity through the cardiac cycle with the precision of a conventional Doppler device. *Because of these limitations, the color flow mapper is often used to identify a flow abnormality that is subsequently characterized by a conventional Doppler approach.*

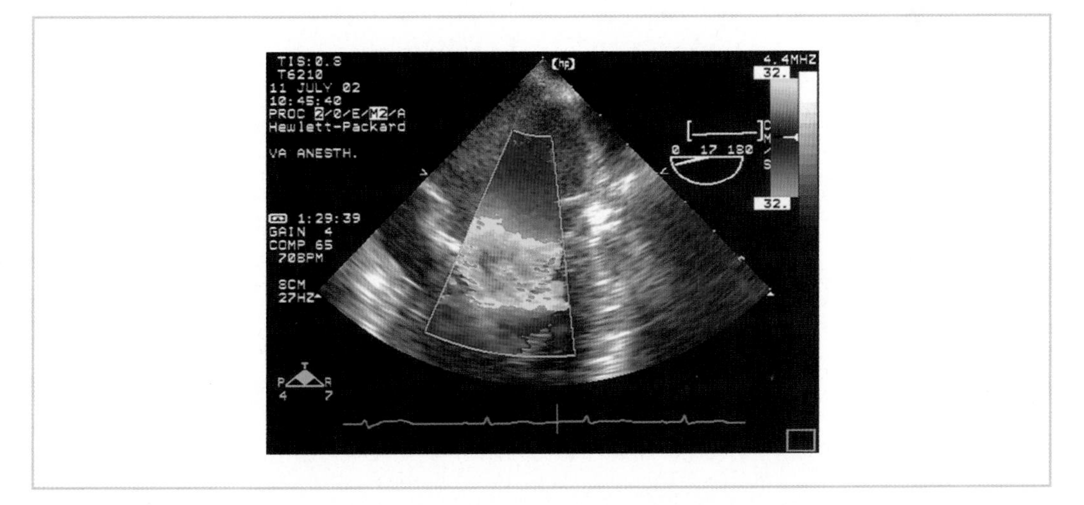

Figure 5.14. Aliasing of color display. Blood flow through the mitral valve (midesophageal four-chamber view) during early diastole results in aliasing in the color flow mapper. Flow velocity accelerates in the left atrium as blood is funneled to the mitral valve orifice, shown as the color code of dark blue transitioning to light blue, and reaches 32 cm/s (the Nyquist limit), as seen on the color bar. As a result, aliasing signals are coded bright yellow, then red, as the velocity reaches a maximum at the level of the leaflet tips. Once in the left ventricle, the blood flow decelerates to fall below the Nyquist limit and is again appropriately coded blue by the echocardiographic system.

SUMMARY

Doppler echocardiography has greatly expanded the diagnostic capabilities of clinical echocardiography. Quantitative measurements of blood velocity derived from the spectral display of pulsed wave and continuous wave Doppler signals are widely used to characterize systolic and diastolic cardiac performance and valve function. Color flow mapping allows the visualization of cardiac blood flow. The broad clinical applications of Doppler echocardiography are described in detail in the next chapters. The clinician must remain mindful of the underlying principles of good technique to obtain optimal Doppler signals and avoid incorrect diagnoses related to erroneous measurements.

SUGGESTED READINGS

Hatle L, Angelsen B. *Doppler ultrasound in cardiology*. Philadelphia: Lea & Febiger, 1985.

Nishimura RA, Miller FA, Callahan MJ, et al. Doppler echocardiography: theory, instrumentation, technique, and application. *Mayo Clin Proc* 1985;60:321–343.

Quinones MA, Otto CM, Stoddard M, et al. Recommendations for the quantification of Doppler echocardiography: a report from the Doppler Quantification Task Force of the Nomenclature and Standards Committee of the American Society of Echocardiography. *J Am Soc Echocardiogr* 2002;15:167–184.

Weyman A. *Principles and practice of echocardiography*. Philadelphia: Lea & Febiger, 1994.

QUESTIONS

1. **All of the following statements about Doppler echocardiography are true except**
   a. The received Doppler signal is stronger than the two-dimensional signal.
   b. Christian Doppler was a Swedish echocardiographer.
   c. Doppler velocity measurements are based on changes in signal frequency.
   d. Doppler velocity measurements are based on reflections from plasma.

2. **In clinical practice, the Doppler frequency shift is**
   a. Typically 2.5 to 7.5 MHz.
   b. Less than 1 MHz.
   c. Not relevant to the Nyquist limit.
   d. Negative for flow directed perpendicular to the ultrasound beam.

3. **The Doppler frequency shift is affected by all of the following except**
   a. Transmitted frequency
   b. Blood velocity
   c. Incident angle of the ultrasound beam
   d. Distance of the target from the transducer

4. **Fast Fourier analysis is applied to**
   a. Pulsed wave but not continuous wave Doppler signals.
   b. Identify the Doppler frequency shift.
   c. Identify the component frequencies of the Doppler frequency shift.
   d. Extract noise from weaker Doppler signals.

5. **All of the following statements are true of pulsed wave Doppler except**
   a. It requires two separate crystals.
   b. It is useful to identify blood flow in a particular area.
   c. It has a limited maximal velocity that can be measured.
   d. It is the basis for color flow Doppler.

6. **Techniques useful to correct an alias signal include all of the following except**
   a. Adjusting the baseline
   b. Positioning the transducer closer to the target
   c. Increasing the transmitted frequency
   d. Using high-frequency pulsed Doppler

7. **The Nyquist limit is directly related to**
   a. Blood flow velocity.
   b. Pressure gradient.
   c. Pulse repetition frequency.
   d. Red cell mass.

8. **Which of the following statements about color flow Doppler is true?**
   a. It is susceptible to aliasing.
   b. It is a good choice for measuring high-velocity blood flow.
   c. It is based on continuous wave technology.
   d. It provides nonquantitative information.

9. **Demodulation**
   a. Filters out noise in the Doppler signal
   b. Identifies the Doppler shift

c. Is not necessary for color flow Doppler
d. Is not necessary for continuous wave Doppler

10. A spectral display with sharp, dense edges
a. Is diagnostic of stenotic lesions
b. Suggests echoes from a strong reflector, such as a nearby calcified valve
c. Ensures that the beam is parallel to the blood flow
d. Suggests proper interrogation of blood flow

Answers appear at the back of the book.

6 Quantitative Doppler and Hemodynamics

Andrew Maslow and Albert C. Perrino, Jr.

> When you can measure what you are speaking about, and express it in numbers, you know something about it; but when you cannot express it in numbers, your knowledge is of a meagre and unsatisfactory kind.
>
> —*Lord Kelvin*

Hemodynamics is the study of blood flow and its associated forces. The objective of this chapter is to describe the use of Doppler echocardiography for the quantitative assessment of hemodynamics. Although two-dimensional echocardiography displays cardiac dimensions and motion, it does not readily assess cardiac blood flow and pressures. Doppler echocardiography provides excellent assessments of hemodynamics that compare favorably with more invasive measurements. Accordingly, a quantitative Doppler assessment of blood flow, chamber pressures, valvular disease, pulmonary vascular resistance (PVR), ventricular function (systolic and diastolic), and anatomic defects is an essential component of the echocardiographic examination.

The accuracy of the Doppler evaluation depends on the ability to minimize interference from neighboring blood flows and align the ultrasound beam parallel to the blood flow of interest. Traditionally, transthoracic echocardiography was a superior approach because it offered multiple windows and angles from which blood flow could be interrogated. The introduction of multiplane transesophageal echocardiography (TEE) has increased the number of imaging windows and angles from which the heart can be evaluated with TEE and has greatly facilitated accurate hemodynamic evaluation.

VOLUMETRIC FLOW CALCULATIONS

Doppler Measurements of Stroke Volume and Cardiac Output

PRINCIPLES

In many instances, knowledge of the *volume* of blood flow is desired. Cardiac output (CO) and stroke volume (SV) are familiar examples. It is important not to confuse blood flow velocity, which is the speed at which blood flows (expressed in centimeters per second), with volumetric flow, which is the amount of blood that flows (expressed in cubic centimeters per second). The volumetric flow (Q) at any point in time equals the blood flow velocity (v) times the cross-sectional area (CSA) of the conduit

$$Q = \mathrm{v} \times \mathrm{CSA}$$

To determine the volumetric flow with echocardiography, a Doppler measurement of the instantaneous blood flow velocities and a two-dimensional measurement of the CSA are required.

In the clinical setting, the volume of blood produced during each cardiac cycle, known as the *SV*, is an important parameter of cardiac performance. To calculate the SV, the instantaneous velocities during systole are traced from the spectral display, and the internal software package of the echocardiographic system calculates the time-velocity integral (TVI), which is expressed in centimeters (Figure 6.1). Conceptually, the TVI

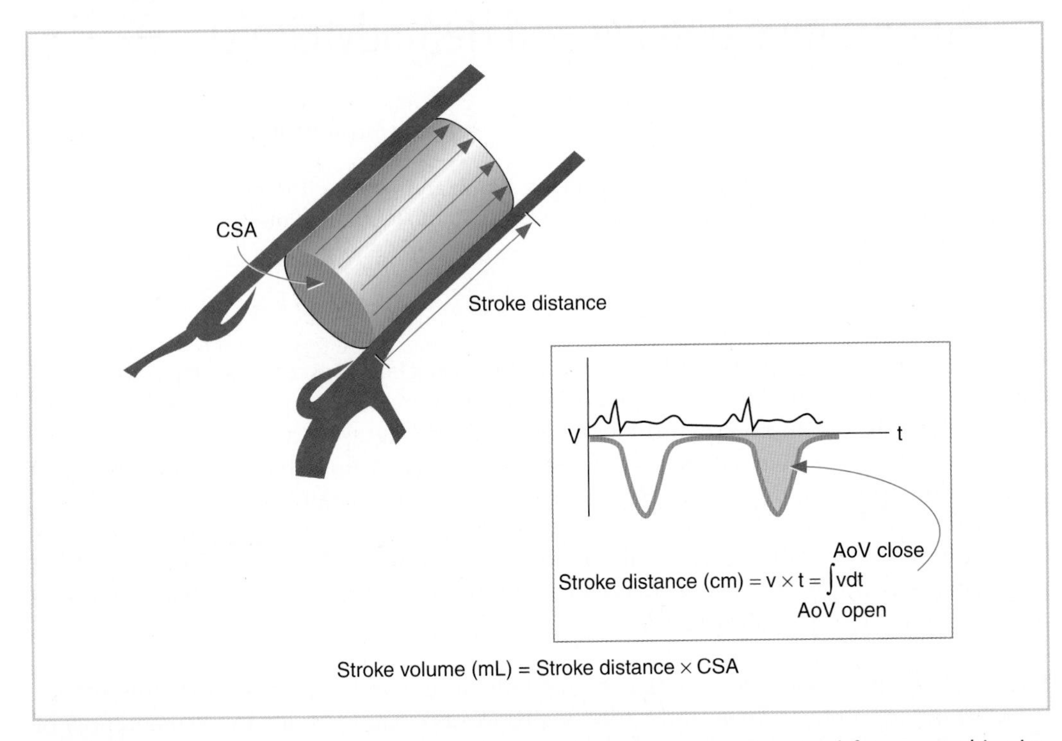

Figure 6.1. Determination of stroke volume. Volumetric flow can be determined from a combination of area and velocity measurements. In this example, flow through the ascending aorta is used to determine the stroke volume. Integrating the Doppler-derived flow velocities over time (known as the *time-velocity integral*) during a single cardiac cycle calculates the stroke distance. The cross-sectional area measurement is obtained with two-dimensional echocardiography. The product of these two measurements, conceptualized as a cylinder, is the stroke volume. CSA, cross-sectional area; AoV, aortic valve.

represents the cumulative distance, commonly referred to as the *stroke distance*, that the red cells have traveled during the systolic ejection phase. When the stroke distance is multiplied by the CSA (in square centimeters) of the conduit (e.g., aorta, mitral valve [MV], pulmonary artery [PA]) through which the blood has traveled, the SV (in cubic centimeters) is obtained (1–7). CO, which expresses volumetric flow in cubic centimeters per minute, is estimated from the product of the SV and the heart rate (HR).

ECHOCARDIOGRAPHIC TECHNIQUE FOR DOPPLER MEASUREMENTS OF STROKE VOLUME

The SV and CO are best measured with TEE at the left ventricular outflow tract (LVOT) or aortic valve (AoV) (1–7). These locations offer several advantages to the clinical echocardiographer. First, the entire ejected SV traverses these structures, whereas it does not in more distant vessels, so that the total SV can be calculated. Second, Doppler interrogation typically assesses blood flow from only a small fraction of the total CSA of the vessel, and therefore SV calculations assume that the measured velocity reflects the mean flow velocity throughout the cross section of the vessel. This assumption is most accurate when blood flow is laminar and has the same velocity across the entire vessel, a situation known as a *blunt* or *flat flow profile* (Figure 6.2). Because the blood is accelerated along the truncated LVOT during systole, the velocity profile has a blunt, uniform pattern rather than the parabolic pattern seen in the ascending aorta or PA. Consequently, the LVOT and AoV are attractive because the risk for sampling blood velocities that are not

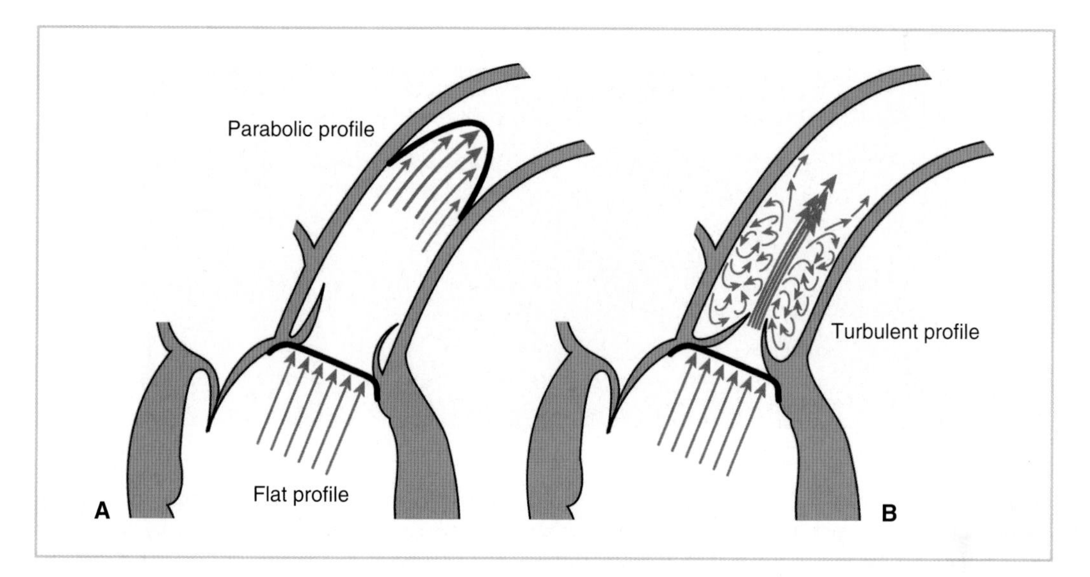

Figure 6.2. Common flow profiles. **A:** The acceleration of the blood flow as it enters the truncated left ventricular outflow tract leads to a "flat" profile in which velocities are uniform. As blood travels in the ascending aorta, the effects of wall friction and a curved conduit result in an asymmetric and parabolic flow profile. **B:** When blood is forced through a narrow opening, laminar flow is replaced with turbulence. In this illustration, aortic stenosis has created a narrow, high-velocity jet encased by turbulent flow.

reflective of the average blood flow velocity is reduced. Third, the LVOT and ascending aorta are more circular and the CSA changes less during the cardiac cycle. Multiplane TEE offers excellent windows at these sites for both Doppler blood flow measurements and two-dimensional echocardiographic measurements of the CSA. Several clinical studies have confirmed that the CO measurements obtained by TEE compare favorably with those obtained by thermodilution (1–3,5–7).

LVOT or transaortic valvular flows are most reliably obtained from the transgastric (TG) long-axis and the deep TG long-axis views because the blood flow is nearly parallel to the ultrasound beam. It is critical to interrogate blood flow carefully through minor alterations in the probe position and multiplane angle to obtain the optimal Doppler spectral signal. The maximal velocity profile with a dense spectral signal is sought.

Calculation of the left ventricular outflow tract stroke volume

1. The pulsed wave Doppler sample volume is positioned in the LVOT immediately proximal to the AoV (TG long-axis and deep TG long-axis views).
2. The CSA for the LVOT is best obtained from the midesophageal (ME) LVOT view. The CSA is calculated from a measurement of the LVOT diameter as follows:
   $\text{CSA}_{\text{LVOT}} = \pi\ (\text{diameter}/2)^2$

Calculation of the transaortic valve stroke volume

1. The continuous wave Doppler beam is directed through the AoV orifice from the TG long-axis or deep TG long-axis view (Figure 6.3).
2. The CSA of the valve is best estimated by planimetry of the equilateral triangle—shaped orifice observed in midsystole (6). The AoV is viewed in cross section from the ME AoV short-axis window, and frame-by-frame review is used to capture the valve in midsystole. Planimetry of the triangle-shaped orifice yields the effective CSA.

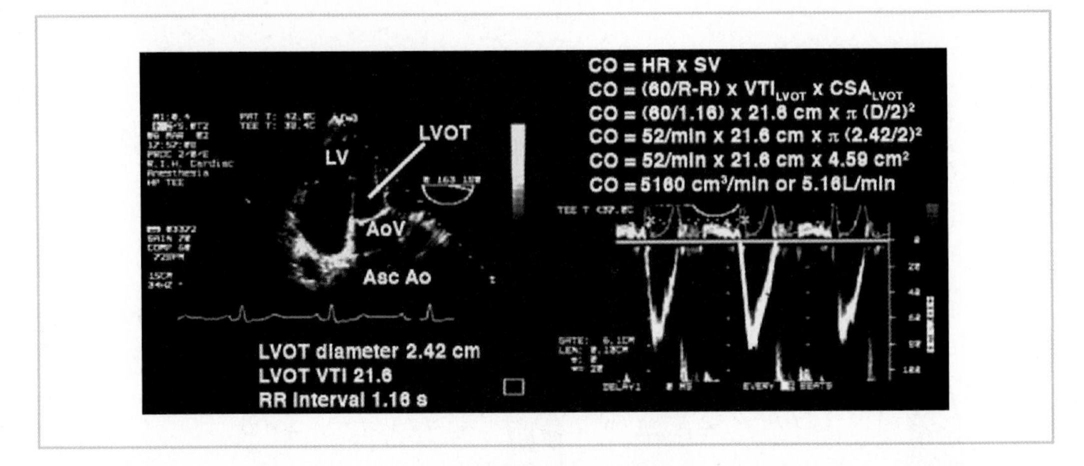

Figure 6.3. Calculation of cardiac output: LVOT approach. The cardiac output (CO) through the left ventricular outflow tract (LVOT) was calculated from the product of the heart rate (HR) by the stroke volume (SV). The latter was calculated from the product of the cross-sectional area or the LVOT (CSA_{LVOT}) and the time-velocity integral of the LVOT (TVI_{LVOT}). The HR was obtained by dividing 60 by the time distance between tow cardiac cycles or the R-R interval. The CSA was measured by assuming a circular orifice ($\pi[D/2]^2$). The LVOT diameter was measured from the midesophageal long-axis view of the LVOT. The time-velocity profile was obtained from the deep transgastric light ventricular outflow window, which can be obtained by rotating the transesophageal echocardiographic probe and transducer from 0 to 165 degrees. LV, left ventricle; AoV, aortic valve; As Ao, ascending aorta.

Calculation of the stroke volume of the right side of the heart

Alternatively, right-sided flows and diameters can be analyzed from the main PA or the MV. Pulsed wave or continuous wave Doppler analysis proceeds after the main PA is imaged from high esophageal windows at the level of the superior mediastinal vessels (Figure 6.4) or the right ventricular outflow tract (RVOT) is imaged from TG windows at 110- to 150-degree rotation of the transducer and rightward turn of the TEE probe (Figure 6.5). In all cases, the maximal velocity profile is sought. Flow across the MV is measured by placing the sample volume at the level of the mitral annulus to obtain the transmitral TVI, which is then multiplied by the area of the MV annulus. Compared with the diameters of the LVOT and ascending aorta, the diameters of the main PA and MV fluctuate more during the cardiac cycle, and these measurements are less reliable than those from the LVOT and AoV (4). In addition, the MV orifice is not circular, and its size changes during diastole.

Regurgitant Volume

Regurgitant volume is the quantity of blood that flows back through a regurgitant lesion in a single cardiac cycle. The total SV traversing a regurgitant valve during systole is greater than that in a normal valve. For a regurgitant valve, the total SV equals the regurgitant volume plus the SV delivered to the peripheral circulation. The regurgitant volume can be calculated as the difference between the total forward flow through the regurgitant valve and the total forward flow through a reference valve

$$\text{Regurgitant Volume} = \text{forward flow through regurgitant valve} - \text{forward flow through reference valve}$$

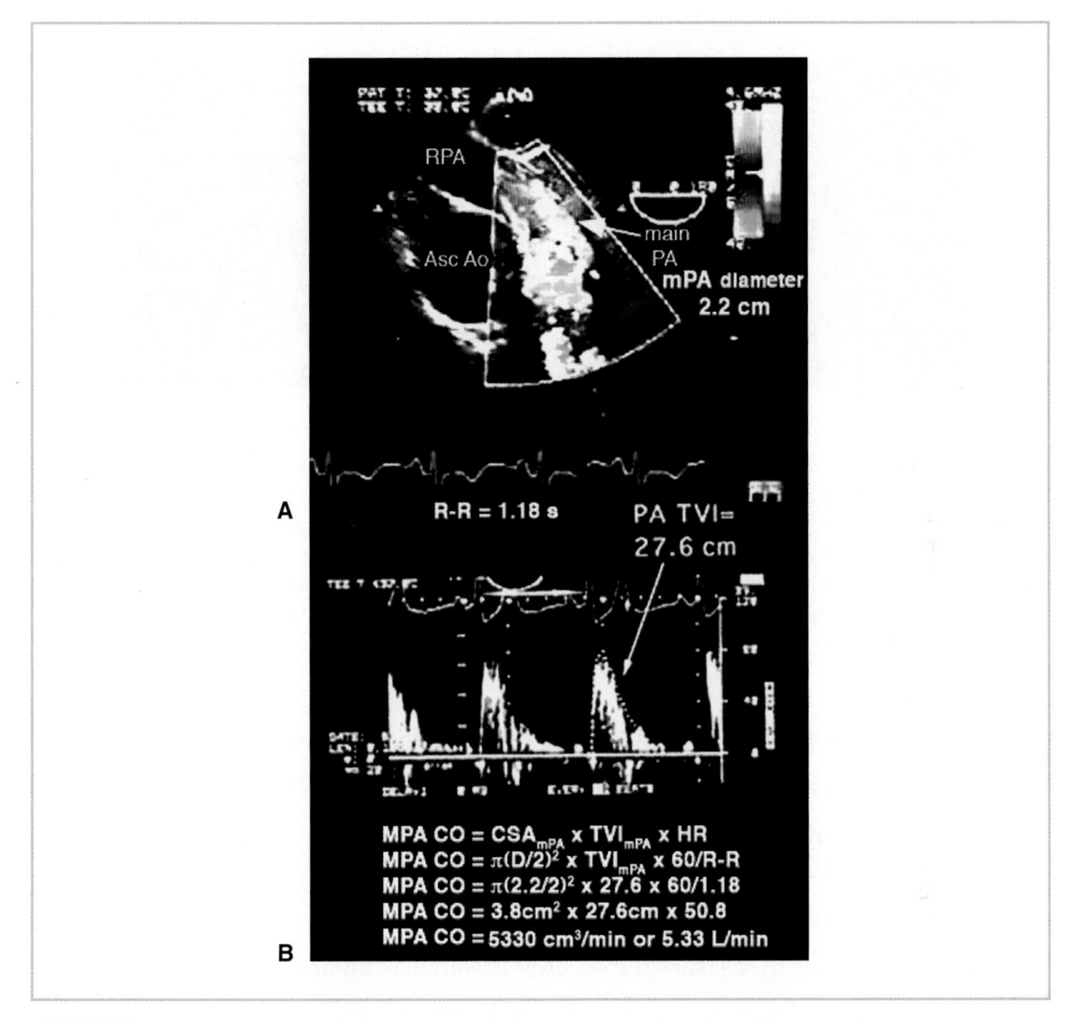

Figure 6.4. A, B: The cardiac output (CO) through the main pulmonary artery (main PA; MPA) was calculated from the product of the heart rate (HR) by the stroke volume (SV). The latter was calculated from the product of the cross-sectional area or the MPA (CSA_{mPA}) and the time-velocity integral of the MPA (TVI_{mPA}). The HR was obtained by dividing 60 by the time distance between tow cardiac cycles or the R-R interval. The CSA was measured by assuming a circular orifice ($\pi[D/2]^2$). The time-velocity profile and mPA diameter were obtained from the transesophageal superior mediastinal view as depicted in A. RPA, right pulmonary artery; As Ao, ascending aorta; mPA, main pulmonary artery.

In the case of mitral regurgitation (MR) (in the absence of significant AoV disease), the SV across the AoV can be used as the true SV

$$\text{Regurgitant volume}_{\text{MV}} = \text{forward flow through MV} - \text{flow through AoV}$$
$$\text{RV}_{\text{MV}}(\text{mL}) = \text{SV}_{\text{MV}} - \text{SV}_{\text{AoV}}$$

However, there is a significant potential for error in the mitral flow measurements because the MV orifice is not circular (4), and its diameter changes during the cardiac cycle.

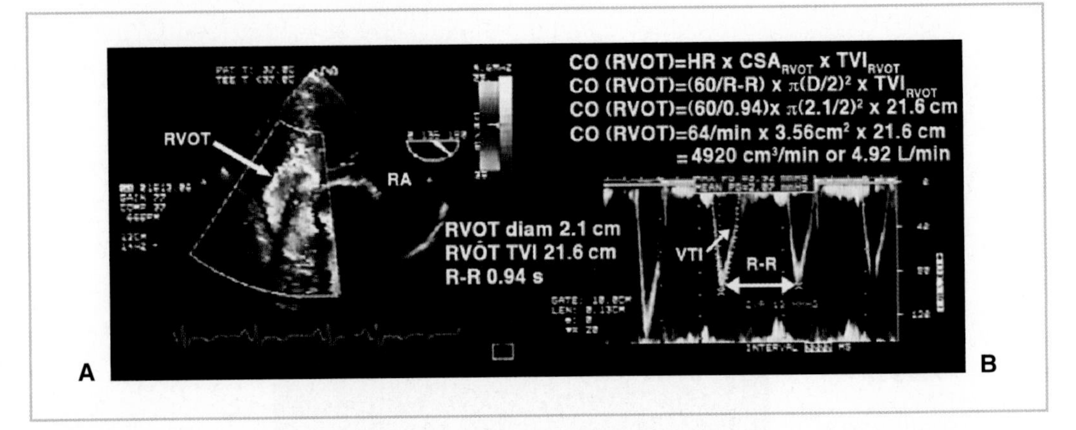

Figure 6.5. A, B: The cardiac output (CO) through the right ventricular outflow tract (RVOT) was calculated as the product of the heart rate (HR) by the stroke volume. The latter was calculated from the product of the cross-sectional area of the RVOT (CSA_{RVOT}) and the time-velocity integral of the RVOT (TVI_{RVOT}). The HR was obtained by dividing 60 by the time distance between tow cardiac cycles or the R-R interval. The CSA was measured by assuming a circular orifice ($\pi[D/2]^2$). The time-velocity profile and RVOT diameter were obtained from the transgastric right ventricular inflow/outflow window. RA, right atrium.

Similarly, the aortic regurgitant volume can be calculated as follows:

$$\text{Regurgitant volume}_{AV} = \text{forward flow through AoV} - \text{flow through MV}$$

The regurgitant fraction is simply the ratio of the regurgitant volume to the total SV through the diseased valve and is typically expressed as a percentage:

$$\text{Regurgitant fraction (\%)} = \text{regurgitant volume/forward flow}$$

Alternative techniques to measure the severity of valvular regurgitation are discussed in Chapters 8 and 11.

Intracardiac Shunts

The ratio of pulmonic to systemic SV, Q_p/Q_s, is important in assessing the severity of shunts and in guiding treatment. Intracardiac shunts are assessed by calculating the SV (8). By measuring the left-sided (LVOT or AoV) and right-sided (PA or RVOT) SVs, one can determine Q_p/Q_s:

$$Q_p/Q_s = SV_{\text{Right Heart (e.g., PA, RVOT)}}/SV_{\text{Left Heart (e.g., LVOT, AOV)}}$$

These measurements are often combined with two-dimensional and color Doppler data to provide a complete assessment of congenital lesions.

Valve Area: The Continuity Equation

The principle of conservation of mass is the basis of the *continuity equation*, which is commonly used to measure the AoV area (9) (Figure 6.6B). The continuity equation simply states that the volume of blood passing through one site (e.g., the LVOT) is equal to the mass or volume of blood passing through another site (e.g., the AoV). Of course, there must be no intervening channels for this principle to apply. By using the principle of volumetric flow, discussed earlier, the continuity equation can be applied clinically.

$$\text{Volumetric Flow}_1 = \text{Volumetric Flow}_2$$
$$\text{CSA}_1 \times \text{TVI}_1 = \text{CSA}_2 \times \text{TVI}_2$$
$$\text{CSA}_1 = \text{CSA}_2 \times \text{TVI}_2/\text{TVI}_1$$

To calculate the area of the aortic valve (AoV):

$$\text{Area}_{\text{AoV}} = \text{Area}_{\text{LVOT}} \times (\text{V}_{\text{LVOT}}/\text{V}_{\text{AoV}})$$
$$\text{Area}_{\text{AoV}} = \pi(\text{D}_{\text{LVOT}}/2)^2 \times (\text{V}_{\text{LVOT}}/\text{V}_{\text{AoV}})$$

where D_{LVOT} is the diameter of the LVOT and V_{LVOT} is the velocity in the LVOT.

TEE assessments of LVOT and aortic flows and of LVOT diameter were described earlier in the section "Doppler Measurements of Stroke Volume and Cardiac Output." The continuity equation is the basis for assessments based on the proximal isovelocity surface area method (10–12), which is described in detail in Chapter 9.

INTRACARDIAC PRESSURES AND PRESSURE GRADIENTS: THE BERNOULLI EQUATION

Pressure gradients are used to estimate intracavitary pressures and to assess conditions such as valvular disease (e.g., aortic stenosis), septal defects, outflow tract abnormalities (e.g., LVOT obstruction), and major vessel pathology (e.g., coarctation). As blood flows across a narrowed or stenotic orifice, blood flow velocity increases. The increase in velocity is related to the degree of narrowing. The Bernoulli equation describes the relation between the increases in blood flow velocity and the pressure gradient across the narrowed orifice (13):

$$\Delta P = \underbrace{1/2\rho({v_2}^2 - {v_1}^2)}_{\text{Convection acceleration}} + \underbrace{\rho(dv/dt)dx}_{\text{Flow acceleration}} + \underbrace{R(v)}_{\text{Viscous friction}}$$

where P is the pressure gradient across the area of interest (mm Hg), ρ is the density of blood (1.06×10^3 kg/m^3), v_1 is the peak velocity of blood flow proximal to area of interest (m/s), and v_2 is the peak velocity of blood flow across the area of interest (m/s).

In clinical practice, the Bernoulli equation is simplified by ignoring the effects of flow acceleration, viscous friction, and the velocity proximal to the area of interest (v_1) because:

1. Peak flows are of interest in clinical measurements. During peak flow, the flow acceleration is virtually nonexistent and thus can be ignored.
2. Viscous friction contributes significantly only in discrete orifices with an area of less than 0.25 cm^2. Blood flow is thought to be constant for orifices with an area greater than this, so that viscous friction is also eliminated in the Bernoulli calculation.
3. For clinically significant lesions, v_2 is substantially greater than v_1, such that ${v_2}^2 - {v_1}^2$ is approximated by just ${v_2}^2$

The elimination of these factors yields the simplified Bernoulli equation:

Simplified Bernoulli equation: $\Delta P = 4{v_2}^2$

Therefore, a pressure gradient is obtained in clinical echocardiography by the straightforward process of measuring the peak velocity of blood flow across the lesion of interest (Figure 6.6A)

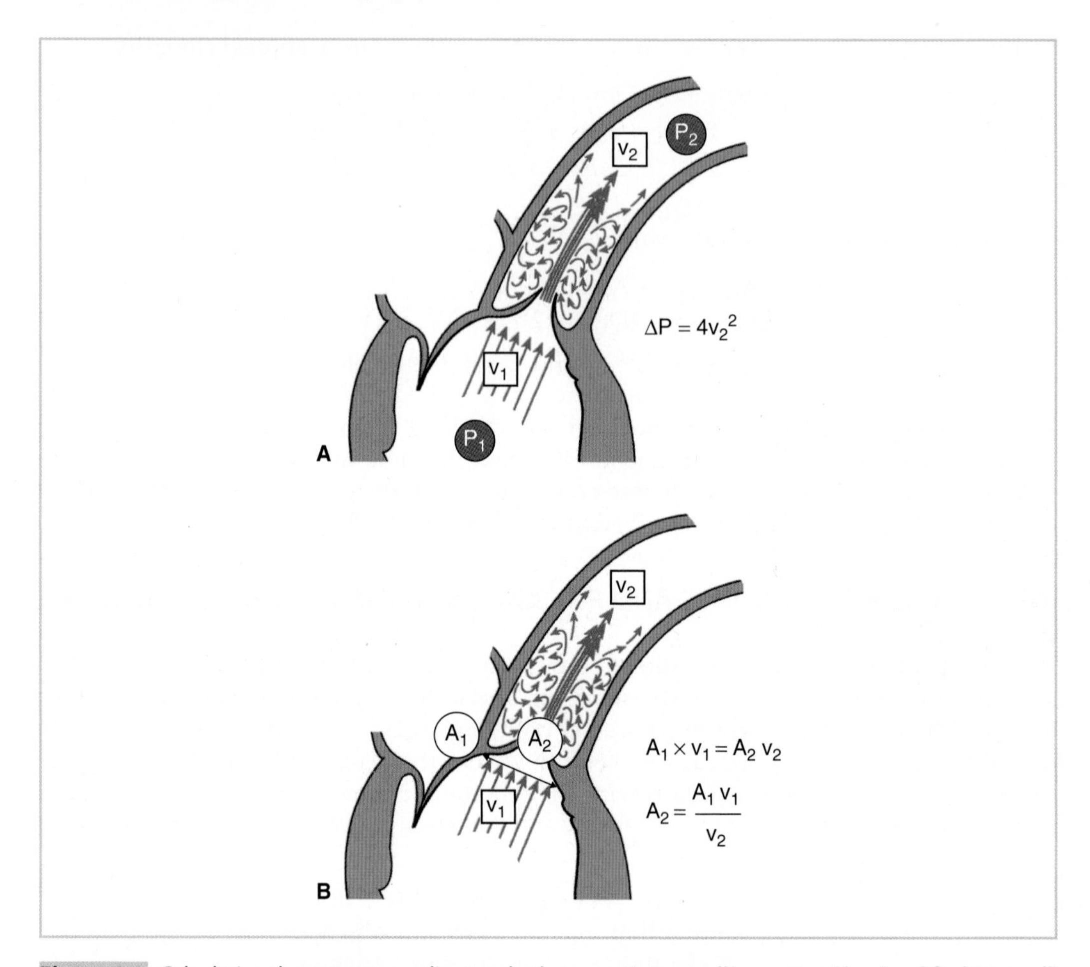

Figure 6.6. Calculating the pressure gradient and valve area. **A:** Bernoulli equation. The simplified Bernoulli equation states that the pressure drop ($P_2 - P_1 = \Delta\ 4P$) across a stenotic orifice is four times the square of the velocity of the high-velocity jet. P_1, blood pressure proximal to stenosis; v_1, flow velocity proximal to stenosis; P_2, blood pressure distal to stenosis; v_2, flow velocity through stenosis. **B:** Continuity equation. The continuity equation is often described as the principle of "what goes in must come out." Accordingly, flow proximal to the stenosis ($A_1 \times v_1$) should equal flow through the stenosis ($A_2, \times v_2,$). A_1, cross-sectional area proximal to stenosis; v_1, flow velocity proximal to stenosis; A_2, cross-sectional area of stenosis; v_2, flow velocity through stenosis.

To calculate the pressure gradient, the pulsed wave Doppler sample volume or continuous wave Doppler beam is directed across the region of interest. The measured peak velocity is then entered into the simplified Bernoulli equation ($\Delta P = 4v_2^2$) to estimate the pressure gradient. When blood flow velocities are high ($\geq$1.4 m/s), continuous wave Doppler is preferred to avoid the aliasing that may occur with pulsed wave Doppler. It is imperative that the Doppler beam be positioned so that it interrogates the jet with the highest velocity; otherwise, the pressure gradient will be significantly underestimated. To obtain the highest velocity flow, interrogation from multiple windows is preferred. Also, accuracy is improved by assessing multiple flow profiles (3–5 for a regular rhythm and 10 for an irregular rhythm) at end-expiration. *The simplified Bernoulli equation is the basis for most pressure gradient calculations in clinical echocardiography.*

Assessment of Valvular Disease

The Bernoulli equation is most commonly used to measure the pressure gradient across a stenotic valve. This application is illustrated in Figure 6.6A. The assessment of valvular stenosis is discussed extensively in Chapters 9 and 12.

In addition, the rate of decline in the pressure gradient across the valve is related to the severity of disease (14). The *pressure half-time* is the time required for the peak transvalvular pressure gradient to decrease by 50%. Typically, a larger orifice has a shorter pressure half-time because pressure can equalize more quickly. The assessment of mitral stenosis and aortic insufficiency can be aided by pressure half-time measurements (see Chapters 9 and 12).

Measurement of Intracavitary Pressures

Intracavitary and pulmonary arterial pressures can be measured by combining a Doppler-derived pressure gradient from a regurgitant jet and a known (or estimated) pressure either proximal or distal to the chamber of interest (Table 6.1). Because accuracy depends on alignment of the ultrasound beam with the blood flow, velocities of central regurgitant jets are more accurately assessed than those of eccentric jets.

RIGHT VENTRICULAR SYSTOLIC PRESSURE AND PULMONARY ARTERY SYSTOLIC PRESSURE

With the simplified Bernoulli equation, the peak velocity of the tricuspid regurgitant (TR) jet is used to calculate the pressure gradient between the right ventricle (RV) and right atrium (RA) (15). The peak TR velocity is obtained by placing the continuous wave Doppler beam parallel to the regurgitant jet. By adding a known or estimated right atrial pressure (RAP) or central venous pressure (CVP) to the RV-RA pressure gradient, the right ventricular systolic pressure (RVSP) is estimated. In patients without significant pulmonic valve stenosis or RVOT obstruction, the RVSP and pulmonary artery systolic pressure (PASP) are similar (Figure 6.7).

$$\text{RVSP or PASP mm Hg} = 4{v_{TR}}^2 + \text{RAP mm Hg}$$

The TEE examination is performed by using the ME RV inflow view with the transducer rotated from 0 to 110 degrees. Interference from left atrial (LA) flows is minimized in many

Table 6.1 Calculation of cardiopulmonary pressures

Pressure	Equation
RVSP or PASP	$= 4({v_{TR}}^2) + \text{RAP}$
PAMP	$= 4(v_{early}\ \text{PI})^2 + \text{RAP}$
PADP	$= 4(v_{late}\ \text{PI})^2 + \text{RAP}$
LAP	$= \text{SBP-}4(v_{MR})^2$
LVEDP	$= \text{DBP-}4(v_{AI\ end})^2$

RVSP, right ventricular systolic pressure; PASP, pulmonary artery systolic pressure; v, peak velocity; TR, tricuspid regurgitation; RAP, right atrial pressure; PAMP, pulmonary artery mean pressure; PI, pulmonic valve insufficiency; PADP, pulmonary artery diastolic pressure; LAP, left atrial pressure; SBP, systolic blood pressure; MR, mitral regurgitation; LVEDP, left ventricular end-diastolic pressure; DBP, diastolic blood pressure; AI, aortic insufficiency.

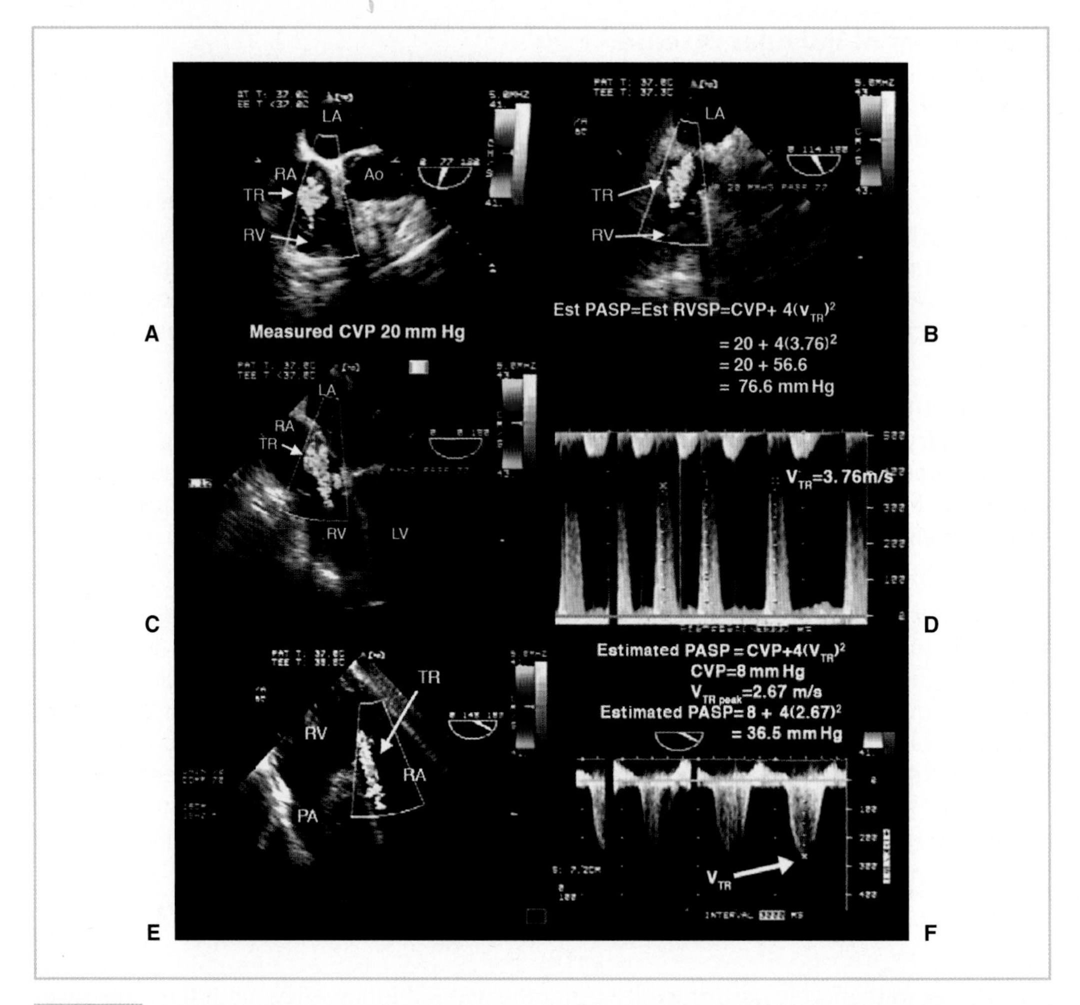

Figure 6.7. **A–D:** Estimation of pulmonary artery systolic pressure (PASP) from the peak velocity of the tricuspid regurgitant (TR; v_{TR}) velocity profile. This was accomplished using the modified Bernoulli equation ($4v^2$), which is then added to the measured central venous pressure (CVP), which, in this patient, was 20 mm Hg. The TR velocity profile was obtained using continuous wave Doppler from different midesophageal echocardiographic windows; **A:** Right ventricular inflow view; **B:** 110 to 120 degrees right ventricular inflow view; and **C:** Four Chamber view. **D:** Doppler display of the time-velocity integrals. **E, F:** Estimation of PASP from the peak velocity of the tricuspid regurgitant (TR; v_{TR}) velocity profile. This was accomplished using the modified Bernoulli equation ($4v^2$), which is then added to the central venous pressure (CVP), which for this patient, was 8 mm Hg. The TR velocity profile was obtained using continuous wave Doppler from the transgastric right ventricular inflow/outflow window. LA, left atrium; RA, right atrium; Ao, aorta; LV, left ventricle; RV, right ventricle; RVSP, right ventricular systolic pressure.

patients by advancing the probe to the level of the coronary sinus, so that the position of the Doppler beam is posterior to the LA.

PULMONARY ARTERY MEAN PRESSURE AND PULMONARY ARTERY DIASTOLIC PRESSURE

These pressures are determined from the pulmonic valve regurgitation (pulmonary insufficiency [PI]) flow profile (15,16) (Figure 6.8). After the continuous wave Doppler beam is placed parallel to the regurgitant jet, the peak early diastolic velocity is obtained to measure the early diastolic gradient between the PA and RV. Using RA pressure as a

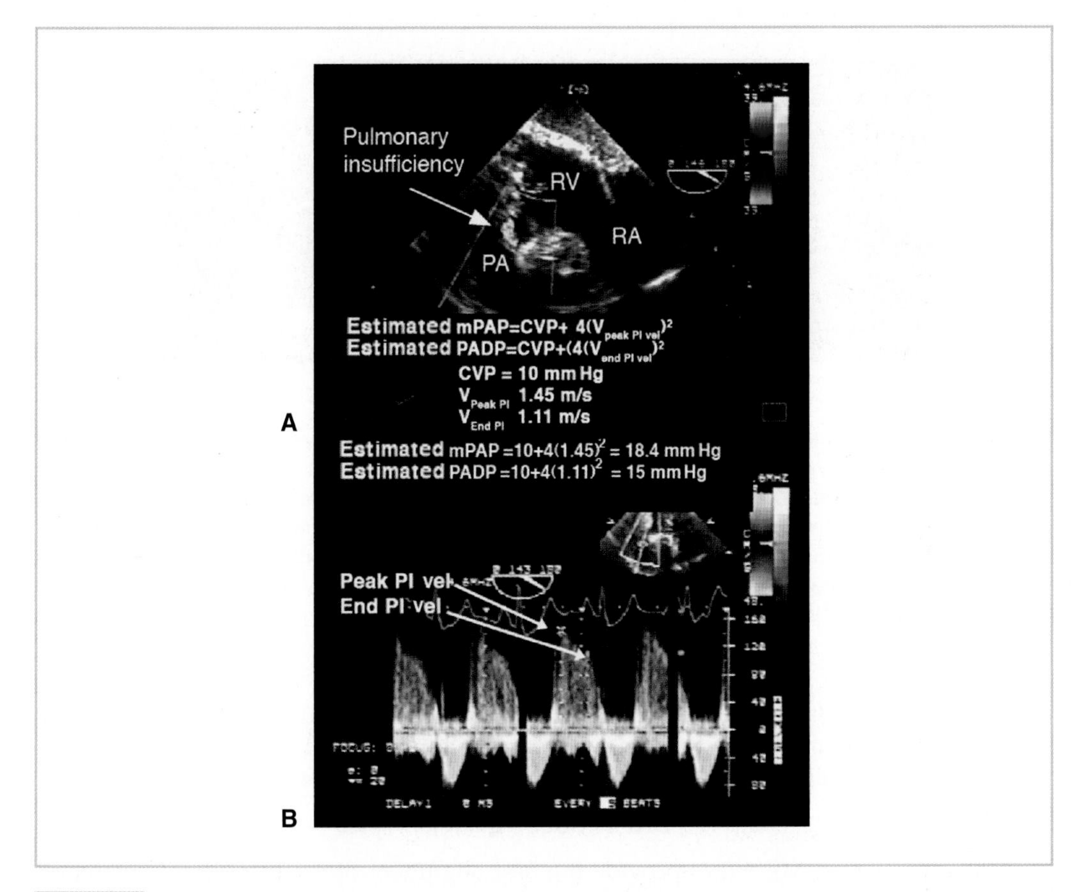

Figure 6.8. **A, B:** Estimation of the pulmonary artery mean and diastolic pressures from the peak and end velocities (vel) from the pulmonary insufficiency (PI) time-velocity integral. This was obtained using Doppler assessment of the pulmonic valve from the transgrastric right ventricular inflow/outflow view typically obtained between 110 and 150 degrees with a rightward rotation of the TEE probe. RA, right atrium; RV, right ventricle; PA, pulmonary artery; CVP, central venous pressure.

substitute for RV pressure in early diastole, this gradient is added to a known or estimated RA pressure to yield the pulmonary artery mean pressure (PAMP).

$$\text{PAMP} = 4(\text{v}_{\text{early}_{\text{PI}}})^2 + \text{CVP}$$

The pulmonary artery diastolic pressure (PADP) can be estimated by using the late peak velocity from the same flow profile.

$$\text{PADP} = 4(\text{v}_{\text{late}_{\text{PI}}})^2 + \text{CVP}$$

The pulmonic valve regurgitant flow is interrogated by using gastric views with rotation of the transducer from 110 to 150 degrees combined with rightward rotation of the TEE probe.

LEFT ATRIAL AND LEFT VENTRICULAR PRESSURES

These pressures are derived by applying the Bernoulli equation or by examining the flow patterns across the MV (17) (Figure 6.9).

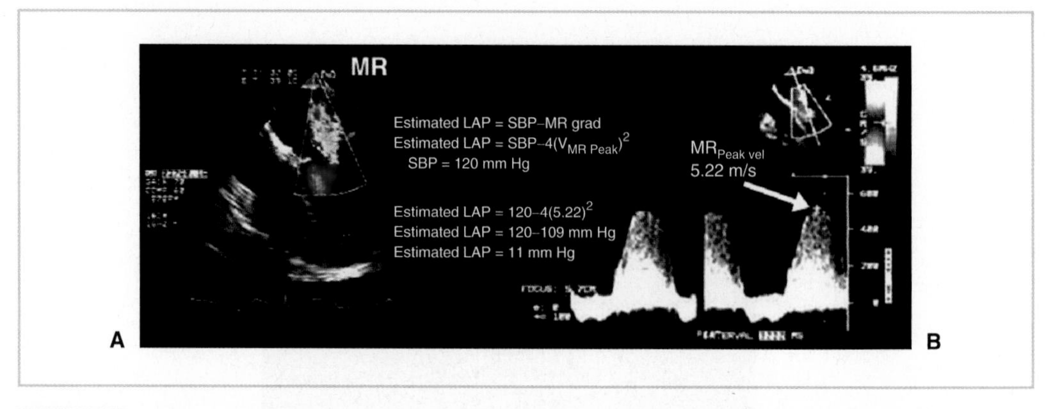

Figure 6.9. **A, B:** Estimation of left atrial pressure (LAP) from the peak velocity ($v_{MR\ Peak}$) of the mitral valve regurgitant (MR) velocity profile. This represents the gradient between the left ventricle and the left atrium (LV-LA Grad) during systole. The LAP was calculated using the modified Bernoulli equation ($4v^2$). This value was then subtracted from the measured systemic systolic blood pressure (SBP). For this patient the measured SBP was 120 mm Hg. The MR velocity profile was obtained using continuous wave Doppler from the midesophageal four-chamber window, however, the MR profile may also be assessed from a number of other midesophageal windows.

To measure the left atrial pressure (LAP), the peak velocity of the MR flow profile is obtained. The calculated pressure gradient is then subtracted from a known systemic systolic blood pressure (SBP), which is similar to left ventricular (LV) systolic pressures in the absence of AoV disease or obstructive outflow tract pathologies.

$$\text{LAP} = \text{SBP} - 4(v_{\text{MR}})^2$$

Most often, standard ME views provide the best alignment of the ultrasound beam and MR flow.

LEFT VENTRICULAR END-DIASTOLIC PRESSURE

The LV end-diastolic pressure (LVEDP) is assessed by using the aortic valve regurgitation (aortic insufficiency [AI]) velocity profile (18) (Figure 6.10). The end-diastolic velocity is obtained by placing the continuous wave Doppler beam parallel to the regurgitant jet. The calculated aortic-ventricular gradient, measured from the peak end-diastolic velocity, is subtracted from the systemic diastolic pressure (DBP) to yield the LVEDP.

$$\text{LVEDP} = \text{DBP} - 4(v_{\text{AIend}})^2$$

The AI flow profile is obtained by using TG windows of the AoV and LVOT, in particular the deep and long-axis views.

LA and LV pressures can also be estimated from the transmitral and pulmonary venous velocity patterns (19–25). This approach is discussed in detail in Chapter 7.

Vascular Resistance

Cardiac function involves a number of functions including preload, contractility, and afterload, the latter being referred to as *resistance*. Although the resistance to flow can be qualitatively determined from measurements of flow and pressures, this does not replace a quantitative assessment. Unfortunately, simple echocardiographic measures of vascular resistance are elusive. There are, however, a number of relatively simple techniques that allow the echocardiographer to determine systemic and PVR.

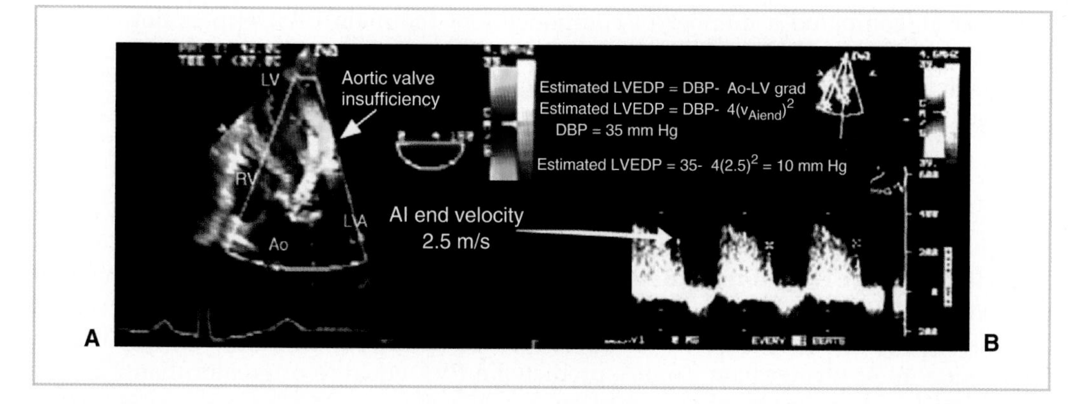

Figure 6.10. **A, B:** Estimation of left ventricular end-diastolic pressure (LVEDP) from the end velocity of the aortic valve regurgitant (AI) velocity profile. This represents the gradient between the aorta and the left ventricle (Ao-LV Grad) during diastole. The LVEDP was calculated using the modified Bernoulli equation ($4v^2$). This value was then subtracted from the measured systemic diastolic blood pressure (DPB). For this patient the measured DBP was 35 mm Hg. The AI velocity profile was obtained using continuous wave Doppler from the deep transgastric light ventricular outflow window. LV, left ventricle; RV, right ventricle; Ao, aorta; LA, left atrium.

Abbas et al. were able to determine **systemic vascular resistance** (SVR; normal 10–14 Wood units [WU]) as either normal or elevated by comparing the ratio of the mitral regurgitant peak velocity (v_{MR} m/s) to the Doppler flow profile of the left ventricular outflow tract (TVI_{LVOT} cm) (26).

$$V_{MR}/TVI_{LVOT}$$

When the v_{MR}/TVI_{LVOT} was greater than 0.27, the SVR was greater than 14 WU. This had a 70% and 77% sensitivity and specificity. When the v_{MR}/TVI_{LVOT} was less than 0.2, the SVR was less than 10 WU, which carried a 92% and 88% sensitivity and specificity. The basis of these measures considers that the v_{MR} may represent systemic velocity, whereas the TVI_{LVOT} represents forward flow. A number of variables may reduce the accuracy of this measure, and include significant mitral and/or AoV disease.

PVR can also be estimated by a number of Doppler techniques. Similar to Abbas et al. for SVR, the PVR may be estimated by calculating the ratio of the tricuspid valve regurgitant peak velocity (v_{TR}) to the Doppler profile of the right ventricular outflow tract (TVI_{RVOT}). The PVR can be obtained by the following equation:

$$PVR = (v_{TR}/TVI_{RVOT}) \times 10 + 0.16 \quad (27)$$

A value of 0.2 was found to be the cutoff for patients above or below 2 WU i.e., less than 0.2 estimated that the PVR was less than 2 WU.

Other methods to obtain the PVR include measuring components of the RVOT Doppler profile (28).

$$PVR = 0.156 + (1.54 \times [(PEP/AcT)/TT]$$

In this equation, the PVR is related to the durations of the pre-ejection period (PEP), the acceleration time (AcT) and the total systolic time (TT) of the RVOT flow profile.

Ebeid et al. compared a number of components of the main PA Doppler flow profile to measured PA pressure and resistance (29). These included the AcT, right ventricular pre-ejection period (RVPEP), the right ventricular ejection time (RVET), and the TVI_{RV}. Analysis included comparisons of the individual components and of a number of ratios.

$$RVPEP/RVET \quad RVPEP/TVI_{RV}$$

Significant correlations were found between these two ratios and PVR. The RVPEP/RVET was able to discern between patients with normal PVR (RVPEP/RVET <0.3) and elevated PVR (RVPEP/RVET >0.4) regardless of PA pressures. More accurate was the correlation between RVPEP/TVI_{RV} and PVR. A value less than 0.4 m/s selected patients with a PVR less than 3 WU. A value between 0.4 and 0.6 m/s correlated with a PVR of 3 to 7.5 WU. A value equal to or greater than 0.6 m/s predicted a PVR equal to or greater than 7.5 WU. These data had a greater than 90% accuracy.

Finally, Shandas et al. combined M-mode and color Doppler echocardiography to assess PVR by measuring the **propagation velocity** of the RVOT (RVOT V_{prop}) or PA outflow (30). After establishing the method in an *in vitro* model the authors tested their hypothesis on 11 patients. The higher the RVOT V_{prop} the lower the PVR. A RVOT V_{prop} greater than 18 cm/s correlated with a PVR less than 6 WU. In the *in vitro* model, this cutoff was found at a RVOT V_{prop} greater than 15 cm/s. In both models it seemed as though a RVOT V_{prop} greater than 20 cm/s was consistent with a PVR less than or equal to 2 WU.

HEART RHYTHM

Pulsed wave Doppler echocardiography is valuable in assessing heart rhythm. In particular, Doppler analysis of transmitral flow and flow in the LA appendage may be useful in assessing rate, rhythm, and atrial function. As discussed in detail in Chapter 7, normal transmitral flow analysis demonstrates early (E wave) and late (A wave) atrial contraction components. The latter describes the contribution of the atrial contraction to the ventricular preload. The presence of both waves indicates that a sinus or atrioventricular rhythm is present. The velocity profile of the LA appendage may also help to diagnose an atrial dysrhythmia. The normal LA appendage profile contains a single positive deflection during atrial contraction.

SUMMARY

Quantitative hemodynamic assessment with Doppler echocardiography offers a range of measurements: valve area, pressure gradients, chamber pressures, blood flow, resistances, and rate/rhythm. These measurements are essential in assessing valvular disease. The echocardiographer should establish a systematic approach to quantitative Doppler that is clinically useful and can be performed reliably and easily on-line. In combination with the two-dimensional echocardiographic examination, these quantitative techniques provide extensive information about cardiac performance.

REFERENCES

1 Savino JS, Troianos CA, Aukburg S, et al. Measurements of pulmonary blood flow with transesophageal two-dimensional and Doppler echocardiography. *Anesthesiology* 1991;75:445–451.
2 Gorcsan J III, Diana P, Ball BS, et al. Intraoperative determination of cardiac output by transesophageal continuous wave Doppler *Am Heart J* 199;13:171–176.

3 Maslow AD, Haering J, Comunale M, et al. Measurement of cardiac output by pulsed wave Doppler of the right ventricular outflow tract. *Anesth Analg* 1996;83:466–471.
4 Stewart WJ, Jiang L, Mich R, et al. Variable effects of changes in flow rate through the aortic, pulmonary, and mitral valves on valve area and flow velocity: impact on quantitative Doppler flow calculations. *J Am Coll Cardiol* 1985;6:653–666.
5 Muhiuden IA, Kuecherer HF, Lee E, et al. Intraoperative estimation of cardiac output by transesophageal pulsed Doppler echocardiography. *Anesthesiology* 1991;74:9–14.
6 Darmon PL, Hillel Z, Mogtader A, et al. Cardiac output by transesophageal echocardiography using continuous-wave Doppler across the aortic valve. *Anesthesiology* 1994;80:796–805.
7 Perrino AC, Harris SN, Luther MA. Intraoperative determination of cardiac output using multiplane transesophageal echocardiography: a comparison to thermodilution. *Anesthesiology* 1998;89:350–357.
8 Valdes-Cruz LM, Horowitz S, Mesel E, et al. A pulsed Doppler echocardiographic method for calculating pulmonary and systemic blood flow in atrial level shunts: validation studies in animals and initial human experience. *Circulation* 1984;69:80–86.
9 Blumberg FC, Pfeifer M, Holmer SR, et al. Quantification of aortic stenosis in mechanically ventilated patients using multiplane transesophageal Doppler echocardiography. *Chest* 1998;114:94–97.
10 Bargiggia GS, Tronconi L, Sahn DJ, et al. A new method for quantitation of mitral regurgitation based on color flow Doppler imaging of flow convergence proximal to regurgitant orifice. *Circulation* 1991;84:1481–1489.
11 Rodriguez L, Thomas JD, Monterroso V, et al. Validation of the proximal flow convergence method: calculation of orifice area in patients with mitral stenosis. *Circulation* 1993;88:1157–1165.
12 Rittoo D, Sutherland GR, Shaw TR. Quantification of left-to-right atrial shunting defect size after balloon mitral commissurotomy using biplane transesophageal echocardiography, color flow Doppler mapping, and the principle of proximal flow convergence. *Circulation* 1993;87:1591–1603.
13 Nishimura RA, Miller FA, Callahan MJ, et al. Doppler echocardiography: theory, instrumentation, technique, and application. *Mayo Clin Proc* 1985;60:321–343.
14 Nakatani S, Masuyama T, Kodama K, et al. Value and limitations of Doppler echocardiography in the quantification of stenotic mitral valve area: comparison of the pressure half-time and the continuity equation methods. *Circulation* 1988;77:78–85.
15 Come PC. Echocardiographic recognition of pulmonary arterial disease and determination of its cause. *Am J Med* 1988;84:384–393.
16 Lee RT, Lord CP, Plappert T, et al. Prospective Doppler echocardiographic evaluation of pulmonary artery diastolic pressure in the medical intensive care unit. *Am J Cardiol* 1989;64:1366–1377.
17 Gorcsan J III, Snow FR, Paulsen W, et al. Noninvasive estimation of left atrial pressure in patients with congestive heart failure and mitral regurgitation by Doppler echocardiography. *Am Heart J* 1991;11: 858–863.
18 Nishimura RA, Tajik AJ. Determination of left-sided pressure gradients by utilizing Doppler aortic and mitral regurgitation signals: validation by simultaneous dual catheter and Doppler studies. *J Am Coll Cardiol* 1988;11:317–331.
19 Oh JK, Appleton CP, Hatle LK, et al. The noninvasive assessment of left ventricular diastolic function with two-dimensional and Doppler echocardiography. *J Am Soc Echocardiogr* 1997;10:46–70.
20 Nishimura RA, Housmans PR, Hatle LK, et al. Assessment of diastolic function of the heart: background and current applications of Doppler echocardiography. Part II Clinical Studies. *Mayo Clin Proc* 1989;64: 181–194.
21 Nagueh SF, Kopelen HA, Quinones MA. Assessment of left ventricular filling pressures by Doppler in the presence of atrial fibrillation. *Circulation* 1996;94:138–145.
22 Temporelli PL, Scapellato F, Corra U, et al. Estimation of pulmonary wedge pressure by transmitral Doppler in patients with chronic heart failure and atrial fibrillation. *Am J Cardiol* 1999;83:724–727.
23 Moller JE, Poulsen SH, Songderfaard E, et al. Preload dependence of color M-mode Doppler flow propagation velocity in controls and in patients with left ventricular dysfunction. *J Am Soc Echocardiogr* 2000;13:902–909.
24 Garcia MJ, Ares MA, Asher C, et al. An index of early left ventricular filling that combined with pulsed Doppler peak E velocity may estimate capillary wedge pressure. *J Am Coll Cardiol* 1997;9:448–454.
25 Gonzalez-Viachez F, Ares M, Ayuela J, et al. Combined use of pulsed and color M-mode Doppler echocardiography for the estimation of pulmonary capillary wedge pressure: an empirical approach based on an analytical relation. *J Am Coll Cardiol* 1999;34:515–553.
26 Abbas AE, Fortuin D, Patel B, et al. Noninvasive measurement of systemic vascular resistance using Doppler echocardiography. *J Am Soc Echocardiogr* 2004;17:834–838.
27 Scapellato F, Temporelli PL, Eleuteri E, et al. Accurate noninvasive estimation of pulmonary vascular resistance by Doppler echocardiography in patients with chronic heart failure. *J Am Coll Cardiol* 2001;37:1813–1819.

28 Bermejo J, Garcia-Fernandez MA, Torrecilla EG, et al. Effects of dobutamine on Doppler echocardiographic indexes of aortic stenosis. *J Am Coll Cardiol* 1996;28:1206–1213.
29 Ebeid MR, Ferrer PL, Robinson B, et al. Doppler echocardiographic evaluation of pulmonary vascular resistance in children with congenital heart disease. *J Am Soc Echocardiogr* 1996;9:822–831.
30 Shanda R, Weinberg C, Ivy D, et al. Development of a noninvasive ultrasound color m-mode means of estimating pulmonary vascular resistance in pediatric pulmonary hypertension. *Circulation* 2001;104:908–913.

QUESTIONS

1. All the statements below are true except

a. Intracardiac pressures can be estimated with Doppler echocardiography.
b. Intracardiac pressures can be indirectly measured with Doppler echocardiography.
c. Intracardiac pressures can be assessed with the Bernoulli equation.
d. Intracardiac pressures can be directly measured with Doppler echocardiography.
e. Intracardiac pressures can be estimated by using blood flow profiles obtained with Doppler echocardiography.

2. The Doppler assessment of stroke volume (SV)

a. Is performed accurately regardless of the orifice shape
b. Is best measured across the mitral valve (MV)
c. Can be used to assess pulmonary-to-systemic blood flow
d. Is measured only with pulsed wave Doppler echocardiography
e. Does not require two-dimensional echocardiographic measurements

3. The following statements regarding Doppler measurement of intracardiac pressures are true except

a. The pulmonary artery (PA) diastolic and mean pressures can be obtained from the pulmonary valve insufficiency flow profile.
b. The PA systolic pressure and right ventricle (RV) systolic pressure may be equal.
c. Pressure gradients are related to known pressures either proximal or distal to the chamber of interest.
d. LV diastolic pressure is measured by using the MV regurgitant flow profile.
e. If the proximal velocity (v_1) is high, then the result obtained with the simplified Bernoulli equation may not be accurate.

4. Doppler measurements of flow velocities must be repeated and averaged to account for

a. Operator error
b. Cor triatriatum
c. Beat-to-beat variability
d. Higher transducer frequencies used in transesophageal echocardiography (TEE)
e. Use of continuous wave Doppler

5. The order of accuracy (best to least) in the measurement of SV is

a. PA, left ventricular outflow tract (LVOT), pulmonary vein
b. LVOT, MV, pulmonary vein
c. LVOT, pulmonary vein, MV
d. LVOT, PA, MV
e. MV, PA, LVOT

6. The direct measurement of central pressures

a. Involves the use of regurgitant flows
b. Involves the peak end-diastolic velocity of the pulmonic valve regurgitant profile
c. Cannot be done with echocardiography
d. Requires a known or estimated pressure
e. Involves two-dimensional echocardiography but not Doppler echocardiography

A 72-year-old, with a known atrial septal defect (Q_p:Q_s = 1.8) and mild RV dysfunction, is undergoing abdominal aortic aneurysm surgery. On release of the aortic cross-clamp, the heart rate (HR) increases to 100 bpm, the blood pressure (BP) decreases to 80/40 (mean 53) mm Hg, and the arterial saturation falls to 91%. The CVP was 15 mm Hg. The TEE exam reveals normal left ventricular (LV) systolic function, moderate RV dysfunction, moderate tricuspid regurgitation (TR peak velocity 3 m/s), mild mitral regurgitation (MR peak velocity 4 m/s), and mild aortic valve (AoV) insufficiency (end AI peak velocity 0.5 m/s; early AI peak velocity 3 m/s). The LV outflow tract (LVOT) diameter is 2.0 cm, the time-velocity integral (TVI) is 10 cm, and the peak velocity is 1.0 m/s. The transaortic valve peak velocity is 1.4 m/s. The main pulmonary artery (MPA) diameter is 2.2 cm, and the TVI is 10 cm.

7. After release of the aortic cross-clamp which of the following are true?

A. The estimated PA systolic pressure is approximately 50 mm Hg.
B. The AoV area is approximately 2.2 cm^2.
C. The Doppler estimate of LV end-diastolic pressure is 15 mm Hg.
D. The Doppler estimate of LV end-diastolic pressure is 4 mm Hg.

a. **A, B** and **C**
b. **A** and **C**
c. **B** and **D**
d. **D**
e. **A, B, C** and **D**

8. All of the following statements regarding the case in Question no. 7 are true except

a. The systemic cardiac output is 3.14 L/min.
b. The systemic stroke volume is 31.4 mL/beat.
c. The Q_p/Q_s is approximately 12.
d. The main pulmonary artery cardiac output is 3.00 L/min.
e. Arterial desaturation and altered hemodynamics may be due increased RV dysfunction and right to left shunt across the atrial septal defect.

A 12-year-old girl undergoing corrective spine surgery for kyphoscoliosis has a decrease in the systemic blood pressure (BP) to 65/40 (mean 48) mm Hg, and an increase in the HR from 90 to 120 bpm. The central venous pressure is 10 mm Hg. TEE exam reveals hyperdynamic RV and LV function, and normal valve function. The LVOT diameter is 2.0 cm, and the TVI is 15 cm. The peak velocity of the tricuspid regurgitation flow profile is m/s.

9. Which of the following statements is false?

a. The patient may be experiencing anaphylaxis.
b. The PA diastolic pressure cannot be obtained from the data presented.
c. The cardiac output is 5.65 L/min.
d. The estimated PA systolic pressure is approximately 6 mm Hg.
e. The patient has had a pulmonary embolism.

A 75-year-old man experiences hypotension after induction of anesthesia (BP 65/40 mm Hg; HR 90 bpm). A TEE exam reveals normal LV function and moderate RV hypokinesis. The LV cavity is small. There is moderate AI and mild mitral regurgitation (MR). The LVOT diameter is 2.0 cm with a peak velocity of 1.0 m/s. The peak velocity across the AoV is 4.0 m/s and the TVI is 30 cm.

10. Which of the following statements is true?

A. The left ventricular outflow tract area is 3.14 cm^2.
B. The aortic valve area is 0.78 cm^2.
C. The systemic cardiac output is. 211 L/min.

D. The systemic stroke volume is 23.4 mL/beat.

a. **A, B** and **C**
b. **A** and **C**
c. **B** and **D**
d. **D**
e. **A, B, C** and **D**

Answers appear at the back of the book.

7 A Practical Approach to the Echocardiographic Evaluation of Ventricular Diastolic Function

Stanton K. Shernan

In comparison to systole, the diastolic phase of the cardiac cycle has only recently acquired appropriate recognition as an important, independent component of overall cardiac performance. Diastole is no longer perceived simply as a passive stage of ventricular filling interposed between each contraction. Adequate ventricular filling is actually dependent upon a complex interaction between ventricular relaxation, compliance and systolic function, in addition to an important late diastolic contribution from atrial contraction.

Following the advent of cardiac catheterization in the 1960s, quantification of ventricular mechanics and ventricular diastolic properties accelerated with the introduction of pulse wave Doppler (PWD) echocardiography in the early 1980s. The relative feasibility, safety, and practicality of echocardiography has helped to delineate diastolic dysfunction over the last several decades, as a major pathophysiologic component of several cardiac disorders including acute and chronic congestive heart failure (CHF) (1). In addition, Doppler echocardiographic modalities have been used to predict functional class and prognosis (2). Recent echocardiographic studies have also suggested that diastolic dysfunction may contribute to perioperative hemodynamic instability and adverse outcomes following cardiac surgery (3). This chapter presents a practical approach to understanding the importance and utility of traditional and newer echocardiographic modalities in assessing ventricular filling and diastolic dysfunction.

CLINICAL RELEVANCE OF DIASTOLIC DYSFUNCTION

CHF is the most common diagnosis amongst inpatients in the United States and accounts for 720,000 hospital admissions annually (4). Nearly half of the patients with CHF have diastolic dysfunction and normal ejection fraction (5). Diastolic dysfunction increases with age, especially amongst elderly patients with hypertensive heart disease (5). Although the prognosis for patients with diastolic heart failure (DHF) is more favorable than for patients with systolic dysfunction, mortality is increased fourfold when compared with age- and gender-matched healthy subjects (6). Therefore, diastolic dysfunction poses an important and clinically relevant challenge to the health care industry.

The relatively high prevalence of DHF in the community is also a concern for the perioperative intensivist because many affected patients will present to the operating room for cardiovascular procedures. Preoperative diastolic dysfunction has been reported in 30% to 70% of cardiac surgical patients and independently associated with difficult weaning from cardiopulmonary bypass (CPB), more frequent inotropic support, and increased morbidity (3,7). Following CPB, acute or progressive diastolic dysfunction associated with ischemia-reperfusion injury, hypothermia, metabolic disturbances or myocardial edema may develop and persist for several minutes to days (8). Identifying high-risk patients preoperatively and monitoring diastolic function intraoperatively may allow for the institution of prophylactic therapeutic strategies, including the administration of pharmacologic agents with direct or indirect lusitropic properties (9) that could facilitate weaning from CPB and reduce perioperative morbidity.

BASICS OF DIASTOLIC PHYSIOLOGY

The diastolic phase of the cardiac cycle is defined as the period from aortic valve (AV) closure to mitral valve (MV) closure (Figure 7.1). Diastole can be further divided into an initial isovolumic relaxation period, followed by early rapid left ventricular (LV) inflow responsible for 80% to 90% of diastolic filling, diastasis and finally, atrial systole (10). LV filling during diastole is dependent on a complex interaction of numerous factors including ventricular relaxation, diastolic suction, viscoelastic forces of the myocardium, pericardial restraint, ventricular interaction, MV dynamics, load heterogeneity, intrathoracic pressure, heart rate/rhythm, and atrial function (11).

Diastolic dysfunction is often defined clinically as an impaired capacity of the ventricles to fill at low pressure and usually involves an abnormality in ventricular relaxation and/or chamber compliance. LV relaxation is associated with resequestration of calcium from the cytosol to the sarcoplasmic reticulum, through a complex energy-dependent process that is required to deactivate the contractile elements and subsequently allow the myofibrils return

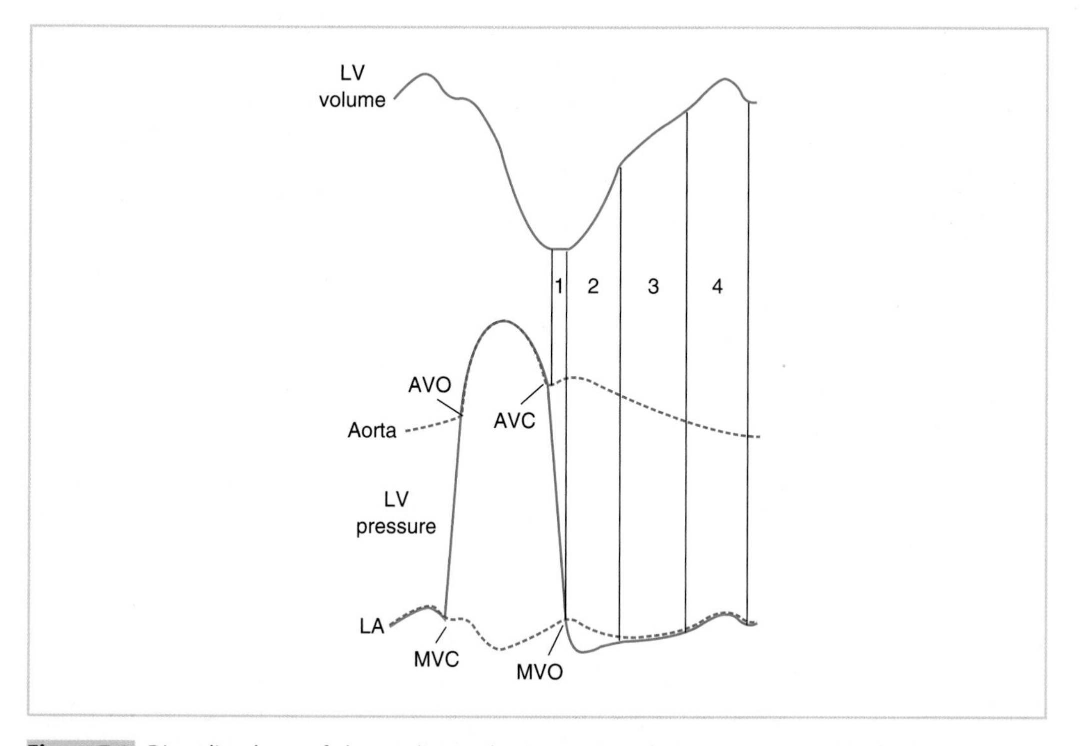

Figure 7.1. Diastolic phase of the cardiac cycle. During isovolumic relaxation (*1*), left ventricular (*LV*) pressure falls rapidly following aortic valve closure (*AVC*). When LV pressure decreases below left atrial (*LA*) pressure, the mitral valve opens (*MVO*) initiating early, rapid LV filling (*2*). Equilibration of LV and LA pressures results in diminished transmitral flow during diastasis (*3*) until atrial contraction (*4*) which normally contributes less than 20% of the total LV end-diastolic volume. Diastole terminates with mitral valve closure (*MVC*) before isovolumic contraction and the aortic valve opening (*AVO*) which permits LV ejection. (Reproduced with permission from Plotnick GD. Changes in diastolic function—difficult to measure, harder to interpret. *Am Heart J* 1989;118:637–641.)

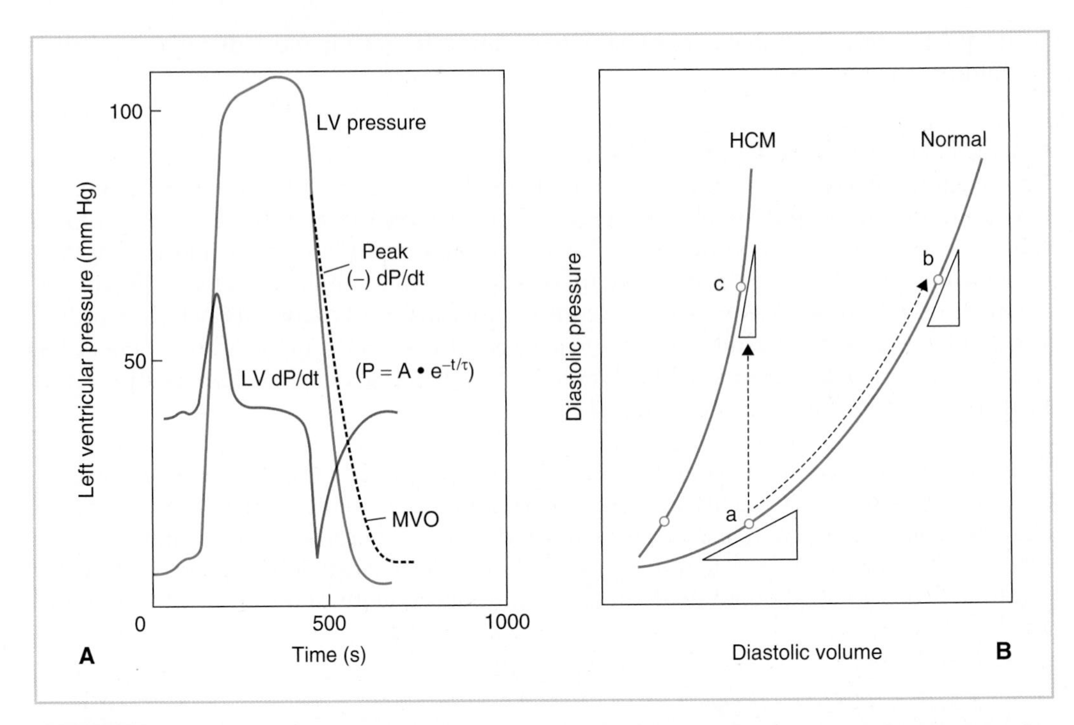

Figure 7.2. **A.** Left ventricular (*LV*) relaxation can be invasively evaluated by measuring the minimum value of the first derivative of ventricular pressure with respect to time ($-dP/dt_{min}$) or preferably, by calculating the time constant time constant (τ) of isovolumic LV pressure decline according to the equation shown. An increase in τ (*dashed line*) generally indicates impaired LV relaxation (myocardial ischemia, hypertrophic heart disease, negative inotropes) which can be associated with decreased LV filling and diminished cardiac performance. P, LV pressure; A, LV pressure at—dP/dt_{min}; t, time after—dP/dt_{min}; e, natural logarithm; MVO, mitral valve opening. (Modified with permission from Zile M, Smith V. Relaxation and diastolic properties of the heart. In: Fozzard H, Haber E, Jennings R, eds. *The heart and cardiovascular system: scientific foundations*, 2nd ed. New York: Raven Press, 1991:353–1367.) **B.** LV pressure-volume (P-V) relationships. LV compliance (*dV/dP*) is described by the tangent drawn to the P-V curve at a particular point. A decrease in LV compliance results in an increase in LV filling pressure depicted as either a shift of the pressure-volume (P-V) curve upward and to the left when myocardial stiffness increases (point *a* → *c*), or to a steeper portion of the curve when volume increases (point *a* → *b*). HCM, hypertrophic cardiomyopathy. (Reproduced with permission from Zile M, Smith V. Relaxation and diastolic properties of the heart. In: Fozzard H, Haber E, Jennings R, eds. *The heart and cardiovascular system: scientific foundations*, 2nd ed. New York: Raven Press, 1991:1353–1367.)

to their original, precontraction length (12). Ventricular relaxation is classically evaluated with high fidelity, manometer-tipped catheters that measure the rate and duration of the LV pressure decrease after systolic contraction during isovolumic relaxation (Figure 7.2A) (13). The time constant of relaxation (τ) is a clinically and experimentally acceptable technique for assessing isovolumic relaxation, although limitations have been described (12). LV chamber compliance is dependent upon the passive properties of the ventricle, and is determined from the exponential relationship between the change in volume and the change in pressure during diastolic filling (dV/dP) (Figure 7.2B) (13).

The left atrial (LA) contribution to left ventricular end-diastolic volume (LVEDV) can also be an important determinant of filling. The LA serves not only as a blood reservoir and passive conduit, but also as an active pump during contraction at end-diastole. The LA contribution to LV diastolic filling is usually less than 20% in young healthy patients, yet may approach 50% in patients with decreased LV filling associated with early diastolic dysfunction.

ECHOCARDIOGRAPHIC EVALUATION OF LEFT VENTRICULAR DIASTOLIC FUNCTION

Conventional, direct assessment of diastolic function requires invasive measurements (high-fidelity, intraventricular, micromanometer catheters) or sophisticated technology (3-D sonomicrometry, cardiac magnetic resonance imaging, ultrafast computed tomography) (12). Pulmonary artery catheterization can be useful for assessing global cardiac performance; however, evaluation of diastolic function is limited by the inability to directly measure LV pressure, volume, or transmitral flow. In contrast, echocardiography provides a relatively safe, practical and noninvasive means to evaluate diastolic function.

Two-Dimensional and M-Mode Echocardiography

Indirect evidence of diastolic function can be obtained during a comprehensive two-dimensional (2-D) echocardiographic examination by assessing LV ejection fraction and LVEDV. Echocardiographic evidence of LV hypertrophy without dilatation and with normal systolic function indicates the presence of DHF in a symptomatic patient. LA enlargement (>4 cm) is often associated with elevated LV filling pressures (14).

Doppler Echocardiographic Evaluation of Left Ventricular Filling: Transmitral Inflow

The utilization of Doppler echocardiography to measure transmitral blood flow (transmitral Doppler flow [TMDF]) velocities provides valuable information towards the assessment of diastolic function. The PWD recording of TMDF velocities is obtained by placing the sample volume at the MV leaflet tips (Figure 7.3). A typical TMDF velocity profile has a biphasic pattern. An initial peak flow velocity (E-wave) occurs during early diastolic filling and a later peak flow velocity (A-wave) occurs during atrial systole. Blood flow during the interposed period of diastasis is usually minimal, because little LV filling occurs during this phase. Several indices of diastolic function have been derived from the TMDF profile and correlated with more classic measures of diastolic function including angiography, radionucleotide techniques and direct measures of intraventricular pressures (Table 7.1) (12,15).

TMDF velocities are determined by the transmitral pressure gradient (TMPG) which is dependent upon several variables including heart rate and rhythm, early filling loads, atrial contractility, MV disease, ventricular septal interactions, the intrinsic LV lusitropic state, and ventricular compliance (6). With normal aging, delayed LV relaxation at any given LV pressure, creates a lower initial TMPG, which results in proportionally less early filling (lower peak E-wave velocity) and a greater, compensatory late filling (higher peak A-wave velocity) accounting for 35% to 40% of LV diastolic inflow. Conversely, more efficient LV relaxation and elastic recoil observed in young adults is associated with predominant early LV filling corresponding with a greater initial TMPG, and a smaller contribution (10%–15%) from atrial contraction. Alternatively, TMPG elevation in patients with decreased LV compliance is primarily due to a progressively increasing left atrial pressure (LAP). Therefore, alterations in LV relaxation and compliance along with consequential changes in LAP alter the TMPG and resulting TMDF profiles. The isovolumic relaxation time (IVRT: the time from cessation of systolic ventricular outflow to the onset LV inflow) is

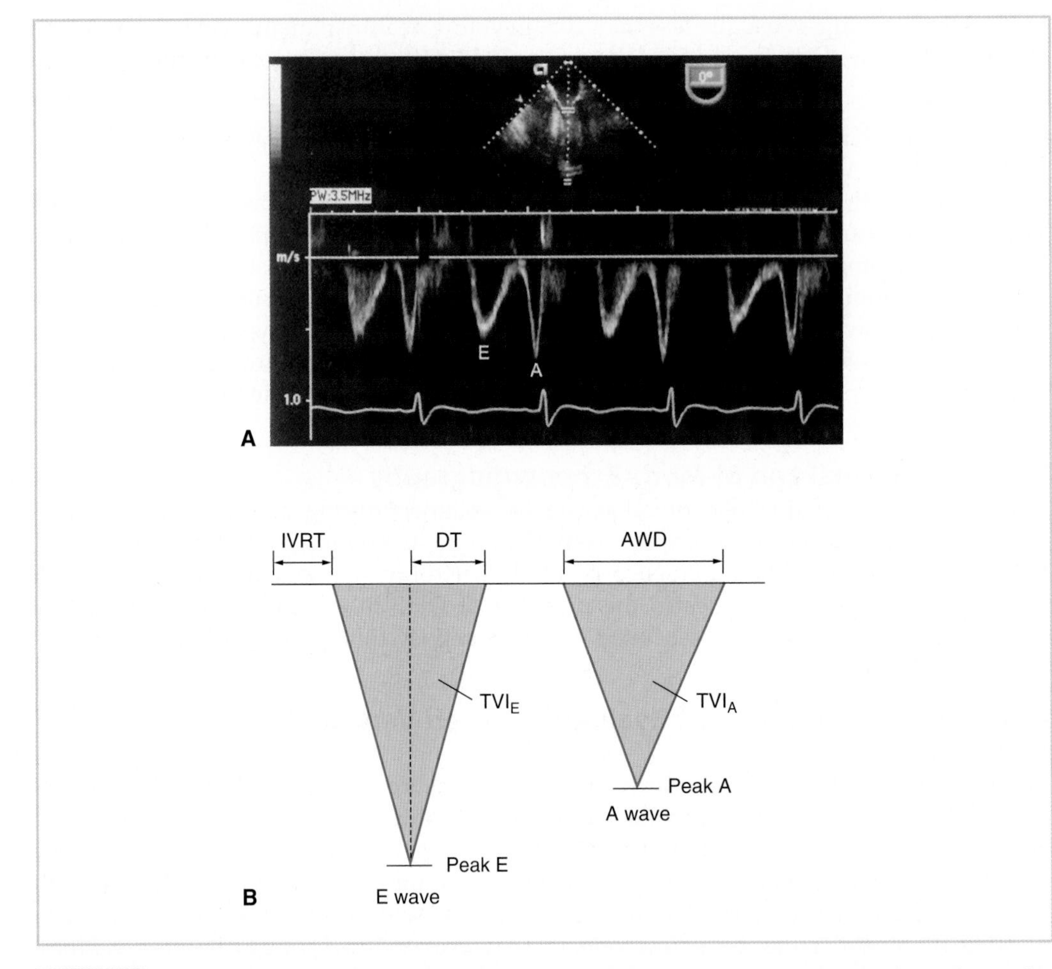

Figure 7.3. A. Transmitral Doppler flow (TMDF) velocity profile using transesophageal echocardiography. The TMDF profile is obtained by placing a pulse wave Doppler sample volume (1–2 mm) at the tips of the mitral valve (*MV*). The initial rapid phase of early left ventricular (*LV*) filling (E) is followed by a variable period of minimal flow (diastasis) and finally late diastolic filling during atrial contraction (A). **B.** Schematic of TMDF profile depicting relevant indices of diastolic function. Several indices of LV diastolic function can be obtained from the TMDF profile including the E- and A-wave peak velocities and ratio, the E- and A-wave time velocity integrals (*TVI*: area under each Doppler envelope) and corresponding E/A TVI ratio, the A-wave duration (*AWD*), the E-wave deceleration time (DT: the time interval from the peak E-wave velocity to the zero baseline), and the isovolumic relaxation time (*IVRT*: the time from cessation of systolic ventricular outflow to the onset of transmitral LV inflow).

also affected by alterations of diastolic function. A shortened IVRT (<60 ms) indicates premature MV opening and can be observed in patients with elevated LAP. Delayed MV opening (IVRT >110 ms) occurs with impaired LV relaxation. The deceleration time (DT; the interval from the peak E-wave velocity to the zero baseline) generally reflects the mean LAP and LV compliance (16). A relatively short DT (<140 ms) can be seen in patients with reduced LV compliance, whereas a prolonged DT is associated with poor LV relaxation.

Changes in LV relaxation and compliance contribute to the spectrum of Doppler LV filling patterns that are observed with progressive diastolic dysfunction. The initial abnormality of

Table 7.1 Left and right ventricular Doppler echocardiographic indices of diastolic function filling dynamics in normal subjects

	Age 21–49 y	Age≥50 y
Left ventricular inflow		
Peak E (cm/s)	72 (44–100)	62 (34–90)
Peak A (cm/s)	40 (20–60)	59 (31–87)
E/A ratio	1.9 (0.7–3.1)	1.1 (0.5–1.7)
DT (ms)	179 (139–219)	210 (138–282)
IVRT (ms)	76 (54–98)	90 (56–124)
Pulmonary Vein		
Peak S (cm/s)	48 (30–66)	71 (53–89)
Peak D (cm/s)	50 (30–70)	38 (20–56)
S/D ratio	1.0 (0.5–1.5)	1.7 (0.8–2.6)
Peak A (cm/s)	19 (11–27)	23 (−5 to 51)
Right ventricular inflow		
Peak E (cm/s)	51 (37–65)	41 (25–57)
Peak A (cm/s)	27 (11–43)	33 (17–49)
E/A	2.0 (1.0–3.0)	1.3 (0.5–2.1)
DT (cm/s)	188 (144–232)	198 (152–244)
Superior vena cava		
Peak S (cm/s)	41 (23–59)	42 (18–66)
Peak D (cm/s)	22 (12–32)	22 (12–32)
Peak A (cm/s)	13 (7–19)	16 (10–22)

Normal reference values for Doppler echocardiographic indices of ventricular diastolic function in two age groups of normal subjects. Data presented are mean values (confidence interval). E, early diastolic flow velocity; A, late diastolic atrial flow velocity associated with atrial contraction; DT, deceleration time; IVRT, isovolumic relaxation time; S, systolic flow velocity; D, diastolic flow velocity.
Reproduced with permission from Cohen G, Pietrolungo J, Thomas J, et al. A practical guide to assessment of ventricular diastolic function using Doppler echocardiography. *J Am Coll Cardiol* 1996;27:1754.

diastolic filling in most disorders of cardiac physiology is impaired myocardial relaxation exceeding that expected with aging alone. Impaired LV relaxation occurs with myocardial ischemia/infarction LV hypertrophy, hypertrophic cardiomyopathy, and in the early stages of infiltrative disorders (17). The TMDF profile associated with *impaired relaxation* is typically characterized by a prolonged IVRT and a decreased initial TMPG (Figure 7.4) (18). Consequently, the peak E-wave velocity decreases relative to the peak A-wave velocity when LV relaxation is impaired (E/A <1), because the MV tends to open before relaxation is complete. In addition, the duration of LV relaxation is prolonged resulting in a prolonged DT (11) because the LA-LV pressure gradient takes longer to equilibrate. There is a subsequent, compensatory flow increase during atrial contraction accounting for the increased peak A-wave velocity, time velocity integral (TVI) and duration due to the relatively high atrial preload. Therefore, the TMDF velocity profile with impaired relaxation is characterized by "E/A reversal" (decreased peak E-wave velocity and increased peak A-wave velocity), prolonged IVRT, and prolonged DT.

Diastolic dysfunction associated with markedly decreased LV compliance and severely increased LAP is often described as a "restrictive" LV filling disorder (17). The TMDF profile associated with a *restrictive pattern* of LV diastolic dysfunction is characterized

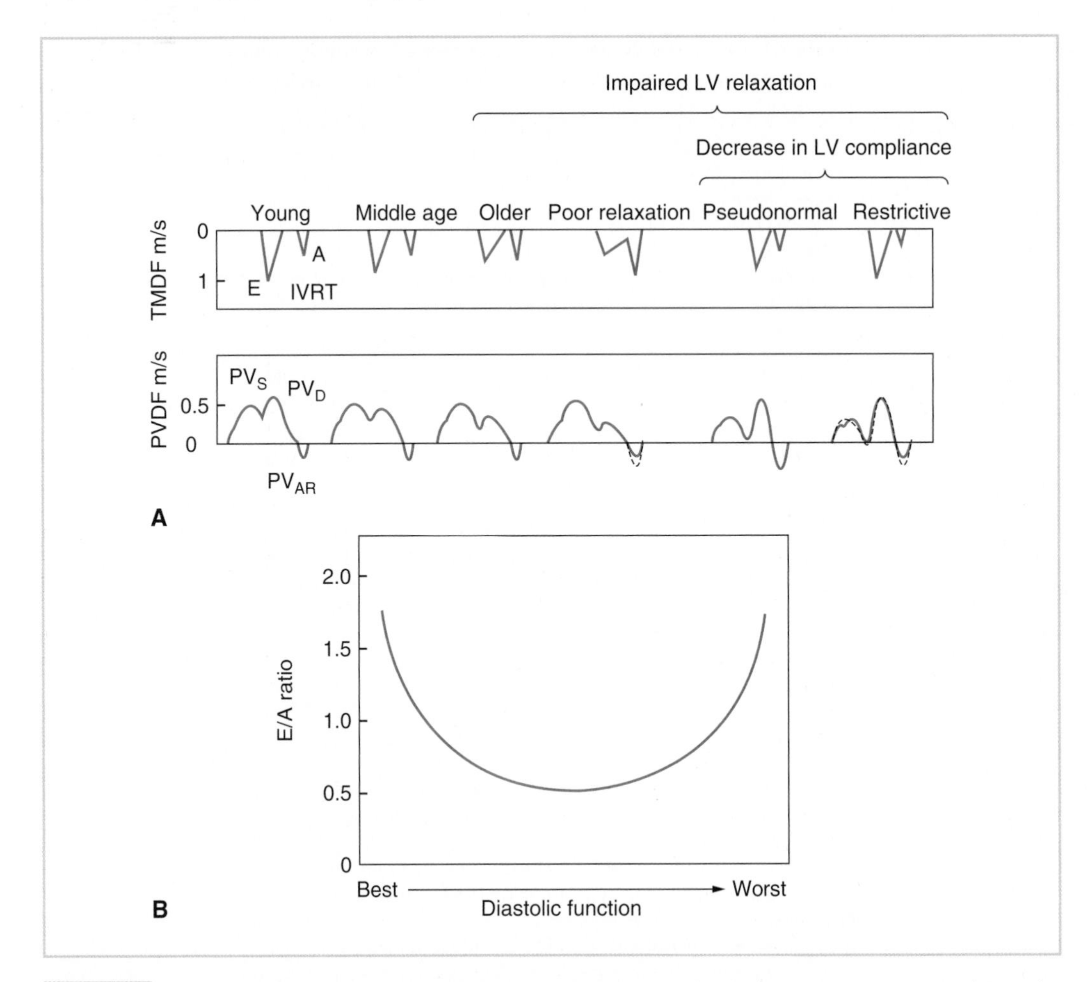

Figure 7.4. A. The impact of progressive left ventricular (*LV*) diastolic dysfunction on transmitral Doppler flow (TMDF) and pulmonary venous Doppler flow (*PVDF*) velocity profiles. Note that all pulsed Doppler indices of the TMDF and PVDF profiles present a parabolic distribution over the progression from normal to advanced diastolic dysfunction. The transmitral pressure gradient is initially elevated in normal, young individuals due to vigorous LV relaxation and elastic recoil, before diminishing when relaxation becomes impaired, and finally increasing again when left atrial pressure increases due to an elevated LV end-diastolic pressure in the restrictive pattern of LV diastolic dysfunction. Respective changes are noted in the pulmonary vein (PV) profile. E, E-wave; A, A-wave; IVRT, left ventricular isovolumic relaxation time; PV_{AR}, late diastolic retrograde velocity; PV_{S1}, first systolic component; PV_{S2}, second systolic component; PV_D, diastolic component. **B.** Parabolic distribution of transmitral E/A velocity ratios associated with progressive diastolic dysfunction. (Modified with permission from Appleton C, Hatle L. The natural history of left ventricular filling abnormalities: assessment by two-dimensional and Doppler echocardiography. *Echocardiography* 1992;9:437–457.)

by an elevated peak E-wave velocity relative to the A-wave velocity due to the elevated LAP (Figure 7.4) (18). Although impaired relaxation coexists with decreased compliance when diastolic dysfunction has progressed, the consequential increase in left ventricular end-diastolic pressure (LVEDP) results in a markedly elevated LAP and an elevated peak E-wave velocity, consistent with very rapid filling during early diastole. The IVRT is shortened as the MV opens prematurely due to the elevated LAP. The DT is also abnormally short, as early transmitral flow into the poorly compliant LV results in rapid equilibration of LA and LV pressures that may even be associated with diastolic mitral regurgitation (MR) (17). Finally, the peak A velocity and duration tend to be compromised by poor atrial contractility and the rapid increase in LV pressure, which can prematurely terminate late mitral inflow. Therefore, a restrictive TMDF velocity profile is characterized by an elevated peak E-wave velocity and decreased peak A-wave velocity (E/A ratio >2.0) along with a shortened IVRT and DT.

Typically, there is a progression of diastolic dysfunction from impaired relaxation to restrictive pathophysiology. During this transition, the TMDF profile may assume a *pseudonormalized pattern* that resembles normal LV filling (Figure 7.4A) (18). The pseudonormalized filling pattern represents a moderate stage of diastolic dysfunction where a "normal" early TMPG is generated by the balance between compromised LV relaxation and gradually increasing filling pressures as LV compliance decreases. Consequently, for varying degrees of diastolic dysfunction, the spectrum of E/A velocity ratios assumes a parabolic shape beginning with a vigorous LV relaxation pattern seen in young, athletic individuals and terminating with a similar-appearing restrictive pattern consistent with severe diastolic dysfunction (Figure 7.4B). The intermediate, pseudonormalized stage of diastolic dysfunction is therefore characterized by normal values for peak E-wave and A-wave velocities, IVRT, and DT. Reducing preload by utilizing reverse Trendelenburg positioning, partial CPB, a Valsalva maneuver (19) or by administering nitroglycerin may also reveal underlying impaired LV relaxation in a patient with pseudonormalized transmitral inflow (20). Healthy individuals usually respond to preload reduction with a more proportional decrease in both E- and A-wave velocities (17). Preload reduction may also be useful in grading the severity of diastolic dysfunction (20). For example, a restrictive pattern is considered "irreversible, end-stage" if it doesn't pseudonormalize in response to preload reduction (10).

Doppler Echocardiographic Evaluation of Left Atrial Filling: Pulmonary Venous Flow

The evaluation of LA filling can provide important insight into the assessment of LV diastolic function especially when combined with data obtained from the TMDF. A typical pulmonary venous Doppler flow (PVDF) profile consists of an antegrade systolic velocity which may appear monophasic, or biphasic, especially in the presence of low LAP probably owing to temporal dissociation of atrial relaxation and mitral annular motion (Figure 7.5) (21). The first systolic component, PV_{S1}, is dependent upon LA relaxation and the subsequent decrease in pressure. The later peaking PV_{S2}, reflects right ventricular (RV) stroke volume, LA compliance, the effects of early ventricular systole on LAP and any concomitant MR. An additional, large antegrade velocity occurs during diastole (PV_D) following early transmitral inflow whereas the LA serves as an open conduit between the PV and LV. The late diastolic retrograde velocity, also known as *pulmonary venous atrial flow reversal* (PV_{AR}), occurs during LA systole and is dependent on LA contractility, heart rate, and compliance of the LA, PV, and LV (6).

Normally, the PV systolic peak amplitude and TVI are equal to or slightly greater than the corresponding PV_D values (Table 7.1) (15). A reduced systolic fraction (systolic TVI divided by the sum of systolic and diastolic TVI) less than 40% has been correlated with increased mean LAP (22). In addition, the normal PV_{AR} (~90–115 ms) duration is the same or less than the transmitral A-wave duration (AWD) (~120–140 ms) (16). In general, LA contraction should result in a greater net forward blood volume and flow toward a normal,

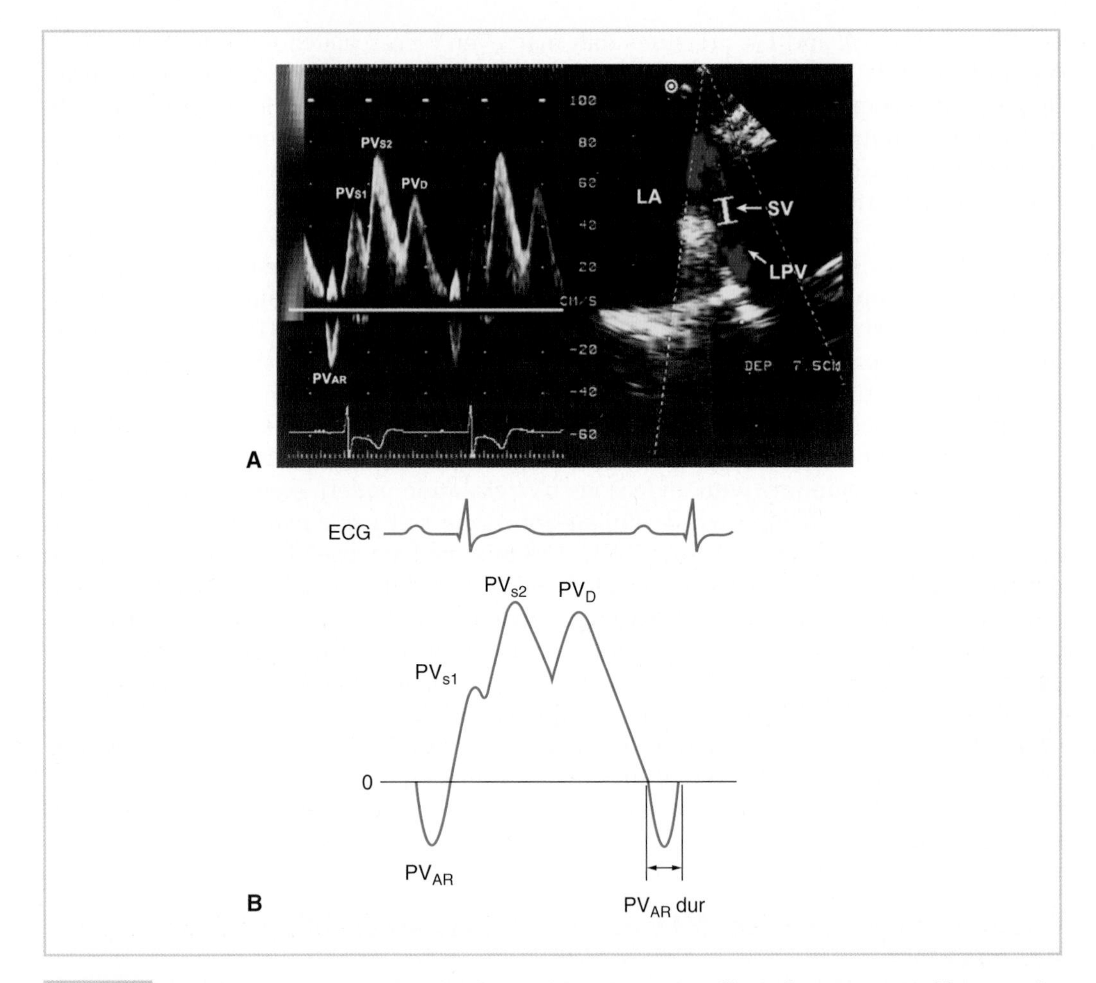

Figure 7.5. A. Pulmonary venous Doppler flow velocity (PVDF) profile. Left atrium (LA) filling can be assessed by placing a pulse wave Doppler sample volume (2–4 mm) approximately 1.0 cm into a pulmonary vein (PV) orifice where it joins the LA. **B.** Schematic of PVDF profile depicting relevant indices of diastolic function. Indices of left ventricular (LV) diastolic function obtained from the PVDF include the peak S/D velocity ratio, as well as the peak A-wave reversal velocity and duration. LPV, left pulmonary vein; SV, sample volume; ECG, echocardiography; PV_{S1}, first systolic component; PV_{S2}, second systolic component; PV_D, diastolic component; PV_{AR}, late diastolic retrograde velocity; PV_{AR} dur, PV_{AR}—wave duration.

compliant LV compared with any retrograde flow back towards the PV. A PV_{AR} velocity that exceeds the mitral A-wave by greater than 35 cm/s or PV_{AR} duration greater than 30 ms longer than the transmitral AWD usually indicates an age-independent elevation in LVEDP (23).

The analysis of PVDF compliments the assessment of TMDF in the evaluation of various stages of diastolic dysfunction (Figure 7.4). The PVDF profile consistent with impaired LV relaxation is characterized by a reduced PV_D velocity that parallels the mitral E-wave velocity, and a compensatory increase in the PV_S velocity, resulting in a pattern of *systolic predominance*. Conversely, the systolic antegrade velocity is reduced when LV filling is restrictive, because of the elevated LAP and decreased LV compliance resulting in a pattern of *systolic blunting*. A greater proportion of antegrade flow occurs during diastole, although the PV_D DT is usually shortened analogous to the rapid deceleration of the transmitral E-wave velocity. The PV_{AR} velocity and duration may be prolonged in the presence of restrictive pathophysiology due to decreased LV compliance and associated increase in LAP, which can promote retrograde flow. Alternatively, the PV_{AR} velocity may be diminished in patients with severe, irreversible restrictive filling, due to atrial mechanical failure (24). The pseudonormalized PVDF velocity profile is often characterized by a pattern of relative systolic blunting and a prolonged PV_{AR} duration and velocity compared with the transmitral AWD depending upon the LAP and degree of reduced LV compliance (Figure 7.4). In this scenario, the PVDF pattern may be helpful in distinguishing a pseudonormal from normal TMDF profile. However, in healthy young adults and athletes who don't rely on a significant LA contribution for LV filling, the LA behaves more like a "passive conduit", and PVs blunting may be commonly observed (24).

Influence of Physiologicl Variables on Left Atrial and Left Ventricular Doppler Flow Profiles

The TMDF and PVDF profiles are considered useful for evaluating LV diastolic function in both nonsurgical and surgical patient populations. The utility of these echocardiographic parameters throughout the perioperative period is limited, however, by the unavoidable effects of changes in preload, afterload, heart rate, and rhythm on peak velocities and proportions of early and late filling (25). Increases in preload will often be associated with a more proportionate increase in the transmitral peak E-wave velocity, a shortened IVRT and steeper DT. The opposite changes will occur with decreases in preload. MR may produce a TMDF velocity profile with an increased E-wave velocity due to the elevated LAP and increased volume flow rate across the MV. Isolated LV systolic dysfunction may be also be associated with an increased transmitral peak E-wave velocity and reduced A-wave because diastolic filling occurs at a steeper portion of the LV pressure-volume curve (26). Finally, the location of the PWD sample volume and respiratory pattern can also affect the TMDF profile (27).

Tachycardia causes fusion of the transmitral E- and A-wave velocities and a pseudo-increase in the A-wave velocity and duration especially if the *E- at A-wave velocity* is greater than 20 cm/s (6). Dysrhythmias and pacing may also be associated with unique alterations in the TMDF and PVDF profiles. For example, atrial flutter may present with "flutter waves" in the TMDF profile. In patients with atrial fibrillation (AF), the transmitral and PV_{AR} waves are absent and the E-wave peak velocity and DT vary with the length of the cardiac cycle. AF may also be associated with a loss of PV_{S1}, and a decreased PV_{S2} relative to the dominant PV_D (28). Peak acceleration rate of the E-wave velocity (29), transmitral E-wave DT shortening, and the duration and initial deceleration slope time of PV_D may still correlate with increased LV filling pressure in the presence of AF (28).

Newer Echocardiographic Techniques for Assessing Left Ventricular Diastolic Function: Mitral Annular Doppler Tissue Imaging and Color M-Mode Transmitral Propagation Velocity

MITRAL ANNULAR MOTION ASSESSED WITH DOPPLER TISSUE IMAGING

Recently, newer echocardiographic techniques for assessing LV diastolic function have been described, which are reportedly less vulnerable to the effects of acute changes in loading conditions. Mitral annular motion is evaluated with Doppler tissue imaging (DTI), a technique which utilizes a low velocity, high amplitude signal to eliminate high velocities associated with blood flow, and provides a signal with high temporal and velocity range resolution (30). Initial studies describing the utilization of DTI to evaluate mitral annular motion used transthoracic echocardiography and a four- or two-chamber apical acoustic window. A midesophageal four-chamber view obtained with a transesophageal echocardiography (TEE) probe is also an appropriate window to position a PWD sample volume (2.5–5 mm) on the lateral corner of the mitral annulus (Figure 7.6). Alternatively, the septal side of the mitral annulus can be evaluated although the tissue velocities tend to be lower and blood flow velocities in the LV outflow tract may obscure the tissue Doppler profile (31). The PWD Doppler beam should be aligned as parallel as possible to the longitudinal axial motion of the LV. It is important to realize that these recorded velocities not only represent the rate of myocardial fiber shortening and lengthening of a specifically selected segment at the level of the mitral annulus, but are also influenced by velocities associated with translation and rotation of cardiac structures (32). The lowest wall filter and minimal optimal gain should be used to eliminate blood flow velocity signals produced by transmitral flow. Finally the Nyquist limit, sweep speed, and size of the Doppler profile should be adjusted for optimal visualization.

The mitral annular DTI profile has a systolic component, which has been shown to correlate with ejection fraction (31), and a biphasic diastolic component that appears as an exact mirror image of the TMDF profile except that the tissue velocities are much lower in magnitude (8–15 cm/s). The initial, early diastolic tissue velocity (E′) begins simultaneously with mitral inflow, yet its peak precedes the peak transmitral E-wave velocity and ends before LV inflow termination (33). In the absence of gross geometric distortion and severe regional wall motion abnormalities, E′ reflects tissue velocities associated with changes in LV volume and is primarily influenced by the rate of myocardial relaxation and elastic recoil. In the healthy patient, the peak E′ velocity is greater than the later diastolic tissue velocity (A′), which tends to reflect LA systolic function (34).

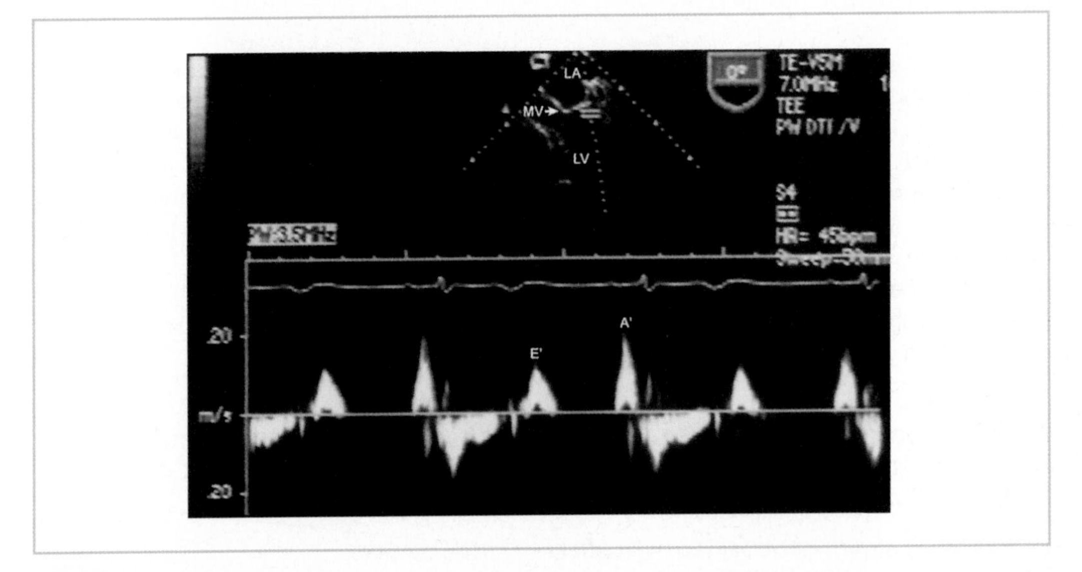

Figure 7.6. Mitral annular motion assessed with Doppler tissue imaging (DTI). The pulse wave Doppler sample volume is positioned at the level of the lateral mitral valve annulus to obtain the DTI profile. The mitral annular DTI profile has a biphasic diastolic component that includes an initial early (E′) and a later (A′) diastolic tissue velocity. LA, left atrium; LV, left ventricle.

E′ has been demonstrated to correlate with τ, supporting its value as an index of LV relaxation (30). E′ and E′/A′ have also been shown to decline with age and are reduced in pathologic LV hypertrophy similar to transmitral inflow velocities (31,32). The concordance between mitral annular motion assessed by DTI and mitral inflow velocities, however, is disrupted with progressive diastolic dysfunction when poor relaxation coexists with an elevated filling pressures. In patients with elevated LVEDP who present with a pseudonormal (32) or restrictive transmitral Doppler inflow velocity profile (33), E′ remains reduced suggesting relative preload independence (Figure 7.7). In fact, E′ has actually been shown to be the best discriminator between normal and pseudonormal patterns when compared to any single or combined index of TMDF or PVDF profiles (30). Furthermore, neither peak E′ velocity nor E′/A′ velocity ratio change significantly after preload alteration with a saline infusion or nitroglycerin (34). Therefore, E′ is a relatively preload-insensitive measure of LV diastolic function that may be particularly useful in the perioperative period when loading conditions can vary considerably.

COLOR M-MODE TRANSMITRAL PROPAGATION VELOCITY

The onset of active LV relaxation is asynchronous, initially starting in apical myocardial segments which serve as a prominent source of recoil during early diastole (35). Early LV relaxation generates a suction force that creates an intraventricular pressure gradient initiated at the level of the mitral orifice. This pressure gradient is maintained in the mid-LV during early diastole and is responsible for accelerating flow and promoting sequential filling towards the apex (35).

The propagation rate of LV peak inflow velocity that is driven by rapid ventricular relaxation can be evaluated using color M-mode Doppler echocardiography. Although standard PWD permits only a temporal distribution of blood flow velocities in a single spatial location, color M-mode Doppler echocardiography provides a spatiotemporal distribution of these velocities, which can be used to delineate the slope of the propagating

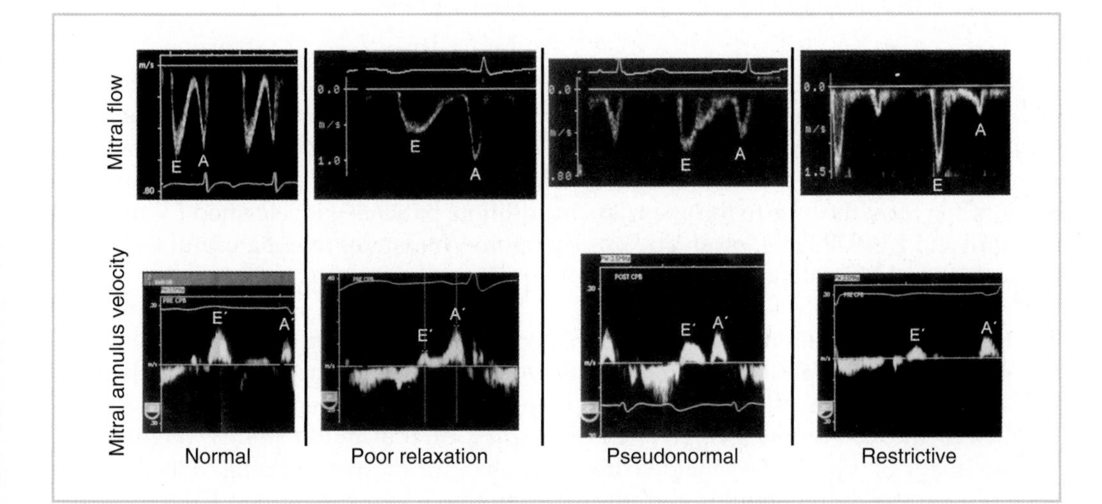

Figure 7.7. Patterns of mitral inflow (E, A) and mitral annular velocities (E′, A′) associated with progressive left ventricular diastolic dysfunction. Although both E/A and E′/A′ decrease with delayed relaxation, the concordance is disrupted with progressive patterns of diastolic dysfunction. E′/A′ remains reduced with the pseudonormalization and restrictive patterns supporting the utility of E′ as a measure of left ventricular (LV) relaxation, and its relative insensitivity to preload compensation.

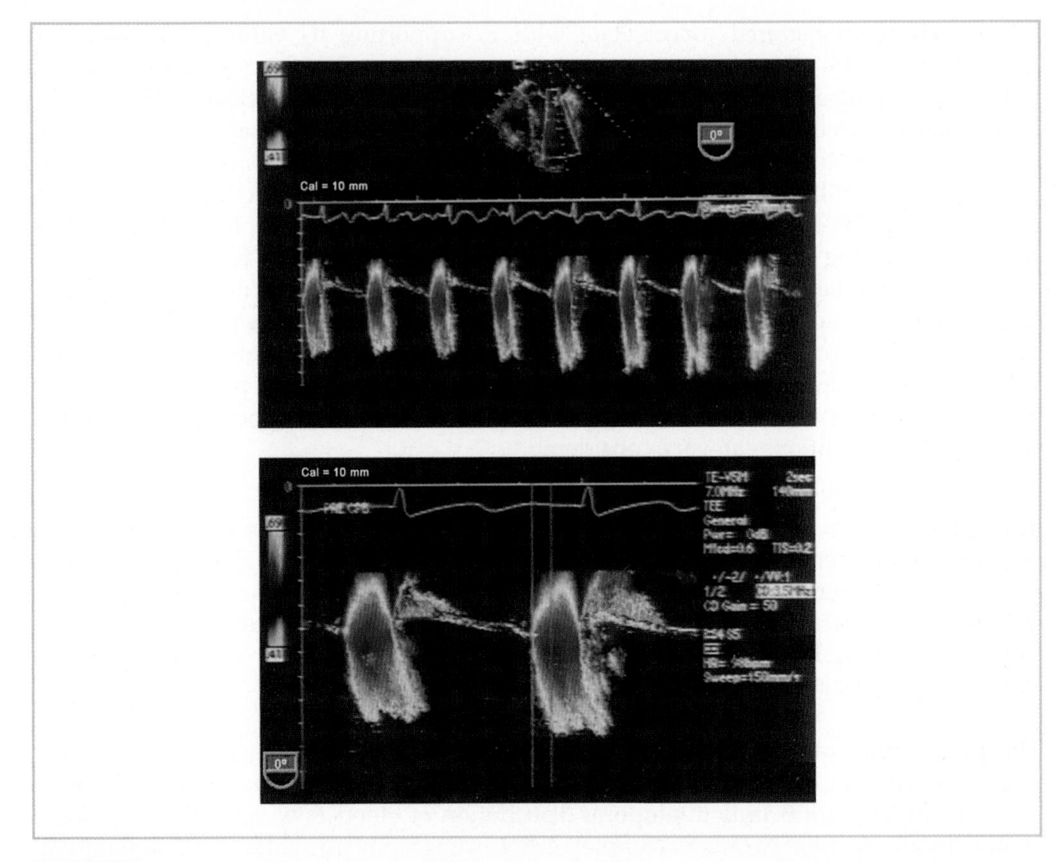

Figure 7.8. Transmitral color M-mode Doppler flow propagation velocity (Vp) is obtained by placing the M-mode cursor through the center of the mitral inflow region in a transesophageal midesophageal four-chamber view, and measuring the slope of the first aliasing velocity.

wave front (Vp) from the mitral orifice toward the LV apex (32). The velocity at which flow propagates within the ventricle (Vp) can be determined from the slope of the color wavefront (Figure 7.8). A significant negative correlation between Vp and τ has been demonstrated and suggests that rapid LV relaxation (short τ) promotes faster propagation of LV filling from the base to the apex (36). In addition, patients with elevated LV minimal pressure and LVEDP have lower Vp (35). Therefore Vp may represent a useful technique for evaluating LV diastolic function.

The technique for obtaining color M-mode Doppler images of LV filling is often described using transthoracic, apical long-axis acoustic windows. A midesophageal, four-chamber TEE view also permits visualization of Vp when an M-mode Doppler beam is aligned parallel to the color flow Doppler (CFD) display of transmitral inflow (Figure 7.8). Measurement of Vp can be obtained from the slope of the first aliasing velocity slope beginning at the mitral annulus and ideally extending 3 to 4 cm into the LV toward the apex (32). Visualization of the color wave front can be optimized by shifting the baseline towards the direction of flow, maximizing sweep speed and adjusting the depth.

In young healthy individuals, color M-mode Vp has been reported between 55 and 100 cm/s (36). Impaired LV relaxation results in a diminished ventricular minimal

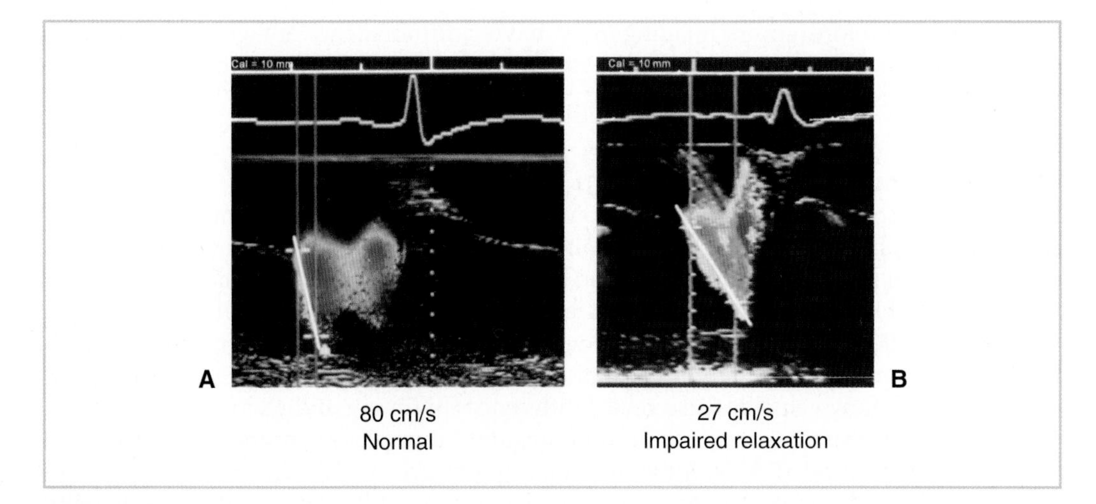

Figure 7.9. In comparison to the normal patient (**A**), the transmitral color M-mode propagation velocity (Vp) is reduced when left ventricular relaxation is impaired (**B**).

pressure, thereby compromising the propagation of early filling (Figure 7.9). In contrast to standard Doppler filling indices, Vp is relatively independent of preload, yet responds to changes in lusitropic conditions (37) and systolic performance (38). Consequently, while TMDF and PVDF tend to show a parabolic distribution from normal through progressive diastolic dysfunction, Vp remains reduced with pseudonormal or restrictive LV filling. Furthermore, altering preload by utilizing various techniques (partial CPB, inferior vena cava (IVC) occlusion, intravenous nitroglycerin, amyl nitrate inhalation, Valsalva maneuver, Trendelenburg positioning, leg lifting) is associated with changes in transmitral peak E-wave velocity, E/A-wave velocity and E-wave deceleration, but has little affect on Vp (38–40). Interestingly, the ratio of peak E-wave velocity/propagation velocity (E/Vp) may be useful to predict LAP (38) and also relates directly with LV filling pressures in patients with AF (29). Vp has also been shown to improve significantly after both on-pump and off-pump coronary artery bypass graft surgery (41). Therefore, like E′, Vp is a relatively preload-insensitive measure of LV diastolic function that may be particularly useful in the perioperative period when loading conditions can vary considerably (7).

STRAIN AND STRAIN RATE

Strain imaging is a relatively new echocardiographic modality derived from DTI, which uses low velocity and high amplitude signals to determine velocity gradients between two myocardial point locations (42,43). Strain (S) is the deformation of tissue as a function of applied forces (stress), while strain rate (SR) is a measure of the rate of tissue deformation. Diastolic deformation of the LV can be analyzed with strain imaging and Vp to describe both early and late filling. In a series of 26 patients with hypertension, normal systolic function and impaired diastolic function, Stoylen et al. demonstrated that both the peak diastolic SR and Vp are reduced (44). In addition Hoffman et al. demonstrated in patients with ischemic LV dysfunction, that SR analysis can detect differences in diastolic function between viable and nonviable myocardial segments (45). Both SR and S imaging are angle dependent. However, they are generally used in long-axis views to measure longitudinal shortening (systolic function) or lengthening (diastolic function) of the LV along the ultrasound beam. Consequently, unlike DTI, both S and SR are relatively independent of translational or rotational movement. Therefore strain imaging may have additional advantages over conventional echocardiography techniques for evaluating diastolic function in the perioperative period.

Right Ventricular Diastolic Function

Indirect evidence of RV diastolic function can be obtained from a comprehensive 2-D echocardiographic examination by examining RV mass or volume. A thorough assessment of RV diastolic function, however, requires a Doppler echocardiographic evaluation of transtricuspid blood flow velocities (Figure 7.10A). Transtricuspid Doppler flow (TTDF) velocities are affected by the same physiologic variables that affect LV filling although they tend to be lower due to the larger tricuspid valve (TV) annular size. Direct comparisons of RV and LV inflow velocities also reveal differences in timing and reciprocal respiratory variation. During spontaneous inspiration, negative intrapleural pressure results in an increase in right atrial (RA) volume and subsequent greater RV diastolic filling velocities up to 20% compared to end-expiratory values (26). LA and LV filling is actually reduced during spontaneous inspiration relative to end-expiration. These reciprocal patterns of respiratory variation become exaggerated in patients with diastolic dysfunction. Although not thoroughly investigated, positive pressure ventilation (PPV) would presumably have an opposite effect on TTDF velocity patterns in comparison to spontaneous ventilation.

The echocardiographic evaluation of RV diastolic function also includes an assessment of RA inflow velocities including the hepatic venous (HV) IVC and superior vena cava (SVC) Doppler profiles, all of which have similar contours and components. The HVs join the intrahepatic IVC tangentially, and can be visualized by advancing and turning the TEE probe rightward from a midesophageal, bicaval acoustic view. The normal HV Doppler profile (Figure 7.10B) is characterized by (a) a small reversal of flow following atrial contraction (*AR-wave*), (b) an antegrade systolic phase during atrial filling from the SVC and IVC (*S-wave*) that is influenced by TV annular motion, RA relaxation, and tricuspid regurgitation (TR), (c) a second small flow reversal at end-systole (*V-wave*) that is influenced by RV and RA compliance, and (d) a second antegrade filling phase while the RA acts as a passive conduit during RV filling (*D-wave*) (26).

Diastolic RV dysfunction can manifest with the same relative changes in transtricuspid peak E- and A-wave velocities, E/A wave ratios and DT that occur with TMDF profiles associated with alterations in LV relaxation and compliance (46,47). The ratio of the total hepatic reverse flow integral/total forward flow integral ($TVI_A + TVI_V/TVI_S + TVI_D$) increases with either RV diastolic dysfunction or significant TR, but appears to be more affected by the former (48). In addition, a marked shortening of the transtricuspid DT and diastolic predominance of HV flow with prominent V- and A-wave reversals during spontaneous inspiration, indicates significant decreases in RV compliance and increased diastolic filling pressures (Figure 7.10C) (6). Changes in IVC diameter during spontaneous inspiration also reflect right atrial pressure (RAP). In general, low RAP (0 to 5 mm Hg) is associated with a small IVC (<1.5 cm diameter) and a spontaneous inspiratory collapse greater than 50% of the original diameter. In contrast, significant increases in RAP (>20 mm Hg) are associated with dilated IVC and HVs, with little respiratory variation (26). Diastolic RV dysfunction (lower TV peak E-wave velocity, lower E/A ratios, and prolonged RV IVRT) has also been demonstrated in patients with pulmonary hypertension (PHT) and in those with symptomatic CHF even in the absence

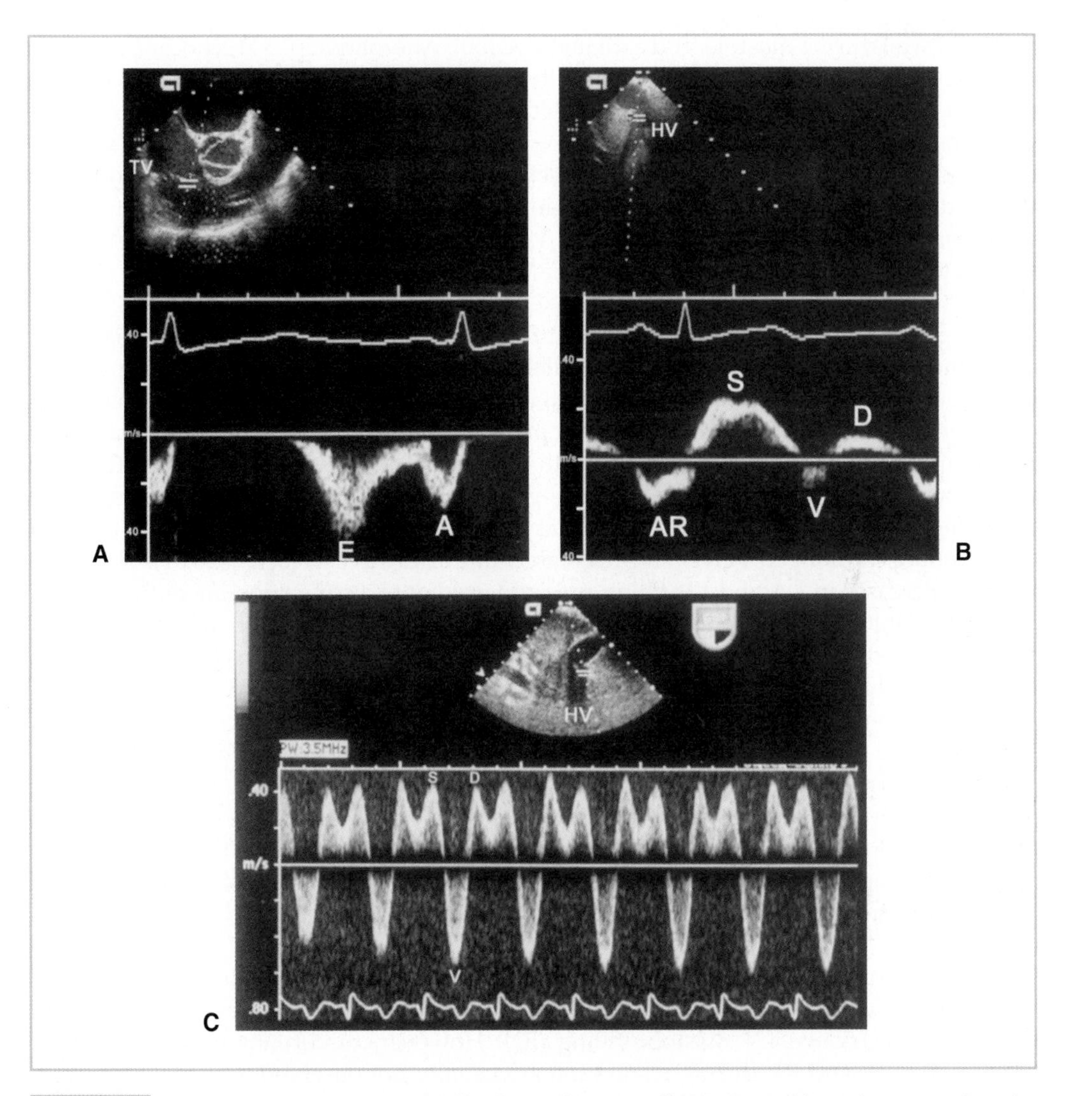

Figure 7.10. **A.** Normal transtricuspid Doppler flow velocity profile. **B.** Normal hepatic venous Doppler flow velocity profiles. **C.** Prominent hepatic flow reversal at end-systole (V) in a patient with decreased right ventricular compliance. TV, tricuspid valve, HV, hepatic vein; S, antegrade early systolic flow; D, antegrade flow during right ventricular filling; E, early diastolic velocity; A, late diastolic velocity; AR, atrial contraction flow reversal.

of PHT, suggesting a potential role for ventricular interdependence in impaired RV filling (49).

Pericardial Disease: Constrictive Pericarditis and Pericardial Tamponade

Pericardial pathology, including constrictive pericarditis (CP) and pericardial tamponade (PT) from effusions can impede diastolic flow. Although chest radiography and magnetic resonance imaging may be helpful in diagnosing pericardial disease, echocardiography continues to be essential for delineating associated pathophysiology. 2-D echocardiography can be helpful in diagnosing CP by identifying a thickened, fibrotic, and calcified echogenic pericardium together with abnormal ventricular septal motion, flattening of the LV posterior wall during diastole, and a dilated IVC (50). Alternatively, 2-D echocardiographic identification of pericardial effusions usually reveals an echo-free space that may contain thrombi. Although small (<25 mL), loculated effusions can be difficult to visualize, larger effusions associated with PT pathophysiology are usually accompanied by additional 2-D echocardiographic and M-mode features including persistence of the effusion throughout the cardiac cycle, a characteristic "swinging motion" of the heart, early diastolic RV collapse, late diastolic to early systolic RA inversion, and abnormal ventricular septal motion (50).

The diagnosis of CP and PT includes identification of significant respiratory variation in atrial and ventricular Doppler inflow profiles. Normally during spontaneous respiration, intrathoracic pressures are transmitted equally to the pericardial space and intracardiac chambers. The transmission of intrathoracic pressure, however, is shielded by the thickened noncompliant pericardium in patients with CP and by significant pericardial effusions. Consequently, LA and LV filling pressure gradients are decreased during spontaneous *inspiration*, resulting in diminished pulmonary venous forward diastolic velocities, delayed MV opening, prolonged IVRT, and decreased mitral E-wave velocity (28,51). Similarly, relative increases in LA and LV filling pressure gradients during spontaneous *expiration*, are responsible for corresponding increases in LA and LV Doppler inflow velocities. Exaggeration of ventricular interdependence with CP and PT is responsible for reciprocal changes in right-sided intracardiac flows, resulting in increased tricuspid E-wave velocities during spontaneous inspiration. In addition, HV forward velocities decrease and reverse flows increase during expiration (52). Because intrathoracic pressure changes associated with PPV are opposite in direction from those seen with spontaneous breathing, mechanical ventilation reverses the respiratory variation pattern of LA and LV inflow velocities seen with CP (53). Therefore, the demonstration of respiratory variation in atrial and ventricular Doppler inflow profiles can be a useful technique to establish the diagnosis of hemodynamically significant pericardial pathology.

The distinction between restriction and constriction may be difficult to determine from LV and LA Doppler inflow velocities alone because both disorders may present with profiles resembling restrictive LV diastolic filling (51). However, discordant pressure changes between the LV and RV during respiration are usually not observed with restrictive cardiomyopathy. Consequently, CP can be differentiated from restrictive cardiomyopathy by demonstrating respiratory variation in TMDF and PVDF (54). Furthermore, patients with CP and preserved systolic function compared to those with restrictive cardiomyopathy, have more rapid Vp (55) and normal or elevated E′ (56).

SUMMARY

Normal diastolic function is required for optimal cardiac performance. Impaired ventricular filling and increased chamber stiffness are responsible for a significant component of the pathophysiology associated with CHF. Diastolic dysfunction is prevalent amongst cardiovascular surgical patients and may contribute to perioperative morbidity. Echocardiography provides an effective, noninvasive means for diagnosing the presence, extent, and etiology of diastolic dysfunction (Figure 7.11; Table 7.2). Although conventional Doppler echocardiographic measurements of atrial and ventricular inflow velocities are still an important component of a thorough examination, newer techniques including mitral annular DTI and color M-mode transmitral Vp, may be less sensitive to changes in loading conditions. In the near future, the availability of more sensitive, cost-effective

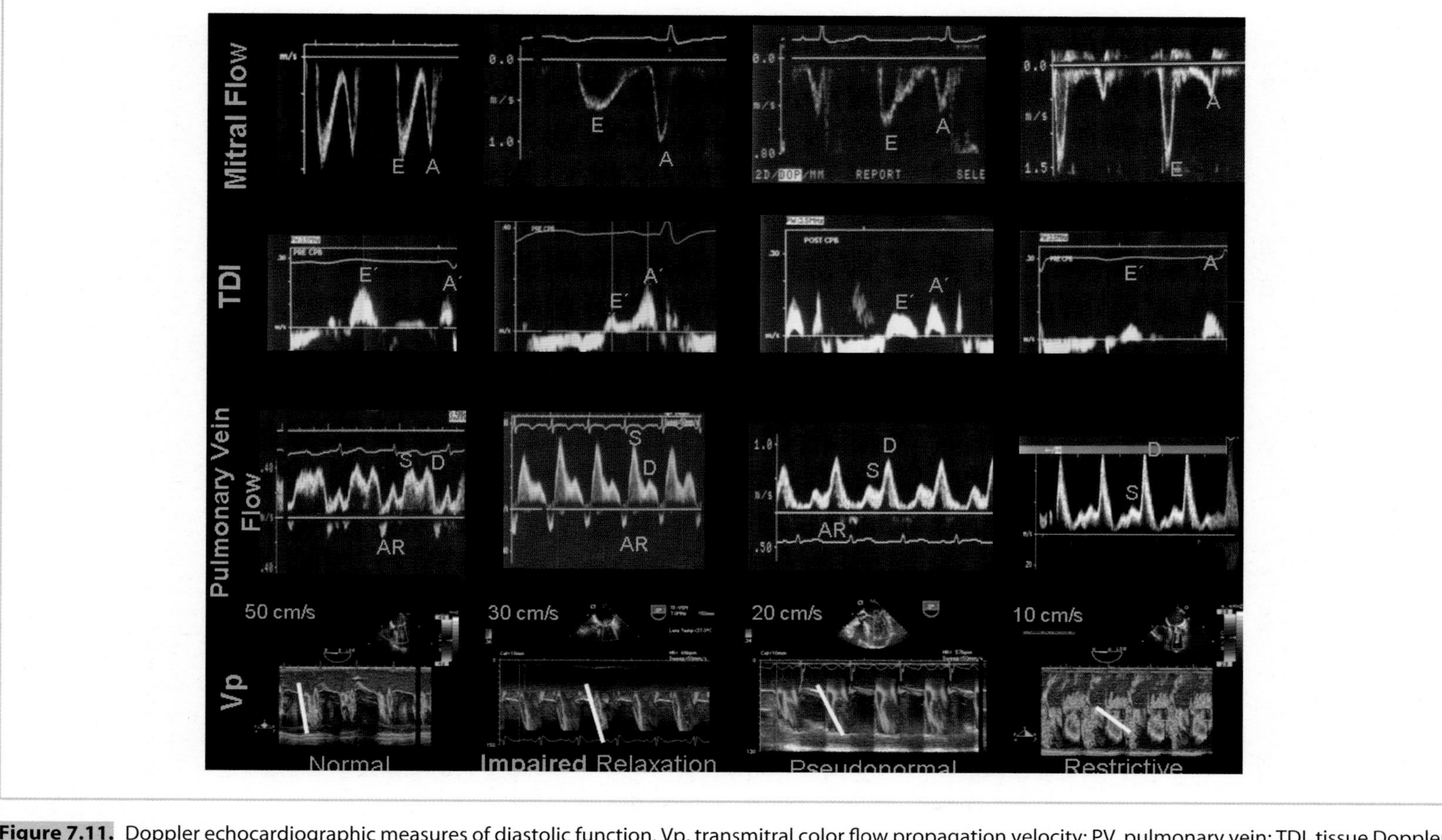

Figure 7.11. Doppler echocardiographic measures of diastolic function. Vp, transmitral color flow propagation velocity; PV, pulmonary vein; TDI, tissue Doppler imaging; E, peak early transmitral Doppler flow velocity; A, peak late transmitral Doppler flow velocity; E′, early diastolic mitral annular tissue velocity; A′, late diastolic mitral annular tissue velocity; AR, pulmonary venous atrial flow reversal; S, systolic pulmonary venous Doppler flow velocity; D, diastolic pulmonary venous Doppler flow velocity.

Table 7.2 Doppler echocardiographic values for indices of left ventricular diastolic dysfunction

	Normal (young)	Normal (adult)	Impaired relaxation	Pseudonormal filling	Restrictive filling
E/A (cm/s)	>1	>1	<1	1–2	>2
DT (ms)	<220	<220	>220	150–200	<150
IVRT (ms)	<100	<100	>100	60–100	<60
S/D	<1	≥1	≥1	<1	<1
PV_{AR} (cm/s)	<35	<35	<35	≥35[a]	≥25[a]
Vp (cm/s)	>55	>45	<45	<45	<45
E′ (cm/s)	>10	>8	<8	<8	<8

[a]Unless atrial mechanical failure is present.
E/A, early-to-late left ventricular (LV) filling ratio; DT, early LV filling deceleration time; IVRT, isovolumic relaxation time; S/D, systolic-to-diastolic pulmonary venous flow ratio; PV_{AR}, pulmonary venous peak atrial contraction reversal velocity; Vp, transmitral color M-mode propagation velocity; E′, peak early diastolic mitral annular velocity.
Reproduced with permission from Garcia M, Thomas J, Klein A. New Doppler echocardiographic applications for the study of diastolic function. *J Am Coll Cardiol* 1998;32:872.

echocardiographic techniques for diagnosing diastolic dysfunction will hopefully facilitate the development of perioperative therapeutic intervention.

REFERENCES

1 Grossman W. Diastolic dysfunction in congestive heart failure. *N Engl J Med* 1991;22:1557–1564.
2 Pinamonti B, Lenarda A, Sinagra G, et al. Restrictive left ventricular filling pattern in dilated cardiomyopathy assessed by Doppler echocardiography: clinical, echocardiographic, and hemodynamic correlations and prognostic implications. *J Am Coll Cardiol* 1993;22:808–815.
3 Bernard F, Denault A, Babin D, et al. Diastolic dysfunction is predictive of difficult weaning from cardiopulmonary bypass. *Anesth Analg* 2001;92:291–298.
4 Yusef S, Thom T, Abbott RD. Changes in hypertension treatment and congestive heart failure mortality in the United States. *Hypertension* 1989;13 Suppl:174–179.
5 Vasan R, Larson M, Benjamin E, et al. Congestive heart failure in subjects with normal versus reduced left ventricular ejection fraction: prevalence and mortality in a population-based cohort. *J Am Coll Cardiol* 1999;33:1948–1955.
6 Appleton C, Firstenberg M, Garcia M, et al. The echo-doppler evaluation of left ventricular diastolic function: a current perspective. In: Kovacs S, ed. *Cardiology clinics.* Philadelphia: WB Saunders, 2000:513–546.
7 Djainani G, Ti L, Mackensen B, et al. Color m-mode propagation velocity identifies patients with diastolic dysfunction during coronary bypass surgery. *Anesth Anlag* 2001;92:SCA74.
8 De Hert S, Rodrigus I, Haenen L, et al. Recovery of systolic and diastolic left ventricular function early after cardiopulmonary bypass. *Anesthesiology* 1996;85:1063–1075.
9 Doolan L, Jones E, Kalman J, et al. A placebo-controlled trial verifying the efficacy of milrinone in weaning high-risk patients from cardiopulmonary bypass. *J Cardiothorac Vasc Anesth* 1997;11:37–41.
10 Plotnick GD. Changes in diastolic function—difficult to measure, harder to interpret. *Am J Heart J* 1989;118:637–641.
11 Nishimura R, Tajik A. Evaluation of diastolic filling of left ventricle in health and disease: doppler echocardiography is the clinician's Rosetta stone. *J Am Coll Cardiol* 1997;30:8–18.
12 Pagel P, Grossman W, Haering J, et al. Left ventricular diastolic function in the normal and diseased heart: perspectives for the anesthesiologist. *Anesthesiology* 1993;79:836–854.
13 Zile M, Smith V. Relaxation and diastolic properties of the heart. In: Fozzard H, Haber E, Jennings R, et al. *The heart and cardiovascular system: scientific foundations*, 2nd ed. New York: Raven Press, 1991:1353–1367.
14 Appleton C, Galloway J, Gonzalez M, et al. Estimation of left ventricular filling pressures using two-dimensional and Doppler echocardiography in adult patients with cardiac disease: additional value of

analyzing left atrial size, left atrial ejection fraction and the difference in duration of pulmonary venous and mitral flow velocity at atrial contraction. *J Am Coll Cardiol* 1993;22:1972–1982.

15 Cohen G, Pietrolungo J, Thomas J, et al. A practical guide to assessment of ventricular diastolic function using Doppler echocardiography. *J Am Coll Cardiol* 1996;27:1753–1760.

16 Little W, Ohno M, Kitzman D, et al. Determination of left ventricular chamber stiffness from the time for deceleration of early left ventricular filling. *Circulation* 1995;92:1933–1939.

17 Oh J, Appleton C, Hatle L, et al. The noninvasive assessment of left ventricular diastolic function with two-dimensional and Doppler echocardiography. *J Am Soc Echocardiogr* 1997;10:246–270.

18 Appleton C, Hatle L. The natural history of left ventricular filling abnormalities: assessment by two-dimensional and Doppler echocardiography. *Echocardiography* 1992;9:437–457.

19 Dumesnil J, Gaudreault G, Honos G, et al. Use of Valsalva maneuver to unmask left ventricular diastolic function abnormalities by Doppler echocardiography in patients with coronary artery disease or systemic hypertension. *Am J Cardiol* 1991;68:515–519.

20 Hurrell D, Nishimura R, Ilstrup D, et al. Utility of preload alteration in assessment of left ventricular filling pressure by Doppler echocardiography: a simultaneous catheterization and Doppler echocardiographic study. *J Am Coll Cardiol* 1997;30:459–467.

21 Nishimura R, Abel M, Hatle L, et al. Relation of pulmonary vein to mitral flow velocities by transesophageal Doppler echocardiography: effect of different loading conditions. *Circulation* 1990;81:488–497.

22 Kuecherer H, Muhiudeen I, Kusumoto F, et al. Estimation of mean left atrial pressure from transesophageal pulsed Doppler echocardiography of pulmonary venous flow. *Circulation* 1990;82:1127–1139.

23 Yamamoto K, Nishimura R, Burnett J, et al. Assessment of end-diastolic pressure by Doppler echocardiography: contribution of duration of pulmonary venous versus mitral flow velocity curves at atrial contraction. *J Am Soc Echocardiogr* 1997;10:52–59.

24 Appleton C, Hatle L, Popp R. Relation of transmitral flow velocity patterns to left ventricular diastolic function: new insights from a combined hemodynamic and Doppler echocardiographic study. *J Am Coll Cardiol* 1988;12:426–440.

25 Nishimura R, Abel M, Hatle L, et al. Assessment of diastolic function of the heart: background and current applications of Doppler echocardiography: Part II Clinical Studies. *Mayo Clin Proc* 1989;64:181–204.

26 Otto C. Echocardiographic evaluation of ventricular diastolic filling and function. In: Otto C, ed. *Textbook of clinical echocardiography*, 2nd ed. Philadelphia: WB Saunders, 2000:132–152.

27 Oka Y, Kato M, Strom J. Mitral valve. In: Oka Y, Goldiner P, eds. *Transesophageal echocardiography.* Philadelphia: JB Lippincott Co, 1992:99–151.

28 Oh J. Assessment of diastolic function. In: Oh J, ed. *The echo manual*, 2nd ed. Philadelphia: Lippincott Williams & Wilkins, 1999:45–57.

29 Nagueh S, Kopelen H, Quinones M. Assessment of left ventricular filling pressures by Doppler in the presence of atrial fibrillation. *Circulation* 1996;94:2138–2145.

30 Farias C, Rodriguez L, Garcia M, et al. Assessment of diastolic function by tissue Doppler echocardiography: comparison with standard transmitral and pulmonary venous flow. *J Am Soc Echocardiogr* 1999;12:609–617.

31 Nagueh S, Middleton K, Kopelen H, et al. Doppler tissue imaging: a noninvasive technique for evaluation of left ventricular relaxation and estimation of filling pressures. *J Am Coll Cardiol* 1997;30:1527–1533.

32 Garcia M, Thomas J, Klein A. New Doppler echocardiographic applications for the study of diastolic function. *J Am Coll Cardiol* 1998;32:865–875.

33 Garcia M, Rodriguez L, Ares M, et al. Differentiation of constrictive pericarditis from restrictive cardiomyopathy: assessment of left ventricular diastolic velocities in longitudinal axis by Doppler tissue imaging. *J Am Coll Cardiol* 1996;27:108–114.

34 Sohn D, Chai I, Lee D, et al. Assessment of mitral annulus velocity by Doppler tissue imaging in the evaluation of left ventricular diastolic function. *J Am Coll Cardiol* 1997;30:474–480.

35 Takatsuji H, Mikami T, Urasawa K, et al. A new approach for evaluation of left ventricular diastolic function: spatial and temporal analysis of left ventricular filling flow propagation by color m-mode Doppler echocardiography. *J Am Coll Cardiol* 1996;27:363–371.

36 Brun P, Tribouilloy C, Duval A, et al. Left ventricular flow propagation velocity during early filling is related to wall relaxation: a color M-mode Doppler analysis. *J Am Coll Cardiol* 1992;20:420–432.

37 Garcia M, Smedira N, Greenberg N, et al. Color M-mode Doppler flow propagation velocity is a preload insensitive index of left ventricular relaxation: animal and human validation. *J Am Coll Cardiol* 2000;35:201–208.

38 Garcia M, Ares M, Asher C, et al. An index of early left ventricular filling that combined with pulsed Doppler peak E velocity may estimate capillary wedge pressure. *J Am Coll Cardiol* 1997;29:448–454.

39 Moller J, Poulsen S, Sondergaard E, et al. Preload dependence of color M-mode Doppler flow propagation velocity in controls and in patients with left ventricular dysfunction. *J Am Soc Echocardiogr* 2000;13:902–909.

40 Garcia M, Palac R, Malenka D, et al. Color M-mode Doppler flow propagation velocity is a relatively preload-independent index of left ventricular filling. *J Am Soc Echocardiogr* 1999;12:129–137.

41 Ng K, Popovic Z, Troughton R, et al. Comparison of left ventricular diastolic function after on-pump versus on-pump coronary artery bypass grafting. *Am J Cardiol* 2005;95:647–650.
42 Sutherland G, Di Salvo G, Claus P, et al. Strain and strain rate imaging: a new clinical approach to quantifying regional myocardial function. *J Am Soc Echocardiogr* 2004;17:788–802.
43 Gilman G, Khanderia B, Hagen M, et al. Strain and strain rate: a step-by-step approach to image and data acquisition. *J Am Soc Echocardiogr* 2004;17:1011–1020.
44 Stolyen A, Slordahl S, Skjelvan G, et al. Strain rate imaging in normal and reduced diastolic function: comparison with pulse Doppler tissue imaging of the mitral annulus. *J Am Soc Echocardiogr* 2001;14:264–274.
45 Hoffmann R, Altiok E, Nowak B, et al. Strain rate analysis allows detection of differences in diastolic function between viable and nonviable myocardial segments. *J Am Soc Echocardiogr* 2005;18:330–335.
46 Klein A, Hatle L, Burstow D, et al. Comprehensive Doppler assessment of right ventricular diastolic function in cardiac amyloidosis. *J Am Coll Cardiol* 1990;15:99–108.
47 Spencer K, Weinert L, Lang R. Effect of age, heart rate and tricuspid regurgitation on the Doppler echocardiographic evaluation of right ventricular diastolic function. *Cardiology* 1999;92:59–64.
48 Nomura T, Lebowitz L, Koide Y, et al. Evaluation of hepatic venous flow using transesophageal echocardiography in coronary artery bypass surgery: an index of right ventricular function. *J Thorac Cardiovasc Anesth* 1995;9:9–17.
49 Yu C, Sanderson J, Chan S, et al. Right ventricular diastolic dysfunction in heart failure. *Circulation* 1996;93:1509–1514.
50 Feigenbaum H. Pericardial disease. In: Feigenbaum H, ed. *Echocardiography*, 5th ed. Baltimore: Williams & Wilkins, 1994:556–588.
51 Klein A, Cohen G, Pietrolungo J, et al. Differentiation of constrictive pericarditis from restrictive cardiomyopathy by Doppler transesophageal echocardiographic measurements of respiratory variations in pulmonary venous flow. *J Am Coll Cardiol* 1993;22:1935–1943.
52 Burstow D, Oh J, Bailey K, et al. Cardiac tamponade: characteristic Doppler observations. *Mayo Clin Proc* 1989;64:312–324.
53 Abdalla I, Murray D, Awad H, et al. Reversal of the pattern of respiratory variation of Doppler inflow velocities in constrictive pericarditis during mechanical ventilation. *J Am Soc Echocardiogr* 2000;13:827–831.
54 Schiavone W, Calafiore P, Salcedo E. Transesophageal Doppler echocardiographic demonstration of pulmonary venous flow velocity in restrictive cardiomyopathy and constrictive pericarditis. *Am J Cardiol* 1989;63:1286–1288.
55 Rodriguez L, Ares M, Vandervoort P, et al. Does color M-mode flow propagation differentiate between patients with restrictive vs. constrictive physiology? [Abstract] *J Am Coll Cardiol* 1996;27:268A.
56 Rajagopalan N, Garcia M, Rodriguez L, et al. Comparison of Doppler echocardiographic methods to differentiate constrictive pericarditis from restrictive cardiomyopathy [Abstract]. *J Am Coll Cardiol* 1998;31:164A.

QUESTIONS

1. **Which one of the following patterns of left ventricular diastolic dysfunction occurs most commonly with acute myocardial ischemia?**
   a. Restrictive
   b. Pseudonormal
   c. Constrictive
   d. Poor relaxation

2. **During spontaneous inspiration, patients with pericardial tamponade will most likely demonstrate which one of the following changes in the peak E-wave velocity of the transtricuspid and transmitral Doppler flow profiles?**

	Peak E-wave velocity	
	Transtricuspid	**Transmitral**
a.	Increase	Decrease
b.	Decrease	Decrease
c.	Decrease	Increase
d.	Increase	Increase

3. **In comparison to the poor relaxation pattern of left ventricular diastolic dysfunction, the restrictive pattern is characterized by which of the following changes in the transmitral Doppler flow velocity isovolumic relaxation and E-wave deceleration times?**

	Transmitral Doppler flow velocity	
	Isovolumic relaxation	**E-wave deceleration**
	Time	Time
a.	Increase	Increase
b.	Increase	Decrease
c.	Decrease	Increase
d.	Decrease	Decrease

4. **An increased pulmonary AR-wave/mitral A-wave duration ratio is consistent with which one of the following conditions?**
   a. Increased left atrial compliance
   b. Decreased left atrial pressure
   c. Increased left ventricular end-diastolic pressure
   d. Decreased pulmonary venous compliance

5. **A pulmonary venous Doppler flow velocity profile with a biphasic systolic component, has an initial antegrade velocity (PV_{S1}) that is most related to which one of the following cardiac cycle components?**
   a. Left atrial relaxation
   b. Left ventricular contraction
   c. Left atrial contraction
   d. Left ventricular compliance

6. **In comparison to normal adult values, the restrictive pattern of left ventricular diastolic function exhibits which one of the following sets of relative changes in Doppler echocardiographic velocities?**

	Pulmonary vein systolic/diastolic ratio	Mitral annular Doppler tissue imaging	Transmitral color M-mode
	Velocity ratio	Peak E velocity (E′)	Propagation velocity (Vp)
a.	Increased	Increased	Decreased
b.	Decreased	Decreased	Decreased
c.	Increased	Increased	Increased
d.	Decreased	Decreased	Increased

7. **Which one of the following Doppler echocardiographic measurements is the best predictor of increased left ventricular filling pressure in patients with atrial fibrillation?**
   a. Increased PV_{AR}/MV_A duration ratio
   b. Decreased pulmonary venous diastolic flow
   c. Increased transmitral peak E-wave velocity
   d. Decreased transmitral E-wave deceleration time

8. **The use of a Valsalva maneuver will convert a pseudonormalized left ventricular inflow pattern to which one of the following transmitral Doppler flow velocity patterns?**
   a. Normal
   b. Restrictive
   c. Poor relaxation
   d. Constrictive

9. **The transmitral color M-mode propagation velocity (Vp) is most likely to decrease during which one of the following conditions?**
   a. Administration of esmolol
   b. Reverse Trendelenburg positioning
   c. Administration of nitroglycerin
   d. Valsalva maneuver

10. **In comparison to other conventional Doppler echocardiographic measures of diastolic function, which of the following is most unique for strain imaging?**
   a. Angle dependence
   b. Independent of rotational and translational movement of the heart
   c. Uses measures of tissue velocity
   d. Can also be used to evaluate systolic function

11. **Which one of the following echocardiographic measurements made during spontaneous inspiration is most consistent with a diagnosis of decreased right ventricular compliance and increased filling pressures?**
   a. Prolonged transtricuspid E-wave deceleration time
   b. Diastolic predominance of hepatic vein flow
   c. Diminished hepatic AR-wave velocity time integral
   d. Greater than 50% inspiratory collapse of the inferior vena cava (IVC)

Answers appear at the back of the book.

Transesophageal Echocardiography in Valvular Disease and Surgery

8 Mitral Regurgitation

A. Stephane Lambert

Transesophageal echocardiography (TEE) has become a standard of care in the cardiac operating room, allowing the anesthesiologist to play an important part in the surgical decision-making process. In that role, few areas are as challenging as the assessment of intraoperative mitral regurgitation (MR). Yet few applications of intraoperative TEE have as much impact on the course of surgery and on patient outcome as the evaluation of MR.

ANATOMY

The mitral valve is bicuspid and consists of a large anterior leaflet and a smaller posterior leaflet (Figure 8.1). The anterior leaflet covers about two thirds of the surface area of the valve. The posterior leaflet is C-shaped and wraps around the anterior leaflet accounting for about two thirds of the circumference of the valve. The leaflets join at the anterolateral and posteromedial commissures. The posterior leaflet is further divided anatomically into three scallops whereas the anterior leaflet does not have scallops *per se*. It is important to keep in mind when considering the various TEE imaging planes of the mitral valve that coaptation of the two leaflets forms a semicircular, not linear, path. The valve is encircled by a dynamic fibromuscular ring, the mitral annulus. It is saddle shaped and plays an important role in proper valve closure by reducing its diameter in systole. In various disease states the mitral annulus dilates and tends to flatten, causing increased stress on the mitral leaflets and impairs its function (1). The mitral valve attaches to two papillary muscles, anterolateral and posteromedial, through chordae tendinae. Each papillary muscle sends off chordae tendinae to both mitral leaflets. In systole, the papillary muscles contract to keep the chordae tendinae taut and prevent prolapse of the leaflets into the left atrium. There are three types of chordae tendinae. First-order (or primary) chordae attach to the edge of the leaflets, second-order (or secondary) chordae attach to the body of the leaflets and third-order (or tertiary) chordae attach to the base of the posterior leaflet. The anterior leaflet of the mitral valve shares the same fibrous attachment as the aortic valve, an area sometimes referred to as the *fibrous body* or *crux of the heart*. This relationship is important to consider and surgery to one valve can result in impaired function of the other.

NOMENCLATURE

There exist three nomenclatures of the mitral valve in the literature. The classic anatomic nomenclature refers to the three scallops of the posterior leaflet of the mitral valve as anterolateral, middle, and posteromedial, according to their anatomic location (2). The anterolateral scallop is the closest to the left atrial appendage. No specific description is given to any part of the anterior leaflet. *The most commonly used* nomenclature amongst echocardiographers is attributed to Carpentier (3) and defines the three scallops of the posterior leaflet as P1, P2, and P3, where P1 is closest to the left atrial appendage. It also defines three corresponding areas of the anterior leaflet as A1 (opposite P1), A2 (opposite P2), and A3 (opposite P3). This nomenclature was adopted by the American Society of Echocardiography Council for Intraoperative Echocardiography and the Society of Cardiovascular Anesthesiologists Task Force for Certification in Perioperative Transesophageal Echocardiography, in their published "Guidelines for performing a comprehensive intraoperative multiplane transesophageal echocardiography examination" (4).

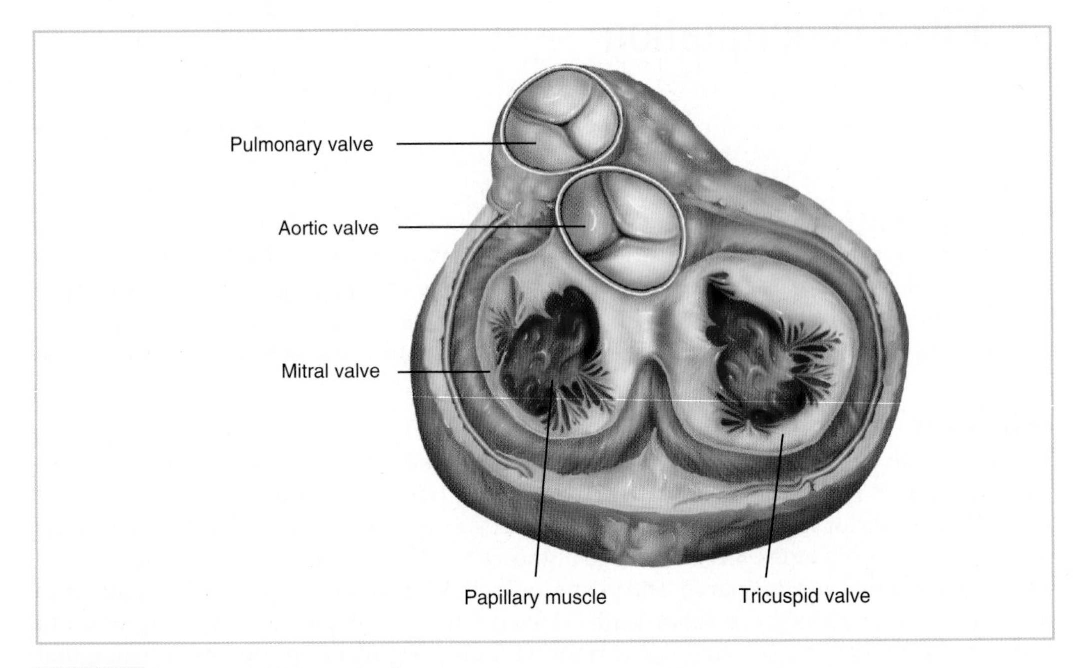

Figure 8.1. Anatomy of the mitral valve.

A third nomenclature, often called the *Duran nomenclature* (5), describes the mitral valve segments according to their attachment to the papillary muscles. It refers to the three scallops of the posterior leaflet as P1, PM (middle), and P2, where P1 is closest to the left atrial appendage. The PM scallop is further subdivided into PM_1 laterally and PM_2 medially. Duran divides the anterior leaflet into two areas, A1 and A2, opposite the corresponding scallops of the posterior leaflet. The two commissural areas of the valve are defined as C1 (between A1 and P1) and C2 (between A2 and P2). The rationale for this nomenclature is that every part of the mitral valve attached to the anterolateral papillary muscle is given the number one and every part of the mitral valve attached to the posteromedial papillary muscle is given the number two. A schematic representation of the three nomenclatures of the mitral valve is shown in Figure 8.2 (6).

Each institution or group of practitioners favors one nomenclature over another and it doesn't matter which one is used, as long as every member of the team agrees on which terminology is used. The reader is encouraged to have a basic understanding of all of them to avoid confusion. For example, P2 refers to a different area of the valve in the Carpentier and Duran nomenclatures.

ETIOLOGY AND MECHANISM OF MITRAL REGURGITATION

MR can be classified according to its etiology (Table 8.1), or more simply, according to the pathophysiologic mechanism leading to the regurgitation. Carpentier proposed the now widely used classification of MR based on leaflet motion (7,8) (Figure 8.3).

- In type 1 lesions, the MR is usually the result of *annular dilatation and the leaflet motion is normal.* In such cases, the MR jet tends to be central. Less common mechanisms of type 1 MR include mitral valve clefts, aneurysms, perforation or destruction, as a result of endocarditis.

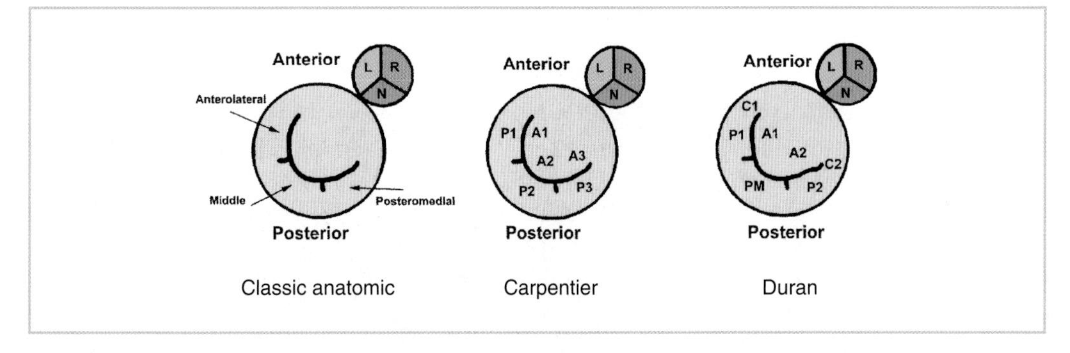

Figure 8.2. Schematic representation of the various nomenclatures of the mitral valve. The mitral valve is shown with its relationship to the aortic valve, viewed from the left atrium. See text for details. (Adapted from Lambert AS, Miller JP, Merrick SH, et al. Improved evaluation of the location and mechanism of mitral valve regurgitation with a systematic transesophageal echocardiography examination. *Anesth Analg* 1999;88:1205–1212, with permission.)

- In type 2 lesions, there is *excessive mitral leaflet motion* and the MR jet is typically directed away from the diseased leaflet. The spectrum of severity of excessive leaflet motion is illustrated in Figure 8.4. Billowing (or scalloping) refers to a situation where part of a mitral leaflet projects above the annulus in systole, but the coaptation point remains below the mitral annulus. Prolapse is used to describe the excursion of a leaflet tip above the level of the mitral annulus during systole, causing regurgitation. The term *flail* is reserved for a situation where a leaflet edge is flowing freely into the left atrium in systole, as a result of one or more ruptured chordae tendinae. The distinction between severe prolapse and flail is sometimes difficult to make because the ruptured chordae may not be visible by echocardiogram. It is also somewhat academic, as the hemodynamic consequences and the surgical treatment of the two are often the same.
- Type 3 lesions refer to *restricted leaflet motion* and are further subdivided into type 3a and 3b. In type 3a, the restriction is "structural" (most often rheumatic) and the leaflet

Table 8.1 Causes of mitral regurgitation

Causes
Congenital
Endocardial cushion defect
Associated with other pathologies (e.g., corrected transposition)
Myxomatous degeneration
Rheumatic (often accompanied by mitral stenosis)
Endocarditis
Bacterial, viral, etc.
Cardiomyopathy
Dilated (ischemic, idiopathic, EtOH, drug related)
Hypertrophic
Other
Systemic lupus
Rheumatoid arthritis
Ankylosing spondylitis

EtOH, ethanol.

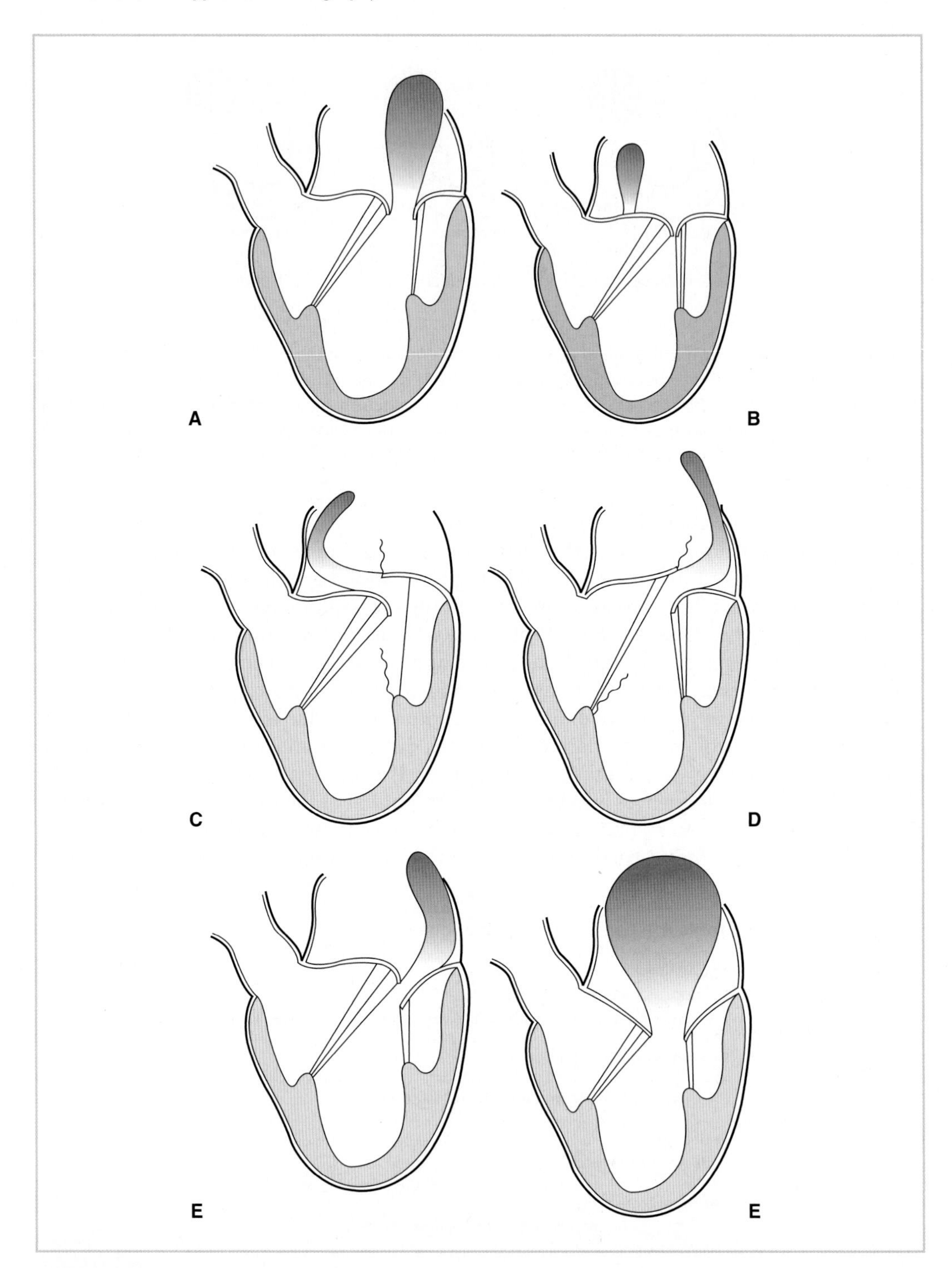

Figure 8.3. Carpentier's classification of mitral regurgitation (MR) based on leaflet motion. In type 1, the leaflet motion is *normal* and the MR jet tends to be central. In type 2, there is *excessive* leaflet motion and the MR jet is typically directed away from the diseased leaflet. In type 3 lesions, the leaflet motion is *restricted* leaflet motion and is further subdivided into type 3a (structural) and type 3b (functional). In type 3 lesions, the regurgitant jet may be directed away from the diseased leaflet if only one leaflet is affected, or it may be central if both mitral leaflets are equally affected. (*Courtesy Dr. Gregory M. Hirsch*).

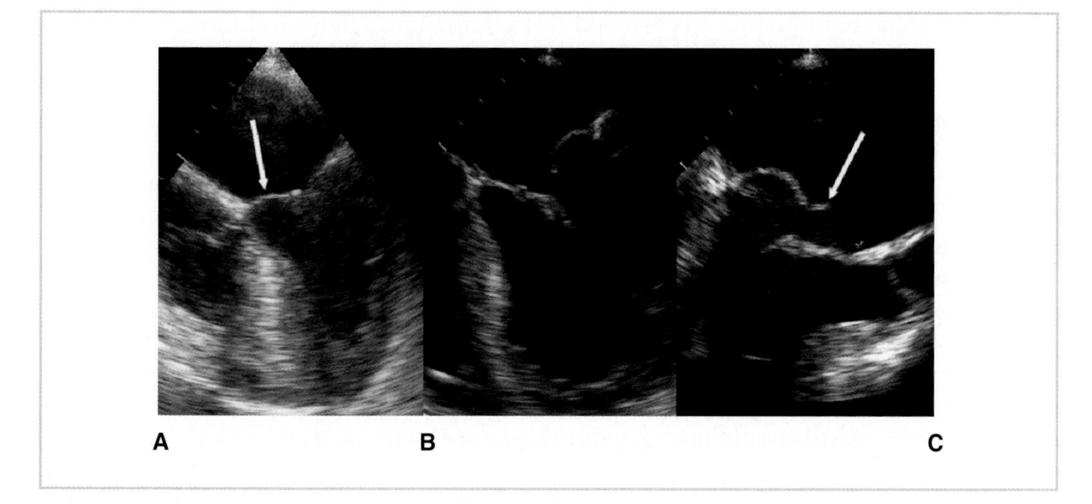

Figure 8.4. Excessive leaflet motion. **A:** Billowing (or scalloping) refers to a situation where part of a mitral leaflet (*arrow*) projects above the annulus in systole, but the coaptation point remains below the mitral annulus. **B:** Prolapse is used to describe the excursion of a leaflet tip above the level of the mitral annulus during systole, causing regurgitation. **C:** The term *flail* is reserved for a situation where a leaflet edge (*arrow*) is flowing freely into the left atrium in systole.

motion is affected in both systole and diastole. In type 3b the restriction is "functional" and proper coaptation is prevented by systolic tethering of the mitral leaflets as a result of a dilated LV and/or displaced papillary muscles. Coronary artery disease is often the etiology of type 3b MR and is referred to as *ischemic MR*. In type 3b, leaflet motion is normal in diastole. Usually in type 3 lesions, the regurgitant jet may be directed away from the diseased leaflet if only one leaflet is affected, but the jet may also be central if both mitral leaflets are equally affected by the disease process. This is often the case in type 3b abnormalities, because each papillary muscle supports both leaflets. Structural restriction of leaflet motion commonly coexists with some degree of mitral stenosis. An ischemic (i.e., stiff) papillary muscle may also temporarily restrict leaflet motion, causing failure of coaptation.

THREE-STEP APPROACH TO THE TRANSESOPHAGEAL ECHOCARDIOGRAPHY EVALUATION OF MITRAL REGURGITATION

In the setting of mitral valve surgery, the intraoperative TEE evaluation of MR requires one to answer three basic questions: (a) How severe is the MR? (b) What is the mechanism of the MR and where on the mitral valve is the lesion? (c) Can the valve be surgically repaired?

Step 1—How Severe Is the Mitral Regurgitation?

The severity of MR is classified as trivial, mild, moderate, or severe. This corresponds to 1+, 2+, 3+ and 4+ by angiography. The basic two-dimensional (2D) examination (see chapter 2 on basic examination) of the heart often provides clues that significant MR may be present. Such clues may be direct, like a large coaptation defect or a structural anomaly of a leaflet, or indirect indicators such as the hemodynamic sequelae of severe MR, like volume overload of the left ventricle and left atrium, or signs of pulmonary hypertension (dilated right ventricle, hypertrophied right ventricle, septal flattening, dilated pulmonary arteries, tricuspid regurgitation). A detailed 2D examination of the mitral valve is extremely valuable for precise localization of lesions and is discussed in the following text.

Color Doppler remains the easiest and best method to screen for MR because of its high sensitivity and specificity. It also provides a semiquantitative assessment of the severity of MR. The general appearance (size and depth of penetration) of the regurgitant jet offers a rough index of the severity of regurgitation, but that appearance is highly dependent on machine settings as well as pressures in the receiving chamber and may lead to confusion. The "experienced eyeball method" tends to only work in mild or severe cases. The ratio of the regurgitant jet area (RJA) over the total left atrial area (LAA) has been reported to correlate better with the severity of MR on cardiac catheterization in almost 94% of a group of 82 patients (9). An RJA/LAA greater than 40% was found in patients with severe MR on cardiac catheterization. However, there are also important limitations to this sign (10–12) and the severity of MR should not be determined only by the size of the Doppler jet.

The narrowest portion of the jet, known as the *vena contracta*, can be measured and diameters of 5.5 mm or more correlate with severe MR on cardiac catheterization (13) (Figure 8.5). The use of 7 mm as the cutoff point for severe MR is useful as it provides more specificity but not surprisingly at the cost of decreased sensitivity (14).

The direction of the MR jet is also important, not only as a clue to its etiology, but also as a sign of its severity. While central jets may result from annular dilatation or ventricular dysfunction, *eccentric jets* (Figure 8.6) *are almost always due to a structural abnormality of the mitral apparatus itself and they are unlikely to improve after revascularization.* Furthermore, eccentric regurgitant jets always warrant a close examination: first, jets that have enough energy to "hug the wall" of the atrium for some distance should be considered hemodynamically significant until proven otherwise (15). Second, wall-hugging jets are

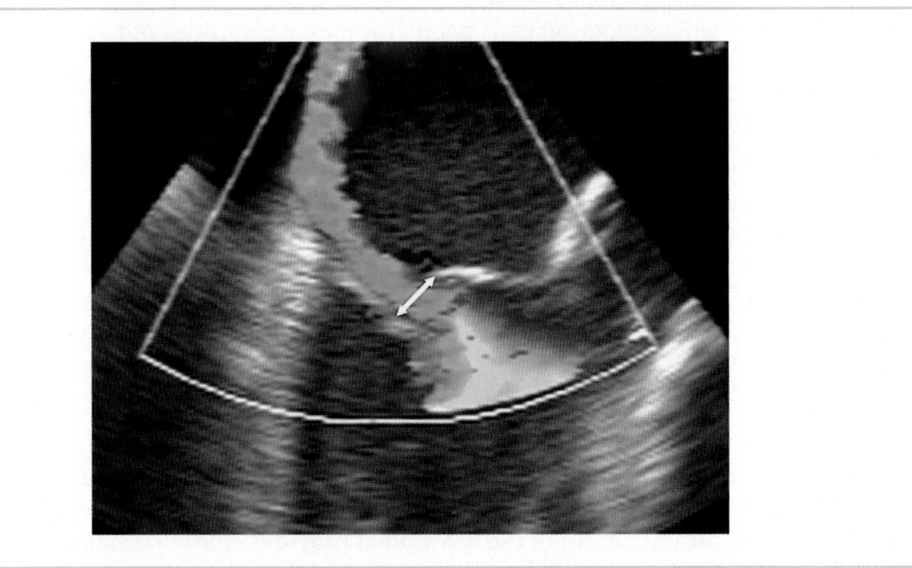

Figure 8.5. Measurement of the vena contracta. This is a color Doppler scan of the mitral valve in the midesophageal four-chamber view. The diameter of the base of the mitral regurgitation (MR) jet correlates with the severity of regurgitation.

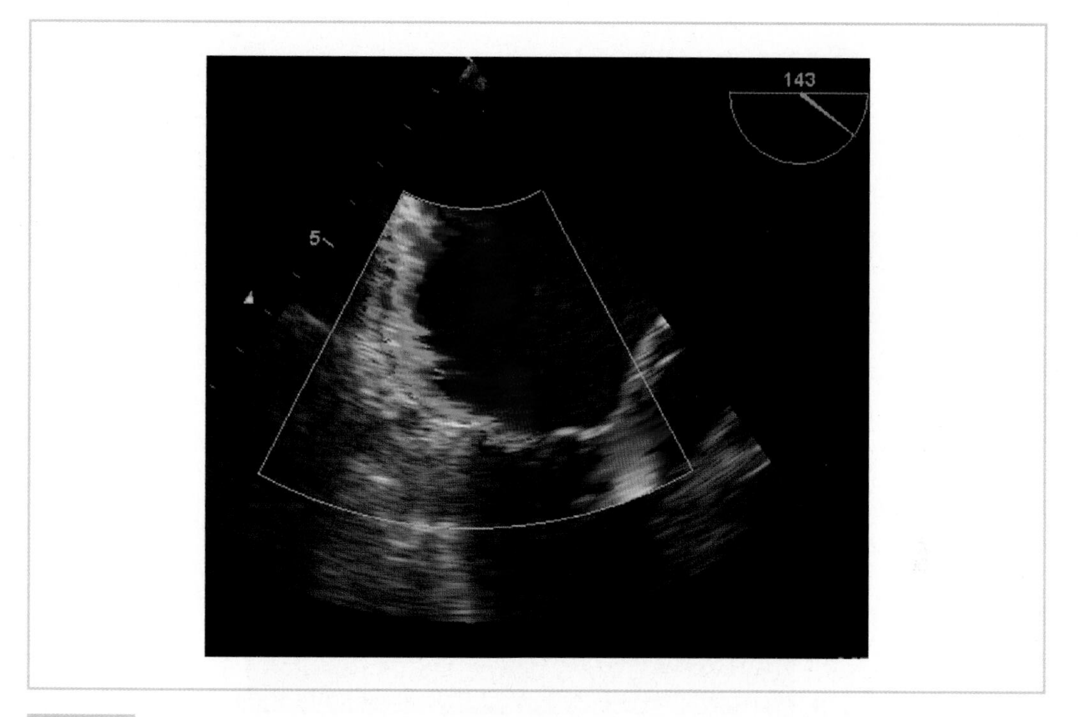

Figure 8.6. Eccentric mitral regurgitation (MR) jet. This is a color Doppler scan of the mitral valve in the midesophageal four-chamber view. Note the severe MR jet which "hugs" the medial wall of the left atrium all the way to the top. Wall-hugging jets should be considered severe until proven otherwise.

subjected to the "coanda effect". This is a physical principle by which a jet of fluids will get "sucked" against the wall, making it appear smaller than it actually is. Consequently, *a wall-hugging jet should be considered severe until proven otherwise.*

As mentioned in the preceding text, it is important to remember that any quantitative assessment made by color Doppler is highly dependent on the settings of the echo machine (aliasing velocity, pulse repetition frequency, frame rate, etc.). This is further discussed in the chapter 5 on color Doppler.

Spectral Doppler adds to the semiquantitative assessment of the valve. While the peak velocity of the regurgitant jet is mostly a function of the systolic gradient between the LV and the LA, the density of the MR signal by continuous wave (CW) Doppler is proportional to the number of blood cells detected by the Doppler beam (see the chapter 5 on Doppler). A dense MR jet with a sharp envelope on CW Doppler suggests that a large fraction of the left ventricular output is going backwards into the left atrium. Conversely, a weaker signal with an incomplete envelope suggests a smaller regurgitant fraction (RF).

The evaluation of pulmonary venous flow by pulsed wave (PW) Doppler is also very important and should be a routine part of any assessment of MR. The normal PW Doppler pattern of pulmonary venous flow is forward in systole and in diastole (Figure 8.7A). Significant regurgitation of the LV stroke volume in systole causes blunting or reversal of the systolic component of pulmonary vein flow and this sign is a reliable indicator of hemodynamically significant MR (Figure 8.7B) (16). However, it is important to remember that although pulmonary venous flow reversal is specific, it is not a particularly sensitive

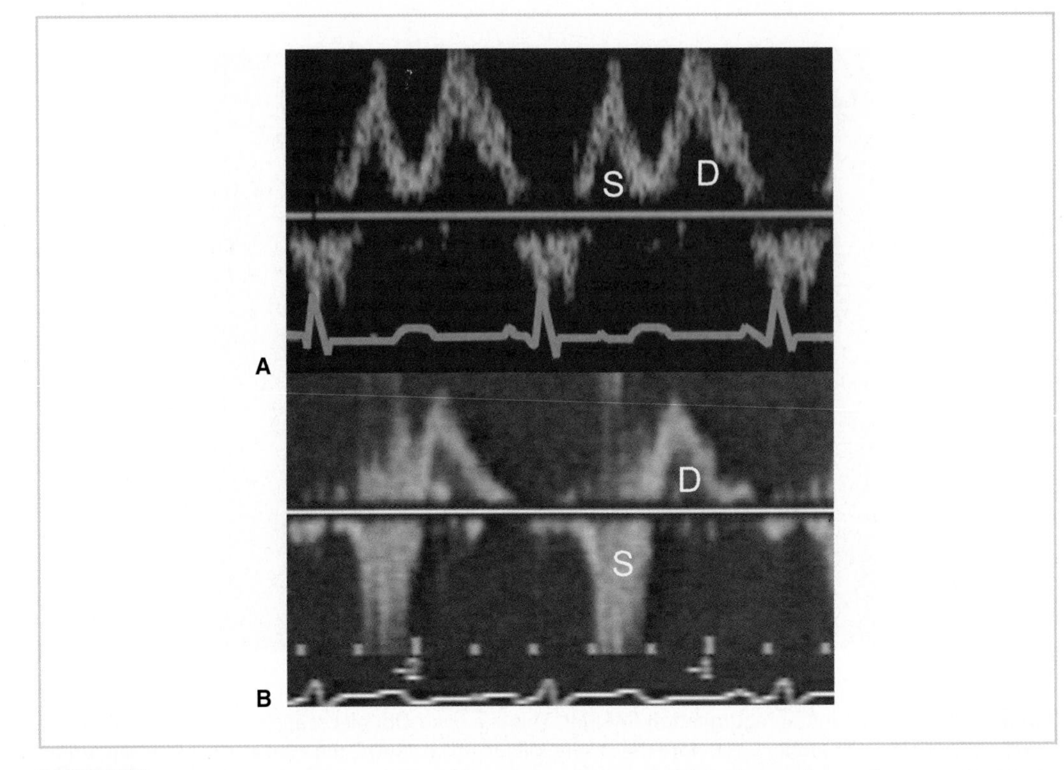

Figure 8.7. Pulsed wave Doppler of the pulmonary vein flow. **A:** The picture shows the normal pattern, forward in systole and diastole. **B:** The picture shows the typical pattern of systolic reversal seen in severe mitral regurgitation. Note the nonlaminar aspect of the flow in the reversed S wave, caused by severe mitral regurgitation

method to detect MR. The absence of systolic pulmonary venous flow blunting or reversal does not rule out severe MR, especially in chronic cases where a large and compliant left atrium may dissipate the energy from the regurgitant jet. Table 8.2 summarizes the Doppler parameters typically found in mild, moderate, and severe MR.

Finally, it is important to remember that none of the signs described in the preceding text are enough by themselves to make a diagnosis of severe MR, but taken as a group they provide much better diagnostic accuracy. Reference 14 provides an excellent review on the use of multiple techniques for assessing MR severity.

More precise quantitative assessments of MR require the use of mathematical calculations, which are described in a later section of this chapter.

Step 2—What Is the Mechanism of Mitral Regurgitation and Where on the Mitral Valve Is the Lesion?

SYSTEMATIC TWO-DIMENSIONAL EXAMINATION OF THE MITRAL VALVE

Once it has been established that there is significant MR, one must determine the mechanism of the MR and the precise location of the lesion, so that an appropriate surgical plan can be formulated. The various mechanisms of MR were discussed in the preceding text. The precise localization of lesions involves a systematic 2-D echo examination of the mitral valve.

Table 8.2 Doppler and quantitative values typically found in mild, moderate, and severe mitral regurgitation

	Mild	Moderate	Severe
Doppler parameters			
Jet area/LA area	<20%	—	>40%
Density of CW	—	—	Dense complete envelope
Pulmonary venous flow	—	Systolic blunting[a]	Systolic reversal[a]
Quantitative parameters			
Vena contracta (mm)	<3	3–6.9	≥7
Regurgitant volume (mL)	<30	30–60	≥60
Regurgitant fraction (%)	<30	30–50	≥50
EROA	<0.20	0.20–0.40	≥0.40

[a] Systolic blunting and reversal are specific but not sensitive signs. See text for details.
LA, left atrial; CW, continuous wave; EROA, effective regurgitant orifice area.

Several approaches have been proposed. Lambert et al. presented a systematic examination of the mitral valve involving a sequence of six views. This sequence of views was tested prospectively on a small number of patients and resulted in 97% accuracy in pinpointing prolapsed mitral valve segments (6). In a retrospective study, Foster et al. also reported a high accuracy in recognizing diseased mitral valve segments on previously recorded biplane TEE studies (17). Finally, in the American Society of Echocardiography/Society of Cardiovascular Anesthesiologists (ASE/SCA) guidelines on how to perform a comprehensive TEE examination, Shanewise et al. recommended an approach based on "transducer rotation" and standardized the terminology (4).

All three approaches advocate a complete, systematic examination of the mitral valve and the reader is strongly encouraged to become familiar with those three references. Ultimately, this author believes that the best approach to the mitral valve examination combines elements from all three methods discussed in the preceding text. The key is to obtain multiple redundant views of all parts of the valve and to identify each mitral segment using internal, recognizable cardiac landmarks. Accordingly, the sequence described in the following text and illustrated in Figure 8.8 is recommended:

1. Begin the examination in the **midesophageal (ME) four-chamber view** at 0 degrees of transducer rotation, with the mitral valve in the center of the screen. The anterior mitral leaflet is medial, adjacent to the aortic valve and the posterior leaflet is lateral. Slight withdrawal (17) or anteflexion (6) of the probe brings the left ventricular outflow tract (LVOT) into the plane of the scan, which demonstrates the anterior segments of the valve (A1/A2, P1/P2). Conversely with slight insertion (17) or retroflexion (6) of the probe, the LVOT disappears from the scanning plane, allowing the examination of the posterior segments of the valve (A2/A3, P2/P3). The entire mitral valve can therefore be seen at 0 degree of transducer rotation, by gently anteflexing or retroflexing the probe. A note of caution: because of anatomic variations this author does not believe

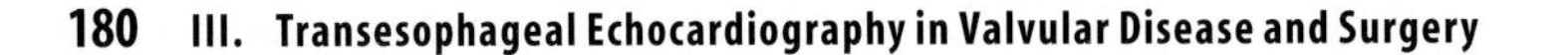

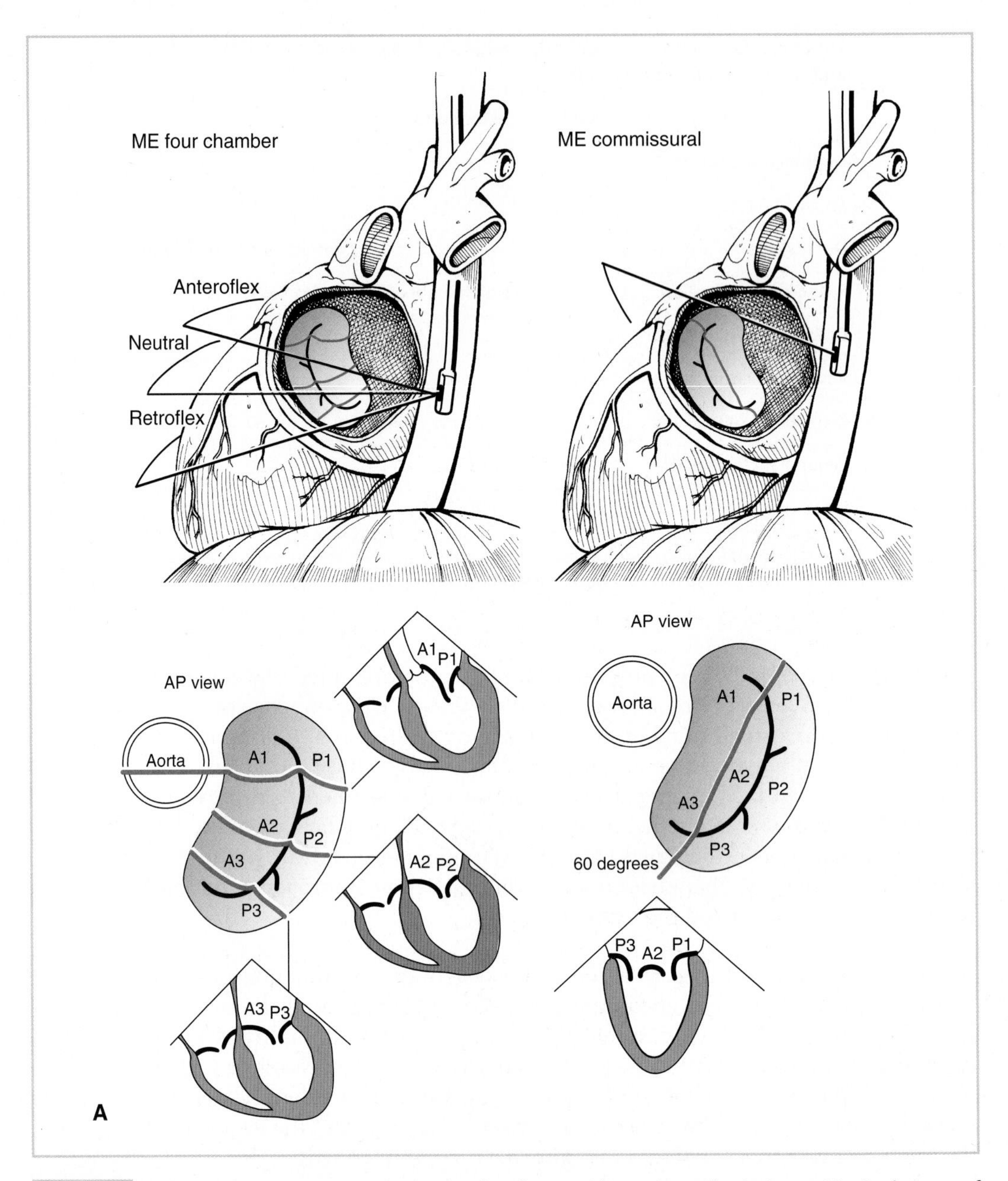

Figure 8.8. Sequential examination of mitral valve from mid-esophageal windows. Manipulations of the probe and imaging angle enhance the assessment of leaflet anatomy. **A:** Atrial view is similar to direct intraoperative visualization. **B:** Anterior view mimics the right-to-left orientation of a clinician facing the patient as well as the echo display from the transverse (0 degree) plane. ME, midesophageal; AP, anteroposterior.

that the average echocardiographer can consistently discriminate between P1 and P2, or between P2 and P3 using only 0-degree views.

2. Obtain an **ME mitral commissural view** by rotating the imaging array to obtain the best possible cut through the commissures. This is usually achieved between 60 and 90 degrees (4). This cross-section typically demonstrates P1 laterally, P3 medially, and

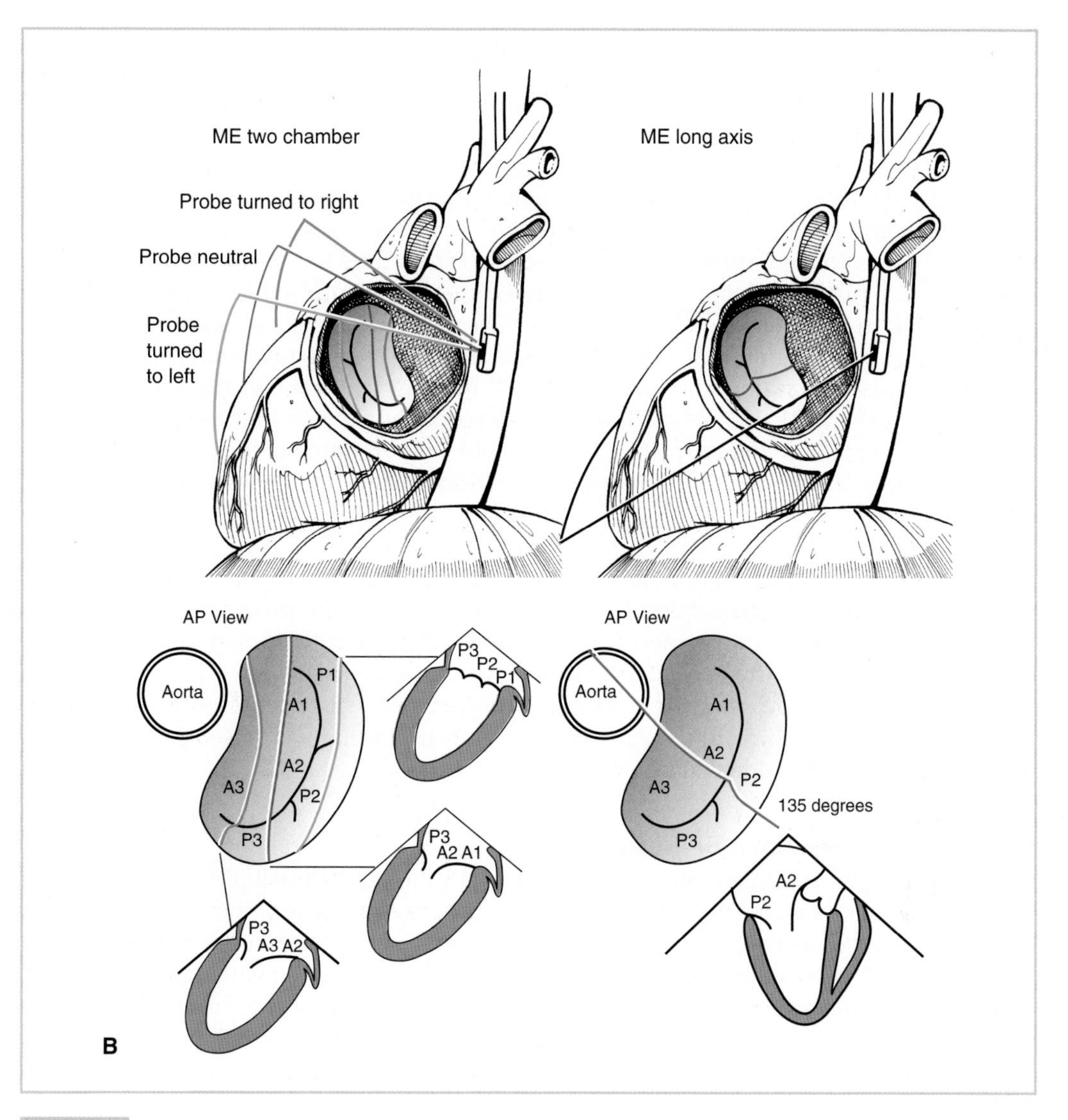

Figure 8.8. *(continued)*

variable amounts of anterior leaflet in the middle. The apparent double orifice stems from the semicircular coaptation between the leaflets of the mitral valve. The presence and severity of disease at the level of the commissures can be evaluated here.

3. Next, the **ME two-chamber view** is obtained by rotating the transducer forward to approximately 80 to 100 degrees. Additionally, by turning the shaft of the probe leftward and rightward three reproducible cross-sections can be obtained, allowing further identification of the valve segments (6,17).
4. Then, the **ME long axis view** is obtained by rotating the transducer to approximately 130 to 150 degrees. This provides a cut through the center of each mitral valve leaflet, which allows reliable identification of A2 and P2 (4). As this view cuts across the saddle-shaped annual plane at its most superior aspect, it is a preferred view for assessing mitral valve prolapse because it avoids the false positives which occur using the ME four-chamber view.

5. Finally, the probe is advanced into the stomach and the **TG basal SAX** view of the mitral valve is obtained (4,6) (Fig 2.18). This cross-section is useful to diagnose clefts and perforations and color Doppler provides additional information on the origin of the regurgitant jet(s).

Technically, it is extremely important to remember that the classic imaging planes described in the preceding text are obtained *only* when the echo scan crosses through the *center* of the mitral valve. Indeed, turning of the probe shaft from the ME commissural or ME long axis views will provide a lot of additional three-dimensional information from transitional images, but it may be misleading to the novice eye. For example, gently turning the probe to the right in the commissural view will reveal more of the anterior leaflet, showing not only A2 but also extending toward A1 and A3. Turning the probe to the left will reveal more of P2, not only P1 and P3 on either side as expected. Likewise in the long axis view, a well-centered scan will demonstrate A2 and P2, but slight rotation of the probe to the right will move the scan toward A3/P3 and slight rotation to the left will move the scan toward A1/P1.

The whole detailed examination can be done very quickly when one becomes familiar with it. The recommended sequence of views mentioned in the preceding text provides sufficient redundancy in the segment identification that in the author's experience results in high accuracy and consistent reliability. Whatever the sequence of views, the examination should be consistent and systematic. As in other aspects of echocardiography, repetition is important, and by learning to recognize the variants of normal and the wide spectrum of pathologies are better appreciated.

Step 3—Can the Valve Be Repaired?

Mitral valve repair has many proven advantages (18,19), but its feasibility depends on the location, extent, and mechanism of MR. Some lesions, like prolapse of the posterior middle scallop, tend to be easier to repair, whereas lesions that involve the anterior leaflet or both leaflets, as well as calcified or fibrosed leaflets, tend to be more challenging (18,20,21). Ultimately, the determination of whether a valve repair should be attempted is surgeon dependent and it is important for the echocardiographer to know the preferences and capabilities of their surgical colleagues. The subject of valve repair is discussed in detail in Chapter 10.

QUANTITATIVE EVALUATION OF THE MITRAL VALVE

Regurgitant volume, RF, and regurgitant orifice area (ROA) can be calculated using the continuity principle. For a detailed discussion of this principle, please see the chapter 6 on hemodynamic assessment.

- The regurgitant volume is the difference between the amount of blood that enters the left ventricle in diastole and the amount of blood that exits through the aortic valve in systole. It is typically obtained by calculating the stroke volume across the LVOT ($VTI_{LVOT} \times Area_{LVOT}$) and subtracting it from the forward stroke volume which crosses the mitral valve in diastole ($VTI_{MV} \times Area_{MV}$). An alternative site such as the pulmonary artery can also be used. Calculation of regurgitant volume is complicated by the fact that the mitral valve opening is oval, not round, and its surface area changes throughout diastole. For these reasons, this author prefers to use the proximal isovelocity surface area (PISA) method to calculate the regurgitant volume, as described in the following text.

- The **RF** (the percentage of left ventricular blood that flows backwards into the left atrium in systole) is the ratio of the regurgitant volume over the volume that flows forward across the mitral valve in diastole (i.e., the total stroke volume).
- Calculation of the **effective regurgitant orifice area (EROA)** is achieved by the PISA method. This method is also used in the evaluation of mitral stenosis and it is described in detail in Chapter 9. In brief, PISA takes advantage of the flow dynamics of blood because it is forced into the regurgitant orifice. Approaching the orifice, the blood cells accelerate along a series of concentric hemispheres which can be visualized by color Doppler. At the aliasing velocity (Nyquist limit) the color turns from red to blue (Figure 8.9) and provides both the velocity and the radius of the hemisphere. By knowing the velocity and radius of the hemisphere, one can calculate the volumetric flow at that radius (= Area × velocity = $2\pi r^2 \times$ Nyquist limit). Then one measures the peak velocity of the MR jet by CW Doppler to calculate the EROA.

$$\text{EROA} = \frac{2\pi r^2 \times \text{Nyquist limit}}{\text{MR velocity}}$$

The PISA method is based on a number of assumptions, which create important limitations (22): first it assumes that the orifice is round, which may not be the case. Also, this method's estimation of cross sectional area as $2\pi r^2$ assumes that the PISA "shells" are true hemispheres, not cones or flattened shells. Utsunomiya et al. established that PISA shells are closest to being true hemispheres when their radius is approximately 11 to 15 mm (23). The Nyquist limit and the color baseline should be adjusted accordingly to minimize error. Also, for eccentric jets, an angle correction must be used, as described in the chapter 9 on mitral stenosis.

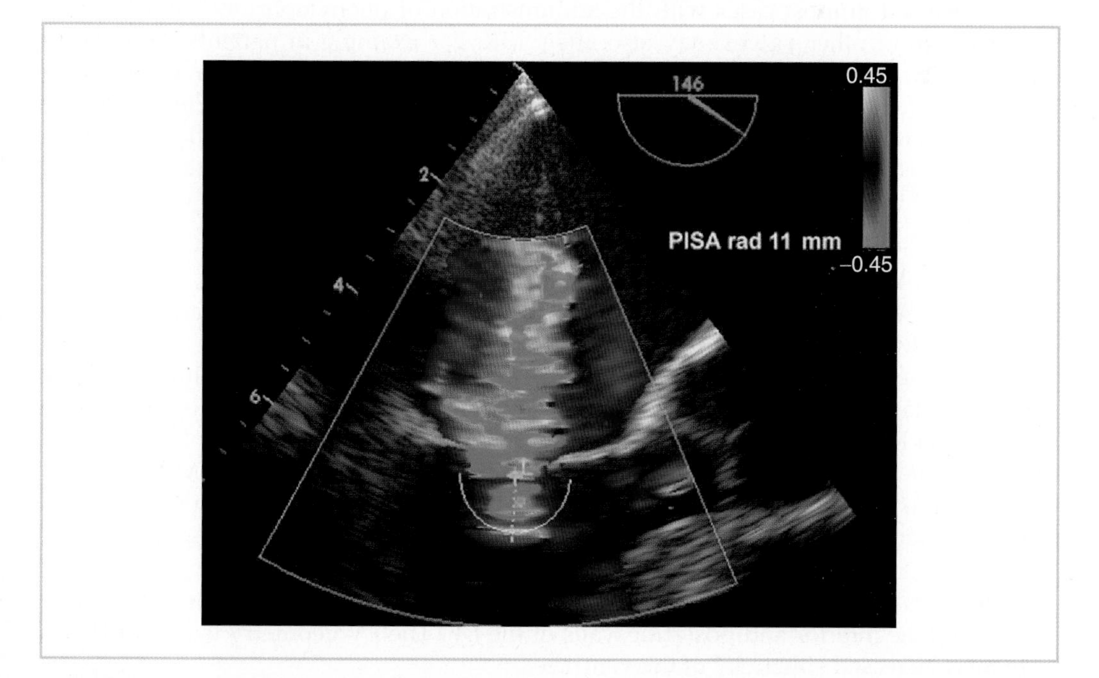

Figure 8.9. Estimated regurgitant orifice area by the proximal isovelocity surface area (PISA) method. The radius of the hemisphere where the cells reach the aliasing velocity is measured and used in the PISA equation.

Finally, when certain clinical conditions are met, a simplified PISA formula can be used. Indeed, when the Nyquist limit is set at 40 cm/s and the gradient across the MR jet is 100 mm Hg, the whole formula simplifies down to:

$$\text{EROA} = \frac{r^2}{2}$$

Regurgitant volume, RF, and regurgitant area are time-consuming measurements and may not always be practical in the busy setting of the operating room. As such, they may not always be required in mild or severe cases. However, they are the only true quantitative measurements of MR that we have and they are important in borderline cases. They are also important research tools.

Table 8.2 summarizes the quantitative values typically found in mild, moderate, and severe MR (14).

PITFALLS IN THE EVALUATION OF MITRAL REGURGITATION

Patients with mitral valve disease often have dilated hearts and distorted cardiac anatomy. This can make the TEE examination challenging because it changes the appearance of the various TEE cross-sections of the mitral valve. Changes in preload, afterload, myocardial contractility, and compliance can have a profound impact on the appearance of MR. In the operating room, all of these are affected by general anesthesia (GA). Several authors have documented that MR improves by at least one grade following induction of anesthesia (24–26). The difference seemed least pronounced in flail mitral valves and most significant in patients with functional MR (25). Gisbert et al. reported that the effect of GA can be reversed in most cases with the administration of phenylephrine (26). Changing the condition of other valves may also affect MR. For example in patients with MR in the presence of significant aortic stenosis, the severity of MR usually improves following aortic valve replacement (AVR) due to lower intraventricular pressures. Finally, any of these factors can change acutely many times during the course of an operation. For these reasons, the echocardiographer must remain cognizant of the clinical conditions present at the time of the examination when assessing the severity of MR.

FUNCTIONAL MITRAL REGURGITATION

MR can also be seen in the absence of structural abnormality of the mitral leaflets. Termed *functional MR*, it typically occurs in the setting of chronic left ventricular dysfunction. Most cases of functional MR fall into the Carpentier type 3b category, although some annular dilatation can also be present as part of the mechanism. The most common cause of functional MR is ischemic cardiomyopathy, but it can also be the result of other forms of dilated cardiomyopathies as well. The clinical importance of functional MR resides in the fact that it is associated with a worse overall prognosis. The mechanism of functional MR is multifactorial. Some of the proposed factors include the following:

1. Regional wall motion abnormalities and dilatation (sometimes frank aneurysm) usually affecting the inferior and posterior walls of the LV. The LV geometry is modified and there is increased sphericity of the ventricle.
2. Distortion in the relationship between the LV and the mitral apparatus can result in increased interpapillary distance and changes in papillary muscle orientation relative to the leaflets.

3. The conditions mentioned in the preceding text can result in tethering of the mitral leaflets, which ultimately leads to failure of coaptation and regurgitation.
4. Annular dilatation may also occur, developing mostly in the anterio-posterior (A-P) diameter.
5. Finally, if ventricular function is depressed, decreased closing forces on the mitral valve during systole may also play some role in the failure of coaptation.

The best time to assess functional MR is preoperatively. As mentioned in the preceding text, GA affects loading conditions and MR is typically underestimated under anesthesia. In cases of structural MR, the jet may look less severe under anesthesia, but the structural abnormality of the mitral valve will still be present. In the case of functional MR, where little structural abnormality in the mitral valve is present, the reduced loading conditions may mislead the clinician not to correct the pathology, which could be detrimental to the patient.

When faced with having to assess functional MR in the operating room, the same general principles apply:

- Anatomy, anatomy, anatomy: Rule out structural causes of MR, for example, leaflet prolapse.
- Carefully look at the mitral leaflets for tethering (leaflets not returning to the annular plane during systole) or other restriction to valve closure, mitral annulus diameter, papillary muscles location and wall motion in areas supporting the papillary muscles.
- Look at overall LV size and shape.

The surgical approach to functional MR is controversial and is discussed at length in the chapter 10 on mitral repair.

CONCLUSION

Intraoperative TEE has become an integral part of the surgical decision-making process in mitral valve surgery, and a standard of care in the evaluation of MR. A thorough and systematic approach to the examination of the mitral valve allows one to define the pathology and to pinpoint its precise location on the valve.

Following the surgical procedure, the immediate results can be determined and further interventions can be undertaken immediately if necessary. This will be discussed in the chapter 10 on mitral repair.

REFERENCES

1 Salgo IS, Gorman JH III, Gorman RC, et al. Effect of annular shape on leaflet curvature in reducing mitral leaflet stress. *Circulation* 2002;106(6):711–717.
2 Cheitlin MD, Finkbeiner WE. Cardiac anatomy. In: Chatterjee K, Cheitlin MD, Karliner J, et al. *Cardiology, an illustrated text*. Philadelphia: JB Lippincott Co, 1991:1.9–1.10.
3 Carpentier AF, Lessana A, Relland JY, et al. Loulmet: the "physio-ring": an advanced concept in mitral valve annuloplasty. *Ann Thorac Surg* 1995;60:1177–1185.
4 Shanewise JS, Cheung AT, Aronson S, et al. ASE/SCA guidelines for performing a comprehensive intraoperative multiplane transesophageal echocardiography examination: recommendations of the American Society of Echocardiography Council for Intraoperative Echocardiography and the Society of Cardiovascular Anesthesiologists Task Force for Certification in Perioperative Transesophageal Echocardiography. *Anesth Analg* 1999;89:870–884.

5 Kumar N, Kumar M, Duran CM. A revised terminology for recording surgical findings of the mitral valve. *J Heart Valve Dis* 1995;4:70–75.
6 Lambert AS, Miller JP, Merrick SH, et al. Improved evaluation of the location and mechanism of mitral valve regurgitation with a systematic transesophageal echocardiography examination. *Anesth Analg* 1999;88:1205–1212.
7 Carpentier AF. Cardiac valve surgery-the "French correction". *Jpn J Thorac Cardiovasc Surg* 1983;86:323–327.
8 Stewart WJ, Currie PJ, Salcedo EE, et al. Evaluation of mitral leaflet motion by echocardiography and jet direction by Doppler color flow mapping to determine the mechanisms of mitral regurgitation. *J Am Coll Cardiol* 1992;20:1353–1361.
9 Helmcke F, Nanda NC, Hsiung MC, et al. Color Doppler assessment of mitral regurgitation with orthogonal planes. *Circulation* 1987;75:175–183.
10 Cape EG, Yoganathan AP, Weyman AE, et al. Adjacent solid boundaries alter the size of regurgitant jets on Doppler color flow maps. *J Am Coll Cardiol* 1991;17:1094–1102.
11 Simpson IA, Valdes-Cruz LM, Sahn DJ, et al. Doppler color flow mapping of simulated *in vitro* regurgitant jets: evaluation of the effects of orifice size and hemodynamic variables. *J Am Coll Cardiol* 1989;13: 1195–1207.
12 Stevenson J. Two-dimensional color Doppler estimation of the severity of atrioventricular valve regurgitation: important effects of instrument gain setting, pulse repetition frequency and carrier frequency. *J Am Soc Echocardiogr* 1989;2:1–10.
13 Tribouilloy C, Shen WF, Quere JP, et al. Assessment of severity of mitral regurgitation by measuring regurgitant jet width at its origin with transesophageal Doppler color flow imaging. *Circulation* 1992;85:1248–1253.
14 Zoghbi WA, Enriquez-Sarano M, Foster E, et al. American Society of Echocardiography. Recommendations for evaluation of the severity of native valvular regurgitation with two-dimensional and Doppler echocardiography. *J Am Soc Echocardiogr* 2003;16(7):777–802.
15 Schiller NB, Foster E, Redberg RF. Transesophageal echocardiography in the evaluation of mitral regurgitation. The twenty-four signs of severe mitral regurgitation. *Cardiol Clin* 1993;11:399–408.
16 Pu M, Griffin BP, Vandervoort PM, et al. The value of assessing pulmonary venous flow velocity for predicting severity of mitral regurgitation: a quantitative assessment integrating left ventricular function. *J Am Soc Echocardiogr* 1999;12:736–743.
17 Foster GP, Isselbacher EM, Rose GA, et al. Accurate localization of mitral regurgitant defects using multiplane transesophageal echocardiography. *Ann Thorac Surg* 1998;65:1025–1031.
18 David TE, Armstrong S, Sun Z, et al. Late results of mitral valve repair for mitral regurgitation due to degenerative disease. *Ann Thorac Surg* 1993;56:7–12.
19 Spencer FC, Galloway AC, Grossi EA, et al. Recent developments and evolving techniques of mitral valve reconstruction. *Ann Thorac Surg* 1998;65:307–313.
20 Alvarez JM, Gray D, Choong C, et al. Repair of the anterior mitral leaflet. *Aust N Z J Med* 1993;23:279–284.
21 Cosgrove DM, Stewart WJ. Mitral valvuloplasty. *Curr Probl Cardiol* 989;14:359–415.
22 Simpson IA, Shiota T, Gharib M, et al. Current status of flow convergence for clinical applications: is it a leaning tower of "PISA"? *J Am Coll Cardiol* 1996;27(2):504–509.
23 Utsunomiya T, Doshi R, Patel D, et al. Calculation of volume flow rate by the proximal isovelocity surface area method: simplified approach using color Doppler zero baseline shift. *J Am Coll Cardiol* 1993;22(1): 277–282.
24 Grewal KS, Malkowski MJ, Piracha AR, et al. Effect of general anesthesia on the severity of mitral regurgitation by transesophageal echocardiography. *Am J Cardiol* 2000;85(2):199–203.
25 Bach DS, Deeb GM, Bolling SF. Accuracy of intraoperative transesophageal echocardiography for estimating the severity of functional mitral regurgitation. *Am J Cardiol* 1995;76(7):508–512.
26 Gisbert A, Souliere V, Denault AY, et al. Dynamic quantitative echocardiographic evaluation of mitral regurgitation in the operating department. *J Am Soc Echocardiogr* 2006;19(2):140–146.

QUESTIONS

1. **Which of the following statements is true, regarding mitral valve anatomy?**
   a. The posterior leaflet has true scallops, whereas the anterior leaflet does not.
   b. The mitral annulus reduces its diameter in systole.
   c. The anterior leaflet is larger than the posterior leaflet.
   d. The anterior leaflet shares a common attachment with the aortic valve.
   e. All of the above statements are true.

2. **Which of the following is anatomically closest to the left atrial appendage (LAA)?**
   a. Carpentier P2
   b. Duran P2
   c. Duran A2
   d. Duran C2

3. **Which of the following mitral valve segments receives chordae tendinae from the anterolateral papillary muscle?**
   a. Duran A2
   b. Duran P2
   c. Duran C2
   d. Carpentier P2

4. **Ischemic heart disease is typically associated with which type of mitral regurgitation?**
   a. Type 1
   b. Type 2
   c. Type 3a
   d. Type 3b

5. **What direction would you expect the mitral regurgitant (MR) jet to be directed in a typical P2 prolapse?**
   a. Central
   b. Anteromedial
   c. Posterolateral
   d. Anterolateral
   e. Posteromedial

6. **Which of the following would you not expect in a patient with severe MR?**
   a. Systolic pulmonary venous (PV) flow reversal
   b. Regurgitant orifice area (ROA) of 0.5 cm^2
   c. Vena contracta 0.4 cm
   d. Jet area/left atrial (LA) area more than 50%

7. **Which of the following is/are recognized pitfalls of the PISA method, when evaluating MR?**
   a. It assumes that the regurgitant orifice is round.
   b. It needs to be angle corrected.
   c. It assumes that the red blood cells accelerate along a series of true hemispheres.
   d. All of the above.

8. **Which of the following best describes the coanda effect?**
   a. A wall-hugging jet appears milder on color flow Doppler (CFD) than it actually is.
   b. A wall-hugging jet appears more severe on CFD than it actually is.

c. A wall-hugging jet appears more eccentric on CFD than it actually is.
d. The vena contracta of a wall-hugging jet appears falsely narrow.

9. Decreasing the aliasing velocity (Nyquist limit) would have which of the following effects, except

a. Larger regurgitant jet
b. Wider vena contracta
c. Larger proximal flow convergence (proximal isovelocity surface area [PISA]) shell
d. Larger calculated ROA

10. What angle of transducer rotation usually provides the best mitral commissural view?

a. 0 to 30 degrees
b. 60 to 90 degrees
c. 90 to 120 degrees
d. 120 to 150 degrees

Answers appear at the back of the book.

9 Mitral Valve Stenosis

Colleen Gorman Koch

The 19th century physician Jean Nicholas Corvisart established the diagnostic value of percussion in the physical diagnosis of cardiac disorders. He described the diastolic thrill of mitral stenosis (MS) as "a peculiar rushing like water, difficult to be described, sensible to the hand applied over the precordial region, a rushing which proceeds apparently from the embarrassment which the blood undergoes in passing through an opening which is no longer proportioned to the quantity of fluid which it ought to discharge" (1). As early as 1898, D. W. Samways discussed the potential for performing cardiac surgery in the most severe cases of MS in an article entitled "Cardiac Peristalsis: Its Nature and Effects," published in *The Lancet* (2). In the modern era of heart disease, cardiac catheterization has provided hemodynamic information and assessed the severity of MS. Popovic et al. (3) investigated time-related trends in the use of preoperative invasive hemodynamic measurements in 1,985 patients with isolated valvular stenosis. During an 8-year study period, cardiac catheterization before valve surgery remained a common practice; however, it was performed primarily to ascertain coronary anatomy. The need for invasive hemodynamic measurements acquired during catheterization dramatically decreased, superseded by noninvasive hemodynamic measurements obtained with echocardiography (3). *Currently, two-dimensional and Doppler echocardiography have supplanted cardiac catheterization in providing a complete evaluation of patients with MS* (4).

MITRAL VALVE ANATOMY

Morphologically, the mitral valve (MV) apparatus is composed of the left atrial (LA) wall, mitral annulus, anterior and posterior MV leaflets, chordal tendons, anterolateral and posteromedial papillary muscles, and left ventricular (LV) myocardium (5,6). The valvular tissue can be divided into two commissural regions, the anterolateral commissure and the posteromedial commissure, and two leaflet areas, the anterior and posterior MV leaflets. The anterior mitral leaflet is somewhat triangular in shape, with an attachment to approximately one third of the circumference of the mitral annulus. It is attached to the fibrous skeleton of the heart, as are the left coronary cusp and half of the noncoronary cusp of the aortic valve. The attachment of the posterior mitral leaflet to the mitral annulus is lengthier than that of the anterior mitral leaflet. Clefts along the free margin of the posterior leaflet allow the identification of individual scallops (5). Although the anterior mitral leaflet base-to-margin dimension is longer than that of the posterior mitral leaflet, and although the basal attachments are different for each leaflet, the two leaflets are nearly identical in overall surface area. Chordal tendons from each papillary muscle attach to both of the MV leaflets. On average, 120 chordal tendons attach to the undersurface of the MV leaflets. The chordal tendons subdivide as they project from the papillary muscles toward the MV leaflets. The spaces between the chordae serve as secondary orifices between the LA and LV (6).

The normal MV orifice area is approximately 4 to 6 cm^2. An orifice area in the range of 2 cm^2 causes a minimal elevation in the transvalvular pressure gradient, whereas a valve area of less than 1.4 cm^2 is associated with a significant transvalvular pressure gradient and the clinical presentation of MS (7–9).

ETIOLOGY OF MITRAL STENOSIS

The causes of MS include the following: rheumatic heart disease, LA myxoma, severe mitral annular calcification, thrombus formation, parachute MV deformity, congenital MS, supravalvular mitral ring, and cor triatriatum (6,10). Figures 9.1 and 9.2 depict a large LA myxoma obstructing mitral inflow.

The most common cause of MS in adult patients is still rheumatic heart disease (3,6,9). Pathologic features of rheumatic MS include fusion of the commissures; contracture, scarring, and diffuse thickening of the leaflet tissue and subvalvular apparatus; and calcium deposition within the mitral leaflets. This process results in a diminished size of the effective valvular orifice, in addition to valve rigidity as a consequence of the leaflet fibrosis and calcification. As the valve area becomes more restricted, increases in the transvalvular pressure gradient and LA pressure may lead to pulmonary hypertension with tricuspid regurgitation and right ventricular dysfunction (6,8–10).

TRANSESOPHAGEAL ECHOCARDIOGRAPHIC EVALUATION OF MITRAL STENOSIS

A discussion of the complete diagnostic evaluation follows, and the chapter concludes with a concise summary of the recommended approach to an accurate diagnosis of MS.

Two-Dimensional Echocardiography

The anatomy of MS can be defined more clearly from multiple imaging planes of two-dimensional transesophageal echocardiography (TEE) than by any other diagnostic modality. On the basis of the pathophysiologic features of rheumatic MS, key features that must be identified echocardiographically include the following: degree of leaflet thickening, amount of calcium deposition, extent of subvalvular involvement, decrement in leaflet mobility, and overall changes in chamber dimensions and function (11). Related issues, such as involvement of other valve structures and pulmonary hypertension, can also be assessed.

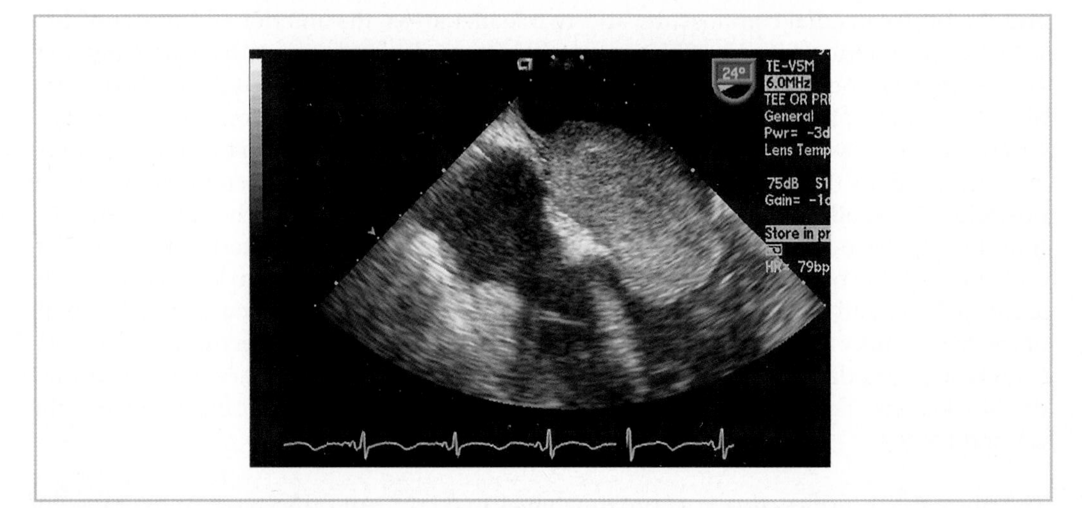

Figure 9.1. A transesophageal echocardiographic midesophageal four-chamber image displays a 3 × 6-cm left atrial myxoma causing symptomatic mitral stenosis. The atrial myxoma is visualized prolapsed through the mitral valve into the left ventricular cavity during diastole.

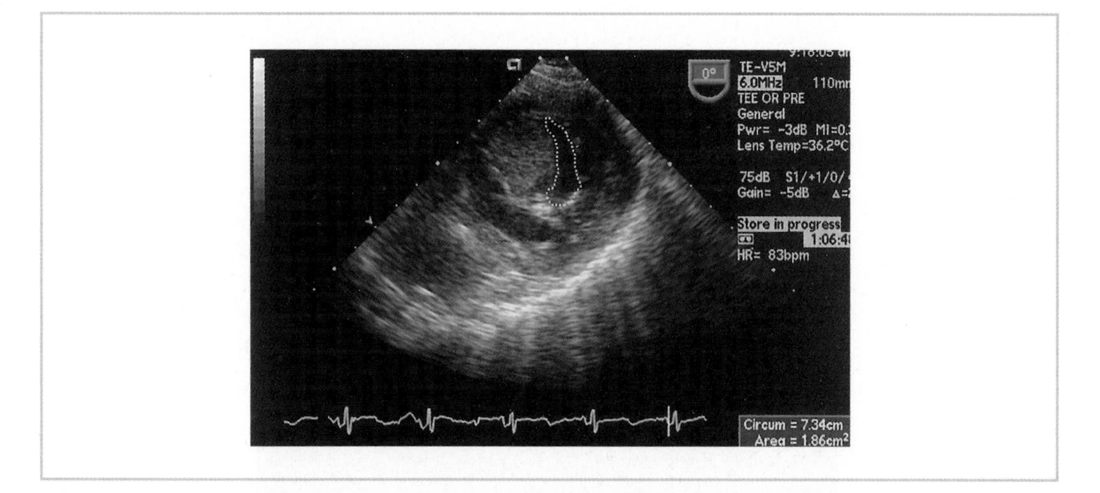

Figure 9.2. An atrial myxoma displayed from a transgastric basal short-axis imaging plane occupies a large portion of the mitral orifice. The mitral valve orifice measures 1.86 cm^2 in diastole.

Mitral leaflet tissue can display varying degrees of thickening and calcium deposition that cause the MV leaflets to appear "enhanced," or echo-bright. The "shadow" cast by calcium may obstruct the view of the distal anatomy; one of the strengths of TEE in this circumstance is the ability to view the structures from another plane, so that the operator can see beyond the "shadow." The standard midesophageal (ME) views (four-chamber, commissural, two-chamber, and long-axis) assist in evaluating the extent of disease. The chordal tendons can display varying degrees of thickening and contracture. The transgastric (TG) long-axis imaging plane provides the best information with regard to the extent of subvalvular involvement in the rheumatic process. The characteristic two-dimensional echocardiographic findings associated with rheumatic MS are represented in Figure 9.3. Rheumatic heart disease results in varying degrees of restricted mitral leaflet motion. In two-dimensional TEE, restricted leaflet motion is characterized by decreased leaflet excursion and by diastolic "doming" of the anterior mitral leaflet. The appearance of "doming" is the result of fusion of the anterior and posterior leaflets along the medial and lateral commissures. The leaflets are restricted or abnormally stenotic at the tips. The maximal amplitude of motion occurs in the mobile midsection, giving the anterior mitral leaflet an arched appearance, convex toward the LV outflow tract in diastole (12,13). Figure 9.3 demonstrates the characteristic "doming" or "hockey stick" deformity of the anterior mitral leaflet in diastole.

ECHOCARDIOGRAPHIC SCORING SYSTEM

In 1988, Wilkins et al. (11) developed an echocardiographic scoring system to assess MV morphology and its relationship to the success of percutaneous balloon dilation of the MV. Each of the four components of the scoring system is graded on a scale of 0 to 4, such that total scores range from 0 to 16. The four components of the scoring system assess the MV for the pathologic changes characteristically associated with rheumatic heart disease: reduced leaflet mobility, leaflet thickening, subvalvular thickening, and calcification. These investigators reported that a high echocardiographic score (>11), which is representative of advanced leaflet deformity, was associated with a suboptimal outcome after balloon dilation of the MV. A low echocardiographic score (<9) was associated with an optimal outcome (11). Table 9.1 presents the scoring system and describes what each grade on the scale represents for each of the four components. Although this scoring system was

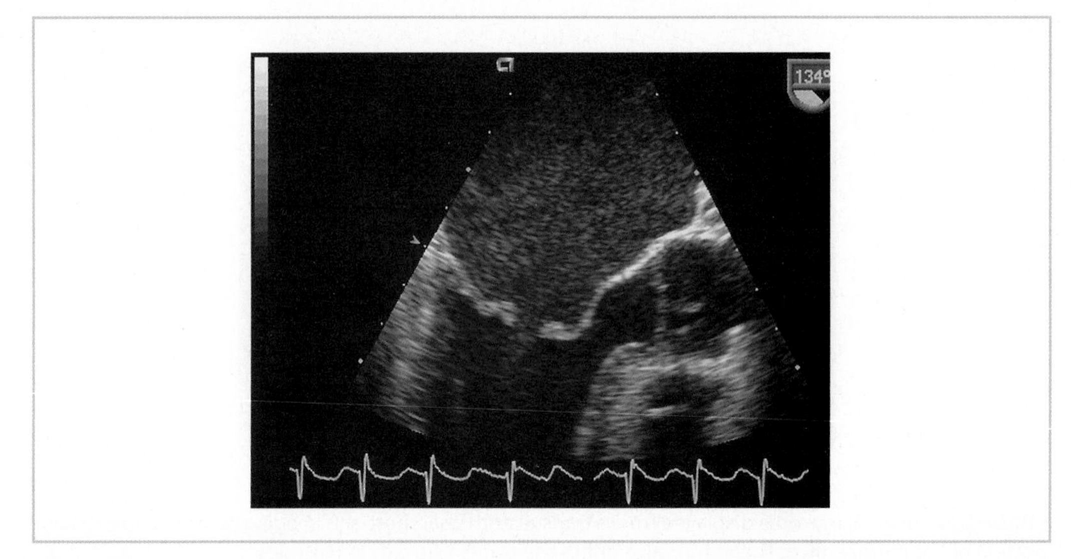

Figure 9.3. A midesophageal long-axis view of rheumatic mitral stenosis displays the characteristic diastolic "doming" of the anterior mitral leaflet in diastole and an enlarged left atrium. The mitral leaflets are thickened, particularly at their margins, and appear echo-bright secondary to calcium deposition.

developed for patients undergoing mitral balloon dilation, it can serve as a useful guide during the TEE examination of patients with rheumatic MS.

Standard chamber dimensions can be altered depending on the duration and degree of MS. Typically, an increase in the LA area is associated with chronic volume and pressure overload. Because of the low-flow state, LA spontaneous echo contrast or thrombus

Table 9.1 Echocardiographic scoring system

Grade	Mobility	Subvalvular thickening	Thickening	Calcification
1	Highly mobile valve with only leaflet tips restricted	Minimal thickening just below the mitral leaflets	Leaflets nearly normal in thickness (4–5 mm)	Single area of increased echo brightness
2	Leaflet mid and base portions have normal mobility	Thickening of chordal structures extending up to one third of chordal length	Mid leaflets normal, considerable thickening of margins (5–8 mm)	Scattered areas of brightness confined to leaflet margins
3	Valve continues to move forward in diastole, mainly from base	Thickening extending to the distal third of chords	Thickening extending through the entire leaflet (5–8 mm)	Brightness extending into midportion of the leaflets
4	No or minimal forward movement of the leaflets in diastole	Extensive thickening and shortening of all chordal structures extending down to papillary muscles	Considerable thickening of all leaflet tissue (>8–10 mm)	Extensive brightness throughout much of the leaflet tissue

From Wilkins G, Weyman A, Abascal A, et al. Percutaneous ballon dilatation of the mitral valve: an analysis of echocardiographic variables related to outcome and the mechanism of dilatation. *Br Heart J* 1988;60:300, with permission.

formation may be present. Daniel et al. (14) characterized LA spontaneous echo contrast as "dynamic clouds of echoes curling up slowly in a circular or spiral shape within the left atrium." They found that LA spontaneous echo contrast is useful in identifying those patients with MS who are at increased risk for thromboembolic events. TEE is more sensitive than transthoracic echocardiography in detecting LA spontaneous echo contrast. Because LA spontaneous echo contrast indicates blood stasis and may be a warning of thrombus formation, it is critical to scan the LA completely to exclude thrombus formation (14,15). Figure 9.4 displays an ME view of the LA with a thrombus in the LA appendage.

Diastolic properties of the LV are also affected in rheumatic MS. In patients with severe isolated rheumatic MS, Liu et al. (16) demonstrated reduced LV diastolic compliance. The reduction in compliance appeared to be related to a functional restriction resulting from chordal tethering to a rigid valve apparatus, a finding that was immediately reversed after balloon mitral valvuloplasty. LV systolic performance in patients with severe isolated MS was nearly identical to that in age-matched controls. Chronic elevation in LA pressure can cause structural alterations in the pulmonary vasculature, leading to pulmonary hypertension and ultimately right-sided heart failure (8,9). TEE evaluation of the right side of the heart may demonstrate varying degrees of right ventricular dysfunction and tricuspid regurgitation. *A comprehensive two-dimensional and Doppler TEE examination of the heart should be performed to exclude these associated findings and other valvular pathology.*

Physiologic Assessments

DETERMINATION OF THE PRESSURE GRADIENT

Normal flow velocity across the MV is less than 1.3 m/s. The pressure drop across a stenotic valve can be calculated from the instantaneous flow velocity by means of the simplified Bernoulli equation (17,18):

$$\text{Pressure gradient (mm Hg)} = 4v^2$$

where v represents the instantaneous velocity.

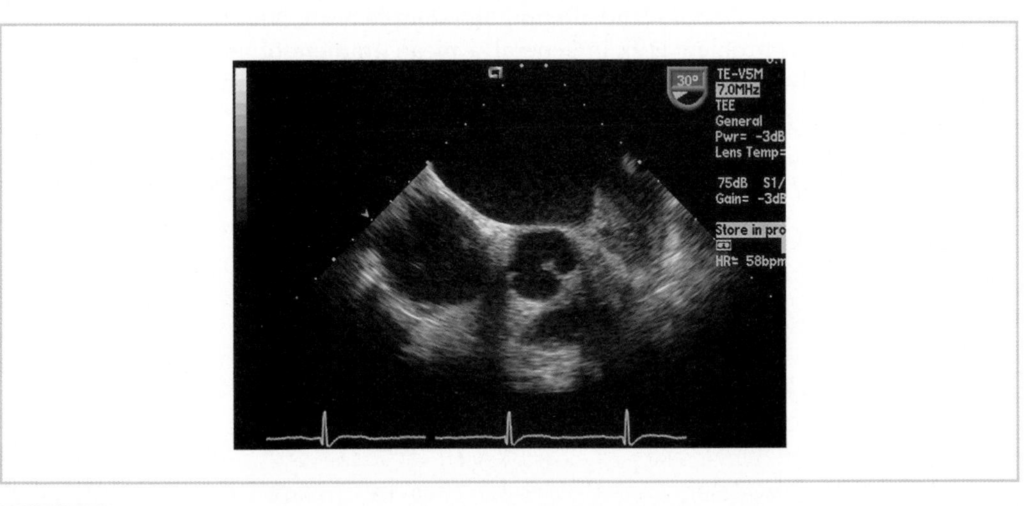

Figure 9.4. A left atrial appendage thrombus (*arrow*) is visualized from a short-axis imaging plane of the left atrium.

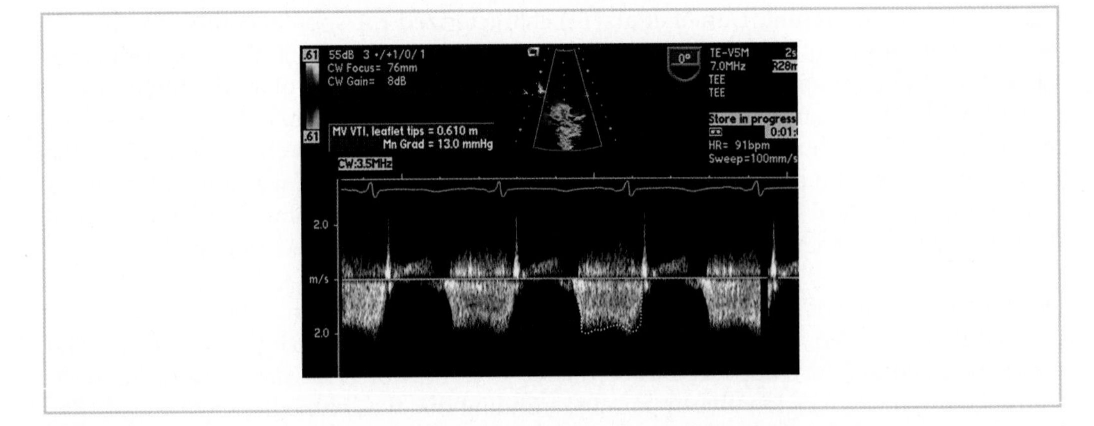

Figure 9.5. A diastolic spectral profile of mitral inflow has been obtained with continuous wave Doppler in this patient with mitral stenosis. The profile has been traced out, and a mean pressure gradient of 13 mm Hg has been calculated with the software available within the machine. Note that the inflow velocities are close to 2 m/s.

The equation is modified from the original in that the terms that account for viscous friction and flow acceleration have been eliminated. Because the velocity distal to the obstruction is significantly greater than the velocity proximal to the obstruction, the proximal velocity term can be ignored (17,18). Continuous wave Doppler interrogation of the inflow velocities across the valve is performed with use of the ME four-chamber, two-chamber, or long-axis view. Following manual tracing of the diastolic spectral profile, the echocardiographic machine software provides a mean gradient in millimeters of mercury. Figure 9.5 displays a mean gradient measurement across the MV in a patient with MS obtained with continuous wave Doppler and the ME four-chamber view. *It is important to note that an increase in forward flow through the mitral orifice, such as occurs in severe mitral valvular regurgitation, can result in a high transmitral gradient although the valve is only mildly stenotic. One therefore must be aware that the degree of MS can be overestimated in the face of significant mitral regurgitation* (4). Pressure gradients are underestimated if the angle between the sampling beam and the flow vector is large (>20 degrees) (17,19). Visualizing the inflow jet with color Doppler and aligning the sample beam with the color inflow can help to minimize this problem (19). In general, a mean gradient of more than 10 mm Hg across a stenotic valve is considered to indicate severe stenosis (20) (Table 9.2).

CALCULATIONS OF VALVE AREA

The severity of MS is also estimated by determining the reduction in MV area. This can be done with the use of two-dimensional and Doppler echocardiographic techniques.

Table 9.2 Severity of mitral stenosis

	Grade		
	Mild	**Moderate**	**Severe**
Mean gradient (mm Hg)	6	6–10	>10
PHT (ms)	100	200	>300
MVA (cm^2)	1.6–2.0	1.0–1.5	<1.0

PHT, pressure half-time; MVA, mitral valve area.

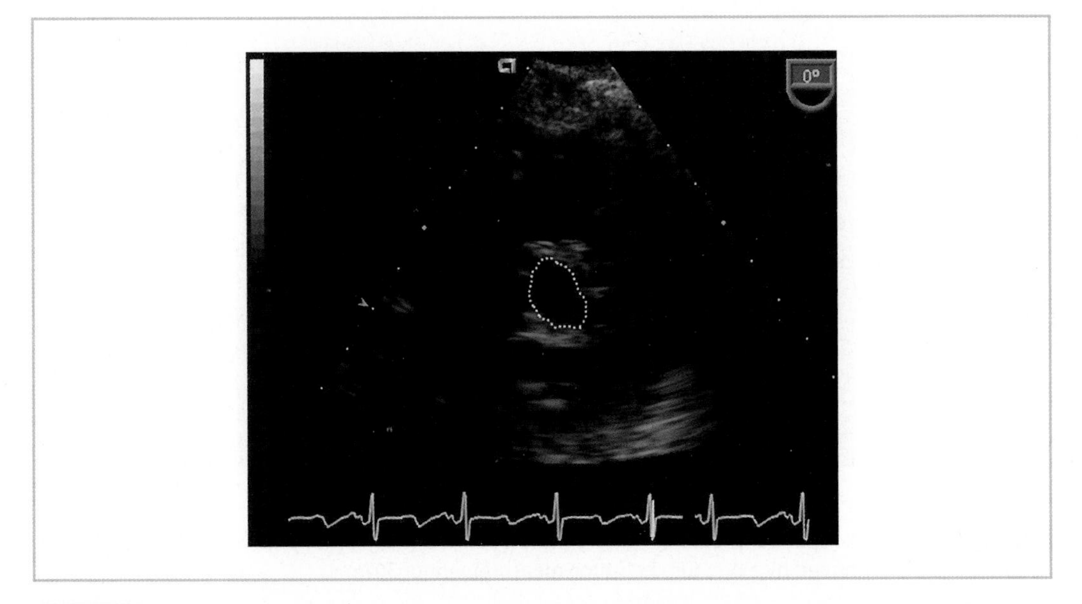

Figure 9.6. The mitral valve orifice assumes a "fish mouth" appearance in a transgastric basal short-axis imaging plane in a patient with rheumatic mitral stenosis. Tracing of the orifice margins of the mitral valve during diastole resulted in a mitral valve area measurement of 1.25 cm^2.

Planimetry valve area

Planimetry is a conceptually simple two-dimensional technique used to calculate the MV area. It involves directly visualizing the MV orifice in diastole from a TG basal short-axis imaging plane and tracing the orifice margins to acquire a valve area measurement in square centimeters (Figure 9.6). The results obtained with technique have been shown to correlate well with valve area measurements acquired invasively (3,12,21). Figure 9.6 demonstrates the use of planimetry in calculating the MV area from the TG basal short-axis imaging plane in a patient with rheumatic MS. A number of operator "pitfalls" should be recognized when this technique is used to optimize its accuracy. Instrumentation factors are critical in obtaining adequate images for planimetry. For example, if the receiver gain settings are too low, the edges of the valve may be obscured, resulting in "echo dropout," and the valve area will be overestimated (12). The opposite occurs when the gain settings are set too high, with resultant image saturation and a falsely narrowed valve orifice (23). Inadequate imaging plane orientation is another important measurement error with this technique. The stenotic MV looks like a funnel in diastole, the narrowest part being the commissural tip of the valve. *It is critical to scan the MV orifice superiorly to inferiorly to acquire the smallest orifice area.* Measuring too superiorly, in the body of the leaflets, can overestimate the valve area (21–23). In patients who have undergone mitral valvuloplasty, the valve area may be underestimated because of the inability to measure the extent of the commissural fractures with planimetry.

Pressure half-time

The pressure half-time describes the pressure difference between the LA and LV and can be quantitatively related to the degree of MS. As MS becomes more severe, the rate of pressure decline between the LA and LV is proportionally slower, and consequently the gradient between the LA and LV is maintained for a longer period of time. The pressure half-time is the time required for the atrioventricular pressure difference to decrease from the maximum to one half that value. To calculate the pressure half-time, the peak

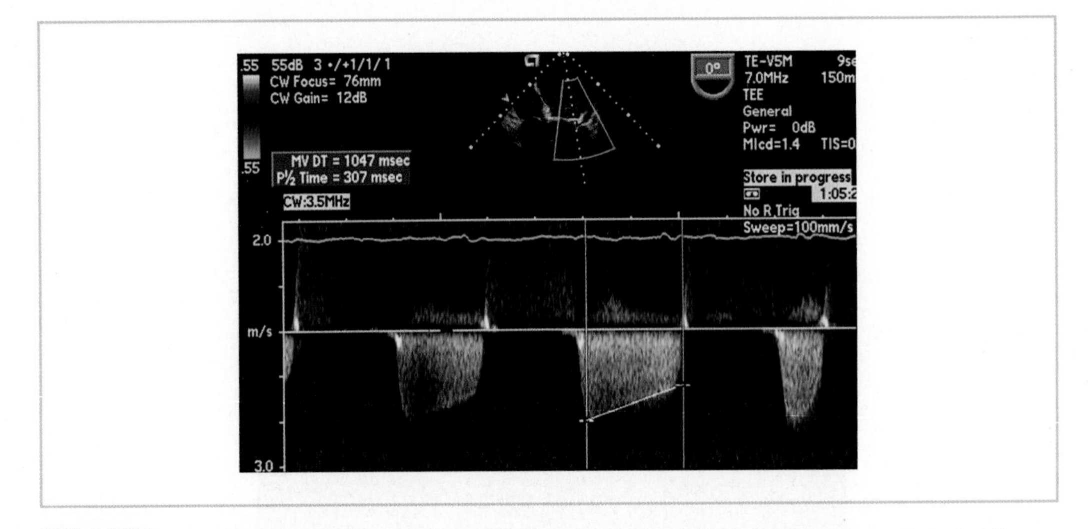

Figure 9.7. A diastolic spectral profile of mitral inflow obtained with continuous wave Doppler. Severe mitral stenosis is confirmed by a pressure half-time measurement of 307 ms.

transmitral flow velocity is measured by Doppler, and the time it takes to decrease by a factor of the square root of 2 is traced and measured (3,20,24). Figure 9.7 displays the pressure half-time measurement in a patient with MS. The signal is acquired by aligning the continuous wave Doppler beam with the mitral inflow and acquiring a transmitral flow velocity signal. The machine software automatically calculates the pressure half-time after the operator labels the maximal and minimal velocities. The pressure half-time increases as the severity of MS increases (20,24–26). In a normal MV, the pressure half-time is generally less than 60 ms. In mild MS, the average pressure half-time is approximately 100 ms; in moderate MS, it is approximately 200 ms, and in severe MS, the average pressure half-time measurement is more than 300 ms (3,24,25) (Table 9.3).

Pressure half-time mitral valve area

The MV area can be calculated from the pressure half-time measurement by using the following formula, originally described by Hatle and Angelsen (27):

$$\text{MV area (cm}^2\text{)} = 220/\text{pressure half-time (ms)}$$

They noted that the rate of pressure decline across a stenotic MV depends on the cross-sectional area of the valvular orifice. Hence, the tighter the orifice (smaller cross-sectional area), the slower the rate of pressure decline.

Table 9.3 Methods of determining mitral valve area

Planimetry	**Trace frozen short-axis view in diastole**
Pressure half-time (PHT, ms)	MVA = 220/PHT
Deceleration time (DT, ms)	MVA = 759/DT
Continuity equation	MVA = (LVOT area × LVOT TVI)/(MV TVI)
PISA	$\text{MVA} = 2\pi r^2 \times \alpha/180 \times v_a/v_p$

ms, milliseconds; MVA, mitral valve area (cm^2); α, funnel angle; v_a, aliasing velocity; v_p, peak transmitral velocity; LVOT, left ventricular outflow tract; TVI, time-velocity integral; PISA, proximal isovelocity surface area.

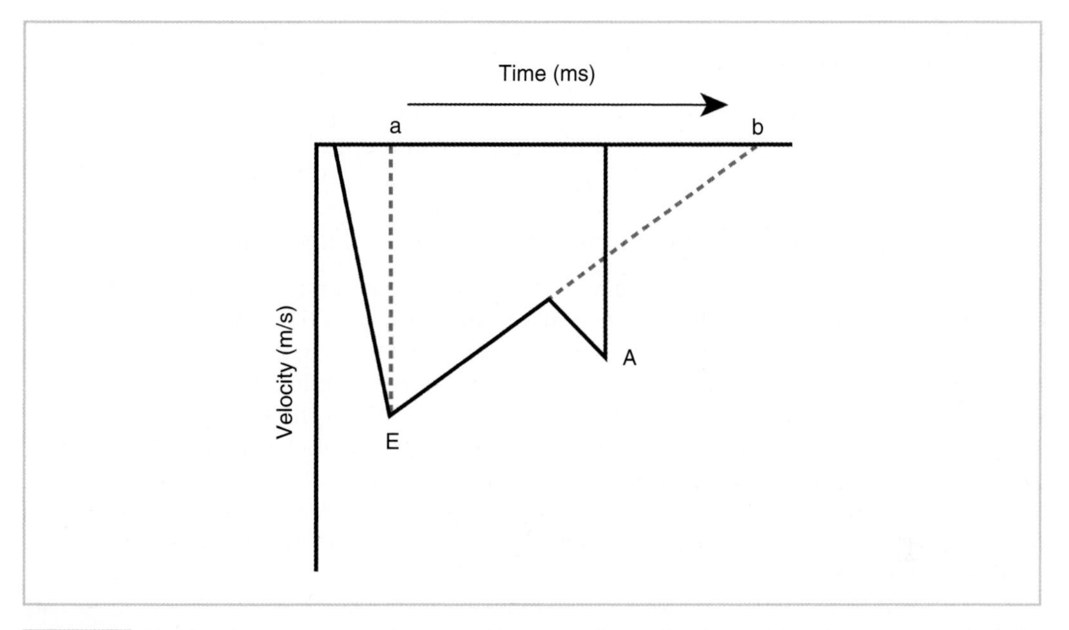

Figure 9.8. The deceleration time is the interval between the peak velocity (*a*) and the time at which the extrapolated inflow velocity reaches baseline (*b*).

The measurements obtained with the pressure half-time method are influenced by hemodynamic factors and depend on the compliance of the LA and LV. These factors must be taken into consideration when the pressure half-time method is applied to a stenotic MV. For example, *decreased LV compliance and severe aortic regurgitation can cause a rapid rise in the LV diastolic pressure, with a resultant shortening of the pressure half-time measurement and an overestimation of the MV area* (28,29). Braverman et al. (28) demonstrated the dependence of the pressure half-time method for calculating the MV area on hemodynamic variables such as peak transmitral gradient and atrioventricular compliance. Conditions such as previous mitral valvuloplasty, atrial septal defect, atrial tachycardia, and restrictive cardiomyopathy also affect the accuracy of the pressure half-time method (20,30–32).

DECELERATION TIME

The deceleration time is another simple means of evaluating the MV area, in which decay of the mitral inflow profile through a stenotic MV is examined. The following formula describes the relationship of the deceleration time to the MV area (19):

$$\text{MV area (cm}^2) = 759/\text{deceleration time (ms)}$$

The deceleration time is the interval between the peak velocity and the time at which the extrapolated inflow velocity reaches baseline. Figure 9.8 graphically displays the measurement of deceleration time. For profiles in which the decay is linear, the pressure half-time is equal to 29% of the deceleration time (20,26).

Advanced Concepts That May Be Helpful in Difficult Cases

CONTINUITY EQUATION

The continuity equation for calculating the area of a valve is based on the law of conservation of mass in hydrodynamics. In the absence of valvular regurgitation or shunts, flow volume at the MV should equal that at another valve according to the following equation (26,29):

$$\begin{aligned}\text{Volumetric flow} &= \text{area}_1 \times \text{time-velocity integral}_1 \\ &= \text{area}_2 \times \text{time-velocity integral}_2\end{aligned}$$

Therefore,

$$\text{Area}_2 = (\text{area}_1 \times \text{time-velocity integral}_1)/\text{time} - \text{velocity integral}_2$$

Flow through the MV can be calculated based on measurements made by Doppler echocardiography as the product of the valve orifice area and the time-velocity integral of the mitral inflow. $\text{Area}_1 \times$ time-velocity integral_1 represents volumetric flow through the reference valve. The reference area (area_1) is a cross-sectional area measurement that assumes the geometric model of a circle: πr^2. The LV outflow tract or pulmonary artery is commonly used for the reference area and time-velocity integral measurements. The equation is rearranged to solve for the MS area, area_2, as previously discussed. *The continuity equation is theoretically independent of transvalvular pressure gradients, LV compliance, and changing hemodynamic conditions, such as the increased forward flow that occurs during exercise* (3,28,29). *The continuity equation does not apply in circumstances of regurgitation in the reference valve or the MV because the forward volumetric flows are not equal, so that significant error is introduced* (29,33).

PROXIMAL ISOVELOCITY SURFACE AREA METHOD

The proximal isovelocity surface area (PISA) method, or flow convergence method, applies the continuity principle to color flow Doppler mapping in the region of the MV orifice where flow is converging from the LA. Figure 9.9 displays a color flow Doppler example of proximal flow convergence in a patient with rheumatic MS. When blood flow converges on an orifice that is small relative to the proximal chamber, it may be considered to form isovelocity "shells" with the shape of a hemisphere. The velocity of blood flow increases as blood approaches the small orifice, resulting in aliasing of the color flow signal and the

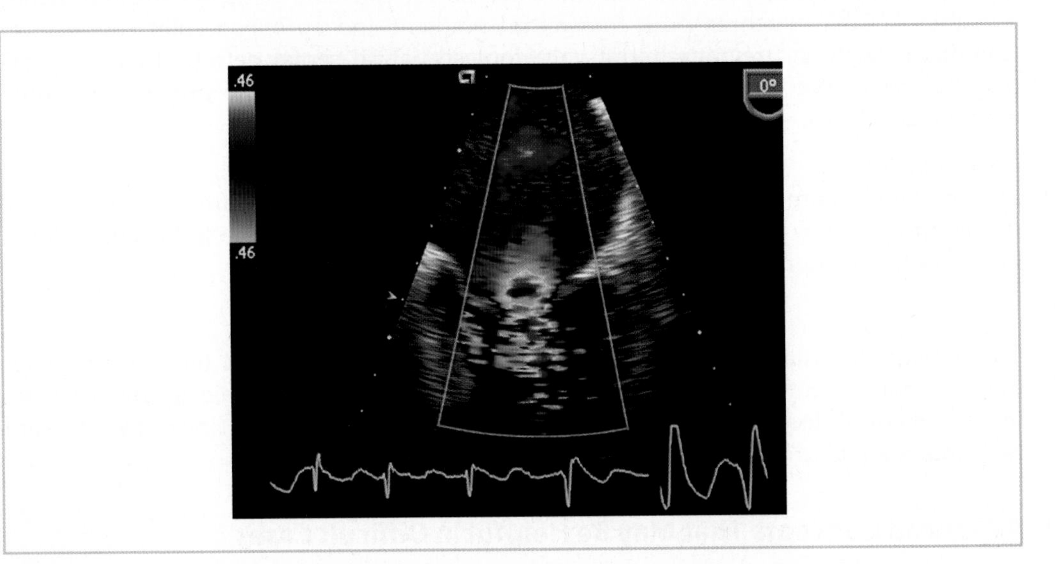

Figure 9.9. Color Doppler imaging from this midesophageal four-chamber view of the mitral valve demonstrates proximal isovelocity surface area or flow convergence on the left atrial side of the mitral valve.

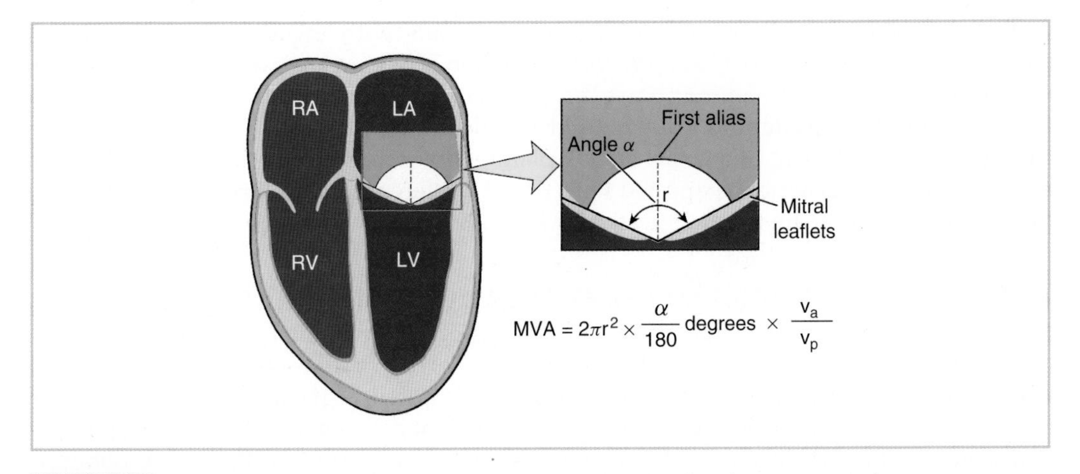

Figure 9.10. Midesophageal four-chamber view of the mitral valve demonstrates the measurements needed to calculate the mitral valve area by the proximal isovelocity surface area method. $\alpha/180$ degrees, angle correction factor; v_a, aliasing velocity; v_p, peak transmitral inflow velocity; RA, right atrium; RV, right ventricle; LA, left atrium; LV, left ventricle; MVA, mitral valve area. (Adapted from Rodriguez L, Thomas JD, Monterroso V, et al. Validation of the proximal flow convergence method: calculation of orifice area in patients with mitral stenosis. *Circulation* 1993;88:1157–1165, with permission.)

creation of a large proximal flow convergence region or shell. As blood approaches the orifice, its increasing velocity is pictured by color flow imaging as progressively smaller shells. The radius of the first aliasing velocity shell is measured from the tips of the MV leaflets to the aliasing boundary (19,34–37) (Figure 9.10). The volumetric flow rate can be calculated as the product of the surface area of the hemisphere of flow and the aliasing velocity. The mitral inflow velocity profile (at the orifice) is obtained with continuous wave Doppler. The basic elements of the continuity equation can therefore be identified by this straightforward color mapping, but the calculation of a valve area requires a correction for the true shape of the mitral orifice. Truly hemispheric shells would occur if the surface of the valve were flat with the leaflets apposed at 180 degrees. The angle α subtended by the mitral leaflets creates a funnel-shaped surface; an angle correction factor (α / 180 degrees) adjusts the hemispheric surface area pictured by color flow mapping to calculate the volumetric flow rate more accurately. The instantaneous volumetric flow rate (Q) in this region can be calculated as the product of the surface area of a hemisphere ($2\pi r^2$) and the aliasing velocity at the shell (v_a):

$$Q = 2\pi r^2 \times \alpha/180 \text{ degrees} \times v_a$$

Flow through this region should equal flow through the restricted orifice based on the continuity principle (34–36). Once the flow rate (Q) is calculated, the MV area can be obtained with the use of the continuity equation:

$$\text{MV area (cm}^2) = Q/v_p \text{ (cm/s)}$$

where Q is the volumetric flow rate and v_p is the peak transmitral inflow velocity.

Figure 9.10 illustrates the use of the flow convergence method in the calculation of MV area.

The MV area can be measured accurately with this method in the presence of mitral insufficiency. Several investigators have validated the use of the flow convergence method in the calculation of MV area by direct comparisons with anatomic and calculated measurements of orifice size (34,36,38,39). Calculation of MV area by the flow convergence method can be time consuming; however, its accuracy is not influenced by associated mitral or aortic regurgitation. This method of calculating MV area may be best under circumstances in which two-dimensional planimetry is technically limited, when the continuity equation cannot be applied with use of a reference volumetric flow, and when the pressure half-time method is affected by hemodynamic changes (35).

A PRACTICAL APPROACH TO THE EVALUATION OF MITRAL STENOSIS

Step 1. A two-dimensional evaluation of the MV is performed with a focus on answering the following questions: What is the appearance of the valve—that is, is the valve disfigured? Are the leaflets of normal thickness and mobility? If not, further assessment of the valve is needed to determine whether it is stenotic or regurgitant (see Chapter 8). Planimetry of the MV in the TG basal short-axis view is initially performed to obtain a rough estimate of the MV area.

Step 2. After completion of the two-dimensional examination, MV inflow interrogation with continuous wave Doppler is performed. The diastolic mitral inflow velocity profile is traced (Figure 9.5), and the mean pressure gradient is determined with the internal software of the echocardiography machine. In addition, the pressure half-time method is used to calculate the MV area (Figure 9.7). Most TEE machines also extrapolate the flow decay and calculate the deceleration time.

If the measurements are in agreement according to Table 9.2, no further evaluation is required.

Step 3. The advanced methods (continuity equation and PISA) are reserved for those patients for whom the pressure half-time method is unreliable or unavailable.

SUMMARY

Table 9.3 summarizes the techniques used to calculate the MV area, and Table 9.2 presents the scores for the various degrees of MS obtained with each of these techniques. In general, an MV area of 1.6 to 2.0 cm^2 is considered to indicate mild MS, 1.0 to 1.5 cm^2 moderate MS, and less than 1.0 cm^2 severe MS (9,20). Each technique has its limitations. *Agreement between the various methods of evaluating the valve together with clinical correlation will enhance accuracy and overall judgment.*

REFERENCES

1 Acierno LJ. Physical examination. In: *The history of cardiology*. London: Parthenon Publishing Group, 1994:461–462.
2 Acierno LJ. Surgical modalities. In: *The history of cardiology*. London: Parthenon Publishing Group, 1994:627.
3 Popovic AD, Thomas JD, Neskovic A, et al. Time-related trends in the preoperative evaluation of patients with valvular stenosis. *Am J Cardiol* 1997;80:1464–1468.
4 Bruce CJ, Nishimura RA. Clinical assessment and management of mitral stenosis, valvular heart disease. *Cardiol Clin* 1998;16:375–403.
5 Ranganathan N, Lam JH, Wigle ED, et al. Morphology of the human mitral valve: the valve leaflets. *Circulation* 1970;41:459–467.
6 Roberts WC, Perloff JK. Mitral valvular disease: a clinicopathologic survey of the conditions causing the mitral valve to function abnormally. *Ann Intern Med* 1972;77:939–974.

7 Kennedy JW, Yarnall SR, Murray JA, et al. Quantitative angiocardiography: IV. Relationships of left atrial and ventricular pressure and volume in mitral valve disease. *Circulation* 1970;41:817–824.
8 Schlant RC, Alexander RW, O'Rourke RA, et al. eds. Mitral valve disease. In: *Hurst's the heart*, 8th ed. New York: McGraw-Hill, 1994;1483–1518.
9 Selzer A, Cohn K. Natural history of mitral stenosis: a review. *Circulation* 1972;45:878–890.
10 Olson LJ, Subramanian R, Ackermann DM, et al. Surgical pathology of the mitral valve: a study of 712 cases spanning 21 years. *Mayo Clin Proc* 1987;62:22–34.
11 Wilkins G, Weyman A, Abascal V, et al. Percutaneous balloon dilatation of the mitral valve: an analysis of echocardiographic variables related to outcome and the mechanism of dilatation. *Br Heart J* 1988;60:299–308.
12 Otto C, ed. Valvular stenosis: diagnosis, quantitation, and clinical approach. In: *Textbook of clinical echocardiography*, 2nd ed. Philadelphia: WB Saunders, 2000:229–264.
13 Nichol PM, Gilbert BW, Kisslo JA. Two-dimensional echocardiographic assessment of mitral stenosis. *Circulation* 1977;55:120–128.
14 Daniel W, Nellessen U, Schroder E, et al. Left atrial spontaneous echo contrast in mitral valve disease: an indicator for an increased thromboembolic risk. *J Am Coll Cardiol* 1988;11:1204–1211.
15 Chen YT, Kan MN, Chen JS, et al. Contributing factors to the formation of left atrial spontaneous echo contrast in mitral valvular disease. *J Ultrasound Med* 1990;9:151–155.
16 Liu CP, Ting CT, Yang TM, et al. Reduced left ventricular compliance in human mitral stenosis: role of reversible internal constraint. *Circulation* 1992;85:1447–1456.
17 Hatle L, Brubakk A, Tromsdal A, et al. Noninvasive assessment of pressure drop in mitral stenosis by Doppler ultrasound. *Br Heart J* 1978;40:131–140.
18 Oh JK, Seward JB, Tajik AJ. Hemodynamic assessment. In: *The echo manual*, 2nd ed. Philadelphia: Lippincott Williams & Wilkins, 1999:59–71.
19 Weyman AE, ed. Left ventricular inflow tract I: the mitral valve. In: *Principles and practice of echocardiography*, 2nd ed. Philadelphia: Lea & Febiger, 1994:391–497.
20 Oh JK, Seward JB, Tajik AJ. Valvular heart disease. *The echo manual*, 2nd ed. Philadelphia: Lippincott Williams & Wilkins, 1999:103–132.
21 Henry WL, Griffith JM, Michaelis LL, et al. Measurement of mitral orifice area in patients with mitral valve disease by real-time, two-dimensional echocardiography. *Circulation* 1975;51:827–831.
22 Wann LS, Weyman AE, Feigenbaum H, et al. Determination of mitral valve area by cross-sectional echocardiography. *Ann Intern Med* 1978;88:337–341.
23 Martin RP, Rakowski H, Kleiman JH, et al. Reliability and reproducibility of two-dimensional echocardiographic measurement of the stenotic mitral valve orifice area. *Am J Cardiol* 1979;43:560–568.
24 Libanoff AJ, Rodbard S. Atrioventricular pressure half-time: measure of mitral valve orifice area. *Circulation* 1968;38:144–150.
25 Hatle L, Angelsen B, Tromsdal A. Noninvasive assessment of atrioventricular pressure half-time by Doppler ultrasound. *Circulation* 1979;60:1096–1104.
26 Bruce C, Nishimura R. Newer advances in the diagnosis and treatment of mitral stenosis. *Curr Probl Cardiol* 1998;23:127–184.
27 Hatle L, Angelsen B, eds. Pulsed and continuous wave Doppler in the diagnosis and assessment of various heart lesions. In: *Doppler ultrasound in cardiology: physical principles and clinical applications*. Philadelphia: Lea & Febiger, 1982:76–89.
28 Braverman AC, Thomas JD, Lee R. Doppler echocardiographic estimation of mitral valve area during changing hemodynamic conditions. *Am J Cardiol* 1991;68:1485–1490.
29 Nakatani S, Masuyama T, Kodama K, et al. Value and limitations of Doppler echocardiography in the quantification of stenotic mitral valve area: comparison of the pressure half-time and the continuity equation methods. *Circulation* 1988;77:78–85.
30 Thomas JD, Wilkins G, Choong CYP, et al. Inaccuracy of mitral pressure half-time immediately after percutaneous mitral valvotomy: dependence on transmitral gradient and left atrial and ventricular compliance. *Circulation* 1988;78:980–993.
31 Thomas JD, Weyman AE. Doppler mitral pressure half-time: a clinical tool in search of theoretical justification. *J Am Coll Cardiol* 1987;10:923–929.
32 Wranne B, Msee PA, Loyd D. Analysis of different methods of assessing the stenotic mitral valve area with emphasis on the pressure gradient half-time concept. *Am J Cardiol* 1990;66:614–620.
33 Karp K, Teien D, Eriksson P. Doppler echocardiographic assessment on the valve area in patients with atrioventricular valve stenosis by application of the continuity equation. *J Intern Med* 1989;225:261–266.
34 Rodriguez L, Thomas JD, Monterroso V, et al. Validation of the proximal flow convergence method: calculation of orifice area in patients with mitral stenosis. *Circulation* 1993;88:1157–1165.
35 Deng Y, Matsumoto M, Wang X, et al. Estimation of mitral valve area in patients with mitral stenosis by the flow convergence region method: selection of aliasing velocity. *J Am Coll Cardiol* 1994;24:683–689.

36 Rifkin R, Harper K, Tighe D. Comparison of proximal isovelocity surface area method with pressure half-time and planimetry in the evaluation of mitral stenosis. *J Am Coll Cardiol* 1995;26:458–465.
37 Vandervoort PM, Rivera M, Mele D, et al. Application of color Doppler flow mapping to calculate effective regurgitant orifice area: an *in vitro* study and initial clinical observations. *Circulation* 1993;88:1150–1156.
38 Degertekin M, Basaran Y, Gencbay M, et al. Validation of flow convergence region method in assessing mitral valve area in the course of transthoracic and transesophageal echocardiographic studies. *Am Heart J* 1998;135:207–214.
39 Faletra F, Pezzano A, Fusco R, et al. Measurement of mitral valve area in mitral stenosis: four echocardiographic methods compared with direct measurement of anatomic orifices. *J Am Coll Cardiol* 1996;28:1190–1197.

QUESTIONS

1. What is the most common cause of mitral stenosis (MS) in the adult patient?
a. Left atrial (LA) myxoma
b. Severe mitral annular calcification
c. Rheumatic heart disease
d. Thrombus formation

2. Which definition of the modified Bernoulli equation is correct?
a. It is a method to calculate mitral valve area.
b. It converts peak pressure gradients to mean pressure gradients.
c. It converts instantaneous velocities to instantaneous pressures.
d. None of the above.

3. Which of the following statements about planimetry imaging "pitfalls" is/are correct?
a. Inadequate imaging plane orientation can introduce measurement error.
b. Gain settings that are too high can result in image saturation and a falsely narrow measurement of area.
c. Gain settings that are too low can result in image dropout and introduce error into the valve area measurement.
d. All of the above.

4. The use of the continuity equation to calculate valve area in patients with MS is invalidated in which of the following clinical circumstances?
a. After mitral valvuloplasty
b. Left ventricular (LV) hypertrophy
c. Mitral regurgitation
d. None of the above

5. Which of the following valve areas is closest to normal?
a. Less than 1 cm^2
b. 4 to 6 cm^2
c. More than 7 cm^2
d. None of the above

6. Which of the following pressure half-time measurements corresponds to severe mitral valve (MV) stenosis?
a. More than 220 ms
b. 60 to 80 ms
c. Less than 60 ms
d. 100 ms

7. Which of the following is not a component of the echocardiographic scoring system?
a. Leaflet mobility
b. Subvalvular involvement
c. Chamber enlargement
d. Calcium deposition

8. Which of the following is the best description of diastolic doming in patients with rheumatic MS?
a. Bowing of the interatrial septum toward the right atrium in diastole
b. The movement of the subvalvular apparatus in diastole

c. The movement of the anterior mitral leaflet in diastole in which it becomes arched, with convexity toward the LV outflow tract
d. None of the above

9. In which of the following clinical circumstances is error introduced into the pressure half-time method?
a. Severe aortic regurgitation
b. Decreased LV compliance
c. Immediately after mitral balloon valvuloplasty
d. All the above

10. Which of the following statements is correct with regard to the benefits of using the flow convergence method in calculating MV area?
a. The flow convergence method can be used accurately when mitral regurgitation is present.
b. Maximal flow rate is calculated from the product of the aliasing velocity and the area of a hemisphere.
c. An angle correction factor is introduced to account for the inflow angle created by the mitral leaflets.
d. All the above.

Answers appear at the back of the book.

10 Mitral Valve Repair

Kristine Johnson Hirsch and Gregory M. Hirsch

HISTORY OF MITRAL VALVE REPAIR

Mitral Stenosis

The first successful mitral valvotomies were performed in the 1920s by Cutler and Levine in Boston (1) and Souttar in England (2). Subsequent attempts by both groups were disappointing, likely in part owing to the lack of such basic resources as blood transfusion, antibiotics, and safe anesthesia. After 25 years had elapsed, Charles P. Bailey, Dwight Harken, and Russell Brock had each devised successful methods of closed mitral valvotomy. Despite the development of safe cardiopulmonary bypass techniques, pioneered by Gibbon at Thomas Jefferson and refined by Kirklin at the Mayo Clinic, continued success with closed approaches delayed the widespread acceptance of "open heart" approaches to mitral commissurotomy until the 1970s.

Mitral Regurgitation

Early attempts were made to repair regurgitant mitral valves (MVs) with ingenious closed approaches, such as circumferential annular sutures. With the advent of reasonably safe cardiopulmonary bypass, Lillehei et al. (3) first carried out direct repair in 1957. In 1961, Starr and Edwards (4) reported the first successful MV replacement, and after this, enthusiasm for mitral repair waned. In Europe, Carpentier, Duran, et al. developed effective and reproducible methods to repair regurgitant MVs and were ultimately able to demonstrate the superiority of these methods over mitral replacement, stimulating renewed interest in mitral repair worldwide.

INDICATIONS FOR MITRAL VALVE REPAIR AND TIMING OF INTERVENTION

Historically, MV replacement was delayed until nearly intractable heart failure and often marked deterioration of LV function developed. This strategy was based on the morbidity and mortality of the surgery in addition to further loss of LV function postoperatively as a consequence of detachment of the chordal apparatus from the papillary muscles. *The advantages of mitral repair over mitral replacement include the preservation of LV function through preservation of the chordal attachments, low rates of thromboembolism and endocarditis, the lack of a requirement for anticoagulants beyond aspirin, and excellent durability.* Given the excellent long-term results of modern mitral repair techniques, the threshold for surgical intervention has been appreciably lowered.

Mitral Stenosis

The normal MV area is 4 to 5 cm^2. Narrowing of the mitral orifice below 2.5 cm^2 is required before the onset of dyspnea in the face of exercise, infection, stress or atrial fibrillation. Symptoms at rest rarely develop with a valve area greater than 1.5 cm^2. Surgically significant mitral stenosis (MS) is almost entirely due to rheumatic mitral disease with anatomic changes that include leaflet thickening and fibrosis, commissural fusion, chordal fusion and shortening. Leaflet and annular calcification may also be seen in longstanding rheumatic disease. The indications for surgical repair of MS include patients with New York Heart Association (NYHA) functional class III or IV with a valve area of 1.5 cm^2 or less. Patients with class II symptoms and with moderate or severe stenosis may be considered for mitral balloon valvotomy if they have suitable MV morphology. Pliability of the anterior leaflet and chordae tendineae are key elements of a repairable valve. Wilkins et.al described a scoring system using echocardiographic variables including leaflet mobility and thickening, chordal fusion and thickening and calcification on a grading scale (see Chapter 9 for detail). A lower cumulative score (<9) confers an increased likelihood of successful valve repair whereas a cumulative score of greater than 11 is associated with a suboptimal outcome.

Surgical intervention for other causes of MS, such as left atrium (LA) myxoma, severe mitral annular calcification (MAC), thrombus formation, congenital MS, supravalvular ring, parachute MV, and cor triatriatum will also require thorough transesophageal echocardiographic (TEE) evaluation of the MV and may incorporate mitral valve repair (MVR) techniques.

Mitral Regurgitation

The American College of Cardiology/American Heart Association Task Force on Practice Guidelines in Valvular Heart Disease recommends that patients with functional class II symptoms or higher and severe mitral regurgitation (MR) and asymptomatic patients with severe MR and echocardiographic evidence of LV dysfunction (left ventricular ejection fraction [LVEF] 0.30 to 0.60 and/or LV end-systolic dimension ≥40 mm) undergo repair. When a successful repair is probable, the weight of evidence favors surgical intervention in asymptomatic patients with severe MR and normal LV function (5).

STRUCTURAL MITRAL REGURGITATION

Structural lesions of the MV resulting in excessive leaflet motion (Carpentier type II) are commonly due to degenerative processes such as elongated or ruptured chordae or papillary muscles with or without annular dilation. Myxomatous degeneration makes up the bulk of the successfully repairable valves with other etiologies being less common and less likely to result in successful repair. Specific lesions lend themselves to established repair techniques such as P2 prolapse, and small anterior leaflet pathologies. As the complexity of the lesions increase, such as bileaflet prolapse, multiple segmental prolapses, and lesions with combined type II and type III (restrictive) abnormalities, the less likelihood of successful, durable repair. However, in centers with extensive experience with mitral repair techniques combined with accurate intraoperative echocardiographic imaging and diagnosis, these pathologies are frequently managed with reasonable success. Rupture papillary muscle due to acute MI is rarely amenable to repair and is most successfully managed with replacement of the MV.

FUNCTIONAL MITRAL REGURGITATION

Functional mitral regurgitation (FMR) is a broad term connoting incomplete closure of structurally normal leaflets in the context of chronically impaired ventricular function. It typically occurs in either segmentally damaged or globally dilated, hypokinetic ventricles with resultant annular dilation or apical tethering of the subvalvular apparatus preventing leaflet coaptation at the level of the MV annulus. Ischemic etiologies make up the largest subset of this group but nonischemic cardiomyopathies may lead to FMR through annular dilation, displacement of papillary muscles and leaflet tethering (Figure 10.1). It occurs in roughly 20% to 25% of patients after MI and 50% of those with congestive heart failure (CHF). FMR due to ischemic heart disease is essentially postinfarction MR, caused by progressive LV remodeling rather than reversible ischemia. The effects of LV remodeling on the mitral apparatus may result in leaflet restriction (Carpentier type III) with or without annular dilation (Carpentier type I).

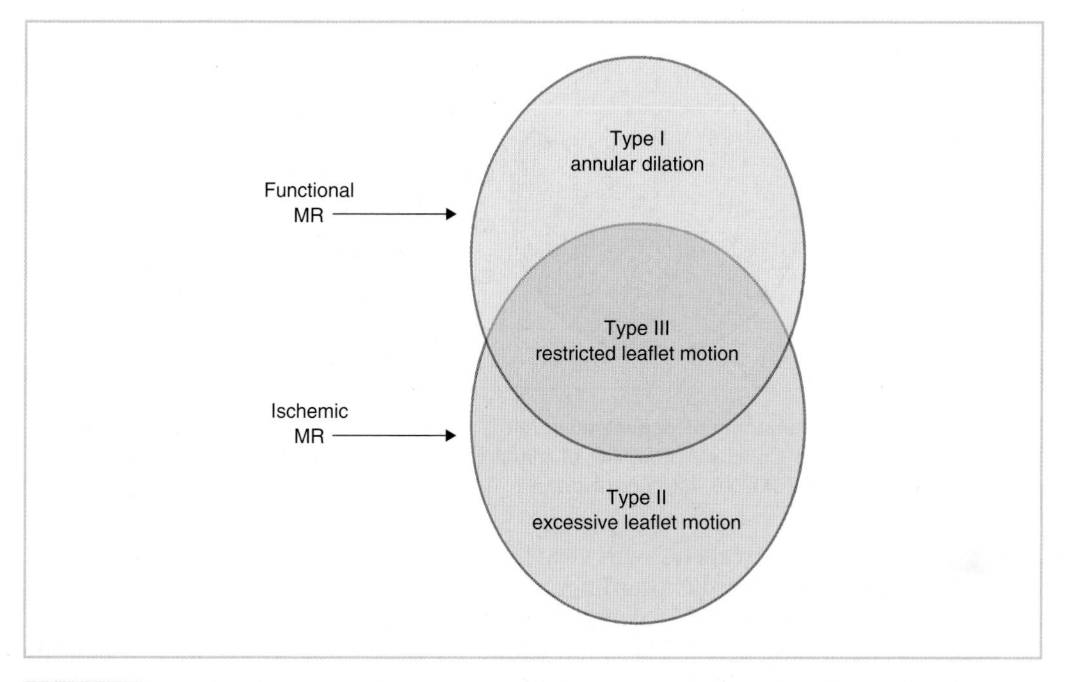

Figure 10.1. Venn diagram depicting causes of functional versus ischemic mitral regurgitation (*MR*).

The problem of FMR is not insignificant. *Up to 40% of coronary artery bypass grafting (CABG) candidates have some degree of chronic ischemic MR and the combined CABG/MVR or repair significantly increases hospital mortality over CABG alone, especially in the older than 80-year patient population.* Although the indications for surgical intervention in patients with FMR are unclear at the present time, arguments for intervention include: (a) concern that FMR may impose a secondary remodeling stimulus on a compromised LV that has previously suffered myocardial damage, (b) strong evidence that even mild MR is a poor prognostic sign in patients with CHF or postacute MI, (c) dramatic clinical improvement in patients post-MVR who had structural MV lesions, and (d) limited medical and surgical options for patients with end-stage CHF.

RESULTS OF MITRAL VALVE REPAIR

Mitral Stenosis

Patients with rheumatic disease had significantly worse repair results than patients with structural MV disease causing MR (76% freedom from reoperation at 15 years) (6). Yau et al. (7) demonstrated improved risk-adjusted, long-term survival in patients with rheumatic disease undergoing mitral repair in comparison with mitral replacement. Although surgically challenging, some centers report a 65% successful repair rate for rheumatic disease of the MV (8).

Mitral Regurgitation

STRUCTURAL MITRAL REGURGITATION

With the development of standardized techniques for MV reconstruction, Deloche et al. (6) demonstrated that MVR was feasible in 95% of patients with degenerative valve disease, 70% with rheumatic valve disease, and 75% with ischemic valve disease. The long-term

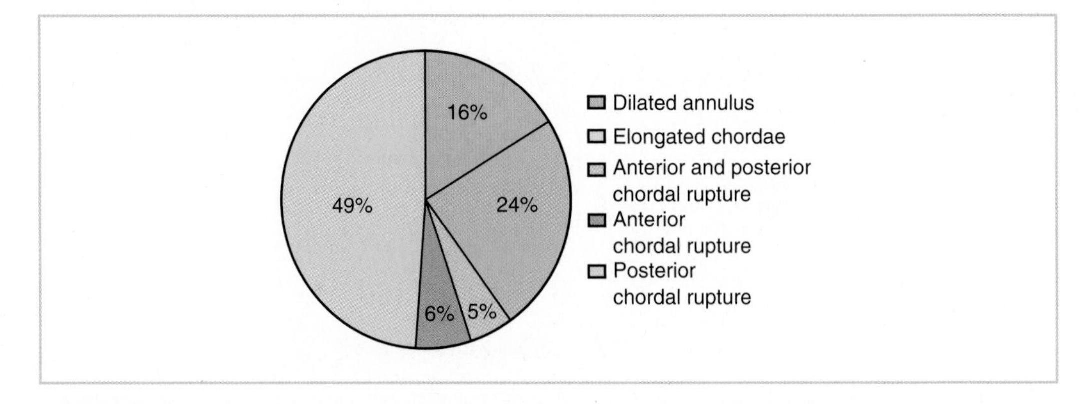

Figure 10.2. Pathologic anatomy of degenerative mitral valve disease (n = 1,072). (From Gillinov AM, Cosgrove DM, Blackstone EH, et al. Durability of mitral valve repair for degenerative disease. *J Thorac Cardiovasc Surg* 1998;116:734–743, with permission.)

results after MVR were excellent, with very low rates of thromboembolism, reoperation, and valve-related mortality. Echocardiographic follow-up analysis revealed no or mild MR in 92% of patients. Gillinov et al. (9) analyzed 1,072 patients undergoing mitral repair for degenerative disease at the Cleveland Clinic. Although this study corroborated the excellent long-term results of Deloche et al. (92.9% freedom from reoperation at 10 years), the results varied when analyzed by anatomic subgroup (Figure 10.2).

Optimal results (97% freedom from reoperation at 10 years) were observed in patients with isolated posterior leaflet (PL) *prolapse* for which the surgical repair included posterior resection and ring annuloplasty. An isolated anterior leaflet repair, chordal-shortening techniques, PL resection without annuloplasty, and annuloplasty alone all significantly decreased durability (9). *In addition, residual MR of grade 2+ or higher at the termination of the procedure was shown to decrease the durability of repair* (10).

FUNCTIONAL MITRAL REGURGITATION

The remarkable prevalence of this condition and its associated adverse long-term outcomes in terms of both CHF and death has resulted in considerable enthusiasm for surgical correction. A number of surgical techniques have been developed, particularly for ischemic MR, but to date none of these procedures has clearly demonstrated improved patient outcomes. Retrospective analyses (11) indicate that severe ischemic MR should be addressed at the time of surgery but that outcomes of patients with coronary artery disease (CAD) and moderate (3+) MR treated with either CABG alone or CABG plus mitral repair had similar medium-term survival. An important consideration is the increase in procedural mortality associated with concomitant mitral valvular procedures at the time of CABG (12). Nevertheless, the symptomatic state of patients postrevascularization with moderate MR appears to be worse with increased CHF symptoms (12). To date, definitive randomized trial data in MVR for FMR are lacking.

ASSESSMENT OF THE PATIENT FOR MITRAL VALVE REPAIR

Preoperative Clinical Assessment

The cardiology referral for MVR is based on clinical signs and symptoms and on echocardiographic and cardiac catheterization findings. Preoperative transthoracic echocardiographic imaging often provides satisfactory information regarding the degree of MR or MS, annular size, involvement of anterior or PLs, chordal and papillary muscle structural integrity, LV dimensions, and systolic and diastolic function. When more detailed anatomic information is required for surgical planning, a preoperative TEE evaluation or three-dimensional echocardiography may be useful. In some patients, particularly in those with clinical symptoms suggestive of chronic heart failure, the use of exercise Doppler echocardiography to elicit changes in valve function under stress may be helpful in determining the degree of FMR. Understanding the patient's entire clinical situation under awake, physiologic conditions may require additional consultation with the cardiologist, radiologist, and surgeon to contextualize the intraoperative TEE examination and guide appropriate surgical management.

Intraoperative Transesophageal Echocardiographic Evaluation

RATIONALE

A detailed intraoperative TEE evaluation of the mitral apparatus is critical for planning surgery, assessing results, and predicting the long-term durability of the MVR (9,13). A comprehensive and systematic approach to evaluating the mitral anatomy is described in Chapter 8.

REPORTING THE TRANSESOPHAGEAL ECHOCARDIOGRAPHIC FINDINGS BEFORE MITRAL REPAIR

1. *Leaflets* should be assessed for perforations, calcifications, excessive length, thickened appearance, and mobility. Abnormal segments as well as areas of normal leaflet coaptation should be fully evaluated and clearly described to the surgeon.
2. The *mitral annulus* should be measured in the five-chamber view with the fibrous anterior annulus providing a fixed reference point from which to measure dilation of the posterior annulus. Normal annular diameter in this view is between 3.0 and 3.8 cm. Diameters greater than 4.0 cm clearly reflect annular dilation. MAC significantly increases the complexity of valve repair procedures and should be specifically noted.
3. The *subvalvular apparatus* often best evaluated in the transgastric (TG) two-chamber view is assessed for chordal changes, such as thickening, shortening, or rupture, and for papillary muscle function. Robust secondary chordae, which may be suitable for transposition to prolapsed leaflets, can often be identified by TEE.
4. The *left ventricle* is assessed for cavitary shape, systolic function, and regional wall motion abnormalities. Tethering resulting from altered subvalvular structural relationships should be evaluated. Findings to note are ventricular volumes, sphericity, and positioning of the mitral annulus relative to the papillary muscles. LV wall motion abnormalities reflecting either active ischemia or scar from previous MI in the inferior and lateral segments will be noted to be more disruptive to the mitral apparatus causing MR than wall motion abnormalities in the anterior and septal walls of the LV which are more notable for causing LV pump dysfunction.
5. A complete evaluation of the heart and great vessels by intraoperative TEE is critical because incidental findings (severe atherosclerotic aortic disease, undiagnosed aortic insufficiency, LA thrombus, and intracardiac masses) often significantly affect surgical planning.
6. *Because the goal of the intraoperative TEE examination before repair is to evaluate the function of the MV, it is critical to assess the valve in a hemodynamic state comparable to that of the awake, ambulatory patient*. The use of inotropes, vasopressors, or volume loading may be necessary to achieve this end.

ASSESSING THE RISK FOR SYSTOLIC ANTERIOR MOTION

Systolic anterior motion (SAM) of the MV with resultant left ventricular outflow tract obstruction (LVOTO) develops in more than 16% of patients following MVR (14–16).

A complete TEE examination after repair will identify this complication. However, intraoperative TEE analysis of the mitral apparatus before bypass can identify the patients in whom this complication is likely to develop. The data allow the surgeon to perform a "sliding leaflet" procedure or modifications of this repair technique and thereby significantly reduce the occurrence of SAM (16–18).

The mechanism of SAM/LVOTO is multifactorial, the major cause being excess mitral leaflet tissue (as in the "floppy MV" of myxomatous disease). Anteriorly displaced papillary muscles, a nondilated LV, and a narrow mitral-aortic angle have also been proposed as contributing factors (16). The incidence of SAM/LVOTO after MVR has been shown to increase in patients with a more anterior position of the leaflet coaptation point. This may be the consequence of a relatively large PL, shifting coaptation closer to the base of the anterior leaflet and causing both anterior displacement of the coaptation line and an increase in the amount of slack leaflet tissue in the outflow tract. An elongated anterior leaflet may cause a similar increase in the amount of slack leaflet available to obstruct LV outflow.

Maslow et al. (15) investigated various prerepair TEE variables to determine the most useful measurements with which to assess the preoperative risk for SAM/LVOTO. These included the anterior leaflet (AL) and PL lengths, used to determine the AL/PL ratio, and the distance from the coaptation point to the septum (C-sept) **(Figure 10.3).** The incidence of postrepair SAM/LVOTO was greater in patients with an AL/PL ratio below 1.0 than in patients with an AL/PL ratio above 3.0. SAM/LVOTO was more likely to develop in

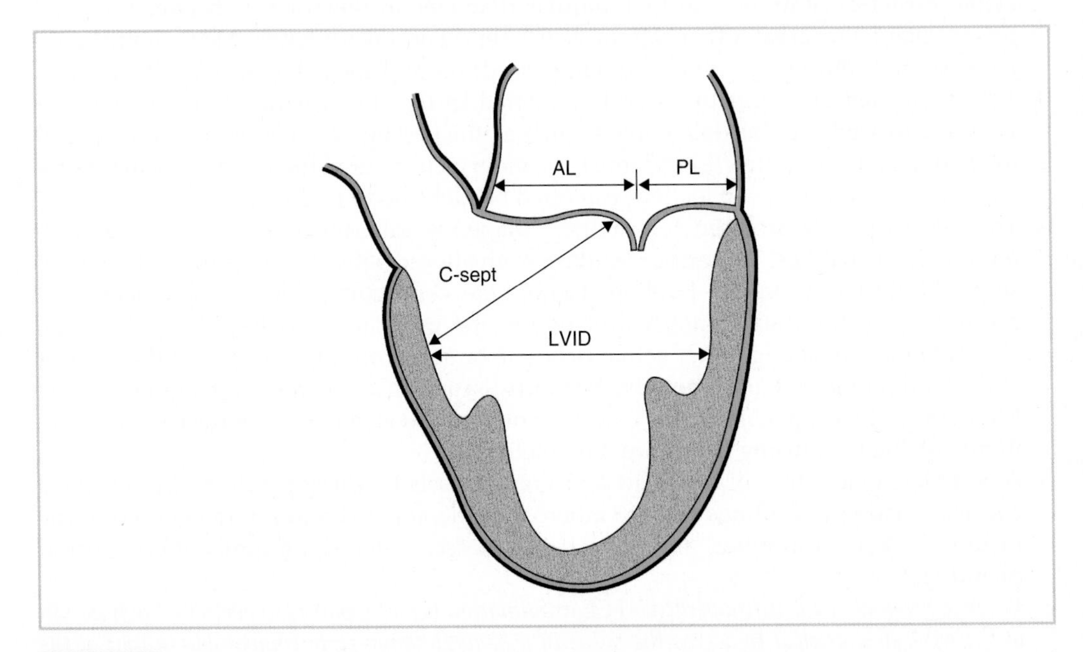

Figure 10.3. Schematic demonstrating the transesophageal echocardiographic measurements used before repair to assess the risk for systolic anterior motion. AL, anterior leaflet length; PL, posterior leaflet length; C-sept, distance from the coaptation point to the septum; LVID, left ventricular internal diameter in systole. (Adapted from Maslow AD, Regan MM, Haering JM, et al. Echocardiographic predictors of left ventricular outflow tract obstruction and systolic anterior motion of the mitral valve after mitral valve reconstruction for myxomatous valve disease. *J Am Coll Cardiol* 1999;34:2096–2104.)

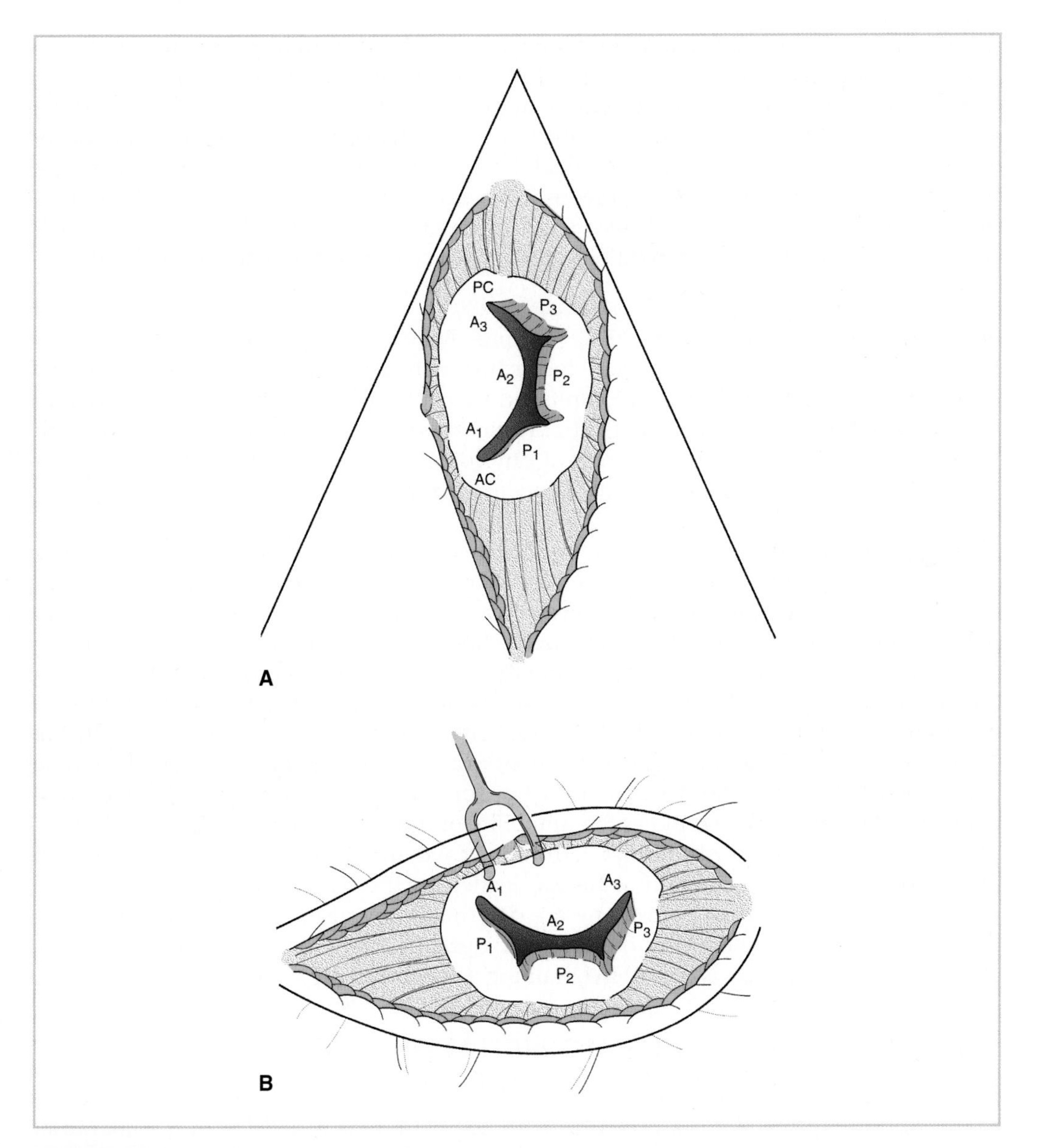

Figure 10.4. Mitral valve leaflet segments. **A:** Echocardiographic short-axis or "fish mouth" view. **B:** Surgeon's view through open left atrium from the patient's right side. The echocardiographic view is rotated 90 degrees counterclockwise relative to the surgeon (tilting one's head to the left.)

patients with a C-sept of 2.5 cm or less than in patients with a C-sept of 3.0 cm or more (15). The identification of patients at high risk for SAM/LVOTO affects the pharmacologic management of hemodynamics after bypass, which is aimed at reducing this complication (discussed later), and alters the surgical techniques described in the preceding text.

TRANSLATING THE TRANSESOPHAGEAL ECHOCARDIOGRAPHIC VIEW INTO THE SURGICAL FIELD

It is extremely useful for the surgeon to be able to correlate the TEE findings with the exposed mitral apparatus in the surgical field **(**Figure 10.4**).** The TG basal short-axis (SAX) view provides the "fish mouth" view of the MV in which the posterior commissure is at the top of the screen and the anterior commissure is at the bottom of the screen with the anterior leaflet to the left and PL to the right. To demonstrate the surgical view, tilting one's head to the left places the posterior commissure at the surgeon's right hand and the anterior commissure at the surgeon's left with the anterior leaflet positioned anteriorly under the aorta and the PL deep in the field. P3 is the leaflet deepest to the surgeon's right hand and P1 is then towards the surgeons left hand. A brief, clear description translating the TEE findings provides invaluable visual information for the surgeon and reduces the confusion around verbal interpretation. "A picture is worth a thousand words."

DIRECT SURGICAL INSPECTION OF THE MITRAL APPARATUS

Before the use of intraoperative TEE became widespread, prerepair valve analysis depended entirely on direct surgical inspection with the heart and mitral apparatus in the "tensed" state. This was accomplished by exposing the valve during ventricular fibrillation, either before application of the aortic cross-clamp or after cross-clamping with infusion of cold blood in the aortic root at physiologic pressure to reduce the risk for air embolization (B. DeVarennes, *personal communication*, 2006).

In the current era, the surgeon plans most of the operation based on the intraoperative TEE findings, so that it is not necessary to evaluate the valve before the administration of cardioplegia. Although in the empty, flaccid heart nearly all leaflet edges can be shown to prolapse above the annular plane, direct inspection after cardioplegia remains a vital step in confirming the location of pathology and the suitability of the various valve structures for the planned repair (19). Leaflet prolapse or restriction is identified by the application of nerve hooks to the leaflet edge and comparison with "normal" leaflet segments, usually the P1 segment. Direct inspection allows the identification of ruptured or elongated chordae and of robust secondary chordae that can be transposed to prolapsing segments. Inspection of the papillary muscles determines the suitability of chordal-shortening approaches or the placement of artificial chords. Leaflet perforations and annular calcification are identified. In MS, the degree of commissural fusion, leaflet calcification, and subchordal disease and the suitability of commissurotomy are determined by visual inspection. During the surgical inspection of the valve, the echocardiographers' clarification of normal versus abnormal mitral anatomy is critical in obtaining an optimal surgical result.

SURGICAL REPAIR OF MITRAL REGURGITATION

Exposing the Mitral Valve

Good exposure of the MV is a prerequisite to adequate repair. Incision in the interatrial groove with bicaval cannulation is a widely used approach, with exposure improved by dissecting the left and right atria to allow a more medial incision (20). A transseptal approach with bicaval cannulation through a right atriotomy, with or without extension into the roof of the LA, also provides excellent exposure. If exposure is still difficult, the placement of annuloplasty ring sutures and the application of tension will deliver the valve into the surgical field. Left-sided pericardial traction sutures should be relaxed. Meticulous attention to myocardial protection, either by intermittent antegrade or a combination of antegrade and retrograde cardioplegia, is an absolute necessity to allow for the safe aortic clamp time necessary to perform a complex repair. TEE can assist in the successful placement of a coronary sinus catheter, particularly in redo surgery in which the palpation of posterior structures is limited. Finally, considerable success has been achieved in selected centers with minimally invasive incisions including video and robotically assisted approaches (21).

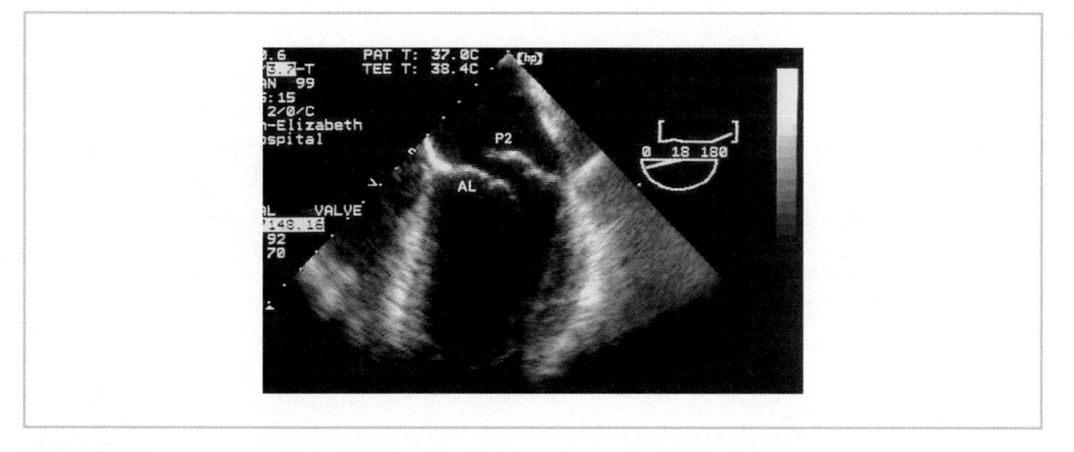

Figure 10.5. Midesohageal four-chamber view of the mitral valve depicting prolapse/flail of the P2 segment of the posterior leaflet. AL, anterior leaflet.

Repair Techniques

This section is intended to give the echocardiographer an appreciation of the common surgical procedures used in MVR. Understanding the suitability of the repair techniques to the pathologic condition can greatly assist in the surgical planning. Familiarity with these techniques also allows appropriate assessment of the surgical result postmitral repair.

REPAIR OF LEAFLET PROLAPSE

Isolated P2 prolapse

When resection and ring annuloplasty are performed, a prolapsed P2 segment is the most reliably repaired regurgitant lesion (9) (Figure 10.5). Briefly, the P2 segment is resected from scallop to scallop in a quadrangular fashion. Intact chordae are detached from the papillary muscles (a robust, intact chord may be preserved to repair another prolapsing segment). The annulus is plicated with a horizontal mattress suture, and direct approximation of the leaflet edges is undertaken.

In the case of excessive leaflet length or other factors predisposing to SAM, or in all cases (author preference), a sliding plasty can be carried out (Figure 10.6). In sliding leaflet plasty, after P2 resection, the P1 and P3 segments are partially detached from their hinge line, starting at the P2-facing edge. Horizontal mattress sutures are then placed through the annulus to reduce the gap left by the resection of P2. The leaflets are reattached to the annulus and their edges reapproximated. After leaflet repair, a ring annuloplasty is performed, with the ring sized to the anterior leaflet area and intercommissural distance.

Isolated anterior leaflet prolapse

Resection is not a reliable approach for the larger anterior leaflet, except for repair of a very small, focal prolapsing area by triangular resection (22). The prolapsing anterior leaflet (Figure 10.7) can be repaired by means of chordal transfer, artificial chordal replacement, or chordal-shortening techniques. Chordal transfer involves transferring robust chords either from a secondary position on the anterior leaflet or from an adjacent PL edge (the latter requiring a quadrangular resection, as described earlier). Artificial chords (Gore-Tex) can be placed from the papillary muscle head to the leaflet edge. A major challenge is adjusting the length of the chords, often by judging adjacent, nonprolapsing leaflet segments. Nevertheless, excellent long-term results have been demonstrated with chordal replacement (10). Finally, elongated chords can be shortened. The trenching technique, in

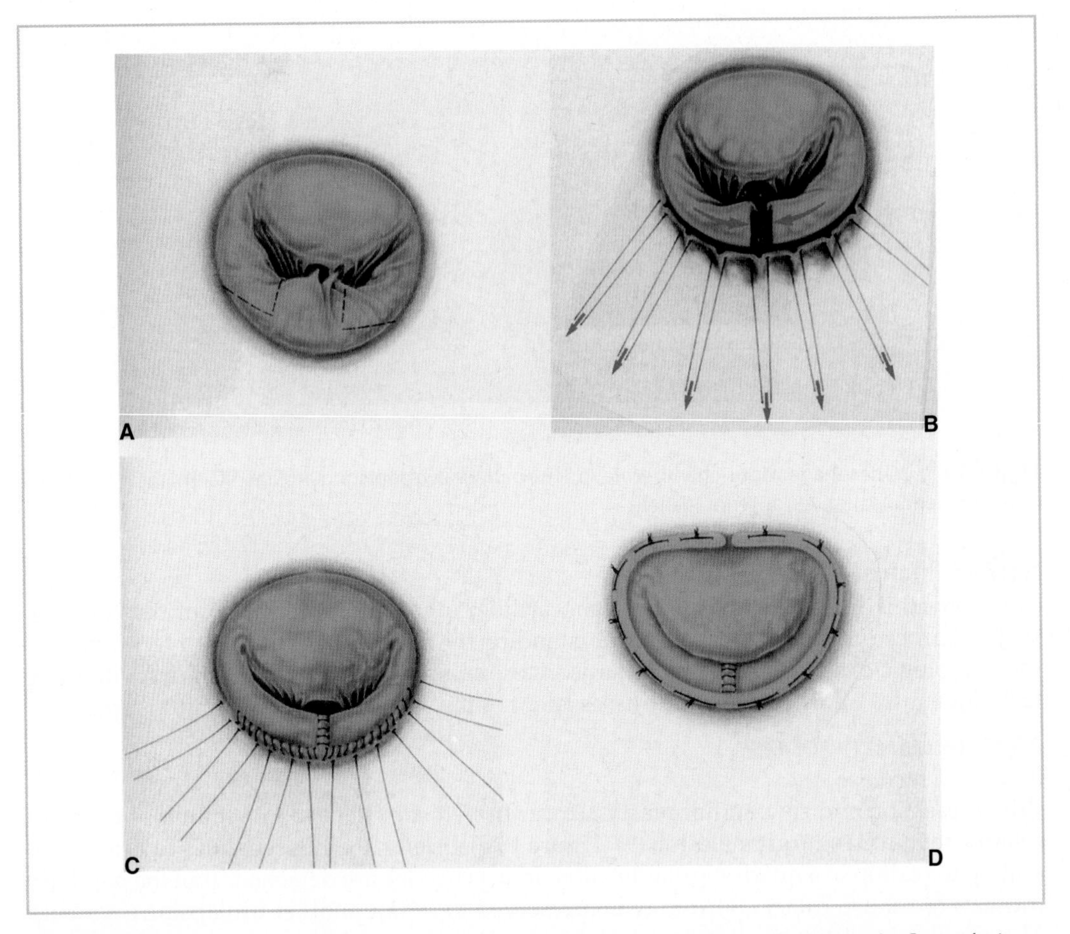

Figure 10.6. Carpentier technique for preventing systolic anterior motion—the sliding leaflet technique. **A:** In cases of excess tissue of the mural leaflet, the quadrangular resection is completed by two triangular resections of the posterior leaflet remnants to correct excess leaflet tissue. **B:** Remnants are translated medially to close the gap. **C, D:** Repair is completed, and the ring is inserted to reinforce the repair. (From Jebara VA, Mihaileanu S, Acar C, et al. Left ventricular outflow tract obstruction after mitral valve repair: results of the sliding leaflet technique. *Circulation* 1992;88:30–34, with permission.)

which elongated chords are buried in a trench cut in the papillary muscle and sutured in place, was previously popular, but long-term durability was unsatisfactory (9,23). Papillary muscle shortening, especially for billowing valves in which multiple chords are elongated, has become popular. The method is efficient because multiple chords are shortened at once; however, exposure can be challenging, and long-term results are not yet available.

Bileaflet prolapse

In cases of prolapse of both the anterior leaflet and PL (Figure 10.8), a systematic approach combining quadrangular resection with chordal transposition, shortening, or replacement is required. If there is dominant posterior prolapse with a myxomatous, prolapsing anterior leaflet, isolated quadrangular resection with ring annuloplasty can be satisfactory (24).

Papillary muscle rupture

Rupture of a papillary muscle complicating an acute myocardial infarction can affect the entire papillary muscle (one third of cases), resulting in bileaflet flail, or only one head

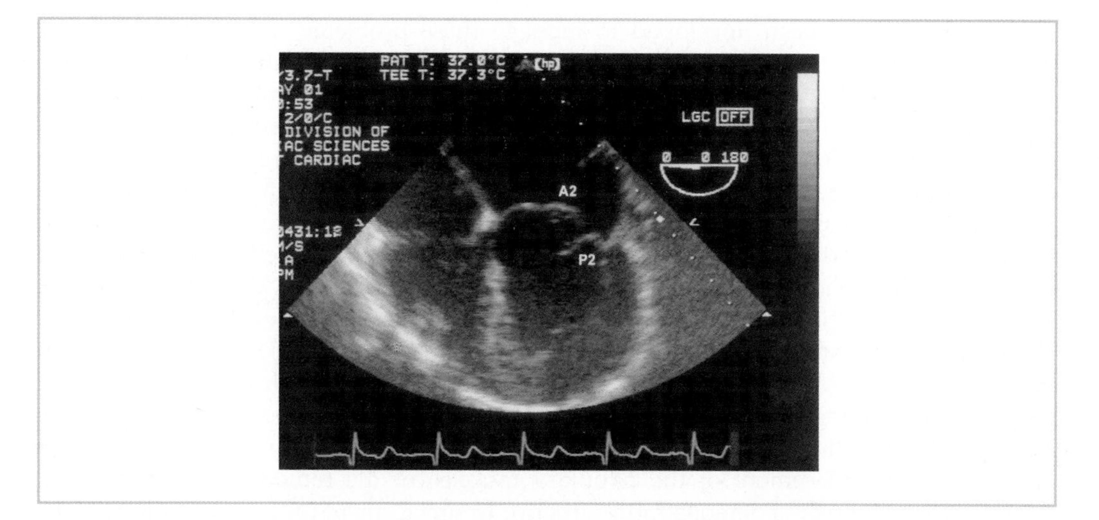

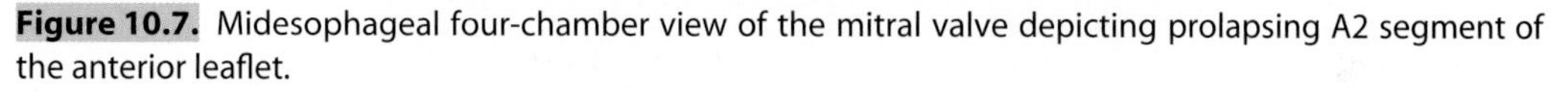

Figure 10.7. Midesophageal four-chamber view of the mitral valve depicting prolapsing A2 segment of the anterior leaflet.

(two third of cases), resulting in flail of either the anterior leaflet or PL. The posteromedial papillary muscle is most often affected (75% of cases) because the coronary circulation to the inferior wall is not redundant. A single ruptured papillary head can be reimplanted in adjacent endocardium. In cases with extensive necrosis of the papillary muscle and adjacent myocardium, an MV replacement with preservation of the remaining intact chords should be carried out (25).

Repair of ischemic mitral regurgitation

Patients with ischemic MR are a diverse group in regard to acuteness of presentation, LV function, and causes of MR (papillary muscle dysfunction, segmental LV wall dysfunction, leaflet restriction, annular dilation, chordal rupture, papillary muscle rupture). A variety

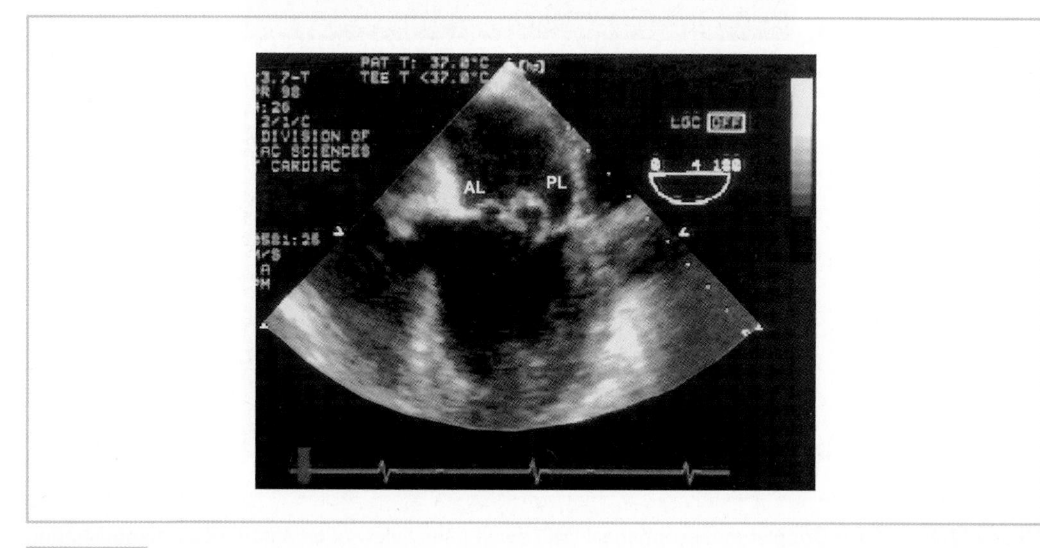

Figure 10.8. Midesophageal five-chamber view of the mitral valve depicting bileaflet prolapse. AL, anterior leaflet; PL, posterior leaflet.

of procedures have been developed to manage these problems. The most commonly performed procedure to date has been undersized mitral ring annuloplasty. In this procedure, the restrictive pathology of FMR, which is largely a ventricular problem, is dealt with by reducing the annular dimensions and forcing coaptation of the downwardly displaced leaflets. Considerable debate exists in terms of ring design and shape, although to date no clear advantage with a particular version of ring has been demonstrated. The literature does suggest that while isolated ring annuloplasty in FMR can be carried out with less procedural mortality than MV replacement, it has been associated with considerable rates of late recurrence of significant MR (26). High rates of recurrent MR with undersized ring annuloplasty have stimulated the development of a host of newer approaches. These include reducing leaflet restriction by cutting second order chords (27) in combination with ring annuloplasty. Alfieri described an edge-to-edge MV leaflet repair for a variety of MV pathologies including FMR, although recurrent MR has been described in cases of ischemic MR treated with Alfieri repair (28) (Figure 10.9). Other approaches include a direct attack on the lateral displacement of the papillary muscles of the remodeled ventricle (29). Although mitral repair is demonstrably superior to replacement for nonischemic MR, the issue remains unresolved for ischemic MR.

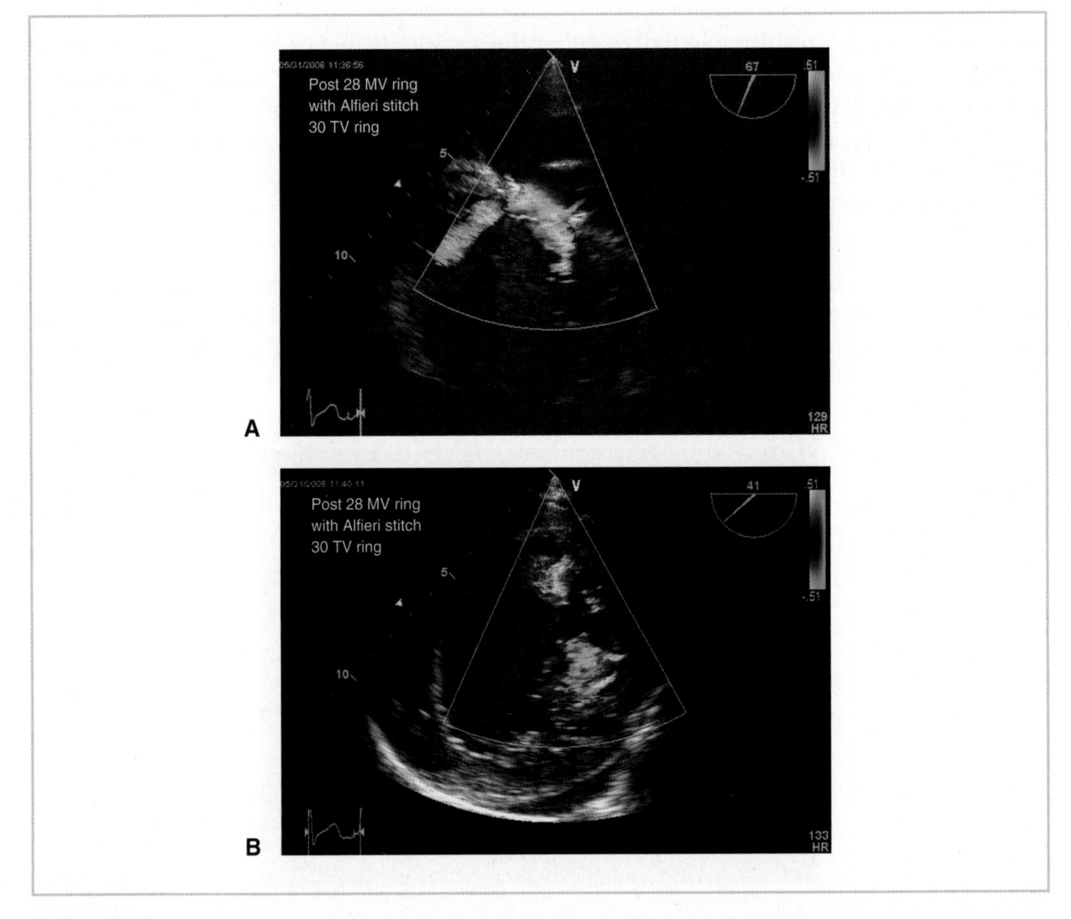

Figure 10.9. **A:** Color Doppler mid esophageal (ME) commissural view of an Alfieri repair demonstrating the classical double mitral valve in flow pattern seen. **B:** Color Doppler transgastric basal short-axis view of an Alfieri repair demonstrating the classical double mitral valve (over and under shotgun) in flow pattern seen. MV, mitral valve; TV, tricuspid valve.

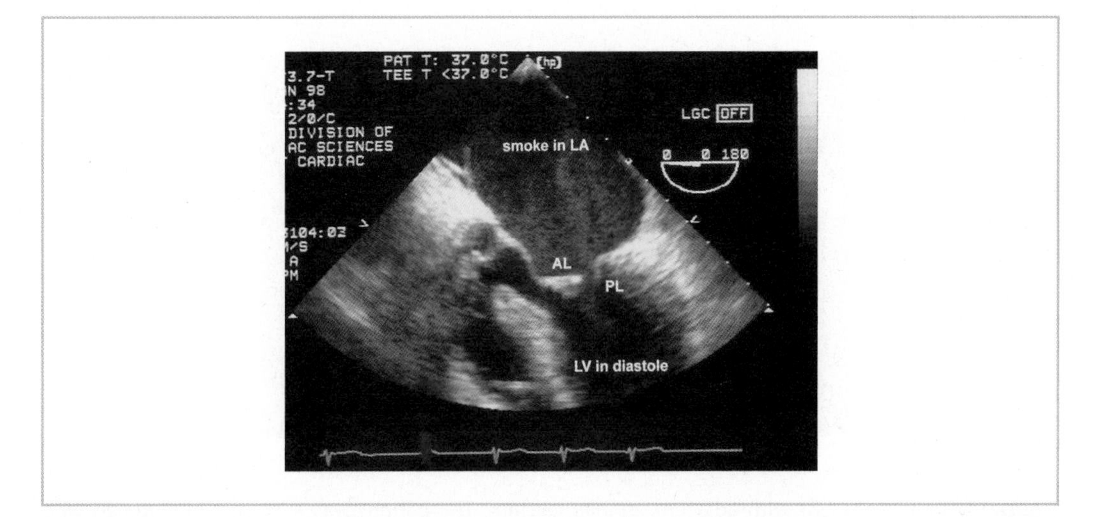

Figure 10.10. Midesophageal five-chamber view of the mitral valve depicting mitral stenosis with "smoke" (spontaneous contrast) in an enlarged left atrium (LA). Note the hockey stick deformity of the anterior leaflet (AL) and marked narrowing of the mitral orifice in diastole. PL, posterior leaflet; LV, left ventricle.

In summary, the issue of replacement versus repair remains uncertain in patients with mild-moderate ischemic MR undergoing CABG. Additionally, the most effective procedure to effect stable resolution of ischemic MR has yet to be determined.

MITRAL REPAIR IN RHEUMATIC DISEASE

Mitral stenosis

Rheumatic mitral disease, as evidenced by decreased leaflet pliability, leaflet thickening and calcification, chordal shortening with "hockey stick" deformity of the anterior leaflet, marked narrowing of the mitral orifice in diastole and often, "smoke" (reflecting stagnant blood flow) in the LA provides a significant surgical challenge (Figure 10.10). The symptoms of patients with some degree of leaflet pliability can be relieved by open commissurotomy and chordal fenestration in lieu of replacement. The anterolateral commissure is often fused to a greater degree than the posteromedial commissure. With a nerve hook distracting either leaflet edge, the fused portions of the leaflets/commissures are divided; great care must be taken to respect the chordal attachments to the papillary muscle heads. This incision can be carried down from the leaflet through the fused chords. In minimally calcified valves with good pliability on echocardiography, comparable results can be achieved with percutaneous balloon valvuloplasty (30).

Mitral regurgitation

Repair of rheumatic MR is a very challenging endeavor. Leaflet restriction can be relieved through aggressive chordal fenestration with fanning of the involved papillary muscle heads. Leaflet decalcification and the transposition of chords from a secondary position back to the leaflet edge can give good results. Ring annuloplasty may be necessary, but care must be taken in mixed lesions that relief of MS is maintained.

Special Surgical Considerations

CALCIFIED MITRAL ANNULUS

The presence of annular calcification considerably complicates mitral repair or replacement, increasing the risk for ventricular rupture, damage to the circumflex coronary artery, and

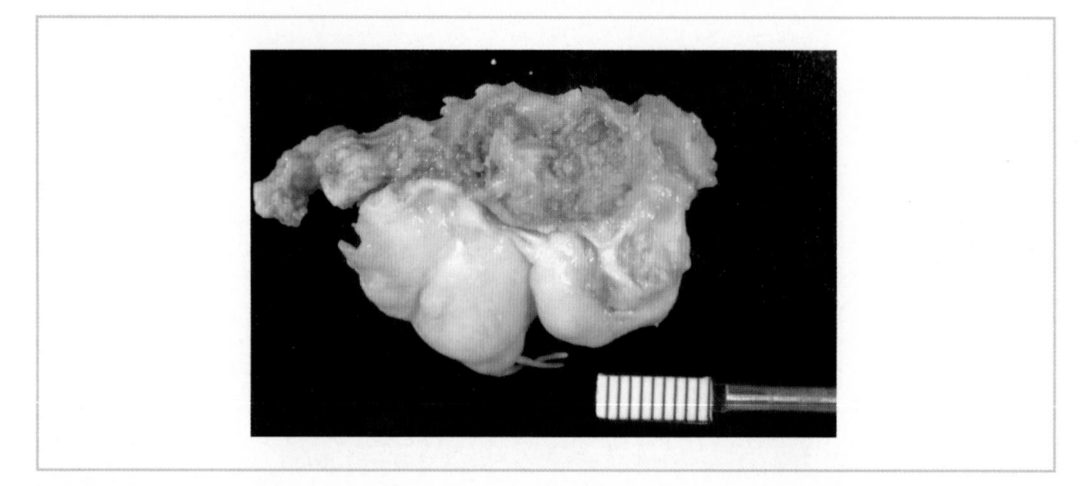

Figure 10.11. P2 segment with adjacent annular calcium. The patient was a 72-year-old woman with marked calcium deposition in the posterior annulus and P2 prolapse with severe mitral regurgitation. En bloc resection was carried out with repair, as described in the text.

postoperative paravalvular MR, and it must be identified in the TEE examination (31). Calcification is most commonly seen in the posterior annulus but can extend into the leaflet tissue or the ventricular myocardium, and rarely to the anterior annulus. It is distinguished from the calcification of rheumatic disease, in which primary leaflet calcification may extend to the annulus with concomitant calcification of subchordal structures. Annular calcification in association with MR occurs most frequently in the elderly and in patients with Marfan syndrome or Barlow disease. Carpentier et al. (32) reported successful en bloc resection of the entire calcium deposit with subsequent repair in 98% of cases, with a 3.3% mortality (Figure 10.11). Once the calcium is resected, the atrioventricular (AV) groove is repaired with vertical mattress sutures. The PL (or its remnants in the case of a P2 resection) is then reattached.

CASES AT HIGH RISK FOR SYSTOLIC ANTERIOR MOTION

The surgical approach to MVR may be modified in cases identified to be at high risk for SAM. In the case of dominant PL prolapse, sliding leaflet plasty can be carried out after P2 resection and the excessive height of the remnants of the PL reduced by the resection of leaflet tissue from the annulus-facing edge (33). If an anteriorly displaced line of coaptation is identified after leaflet resection has been performed, some modification can be achieved by bending a rigid ring so that the anterio-posterior diameter is increased, which reduces the volume of anterior leaflet tissue available to obstruct the left ventricular outflow tract (LVOT). Accurate ring sizing and avoidance of undersizing the annuloplasty ring also reduce the risk for LVOTO secondary to SAM. Finally, postrepair hemodynamic management should be attempted, as outlined later.

ASSESSMENT OF THE MITRAL VALVE AFTER REPAIR

Surgical Valve Assessment

After packs and retraction sutures have been removed to prevent distortion of the valve and ventricle, the passive leak test is performed by forcefully injecting saline solution into the LV. This test remains useful in determining gross inadequacies of repair; a large leak by this test is generally confirmed as severe MR by TEE. Patients with a competent valve following the leak test may still have significant valvular insufficiency by TEE secondary to ischemic wall dysfunction or SAM in the beating, volume-loaded heart (34).

Transesophageal Echocardiographic Assessment of Adequacy of Repair

RESIDUAL MITRAL REGURGITATION

Postrepair assessment by TEE in the physiologically optimized heart is the gold standard in determining the adequacy of MVR. "Immediate failures" are detected in approximately 6% to 8% of patients, who then may undergo further reparative techniques or replacement during the same procedure (35,36). Postrepair MR of grade 1+ or 2+ increases the incidence of late reoperation threefold in comparison with trace or no MR after repair (37). *Therefore, postrepair TEE information is essential in determining whether immediate reintervention is warranted.* Appropriate volume loading, and hemodynamic manipulations may be necessary to adequately evaluate the repaired MV. Immediate repair results by TEE may appear more favorable than subsequent evaluation; therefore, a repeat look at chest closure gives a better indication of the ultimate result.

MITRAL STENOSIS

MS following MVR is a recognized, but rare occurrence more likely to be seen with the Alfieri procedure, commissuroplasties, and small annuloplasty rings. Continuous wave (CW) Doppler gradients displaying a mean gradient greater than 6 mm Hg or peak gradient greater than 16 mm Hg is diagnostic. Although the pressure half-time method is a simple technique to evaluate for MS, the cardiac compliance changes following repair make it a much less reliable indicator of true dysfunction. Evaluation using proximal isovelocity surface area (PISA) measurements (as described in Chapter 9) or the continuity equation are additional methods to reliably diagnosis clinically significant MS.

Transesophageal Echocardiographic Assessment of Complications of Mitral Valve Repair

SYSTOLIC ANTERIOR MOTION/LEFT VENTRICULAR OUTLET TRACT OBSTRUCTION

SAM of the MV leaflets with resultant dynamic LVOTO is a known complication of MVR, as discussed earlier. The echocardiographic findings demonstrate a characteristic systolic bending of the leaflet tips into the outflow tract, turbulent flow in the LVOT and MR as a posteriorly directed jet (Figure 10.12). Gradients across the LVOT (CW shows a dagger-shaped flow pattern) are increased from baseline as a result of dynamic outflow obstruction. When SAM/LVOTO occurs after MVR, hemodynamic maneuvers must be attempted before the results are declared inadequate. Inotropic agents, vasodilators, and low-volume states all exacerbate this condition and perhaps provoke it in susceptible patients. With the discontinuation of these agents and manipulation of the cardiovascular status by volume loading with or without the administration of α-agents, SAM/LVOTO often resolves. In some patients with a significant LVOT gradient, β-blockers may be useful in resolving the LVOTO (38). With persistent SAM/LVOTO, surgical reintervention may be necessary.

CORONARY ARTERY INJURY

The circumflex coronary artery runs in the AV groove deep to the posterior mitral annulus. In MV or mitral ring placement, sutures placed too deeply may compromise this vessel. Of note, the distance of the circumflex coronary artery to the posterior annulus is closest (4.1 mm) in patients with a left-dominant coronary circulation than in either the codominant circulation (5.5 mm) or a right-dominant circulation (8 mm). Injury to the

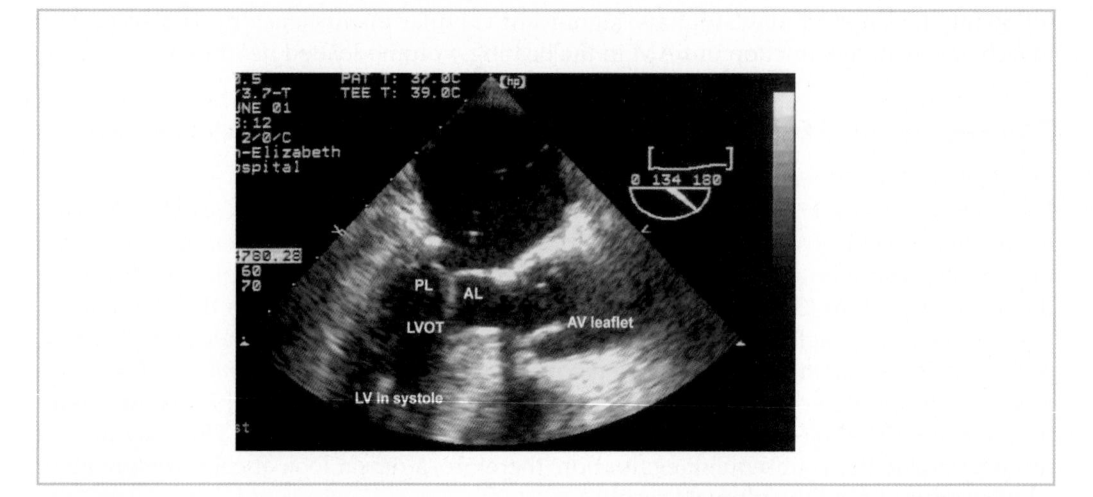

Figure 10.12. Midesophageal long axis view depicting obstruction of the left ventricular outflow tract (LVOT) by leaflet tips during systole (systolic anterior motion with left ventricular outflow tract obstruction). Color Doppler showed turbulence in the left ventricular outflow tract and a posteriorly directed mitral regurgitant jet. PL, posterior leaflet; AL, anterior leaflet; AV, atrioventricular; LV, left ventricle.

circumflex coronary artery is a rare but frequently fatal complication of either mitral repair or mitral replacement (39). Intraoperative TEE findings of new segmental wall motion abnormalities in the lateral wall or inferoposterior regions may suggest circumflex injury, and grafting of the distal coronary artery may be indicated (40).

VENTRICULAR RUPTURE

Disruption of the AV groove or rupture of the LV between the papillary muscle insertions and the AV groove is a feared and devastating complication of MV surgery. Factors predisposing to rupture include female sex, advanced age, annular calcification, and high-profile valve replacement devices in patients with a small LV cavity. Recognition of LV rupture can be aided by TEE, which often demonstrates continuous entrainment of intracardiac air. Repair by placement of an endocardial patch has been shown to be superior to attempts to stem the bleeding by placing external sutures or patches (41).

AORTIC VALVE LEAFLET INJURY

Deep suture placement in the anterior annulus can inadvertently injure the left or non-coronary leaflets of the aortic valve. Massive aortic insufficiency noted either clinically or by TEE alerts the surgeon to this possibility. Simple leaflet tethering may be relieved by suture removal and replacement, whereas tears in the aortic leaflets may require aortic valve replacement or more complex repair (42).

Pitfalls of Transesophageal Echocardiographic Examination after Mitral Valve Repair

UNRELIABILITY OF PRESSURE HALF-TIME RESULTS AFTER REPAIR OF MITRAL STENOSIS

A major limitation of the pressure half-time technique is its dependence on LA and LV compliance. Immediately following MVR, LA and LV compliance is markedly altered and does not reach equilibrium for 24 to 72 hours. Therefore, the pressure half-time method of calculating the MV area after MS repair may not be accurate in the immediate postoperative period.

INADEQUACY OF HEMODYNAMIC STATE INADEQUATE TO EXPOSE MITRAL REGURGITATION

General anesthesia can effectively mask MR by lowering preload, decreasing afterload, and decreasing the inotropic state of the heart. Before TEE assessment of the MV, manipulation (volume loading, administration of an inotrope or α agonist) should be attempted to attain hemodynamics that approximate those of the ambulatory state. This detail is critical in both prerepair and postrepair TEE evaluations.

DECISION TO REINTERVENE

The decision to reintervene because of an imperfect result is a difficult one, in part because of a conflicting literature concerning the significance of mild-moderate residual MR. Fix et al. (36) found no increase in long-term mortality in patients with grade 1 to 2+ MR after repair, although a trend to increased late reoperation was noted. In contrast, Sheikh et al. (43) noted an increase in postoperative morbidity and mortality in patients with grade 2+ or higher residual MR. Interpretation of the postrepair TEE data may reveal the cause of residual MR, and cooperation between the echocardiographer and surgeon will allow a determination of the likelihood of a more successful repair. The decision to reintervene must also take into account the condition of the heart, the potential for injury during a second cross-clamp period, and the potential need for valve replacement with its attendant costs. These decisions must be made in the "heat of battle" and require echocardiographers with a firm and confident grasp of TEE interpretation, surgeons with an awareness of their capabilities, and a clear understanding by the entire team of the short-term implications of reintervention and the long-term implications of residual MR.

SUMMARY

The establishment of intraoperative TEE as the standard of care in MVR places the intraoperative echocardiographer and the surgeon in a close working relationship in which real-time decisions with tremendous implications for the patient are made on a daily basis. Careful assessment of the TEE findings placed within the patient's clinical context along with excellent communication between echocardiographer and surgeon provides the best possible avenue for successful repair of the MV.

REFERENCES

1 Cutler EC, Levine SA. Cardiotomy and valvulotomy for mitral stenosis: experimental observations and clinical notes concerning an operated case with recovery. *Boston Med Surg J* 1923;188:1023–1027.

2 Souttar H. The surgical treatment of mitral stenosis. *Br Med J* 1925;2:603–606.

3 Lillehei CW, Got VL, Dewfall RA, et al. Surgical correction of pure mitral insufficiency by annuloplasty under direct vision. *Lancet* 1957;1:446.

4 Starr A, Edwards ML. Mitral replacement: clinical experience with a ball valve prosthesis. *Ann Surg* 1961;154:726.

5 Bonow RO, Carabello B, Chatterjee K, et al. ACC/AHA 2006 guidelines for the management of patients with valvular heart disease: A report of the American College of Cardiology/American Heart Association Task Force on Practice Guidelines (Writing Committee to Revise the 1998 Guidelines for the Management of Patients with Valvular Heart Disease). *J Am Coll Cardiol* 2006;48:e1–148.

6 Deloche A, Jebara VA, Relland JY, et al. Valve repair with Carpentier techniques. *J Thorac Cardiovasc Surg* 1990;99:990–1002.

7 Yau TM, El-Ghoneimi YA, Armstrong S, et al. Mitral valve repair and replacement for rheumatic disease. *J Thorac Cardiovasc Surg* 2000;119:53–61.

8 Duran CM, Gometza B, De Vol EB. Valve repair in rheumatic mitral disease. *Circulation* 1991;84(III supp 5):125–132.

9 Gillinov AM, Cosgrove DM, Blackstone EH, et al. Durability of mitral valve repair for degenerative disease. *J Thorac Cardiovasc Surg* 1998;116:734–743.
10 David TE, Omran A, Armstrong S, et al. Long-term results of mitral valve repair for myxomatous disease with and without chordal replacement with expanded polytetrafluoroethylene sutures. *J Thorac Cardiovasc Surg* 1998;115:1279–1286.
11 Wong DR, Agnihotri AK, Hung JW, et al. Long term survival after surgical revascularization for moderate ischemic mitral regurgitation. *Ann Thorac Surg* 2005;880:570–578.
12 Malidi HR, Pelletier MP, Lamb J, et al. Late outcomes in patients with uncorrected mild to moderate MR at the time of isolated coronary artery bypass grafting. *Jpn J Thorac Cardiovasc Surg* 2004;127:636–644.
13 Foster GP, Isselbacher EM, Rose GA, et al. Accurate localization of mitral regurgitant defects using multiplane transesophageal echocardiography. *Ann Thorac Surg* 1998;65:1025–1031.
14 Lee KS, Stewart WJ, Lever HM, et al. Mechanism of outflow tract obstruction causing failed mitral valve repair: anterior displacement of leaflet coaptation. *Circulation* 1994;88:24–29.
15 Maslow AD, Regan MM, Haering JM, et al. Echocardiographic predictors of left ventricular outflow tract obstruction and systolic anterior motion of the mitral valve after mitral valve reconstruction for myxomatous valve disease. *J Am Coll Cardiol* 1999;34:2096–2104.
16 Jebara VA, Mihaileanu S, Acar C, et al. Left ventricular outflow tract obstruction after mitral valve repair: results of the sliding leaflet technique. *Circulation* 1993;88:30–34.
17 Perier P, Claunizer B, Mistarz K. Carpentier "sliding leaflet" technique for repair of the mitral valve: early results. *Ann Thorac Surg* 1994;57:383–386.
18 Gillinov AM, Cosgrove DM. Modified sliding leaflet technique for repair of the mitral valve. *Ann Thorac Surg* 1999;68:2356–2357.
19 Shah PM, Raney AA, Duran CMF, et al. Multiplane transesophageal echocardiography: a roadmap for mitral valve repair. *J Heart Valve Dis* 1998;8:625–629.
20 Larbalastier RI, Chard RB, Cohn LH. Optimal approach to the mitral valve: dissection of the interatrial groove. *Ann Thorac Surg* 1992;54:1186–1188.
21 Walther T, Falk V, Mohr FW. Minimally invasive surgery for valve disease. *Curr Probl Cardiol* 2006;31:399–437.
22 Carpentier A. Honored guest's address: cardiac valves surgery—the "French correction". *J Thorac Cardiovasc Surg* 1983;86:323–337.
23 Phillips MR, Daly RC, Schaff HV, et al. Repair of anterior leaflet mitral valve prolapse: chordal replacement versus chordal shortening. *Ann Thorac Surg* 2000;69:25–29.
24 Gillinov MA, Cosgrove DM, Wahli S, et al. Is anterior leaflet repair always necessary in repair of bileaflet mitral valve prolapse? *Ann Thorac Surg* 1999;68:820–824.
25 David TE. Techniques and results of mitral valve repair for ischemic mitral regurgitation. *J Card Surg* 1994;9:274–277.
26 Hung J, Papakostas L, Tahta SA, et al. Mechanism of recurrent ischemic MR after annuloplasty: continued LV remodeling as a moving target. *Circulation* 2004;110(suppl):85–90.
27 Messas E, puzet B, Touchot B, et al. Efficacy of chordal cutting to relieve chronic persistant ischemic MR. *Circulation* 2003;108(Suppl 2):111–115.
28 Bhudia SK, McCarthy MM, Smedira NG, et al. Edge to edge (Alfieri) mitral repair. *Ann Thorac Surg* 2004;77:1598–1606.
29 Borger MA, Alam A, Murphy PM, et al. Chronic ischemic mitral regurgitation: repair, replace, or rethink? *Ann Thorac Surg* 2006;81:1153–1161.
30 Reyes VP, Raju BS, Wynne J, et al. Percutaneous balloon valvuloplasty compared with open surgical commissurotomy for mitral stenosis. *N Engl J Med* 1994;331:961–967.
31 Cammack PL, Edie RN, Edmunds LH. Bar calcification of the mitral annulus: a risk factor in mitral valve operations. *J Thorac Cardiovasc Surg* 1987;94:399–404.
32 Carpentier AF, Pellerin M, Fuzellier JF, et al. Extensive calcification of the mitral valve annulus: pathology and surgical management. *J Thorac Cardiovasc Surg* 1996;111:718–730.
33 Jebara VA, Mihaileanu S, Acar C, et al. Left ventricular outflow tract obstruction after mitral valve repair: results of the sliding leaflet technique. *Circulation* 1993;88:II.30–II.34.
34 Chitwood WR Jr. Mitral valve repair: an odyssey to save the valves! *J Heart Valve Dis* 1998;7:255–261.
35 Saiki Y, Kasegawa H, Kawase M, et al. Intraoperative TEE during mitral valve repair: does it predict early and late postoperative mitral valve dysfunction? *Ann Thorac Surg* 1998;66:1277–1281.
36 Fix J, Isada L, Cosgrove D, et al. Do patients with less than "echo-perfect" results from mitral valve repair by intraoperative echocardiography have a different outcome? *Circulation* 1993;88:II.39–II.48.
37 Gillinov AM, Cosgrove DM, Lytle BW, et al. Reoperation for failure of mitral valve repair. *J Thorac Cardiovasc Surg* 1997;113:467–475.

38 Grossi EA, Galloway AC, Parish MA, et al. Experience with twenty-eight cases of systolic anterior motion after mitral valve reconstruction by the Carpentier technique. *J Thorac Cardiovasc Surg* 1992;103:466–470.
39 Danielson GK, Cooper E, Tweedale DN. Circumflex coronary artery injury during mitral valve replacement. *Ann Thorac Surg* 1967;4:53–59.
40 Travilla G, Pacini D. Damage to the circumflex coronary artery during mitral valve repair with sliding leaflet technique. *Ann Thorac Surg* 1998;66:2091–2093.
41 Karlson KJ, Ashraf MM, Berger RL. Rupture of left ventricle following mitral valve replacement. *Ann Thorac Surg* 1988;46:590–597.
42 Hill AC, Bansal RC, Razzouk AJ, et al. Echocardiographic recognition of iatrogenic aortic valve leaflet perforation. *Ann Thorac Surg* 1997;64:684–689.
43 Sheikh K, DeBruijn N, Rankin J, et al. The utility of transesophageal echocardiography and Doppler color flow imaging in patients undergoing cardiac valve surgery. *J Am Coll Cardiol* 1990;15:363–372.

QUESTIONS

1. **Which of the following is true about ischemic papillary muscle rupture?**
   a. Rupture is caused by fewer chordal attachments to the posteromedial papillary muscle.
   b. Rupture most commonly involves the anterior papillary muscle.
   c. A lack of dual blood supply to the myocardium subtending the posterior papillary muscle makes it the one most commonly involved in ischemic papillary rupture.
   d. Rupture most commonly involves the entire papillary muscle.
   e. Rupture usually results in bileaflet flail.

2. **Mitral ring annuloplasty**
   a. Can increase the risk for systolic anterior motion (SAM) if the ring is oversized
   b. Improves the durability of repair techniques
   c. Decreases the risk for atrioventricular groove disruption
   d. Improves visualization of the mitral apparatus by transesophageal echocardiography (TEE) after mitral valve repair (MVR)
   e. Increases the risk for mitral stenosis (MS) after MVR

3. **After MVR, SAM/left ventricular outflow tract obstruction (LVOTO)**
   a. Can be identified before surgery
   b. Can be successfully treated by increasing the afterload
   c. Should be treated with dopaminergic agents
   d. Can be treated by undersizing the mitral annuloplasty ring
   e. Is more likely in patients with a preoperative anterior leaflet/posterior leaflet (AL/PL) ratio greater than 3

4. **Anterior leaflet prolapse repair**
   a. May involve resection of P2
   b. Is the most durable of all leaflet repairs
   c. Requires at least a small triangular resection of a large anterior leaflet
   d. Results are improved with chordal-shortening procedures
   e. Long-term results are poor after chordal replacement with Gore-Tex

5. **Intraoperative TEE evaluation for mitral repair**
   a. Fails to depict localized leaflet prolapse accurately
   b. Accurately measures postrepair stenosis by the pressure half-time technique after open commissurotomy
   c. Allows inexperienced observers to identify normal and abnormal leaflet segments accurately
   d. Does not correlate well with postoperative TTE findings
   e. Improves the long-term durability of mitral repair

6. **In type III leaflet abnormality**
   a. Of both leaflets, one would expect an eccentric jet of mitral regurgitation (MR).
   b. Of the posterior leaflet, one would expect a posteriorly directed MR jet.
   c. Of the anterior leaflet, one would expect a posteriorly directed MR jet.
   d. Effective resolution of MR by mitral repair does not alter the long-term outcome of patients with severe congestive heart failure (CHF) before surgery.
   e. MR cannot be treated with a mitral annuloplasty ring alone.

7. In MS of rheumatic origin

a. Adequate repair is achieved in more than 90% of cases with good long-term results.
b. Repair is commonly complicated by annular calcification.
c. Balloon mitral commissurotomy may provide adequate treatment.
d. TEE is unable to predict the degree of stenosis accurately before surgery with the pressure half-time method.
e. Chordal fenestration has been shown to improve long-term durability.

8. The surgical view of the mitral valve (MV)

a. Places the P3 and A3 segments to the surgeon's right
b. Allows accurate assessment of leaflet prolapse after the administration of cardioplegia
c. Is most easily replicated with the echocardiographer's head tilted to the right and the TEE image in the fish mouth view
d. Easily demonstrates the continuity of the posterior leaflet with the left ventricular outflow tract (LVOT) and aortic valve apparatus
e. Reliably demonstrates a competent valve if the passive leak test result is negative

9. Late MVR failure

a. Is rarely caused by the progression of valvular disease
b. Is rarely a consequence of procedure-related failures
c. Is most often caused by endocarditis
d. Is more likely with the use of an annuloplasty ring
e. And reoperation are more likely when the trenching technique of chordal shortening is used

10. The American College of Cardiology/American Heart Association practice guidelines recommend MVR

a. For patients with severe MR and marked left ventricle (LV) dysfunction only
b. For asymptomatic patients with severe MR and LV dilation
c. Over percutaneous balloon valvuloplasty for patients with severe MS and pliable leaflets
d. For patients with MS, functional class II symptoms, and an MV area of 2 cm^2
e. For patients with severe MR so long as atrial fibrillation is absent

Answers appear at the back of the book.

11 Aortic Regurgitation

Ira S. Cohen

The exquisite sensitivity of transesophageal echocardiography (TEE) in identifying aortic regurgitation (AR) is manifested by its ability to detect the minute regurgitant jets engineered into the design of the St. Jude prosthetic valve to flush platelet aggregates off the valve surface. Few studies have been performed investigating the assessment of AR primarily using TEE because of its relatively invasive nature. Most assessments of the severity of AR are based on the assumption that transthoracic echocardiographic (TTE) approaches should be equally applicable to TEE. Analysis of the vena contracta is an exception in that it has been investigated for both TTE and TEE.

HEMODYNAMICS OF AORTIC REGURGITATION

AR represents both an increase in preload and afterload to the left ventricle. The increase in preload is a result of the increased end-diastolic volume resulting from the added regurgitant volume. The increase in afterload is a function of the increased radius of the ventricle. Increase in the end-diastolic radius of a ventricle at any wall thickness increases the wall stress and the force needed to eject blood (law of Laplace). The general response of the ventricle to chronic AR is to dilate and become more compliant to accommodate the extra volume and to hypertrophy to reduce wall stress. The hypertrophy occurs both longitudinally as the heart enlarges—so-called eccentric hypertrophy—and concentrically, as evidenced by its maintaining a "normal" wall thickness as it enlarges. Accordingly, the size of the ventricle is an index of the severity and duration of the regurgitation and should be factored into the assessment of the severity of the lesion.

Acute AR, most commonly due to a tear in the valve secondary to endocarditis, to deceleration injury in a motor vehicle accident or to stretching of the annulus secondary to an acute dissection offers a contrasting clinical presentation. Acute aortic insufficiency is one of the least well-tolerated valvular lesions because of the limited ability of the heart to compensate for an acute increase in volume load by the mechanisms mentioned in the preceding text. Consequently, the LV diastolic pressure rises rapidly and is transmitted to the lungs resulting in severe pulmonary congestion. Therefore in acute AR the chamber is often normal in size but with catastrophic hemodynamic consequences. Diagnosis of significant AR in the setting of heart failure is essential as intra-aortic balloon counterpulsation is contraindicated because diastolic pressure augmentation worsens the regurgitation.

The assessment of the severity of valvular insufficiency is complicated by the potentially dramatic effects of even transient changes in loading conditions and peripheral vascular resistance on Doppler indices of AR severity. Because the operating room environment is one in which a multitude of factors affect both the preload and afterload of the ventricle, the potential impact of these changes must be borne in mind when the severity of a valvular lesion is evaluated. Acute increases in peripheral vascular resistance (e.g., following surgical stimulation or the administration of vasopressors) can increase the apparent degree of valvular insufficiency by increasing systemic vascular resistance and impeding peripheral runoff. Conversely, vasodilators (e.g., volatile anesthetics, angiotensin-converting enzyme inhibitors and receptor blockers, calcium channel blockers) reduce peripheral vascular resistance and decrease the apparent degree of insufficiency, both clinically and by Doppler interrogation. The physical properties (e.g., distensibility, elasticity, compliance) of the source (aorta) and recipient (LV) of regurgitant flow, in addition to the size of the regurgitant orifice and the physical properties of the involved valve, are other dynamic variables that further complicate intraoperative assessment. In fact, most clinicians feel it is not possible to definitively assess regurgitant lesions in the operating room environment. *As a result of the multitude of factors influencing any assessment of the severity of AR, the estimate should be based on an integration of the results of all Doppler approaches providing technically adequate data in any given patient.*

Methods for assessing the severity of AR have evolved along with advances in Doppler technology since Ward et al. (1) first described the use of pulsed Doppler in conjunction with motion mode (M-mode) echocardiography and auscultation to detect aortic insufficiency. The general approaches to assessing the severity of AR with TEE will be presented in the order of their relative clinical applicability. Color mapping of the left ventricular outflow tract (LVOT) has traditionally been regarded as the most accurate echocardiographic assessment (2–7). Measurement of the width of the vena contracta, the narrowest cross-sectional area of the regurgitant jet as it traverses the valve plane, is emerging as an attractive approach (8). It appears to be less dependent on loading conditions although its efficacy is not as thoroughly documented (4,6). Most studies of this method have been done either *in vitro* or in the OR with aortic flow probes. The proximity of the TEE probe to the aortic root and LVOT and the ability to interrogate these structures with the higher-frequency TEE signal technically make it possible to delineate the size of these regurgitant jets more accurately than can be done with TTE techniques. The American Society of Echocardiography has recently published its recommendations for assessment of regurgitant valvular lesions (9).

RECOMMENDED VIEWS

In contrast to stenotic lesions, where the velocity of a jet is a critical factor in the assessment of the lesion, in AR interrogation of the leak both parallel *and* perpendicular to the regurgitant jet is critical because its area of distribution in the LVOT is one of the major variables used in the assessment of severity. The most useful views are generally obtained by starting from the standard midesophagus (ME) four-chamber view and changing the angle of interrogation to approximately 120 degrees to visualize the LVOT and proximal aorta in an ME aortic valve long-axis view. Withdrawal from this position and, occasionally, slight rotation are used to optimize the view and allow inspection of the proximal ascending aorta. The ME aortic valve short-axis view at approximately 45 degrees allows excellent resolution of the individual cusps of the aortic valve. This too can be obtained from the four-chamber view by centering the atrioventricular (AV) groove and changing the angle to approximately 45 degrees. Occasionally the probe will need to be withdrawn a few centimeters because the aortic valve is at a slightly higher plane than the AV groove.

Alternatively, but less frequently, good views can be obtained from a deep transgastric (TG) position at an angle close to 0 degrees or greater, subject to individual variation, or from a standard midpapillary TG view at an angle of approximately 120 degrees (TG long-axis view). These approaches have the advantage of aligning the ultrasound beam nearly parallel to the direction of blood flow, which is essential for accurate quantitative Doppler analysis of both the slope of decay of the regurgitant jet and cardiac output. Conversely, this beam orientation and the greater distances traveled reduce spatial resolution making them a poor choice for visualizing the height or cross-sectional area of an AR jet immediately below the valve plane. However, they may be the only means of assessing the outflow tract in the presence of a prosthetic mitral valve (MV), which frequently causes acoustic shadowing of the aortic annulus in more standard views, and occasionally, of an aortic prosthesis when its ring obscures the outflow tract image by acoustic shadowing.

The pressure gradient between the regurgitant and recipient chambers in regurgitant valvular lesions is always high and AR corresponds to the diastolic gradient between the aortic root and the left ventricle. By the simplified Bernoulli equation, the gradient equals four times the square of the peak jet velocity. Again, aligning a Doppler beam parallel to the flow is best accomplished in the TG views in the view that is most parallel to flow. In aortic regurgitant lesions it is the *rate of change in pressure gradients* that provides clinically useful information unlike the peak velocity measurement used to assess stenotic lesions. Fortunately, color Doppler techniques for the assessment of AR lesions provide useful information that is, to a significant degree, independent of the angle of the beam to the regurgitant flow.

When color flow Doppler is used, the appropriate gain setting for mapping is obtained by first setting the gain high enough so that random color pixels appear within or outside the blood pool (on tissue). Gain is then decreased until these random color pixels disappear. Failure to standardize the color examination in this manner leads to invalid data and is the source of the so-called dial-a-jet phenomenon, in which overgaining the Doppler signal can expand the apparent size of the jet. Similarly, using a *standard color velocity scale* is also important because a change in the scale can markedly change the appearance of a jet and its distribution.

APPROACHES TO THE QUANTITATIVE ASSESSMENT OF AORTIC REGURGITATION

Color Flow Mapping

In the initial efforts at quantifying AR, pulsed wave Doppler was used to map the depth of penetration of the regurgitant jet into the LV cavity. This approach entailed several problems related to the effects of a high-pressure gradient crossing a narrow regurgitant orifice (see later discussion). A better approach was developed in which jet mapping from the then newly introduced color flow Doppler technique was used (3,10). Two techniques for color flow mapping are recommended.

RATIO OF JET HEIGHT TO LEFT VENTRICULAR OUTFLOW DIAMETER

Long-axis imaging of the LVOT is used to measure the height of the regurgitant jet *immediately* below (within 1 cm of) the aortic valve plane, which is then compared with the diameter of the LVOT at that same point (3,10). The optimal views are the ME aortic valve long-axis view and the ME five-chamber view (Figure 11.1). The long-axis view that shows the maximal height of the color jet is selected for analysis. The maximal height during diastole is identified during slow motion freeze-frame review. The analysis is performed using the software analysis package of the ultrasound machine. Alternatively, an M-mode cursor can be placed perpendicular to the outflow tract. If color flow mapping is then activated, the regurgitant jet will appear in color in the M-mode view of the outflow tract, and the relative dimensions can be measured from this display by using the caliper function of the ultrasound machine (Figure 11.2). This is generally the easier of the two color methods of analysis to perform (Table 11.1) and has been shown to be effective despite major changes in loading conditions *in vitro* (10).

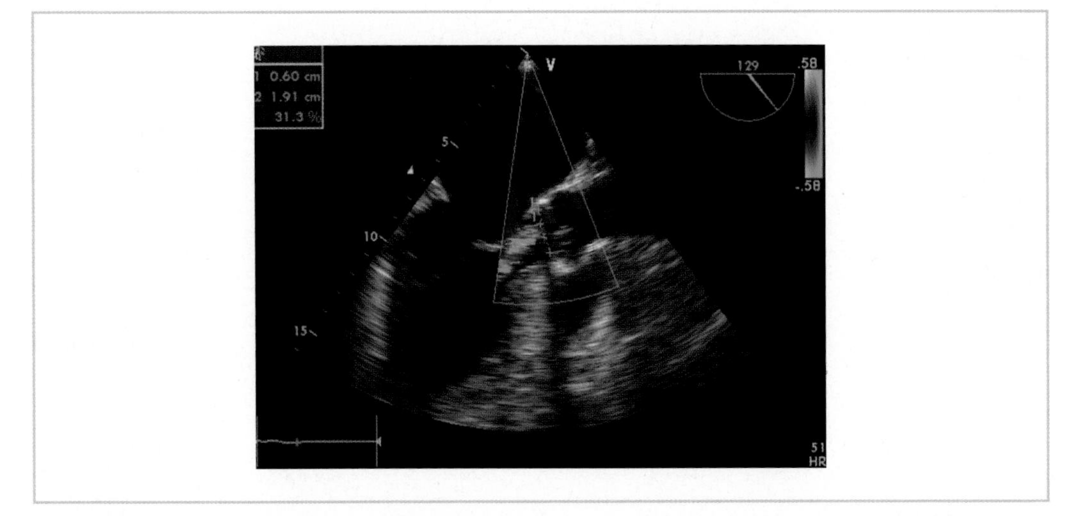

Figure 11.1. Midesophageal aortic valve long-axis view demonstrating calculation of the ratio of aortic insufficiency height to left ventricular outflow tract diameter. The internal caliper on the echocardiography system is used to make these measurements. In this example, the ratio is 31%, indicating mild aortic insufficiency.

RATIO OF JET AREA TO LEFT VENTRICULAR OUTFLOW TRACT AREA

In the second color flow mapping technique, the short axis area of the regurgitant jet in the LVOT is compared with the area of the LVOT at that same level (Figure 11.3). The preferred view for this approach is the ME aortic valve short-axis view, but with the probe advanced to immediately below the valve plane. Again, diastole is evaluated by slow motion freeze-frame review, and the maximal jet area is traced and compared with the

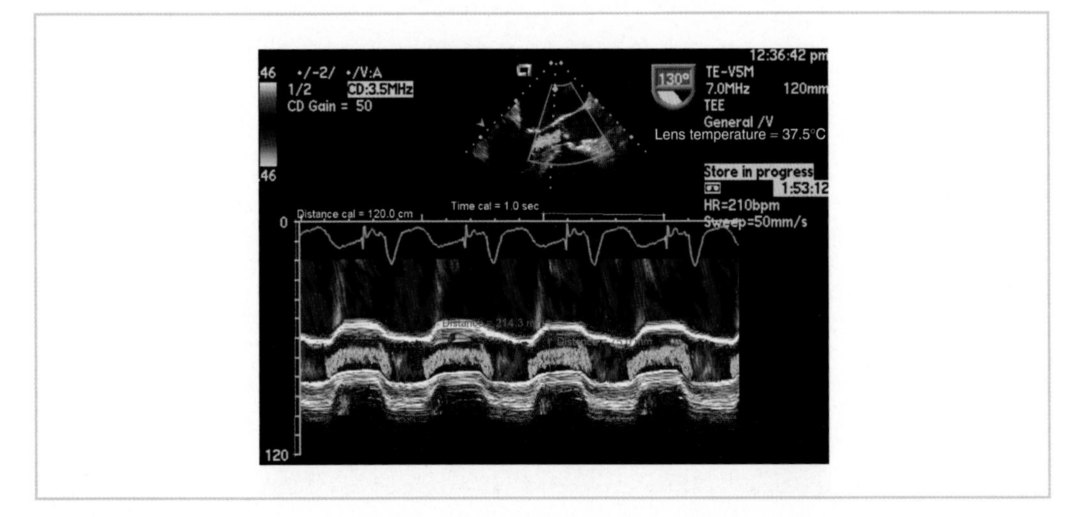

Figure 11.2. Color M-mode assessment of aortic regurgitation. From the midesophageal aortic valve long-axis view, the M-mode cursor is positioned perpendicular to the aortic root as close to the origin of the regurgitant jet as possible. The jet and the outflow tract are well delineated in the color M-mode display. Caliper measurement of the jet height (75 mm) is compared to that of the root (214.3 mm) and the resulting ratio of 35% corresponds to 2+ aortic regurgitation (Table 11.1).

Table 11.1 Scoring of severity of aortic regurgitation

Method of evaluation (view)	Trivial ($0-1^+$)	Mild (1^+-2^+)	Moderate (2^+-3^+)	Severe (3^+-4^+)
AI jet height/LVOT diameter (ME AV LAX)	1%–24%	25%–46%	47%–64%	>65%
AI area/LVOT area (ME AV SAX)	<4%	4%–24%	25%–59%	>60%
Jet depth mapping (ME LAX)	LVOT	Midanterior mitral leaflet	Tip anterior mitral leaflet	Papillary muscle head
Vena contracta mapping (ME LAX, ME AV SAX)	<3 mm	3–6 mm	—	Width >6 mm Area >7.5 mm^2
Aortic diastolic flow reversal (UE aortic arch LAX)	—	—	—	Holodiastolic retrograde flow in the descending aorta
Slope of AR jet decay (TG LAX, deep TG LAX)	—	—	≥2 m/s	≥3 m/s
Pressure half-time (TG LAX, deep TG LAX)	—	>500 ms	200–500 ms	<200 ms

AI, aortic insufficiency; LVOT, left ventricular outflow tract; ME, midesophageal; AV, aortic valve; LAX, long axis; SAX, short axis; UE, upper esophageal; AR, aortic regurgitation; TG, transgastric.

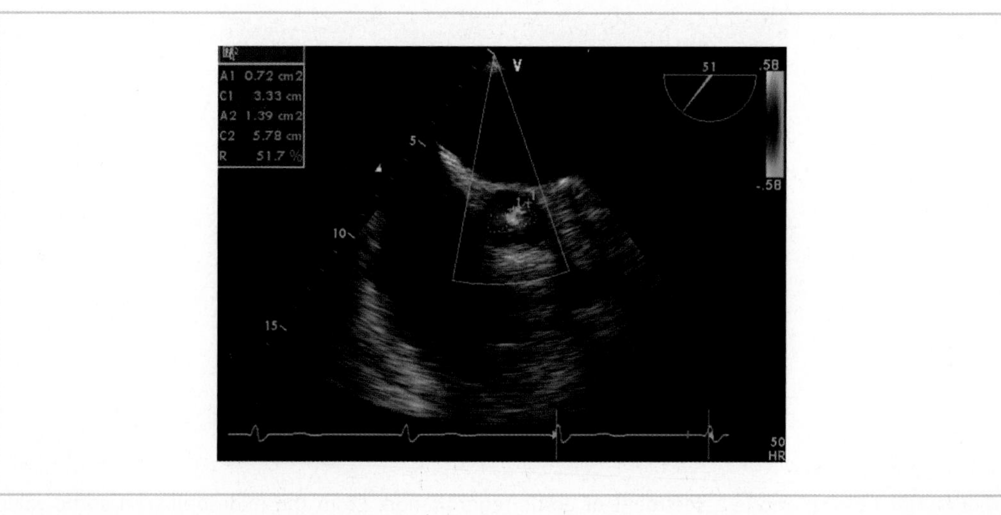

Figure 11.3. Midesophageal aortic valve short-axis view in the same patient as in Figure 11.1 demonstrating the jet area/left ventricular outflow tract area method. The ratio of the areas is 51%, indicating moderate mitral regurgitation. The patient therefore has mild-moderate aortic insufficiency.

area of the LVOT. The process is simplified by using the software analysis package of the ultrasound machine. This method is slightly more accurate than the height-diameter ratio method but is technically more difficult to perform.

CAVEATS

In practice, these approaches provide reliable estimates of severity and have consequently become widely regarded as among the best and most easily applied methods of Doppler assessment (11). They do, however, require technically adequate views and color flow images that cannot always be obtained and may be affected by changes in loading conditions (Table 11.1).

Regurgitant jets have three dimensions. If a jet results from the lack of adequate alignment between two aortic cusps along their line of coaptation (short-axis view) then interrogation at right angles to that jet (long-axis view) may happen to orient perpendicularly to that line. A relatively narrow regurgitant orifice can then appear to be causing regurgitant flow that fills the outflow tract resulting in an overestimation of the severity of the leak. A cursory review of the outflow tract short-axis view of the jet will clarify this.

Eccentric jets that are angled to the plane of the aortic valve are not adequately assessed by this technique. They require the use of a technique similar to that utilized for quantitative assessment of mitral regurgitation based on an application of the conservation of mass. The technique analyzes the proximal isovelocity surface area (PISA) defining the entrance of the jet into its regurgitant orifice and analysis of the volume of flow into the left ventricle to derive the regurgitant orifice. The use of the vena contracta technique (*see subsequent text*) can be helpful in analyzing eccentric jets and is a more practical approach intraoperatively because TEE allows higher resolution definition of this than TTE.

Mapping the Vena Contracta

The *vena contracta* is the narrowest portion of the jet crossing the valve plane and can be identified by first visualizing the convergence zone of color flow (PISA) as it approaches and traverses the valve plane. To optimize visualization, the echo sector is narrowed and the depth decreased to maximize the LVOT size and frame rate. Subtle adjustments of angulation and rotation from this point may be needed to identify the vena contracta (Figure 11.4). In some patients, particularly with very eccentric jets, visualization is not possible. Long- and short-axis views are then obtained from the ME aortic valve long and short-axis views respectively, as outlined earlier. The width of the vena contracta is measured as it passes through and defines the regurgitant orifice to exit the valve plane (6,12). The largest diameter of the vena contracta during any portion of diastole is measured in the long-axis plane of the jet, or planimetry of its area is performed in the short-axis view at the valve plane. In a small series of patients undergoing TEE, a vena contracta width of more than 6 mm or an area of more than 7.5 mm^2 predicted severe AR (6). A vena contracta width of 3 to 6 mm defines moderate valvular insufficiency. When less than 3 mm the insufficiency is mild (Table 11.1). More importantly, and in contrast to observations made during assessments of the severity of mitral regurgitation with this technique (13)), changes in afterload obtained with phenylephrine or volume loading do not change the size of the vena contracta, suggesting this measurement to be relatively load independent (11,14,15). This approach has become the method of choice for intraoperative assessment because of its relative ease of acquisition and apparent load independence. It should be emphasized again that regurgitant jets are three-dimensional and as a consequence multiple views should be obtained and analysis made of the best

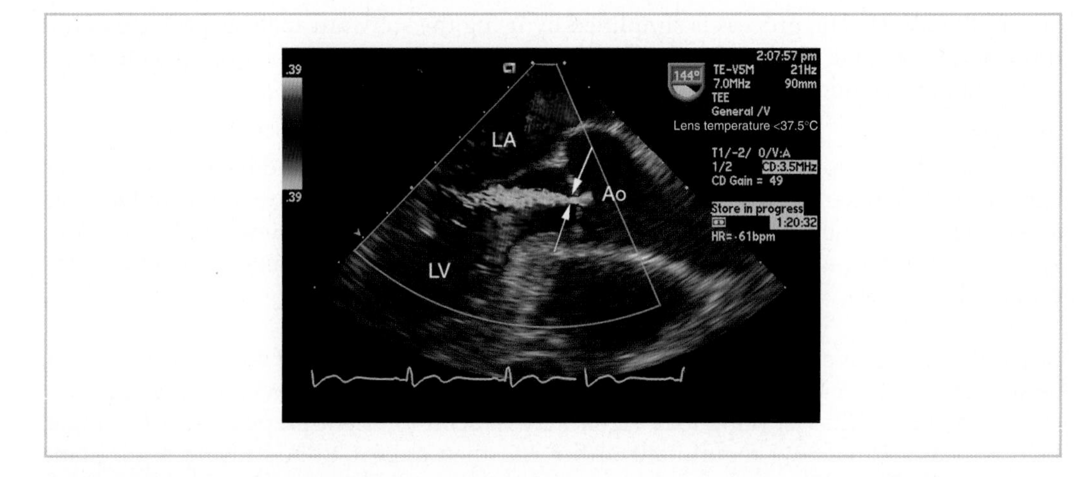

Figure 11.4. Midesophageal long-axis view. Arrows indicate the vena contracta. This often reaches its true (narrowest) dimension slightly below the valve plane at the flow convergence zone. The latter is the point at which flow from the central aorta reaches its narrowest dimension after it is "focused" by entering the regurgitant orifice on the aortic side of the valve. LA, left atrium; Ao, aorta; LV, left ventricle.

defining images. When multiple jets or very eccentric jets are present, the short-axis view may be more helpful in assessing the overall size of the vena contracta (16).

Aortic Diastolic Flow Reversal

Another early index of the severity of aortic insufficiency was based on the demonstration of retrograde diastolic flow in the ascending or, more preferably, the descending aorta or the aortic arch (17). Retrograde flow is best assessed by interrogating the aorta in a plane near the arch (upper esophageal aortic arch long-axis view), as demonstrated in Figure 11.5. This view is obtained by withdrawing the probe from the ME position and rotating it posteriorly to visualize the descending aorta at 0 degree in circular cross section. In patients with a tortuous aorta, the angle necessary for a short-axis view may vary considerably.

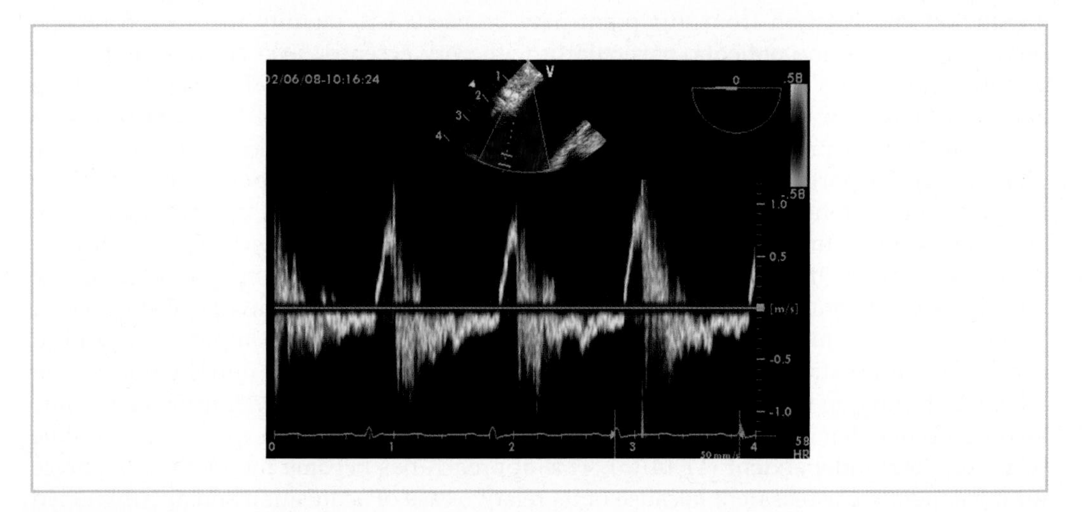

Figure 11.5. Upper esophageal aortic arch long-axis view demonstrating severe aortic regurgitation, evidenced by flow reversal within the distal aortic arch during diastole. Note flow away from the probe, below the baseline, throughout diastole (holodiastolic flow).

As the probe is withdrawn into the upper esophagus, the plane elongates as the arch is cut tangentially at a point slightly deeper than 20 cm from the incisors. Angulation with firm retroflexion from this position generally allows interrogation of the high arch. Images of the ascending and descending portions of the aorta are typically acquired only with significant obliquity and are therefore not generally used in clinical spectral Doppler examinations. However, because the flow abnormality is assessed as the ratio of diastolic to systolic flow as opposed to the absolute flow velocities, the inability to assess true flow velocities is not a limitation. The systolic and diastolic flow curves are traced providing the corresponding velocity time integrals (VTIs) from which the ratio is then calculated. The closer the diastolic VTI is to the systolic VTI, the greater the severity of the leak.

Normally, a minor retrograde flow pattern can be detected in the ascending aorta and proximal descending aorta related to runoff into the great vessels and coronary bed. As aortic insufficiency becomes more severe, the degree of apparent retrograde aortic flow relative to antegrade aortic flow increases (18). In general, the further distally in the aorta (e.g., descending or abdominal aorta) holodiastolic retrograde flow is detected, the more severe the AR.

This assessment remains a useful adjunct for confirming the severity of AR but is less accurate in the presence of coexisting aortic stenosis (7,17,19). *Importantly, the usefulness of the descending aortic diastolic reversal of flow as an index of severe AR intraoperatively has been confirmed in patients in whom the LVOT cannot be adequately imaged on TEE for technical reasons (e.g., interposed MV prosthesis creating an acoustic shadow that obscures the LV outflow). In these patients, color flow mapping of the regurgitant jet is not possible* (5).

Slope of Aortic Regurgitant Jet Decay

Analysis of a continuous wave Doppler wave form of aortic insufficiency from the TG long-axis or deep TG long-axis view is used because the Doppler beam is aligned parallel to the regurgitant jet flow. Basal esophageal views of the LVOT are generally obtained at too great an angle to the flow for an accurate jet to be acquired. It is essential that a smooth waveform with an intact envelope be recorded for analysis to be meaningful.

The principle of this analysis is that the velocity of the regurgitant jet is directly related to the pressure gradient between the aortic root and the LV in diastole, in accordance with the Bernoulli equation. When a large defect in the competence of the valve is present, the pressures equalize more rapidly because more blood leaks through the valve per unit of time. Therefore, the pressure gradient between the aorta and the LV decreases more rapidly in severe regurgitation and, as a result, the velocity of the jet also diminishes more rapidly. The slope of the rate of decay of the velocity is therefore a measure of the severity of regurgitation. A slope of AR velocity decay of 2 to 3 m/s suggests moderately severe or severe (grades 3+ to 4+) AR. Rapid equalization of the pressure gradient can result in premature closure of the MV before the onset of ventricular systole, indicative of severe AR, or in extreme cases, premature opening of the aortic valve in diastole. These latter findings are generally only seen with the acute onset of severe regurgitation. For an analysis of the slope of the AR jet on continuous wave Doppler, the following two technical criteria must be met:

1. A smooth velocity envelope must be defined by continuous wave Doppler.
2. It must be confirmed that the core of the regurgitant jet has been interrogated. With appropriate interrogation, the peak regurgitant jet velocity at the onset of the jet should approximate a value calculated with the Bernoulli equation ($4v^2$) as a reasonable estimate of the gradient between the measured arterial diastolic pressure and an estimate of the

LV diastolic pressure. Typically, jet velocities are high (>4 m/s) in lesser degrees of regurgitation because the initial diastolic pressure gradient between the aorta and LV is generally 60 to 80 mm Hg. The exception is in severe AR, in which the aortic and LV diastolic pressures may be similar. *Otherwise, lower peak velocities on the spectral display suggest that the true regurgitant jet is not being interrogated directly.*

Pressure Half-Time Measurement

Alternatively, a pressure half-time can be calculated. This is defined as the interval between the time when the transvalvular AR pressure gradient is maximal and the time when the pressure gradient is half the maximum. The computer analysis package determines the pressure half-time from the slope of the AR jet decay (Figure 11.6). A pressure half-time of less than 200 ms suggests severe AR (20). *Factors related to LV and aortic compliance and the presence of high LV diastolic pressures (heart failure, restrictive physiology, diastolic dysfunction) all potentially cause the gradient to dissipate more rapidly and artifactually worsen the apparent severity of the lesion by this and slope of regurgitant jet technique approaches.* Accordingly, these two methods of analysis of the decay curve should be used mainly to confirm the color flow findings.

Calculation of Regurgitant Volume

The AR volume can be calculated from the difference between the LV stroke volume and the right ventricular (RV) stroke volume in the absence of other regurgitant lesions (e.g., mitral). The LV stroke volume is calculated by multiplying the cross-sectional area of the LVOT by the VTI of LVOT flow. The RV stroke volume is then estimated from the pulmonary outflow tract diameter and VTI calculated in a similar fashion. Multiplication of the resultant stroke volumes by the heart rate gives the cardiac output for each circuit and allows the quantitative calculation of the regurgitant volume as the difference between the two outputs. However, obtaining accurate measurements of the necessary parameters in an intraoperative situation is time consuming and technically challenging, so that this approach may be impractical in a given patient.

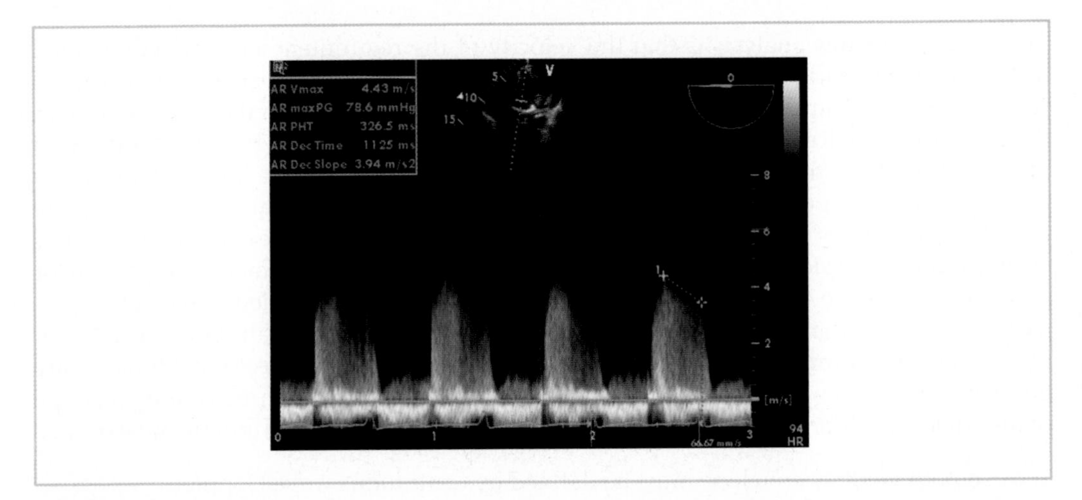

Figure 11.6. Transgastric long-axis view with nearly parallel Doppler beam alignment demonstrating the aortic regurgitant jet velocity profile. The pressure half-time is 218 m/s, with a slope of 3.94 m/s indicating moderate to severe aortic regurgitation.

Color Flow Mapping of the Depth of the Regurgitant Jet

This approach is included for completeness and is no longer used clinically except to screen for the presence of AR.

TECHNIQUE

In the first Doppler approach to quantification of the severity of AR, pulsed wave Doppler was used to map the depth to which the regurgitant jet extended into the LV cavity (18,21,22) (Table 11.1). Color Doppler has supplanted that approach. The maximal depth below the two-dimensional aortic valve plane at which the jet can be detected by color Doppler imaging determines the equivalent angiographic grade of insufficiency. The size of the heart varies with body surface area, so the scale is based on anatomic landmarks instead of depth below the valve plane. Depth is recorded in relation to MV structures because more than 90% of regurgitant jets are oriented toward the anterior mitral leaflet as a result of the Coanda effect. In the less common situation in which the jet is oriented along the interventricular septum, the depth at which it can be detected along the septum is compared with a corresponding depth in relation to MV structures to estimate angiographic severity.

LIMITATIONS

As in any form of valvular insufficiency, a large pressure gradient exists between the two chambers where the leak is occurring. Depending on the location, a pressure head of 60 to 110 mm Hg or greater drives the regurgitant jet through a small orifice. Accordingly, a small regurgitant jet frequently extends far into the recipient chamber despite a leak that is hemodynamically insignificant. *In vitro* analysis of models of AR suggests that the depth is more an index of the gradient between the aorta and LV than of the angiographic grade of severity (10,16).

Use of the color flow map of regurgitant flow as an index of severity is further complicated by the entrainment of blood from a high-velocity jet entering a low-pressure chamber. This leads to color Doppler overestimation of the apparent depth of the regurgitant jet. *Measurements of the apparent depth are more likely to be affected by this phenomenon than are measurements of jet height, which are made close to the aortic valve plane.*

ANCILLARY FINDINGS: ROLE OF THE DOPPLER SIGNAL CHARACTERISTICS IN THE ASSESSMENT OF AORTIC REGURGITATION

Because the blood flow velocity is directly related to the pressure differential, the *diastolic* velocity is always high (4.0–5.0 m/s) in comparison with the *systolic* velocities of 1.0 to 1.7 m/s across normal valves. The to-and-fro systolic and diastolic Doppler signal is easily detected as abnormal by even an untrained ear when heard through the audio system of the ultrasound machine. The sound becomes louder and its tone purer as the alignment of the probe becomes more closely parallel to the core of the jet. High-velocity jets do not *necessarily* mean severe regurgitation is present but rather that the gradient between aorta and left ventricle is higher. If the gain settings are constant, the *intensity* of the spectral Doppler signal is directly related to the severity of the leak. This is because the larger the regurgitant flow, the greater the number of red blood cells contained therein to reflect the ultrasound beam. Consequently, the more severe the regurgitation the more intense the Doppler signals.

In more severe lesions, the velocity of the antegrade flow through the regurgitant valve may be increased in comparison with that in normal subjects. This is a consequence of the increased stroke volume that develops because the heart must eject both the regurgitant and the normal stroke volume through the aortic annulus, which is a fairly rigid structure. The velocity of systolic flow in the LVOT increases with significant insufficiency, and outflow tract velocities equal to or above 1.5 m/s suggest stenosis of the outflow tract relative to the volume of blood flowing through it and support a diagnosis of significant regurgitation. The clinical corollary of this phenomenon is the development of a functional systolic ejection murmur of *relative* aortic stenosis, heard during auscultation of the heart in addition to the diastolic murmur of aortic insufficiency. However, this technique can be misleading in patients with a hyperdynamic state, who can also present with outflow tract flow velocities between 1.5 and 2.0 m/s.

ADDITIONAL USES OF TRANSESOPHAGEAL ECHOCARDIOGRAPHY INTRAOPERATIVELY

The etiology of aortic insufficiency may play a role in the operative approach. The valve most often becomes incompetent due to intrinsic pathology (sclerodegenerative, rheumatic, endocarditis, uni-, bi-, or quadricuspid valve) or changes in the aorta (dissection, aneurysmal dilation as in Marfan syndrome, trauma, lues).

TEE can help delineate potential problems both pre- and postoperatively. The mechanism of AR in cases of aortic dissection can be assessed and used to guide surgery (23–28). For example, the efficacy of resuspension, as opposed to replacement, of a prolapsed aortic valve to correct AR resulting from a Stanford type A dissection is proportional to the percentage of the annulus dissected and, to a lesser extent, the initial diameter of the aortic root (26). The superior resolution of TEE is particularly helpful in defining the anatomic location of regurgitant lesions related to prosthetic heart valves and the suture line of insertion of the valve.

The anatomic continuity of the anterior mitral leaflet with the posterior aortic root creates potential problems in the mitral and aortic valves associated with the debridement of calcification in either annulus or the placement of "overbiting" sutures when a prosthesis is inserted. The potential for poor seating of the valve and paravalvular leaks as well as other complications of surgery can be analyzed with TEE and resolved while the patient is still in the operating room.

The detection of paravalvular leaks is also another valuable screen. The annulus is generally best visualized in the ME aortic valve short-axis view. In addition, seating of the prosthesis can be assessed in the ME aortic valve long-axis view. Here, shadowing by the prosthetic ring can hide small leaks. If neither of these views is acceptable and attempt should be made to check for regurgitation from with a regular deep TG long-axis view. Generally small leaks will seal after heparin effect is reversed with protamine.

SUMMARY

The intraoperative assessment of AR with TEE is generally best accomplished by measuring the width of the vena contracta because this measurement is less load dependent than others. The next most useful is jet height in the LVOT just below the aortic valve plane. The assessment of diastolic flow reversal in the aorta itself remains an important and useful approach that has been reconfirmed. The other approaches discussed in this chapter play an ancillary role, reinforcing the practitioner's confidence in making a definitive assessment.

REFERENCES

1 Ward J, Baker D, Rubenstein S, et al. Detection of aortic insufficiency by pulse Doppler echocardiography. *J Clin Ultrasound* 1977;5:5–10.
2 Meyerowitz C, Jacobs L, Kotler M, et al. Assessment of aortic regurgitation by transesophageal echocardiography: correlation with angiographic determination. *Echocardiography* 1993;10:269–278.
3 Rafferty T, Durkin M, Sittig D, et al. Transesophageal color flow Doppler imaging for aortic insufficiency in patients having cardiac operations. *J Thorac Cardiovasc Surg* 1992;104:521–525.
4 Sato Y, Kawazoe K, Kamata J, et al. Clinical usefulness of the effective regurgitant orifice area determined by transesophageal echocardiography in patients with eccentric aortic regurgitation. *J Heart Valve Dis* 1997;6:580–586.
5 Sutton D, Kluger R, Ahmed S, et al. Flow reversal in the descending aorta: a guide to intraoperative assessment of aortic regurgitation with transesophageal echocardiography. *J Thorac Cardiovasc Surg* 1994;108:576–582.
6 Willett D, Hall S, Jessen M, et al. Assessment of aortic regurgitation by transesophageal color Doppler imaging of the vena contracta: validation against an intraoperative aortic flow probe. *J Am Coll Cardiol* 2001;37:1450–1455.
7 Zarauza J, Ares M, Vilchez F, et al. An integrated approach to the quantification of aortic regurgitation by Doppler echocardiography. *Am Heart J* 1998;136:1030–1041.
8 Yoganathan A, Cape E, Sung H, et al. Review of hydrodynamic principles for the cardiologist: applications to the study of blood flow and jets by imaging techniques. *J Am Coll Cardiol* 1988;12:1344–1353.
9 Zoghbi WA, Enriquez-Sorano E, Foster E, et al. Recommendations for the evaluation of the severity of native valvular regurgitation with two-dimensional and Doppler echocardiography. *J Am Soc Echocardiogr* 2003;16:777–892.
10 Switzer D, Yoganathan A, Nanda N, et al. Calibration of color Doppler flow mapping during extreme hemodynamic conditions *in vitro*: a foundation for a reliable quantitative grading system for aortic incompetence. *Circulation* 1987;75:837–846.
11 Perry J, Helmcke F, Nanda N, et al. Evaluation of aortic insufficiency by Doppler color flow mapping. *J Am Coll Cardiol* 1987;9:952–959.
12 Tribouilloy C, Enriquez-Sarano M, Bailey K, et al. Assessment of severity of aortic regurgitation using the width of the vena contracta: a clinical color Doppler imaging study. *Circulation* 2000;102: 558–564.
13 Kizilbash A, Willett D, Brickner M, et al. Effects of afterload reduction on vena contracta width in mitral regurgitation. *J Am Coll Cardiol* 1998;32:427–431.
14 Ishii M, Jones M, Shiota T, et al. Evaluation of eccentric aortic regurgitation by color Doppler jet and color Doppler-imaged vena contracta measurements: an animal study of quantified aortic regurgitation. *Am Heart J* 1996;132:796–804.
15 Ishii M, Jones M, Shiota T, et al. Quantifying aortic regurgitation by using the color Doppler-imaged vena contracta: a chronic animal model study. *Circulation* 1997;96:2009–2015.
16 Taylor A, Eichhorn E, Brickner M, et al. Aortic valve morphology: an important *in vitro* determinant of proximal regurgitant jet width by Doppler color flow mapping. *J Am Coll Cardiol* 1990;16:405–412.
17 Diebold B, Peronneau P, Blanchard D, et al. Non-invasive quantification of aortic regurgitation by Doppler echocardiography. *Br Heart J* 1983;49:167–173.
18 Quinones M, Young J, Waggoner A, et al. Assessment of pulsed Doppler echocardiography in detection and quantification of aortic and mitral regurgitation. *Br Heart J* 1980;44:612–620.
19 Reimold S, Maier S, Aggarwa l K, et al. Aortic flow velocity patterns in chronic aortic regurgitation: implications for Doppler echocardiography. *J Am Soc Echocardiogr* 1996;9:675–683.
20 Labovitz A, Ferrara R, Kern M, et al. Quantitative evaluation of aortic insufficiency by continuous wave Doppler echocardiography. *J Am Coll Cardiol* 1986;8:1341–1347.
21 Ciobanu M, Abbasi A, Allen M, et al. Pulsed Doppler echocardiography in the diagnosis and estimation of severity of aortic insufficiency. *Am J Cardiol* 1982;49:339–343.
22 Toguchi M, Ichimiya S, Yokoi K, et al. Clinical investigation of aortic insufficiency by means of pulsed Doppler echocardiography. *Jpn Heart J* 1981;22:537–550.
23 Adam M, Tribouilloy C, Mirode A, et al. Contribution of transesophageal and transthoracic echography in the evaluation of the mechanism and quantification of regurgitation in mitral and aortic bioprosthetic valves [in French]. *Arch Mal Coeur Vaiss* 1993;86:1345–1350.
24 Brandstatt P, Carlioz R, Fontaine B, et al. Acute post-traumatic aortic insufficiency: transesophageal echocardiography in the diagnosis and therapy of the lesions [in French]. *Ann Cardiol Angeiol (Paris)* 1998;47:563–567.

25 Hioki J, Shibutani T, Naito T, et al. Aortic valve insufficiency caused by nonpenetrating chest trauma difficult to distinguish from infective endocarditis with transesophageal echocardiography: a case report [in Japanese]. *J Cardiol* 1997;29:143–149.
26 Keane M, Wiegers S, Yang E, et al. Structural determinants of aortic regurgitation in type A dissection and the role of valvular resuspension as determined by intraoperative transesophageal echocardiography. *Am J Cardiol* 2000;85:604–610.
27 Movsowitz H, Levine R, Hilgenberg A, et al. Transesophageal echocardiographic description of the mechanisms of aortic regurgitation in acute type A aortic dissection: implications for aortic valve repair. *J Am Coll Cardiol* 2000;36:884–890.
28 Oda H, Tanaka T, Yamazaki Y, et al. A case of nonpenetrating traumatic aortic regurgitation detected by transesophageal echocardiography. *Tohoku J Exp Med* 1997;182:93–101.

QUESTIONS

1. **Which of the following factors can affect the degree of aortic regurgitation (AR) during an operative examination?**
   a. Administration of vasopressors
   b. Presence of volatile anesthetics
   c. Patient's volume status
   d. All of the above

2. **Which transesophageal echocardiography (TEE) view is most helpful in evaluating the aortic valve in a patient with a St. Jude mitral valve?**
   a. Midesophageal (ME) four-chamber view
   b. ME aortic valve long-axis view
   c. ME aortic valve short-axis view
   d. Transgastric (TG) long-axis view

3. **Which view allows for optimal Doppler beam alignment in a patient with AR?**
   a. ME four-chamber view
   b. ME aortic valve long-axis view
   c. ME aortic valve short-axis view
   d. TG short-axis view
   e. Deep TG long-axis view

4. **When the ratio of the AR jet height to the left ventricular outflow tract (LVOT) diameter is used to quantify the degree of AR, the following is true**
   a. One must optimize the color gain setting.
   b. The ME aortic valve long-axis view is preferred.
   c. The ratio for AR with a grade of 4+ is more than 65%.
   d. All of the above.

5. **When the pressure half-time method is used to quantify the severity of AR, which of the following will not artificially worsen the apparent severity of the AR?**
   a. Congestive heart failure
   b. Restrictive physiology
   c. Diastolic dysfunction
   d. Acute myocardial infarction
   e. Acute hemorrhage

6. **Obtaining diastolic aortic flow reversal in a patient with AR with TEE is difficult. The following statements regarding techniques are true except**
   a. The upper esophageal aortic arch long-axis view is useful.
   b. Obtaining accurate flow velocities is essential.
   c. Holodiastolic flow in the distal aorta indicates severe AR.
   d. AR end-diastolic velocity profiles in the descending aorta correlate better with AR severity than those in the ascending aorta.

7. **Which statement about continuous wave Doppler analysis of AR is true?**
   a. Parallel alignment with the regurgitant jet is essential.
   b. The deep TG long-axis and TG long-axis views are preferred.
   c. ME views are seldom adequate because of poor beam alignment.
   d. A smooth wave form with an intact envelope is necessary.
   e. All of the above.

8. Which principle is not important in an evaluation of the slope of AR jet decay with Doppler?

a. Pulsed wave Doppler is preferred because of "cleaner" envelopes.
b. The velocity of the regurgitant jet is directly proportional to the pressure gradient between the aorta and the LV in diastole.
c. A large regurgitant lesion will equalize the pressure gradient between the aorta and the LV more quickly.
d. The velocity of the AR jet diminishes more quickly as the severity of AR increases.

9. Which of the following observations is useful to remember in an attempt to optimize the Doppler beam alignment in a patient with AR?

a. The velocity should be high (4–5 m/s).
b. AR has a loud and pure audio tone as the jet is entered.
c. The intensity (darkness) of the spectral Doppler signal is proportional to the severity of the leak.
d. Patients with significant AR frequently have LVOT velocities greater than 1.5 m/s.
e. All of the above.

10. All of the following indicate severe AR except

a. Pressure half-time of less than 500 ms
b. Ratio of height of the AR jet in the LVOT to the diameter of the LVOT above 65%
c. Ratio of area of AR jet in LVOT to area of LVOT above 60%
d. Diastolic flow reversal in the descending aorta

Answers appear at the back of the book.

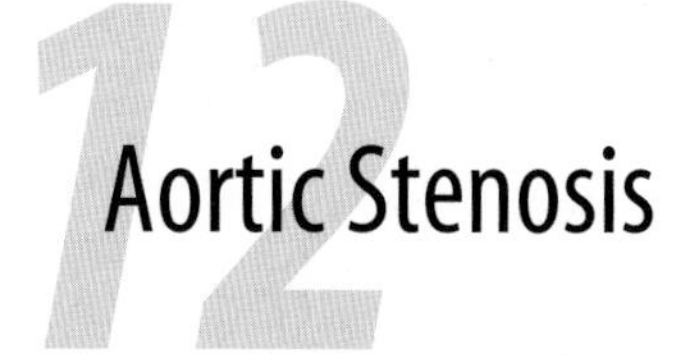

Aortic Stenosis

Ira S. Cohen

Aortic valve replacement for critical aortic stenosis (AS) is probably the most common indication for cardiac surgery in patients past the age of 65 years with the exception of coronary artery bypass grafting procedures. The overwhelming majority of patients in this age-group have atherosclerotic degenerative changes of a tricuspid valve as the pathophysiologic substrate. In contrast, most patients undergoing aortic valve replacement for AS in the 35- to 55-year-old age-group have a bicuspid aortic valve, which typically calcifies early. Aortic valve involvement by rheumatic disease occurs much less frequently than in the preantibiotic era, typically causes commissural fusion, and is almost invariably associated with mitral valve (MV) disease.

In general, critical AS is diagnosed preoperatively. Symptoms of hemodynamically significant AS indicating a clinical need for valve replacement are congestive heart failure (often starting as exertional dyspnea), syncope, and angina. Provided other potential causes of these symptoms have been excluded, their presence is of paramount clinical significance because failure to operate at this point in the course of the disease is associated with a poor prognosis. This is so even if the estimated valve areas are less than "critical." Calculated aortic valve areas are estimates based on assumptions that apply hydraulic principles to a physiologic system and on measurements dependent, to an important degree, on the cardiac output (CO) at the time of measurement. As a result, in patients with poor ventricular function and a low CO, gradients can be quite low despite critical disease.

The rate of progression of stenosis can be fairly rapid and tends to be linear for a given individual, but it is not predictable based on the initial echocardiographic findings (1,2). The issue of whether to replace a noncritically stenotic valve prophylactically is increasingly important. Recently updated guidelines support aortic valve replacement at the time of primary coronary artery bypass surgery in patients with at least moderate AS, even if asymptomatic, in view of the generally progressive nature of this disorder (3). Accordingly, the intraoperative echocardiographer must be adept with the techniques used to assess the severity of AS (Table 12.1).

PATHOPHYSIOLOGY

AS presents a slowly progressive increase in afterload on the ventricle developing over the course of years as the degree of stenosis progresses. The resulting increase in wall stress (force/unit area) induces a variable degree of a concentric hypertrophic response that tends to normalize wall stress. Ultimately this compensatory mechanism fails and typical symptoms develop. The hypertrophied chamber becomes less compliant both because of the stiffness of hypertrophied muscle and concomitant collagen deposition. This results in diastolic dysfunction and increasing preload dependence of the ventricle. Atrial contraction (the "a" kick) can increase from the normal of 3 to 4 mm Hg to levels as high as 30 to 40 mm Hg to stretch the hypertrophied ventricle before each contraction. Loss of atrial contraction by the development of atrial fibrillation can result in the development of acute pulmonary edema. The need for a relatively high preload (i.e., a wedge pressure of approximately 15–18 mm Hg) in these noncompliant ventricles is an important key to effective postoperative management.

Table 12.1 Revised guidelines severity of aortic stenosis

Method of evaluation	Mild	Moderate	Severe
Peak velocity (m/s)	<3.0	3.0–4.0	>4.0
Mean gradient (mm Hg)	<25	25–40	>40
AVA (cm^2)	>1.5	1.0–1.5	<1.0

TVI, time-velocity integral; LVOT, left ventricular outflow tract; AVA, aortic valve area.

AS can cause angina in the absence of significant epicardial coronary artery disease because the tissue turgor of the hypertrophic wall compromises coronary flow reserve by restricting the dilatory capacity of penetrating coronary vessels. Cardiac catheterization is therefore required to exclude critical coronary artery disease (which coexists in ~50% of cases) in patients both with and without angina as silent coronary disease and physical limitation on activity is common at this age. Syncope is a consequence of the inability to increase CO in response to the peripheral vasodilatation associated with exercise, to arrhythmia or to acute heart failure. Pulmonary congestion results from the increasingly high preload required for adequate function in a noncompliant ventricle with diastolic dysfunction.

EVALUATION OF THE AORTIC VALVE

Two-Dimensional Planimetry of the Orifice

The area of the normal aortic valve is between 2.6 and 3.5 cm^2 (Figure 12.1). Newly published guidelines (3), viewing the disease as a continuum based on hemodynamic and natural history data, define severe AS as a valve area less than 1.0 cm^2, a mean gradient greater than 40 mm Hg or peak jet velocity greater than 4.0 m/s (Table 12.1).

Early echocardiographers looked at the characteristics of aortic leaflet motion in an attempt to determine the severity of aortic obstruction. Separation of the aortic leaflets by less than 8 mm in a two-dimensional (2-D) long-axis view suggested critical disease, whereas separation by more than 12 mm suggested noncritical disease (4) (Figure 12.1). In addition, fluttering of an aortic leaflet on motion mode (M-mode) echocardiography was felt to be better than 2-D separation as a discriminator of noncritical disease (5). These findings have been superceded by later techniques.

2-D echocardiography in the midesophageal (ME) aortic valve short-axis view at an approximate angle of 45 degrees images the short-axis plane of the aortic valve and allows planimetry of the aortic valve orifice. Accurate planimetry requires that the imaging plane and machine settings be optimized to identify the minimal total orifice as follows:

1. Obtain a short-axis view of the aortic valve with all three leaflets in view.
2. Use color flow Doppler imaging (with minimal color gain) to aid in adjusting the probe depth and angle of the imaging plane so as to interrogate the *narrowest orifice* and to localize the edges of the orifice.
3. Optimize the 2-D image by adjusting the gain settings to the minimum showing an entire orifice. *Excessive gain leads to an underestimation of valve area because of a "blooming*

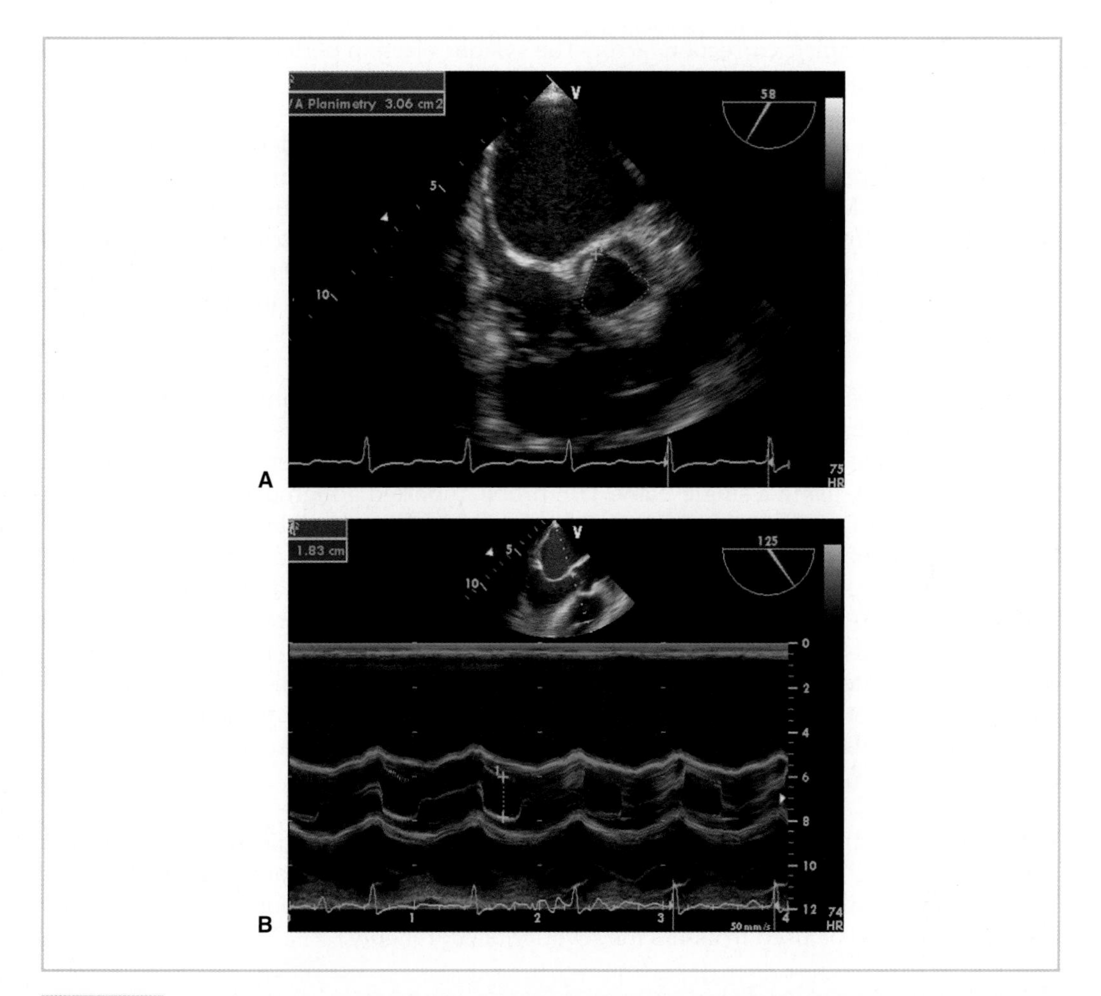

Figure 12.1. **A:** Midesophageal aortic valve short-axis view of a normal aortic valve with a planimetric area of 3.06 cm^2. **B:** Two-dimensional M-mode (motion mode) midesophageal aortic valve long-axis view demonstrating cusp separation of 18 mm in the same patient.

artifact" from the bright echoes of the thickened valve leaflets. Again, slight changes in angulation and in the depth of the probe may be necessary for optimization.

4. Use the electronic tracing caliper of the ultrasound machine to trace the orifice and so obtain its area (Figures 12.1, 12.4A).

All planimetric techniques are limited by an inability to determine whether the actual minimal orifice is being imaged or whether the plane chosen for measurement is at an angle to the true minimal orifice. Errors are minimized using the techniques mentioned earlier. Initial studies of the application of 3-D echocardiography to addressing this problem appear promising.

The accuracy of planimetry has been assessed by comparing it with the "gold standard" reference technique used in the catheterization laboratory to calculate aortic valve area, the Gorlin equation:

$$\text{AVA} = \frac{\text{cardiac output}}{44.3\ (\text{SEP})(\text{HR})\sqrt{\text{mean gradient}}}$$

where 44.3 is an empiric correction factor. The systolic ejection period (SEP) is factored in because we are assessing flow through the valve only in systole.

Because the Gorlin equation–derived aortic valve area is *directly* dependent on the CO and inversely dependent on the *square root* of the gradient, an accurate measurement of the CO is critical. Multiple beats must be averaged when thermodilution estimates of CO are used, especially if the patient is not in normal sinus rhythm. *It also follows that if the CO increases, the mean gradient must increase if the area is to remain constant.* In fact, the Gorlin equation–derived area may increase with output, and its accuracy in these situations is the subject of active debate in the catheterization community.

Although successful measurement by transthoracic echocardiographic (TTE) planimetry has been reported, transesophageal echocardiography (TEE), with its superior resolution, would be expected to be more effective in making this measurement accurately (6). Stoddard et al. (7), using a single-plane TEE probe, reported a high degree of correlation between TEE planimetric aortic valve area and aortic valve area determined by TTE and the continuity equation in both normal and impaired ventricles, and a superior correlation with aortic valve area determined by catheterization and the standard Gorlin formula. Hoffman et al. (8) showed excellent correlation of the planimetric result and the Gorlin formula determined area. The use of multiplane rather than single-plane probes facilitates obtaining adequate studies and is more accurate than biplane techniques (9). Changes in the CO should not cause changes in a planimetric area, so that the technique should be as good in patients with a low *or* normal CO (10), and it has been suggested to be more accurate than the Gorlin equation at low or high output.

TEE is not as accurate in the presence of significant valvular calcification (11), and not all observers have reported uniformly good correlations of TEE planimetric valve areas with Gorlin formula valve areas (12). Consequently, the results of both 2-D and Doppler assessment should be used to assess the severity of AS reliably.

Quantitative Doppler Assessment of Aortic Stenosis

The severity of AS is assessed quantitatively with Doppler echocardiography in two ways: measuring the gradient across the valve with the modified Bernoulli equation or estimating the aortic valve area with the continuity equation (13–15). Both techniques require that the ultrasound beam be parallel to the transvalvular blood flow.

TRANSESOPHAGEAL ECHOCARDIOGRAPHIC DOPPLER VIEWS FOR ASSESSING AORTIC STENOSIS

In AS, aligning the transesophageal transducer parallel to the left ventricular outflow tract (LVOT) and aortic valve can be challenging. The deep transgastric (TG) long-axis and TG long-axis views are commonly used (16). Advancing the probe from a TG short-axis view with continued anteflexion may allow acquisition of the deep TG long-axis view from near the LV apex. Occasionally counterclockwise rotation of the probe and varying the angle of interrogation may facilitate this. The TG long-axis view is obtained with the probe at the midpapillary level and the imaging plane rotated to 120 to 140 degrees. Both techniques offer an excellent approach to aortic valve flow dynamics; however, the patient's anatomy will dictate which view provides the best interrogation of transvalvular blood flow. In a minority of individuals the ME long-axis view (at 120 degrees) allows the best alignment to the transaortic flow, particularly with posteriorly directed jets.

A note of caution is necessary in a discussion of Doppler imaging and the angle of incidence. It is tempting to correct for nonparallel orientation of the Doppler beam to the flow of blood. Many echocardiographic systems provide a means to correct the angle of interrogation visually. The correction is obtained by multiplying the Doppler shift velocity by the cosine of the incident angle of the beam to the aortic flow. *It is generally accepted that this is not a reliable method to use in quantitative Doppler analysis. Because the interaction of beam and blood flow occurs in 3-D, 2-D imaging is unable to determine the true angle of incidence to the jet accurately.* With turbulent jets, as in AS, judging the alignment with flow is particularly difficult (17). Such jets may be very eccentrically directed to the 2-D plane visualized, so that apparent "correction" by looking at a color flow map of the jet can be very imprecise. Obtaining the highest-velocity smooth envelope is a better way to confirm accuracy.

DOPPLER DETERMINATION OF THE AORTIC VALVE GRADIENT: MODIFIED BERNOULLI EQUATION

The Bernoulli equation is used to calculate transaortic valve pressure gradients (Table 12.2). The modified Bernoulli equation states that the maximal pressure gradient equals four times the square of the peak jet velocity and allows calculation of the peak instantaneous gradient across any orifice. Therefore, if the peak blood flow velocity across the aortic valve is 4 m/s, the calculated peak gradient $= 4 \times 4^2 = 64$ mm Hg. The mean gradient is calculated by averaging the instantaneous gradients over time. This function is accomplished by tracing the aortic flow velocity profile and using the analysis program of the ultrasound machine (Figure 12.2). Alternatively, the mean velocity can be estimated from the peak velocity and the mean gradient calculated as $2.4(v_{max})^2$. The mean gradient, in particular, correlates well with invasively determined gradients and is most often used in evaluating the severity of AS (17). It is imperative that a true peak velocity be obtained for this estimate to be valid. A well-defined velocity curve with a smooth envelope is generally a valid one.

Discrepancies often occur between catheterization and echocardiographic pressure gradients in AS. The peak echocardiographic gradient measures the peak *instantaneous* gradient between the LV and aorta. This is often higher than the peak-to-peak gradient (between the peak LV pressure and the generally *later* peak aortic pressure) routinely entered on cardiac catheterization reports (Figure 12.3). Also, a rapid recovery of pressure distal to the stenosis reduces or abolishes the gradient within several centimeters of the valve orifice as the flow becomes more laminar (the phenomenon of "pressure recovery") (18). The peak gradient can be influenced by the flow volume on the ventricular side of the valve plane. Remember that the simplified Bernoulli equation ignores the impact of the LVOT blood flow velocity. *However, the Bernoulli equation must factor in the LVOT blood flow velocity when it exceeds 1.5 m/s, as commonly occurs in associated aortic insufficiency or other high-output states, to avoid overestimation of the pressure gradient* (Table 12.2). For example, if the outflow tract velocity is 1.7 m/s and the peak transvalvular velocity is 4 m/s, the actual gradient is $4 \times (4^2 - 1.7^2) = 4 \times (16 - 2.89) = 4 \times 13.1 = 52.4$ mm Hg, instead of the 64 mm Hg predicted by the simplified Bernoulli equation.

Table 12.2 Equations for aortic transvalvular gradients

Peak gradient (simplified Bernoulli equation)
Peak gradient (mm Hg) $= 4$ (aortic peak velocity)^2
Mean gradient
Mean gradient (mm Hg) $= 4$ (mean velocity)^2 $= 2.4\ (v_{max})^2$
Peak gradient with significant aortic regurgitation (modified Bernoulli equation)
Gradient $= 4$ [(peak aortic velocity)^2 - (LVOT velocity)^2]

LVOT, left ventricular outflow tract.

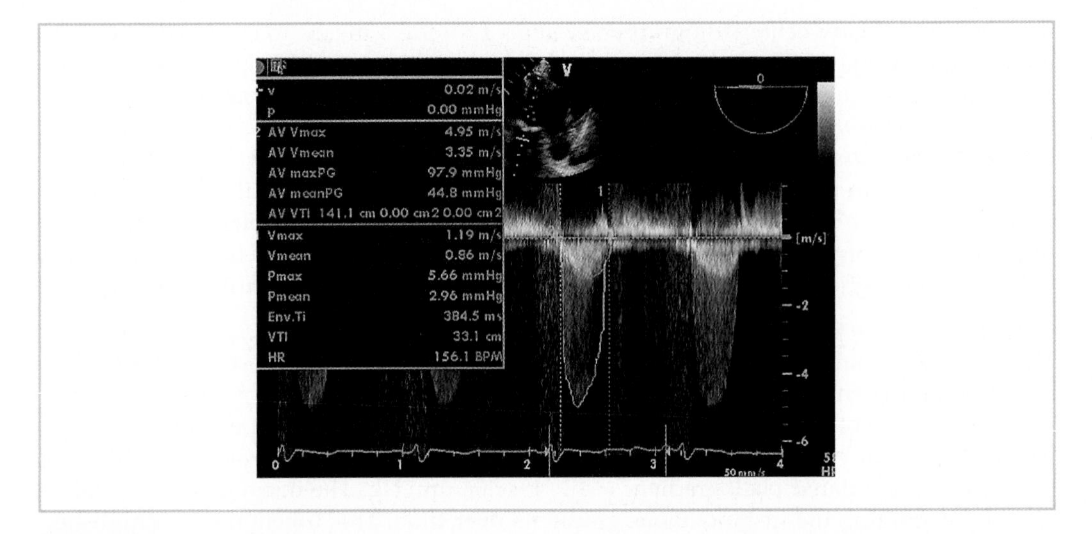

Figure 12.2. Deep transgastric view with parallel continuous wave Doppler beam alignment in a patient with severe aortic stenosis. Aortic stenosis tracing is labeled *2* (*outer envelope*), with a maximal aortic valve velocity of 4.95 m/s and a Bernoulli equation–derived peak aortic valve gradient of 97.9 mm Hg. Aortic valve time-velocity integral (TVI) is 141.1 cm. Tracing *1* is of the left ventricular outflow tract (LVOT) velocity. LVOT maximal velocity is 1.19 m/s, and LVOT TVI is 33.1 cm.

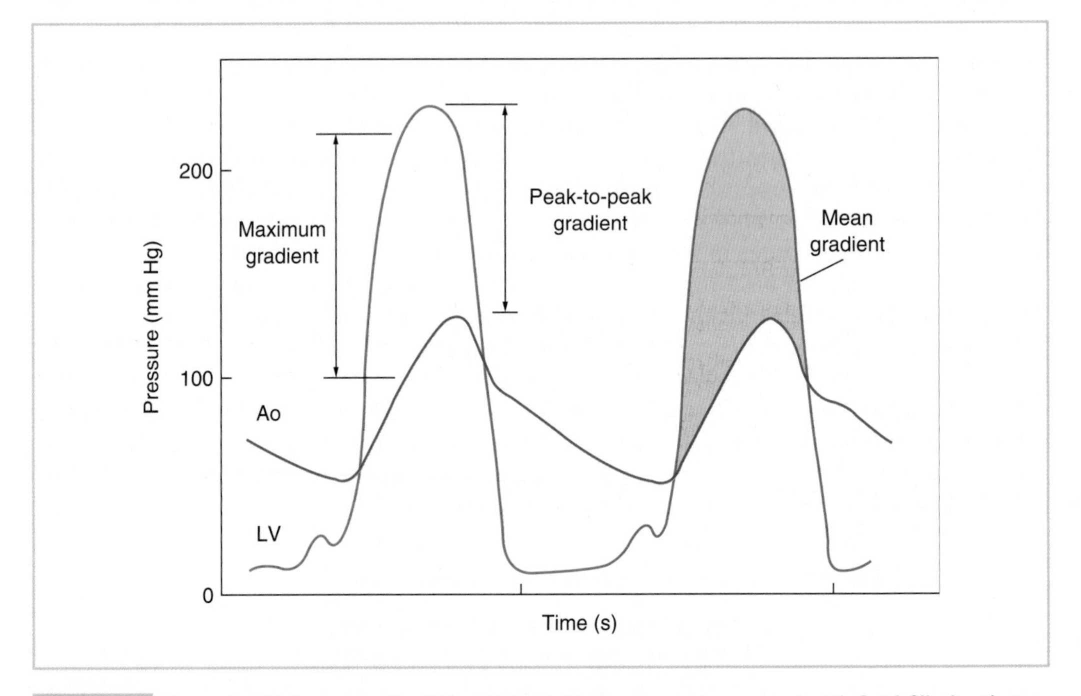

Figure 12.3. Example of left ventricular (LV) and aortic (Ao) pressures measured with fluid-filled catheters in a patient with severe aortic stenosis. The maximal instantaneous gradient is greater than the peak-to-peak gradient. The *shaded area* indicates the mean gradient. (From Otto CM. *Textbook of clinical echocardiography,* 2nd ed. Philadelphia: WB Saunders, 2000:238, with permission.)

Table 12.3 Calculation of aortic valve area with the continuity equation

Continuity Equation ("What goes in must come out.")

LVOT stroke volume = AV stroke volume

Stroke volume = CSA × TVI

Therefore,

$$TVI_{LVOT} \times Area_{LVOT} = TVI_{AV} \times Area_{AV}$$

$$Area_{AV} = \frac{TVI_{LVOT} \times Area_{LVOT}}{TVI_{AV}}$$

Aortic valve area

LVOT velocity (m/s, maximal)

LVOT diameter (cm, inner to inner, mid systole)

LVOT area (cm^2) = πr^2

AV area (cm^2, continuity equation)

LVOT, left ventricular outflow tract; AV, aortic valve; CSA, cross-sectional area; TVI, time-velocity integral.

Hemodynamically significant AS is generally associated with a ***mean*** *gradient of 40 mm Hg or more or a maximal velocity of 4.0 m/s or more* (Table 12.1). The exception is in patients with a low ejection fraction, who may not be able to generate a high gradient. In these patients, peak gradients as low as 20 to 30 mm Hg may be associated with critical stenosis, and the continuity equation *and* planimetry as well as a dobutamine challenge should be used to exclude significant AS (see later discussion).

Doppler Estimation of the Aortic Valve Area: The Continuity Equation

The continuity equation states that the volume of blood that enters the stenotic aortic orifice is equal to the volume of blood that exits it. If we can calculate the volume of flow entering a stenotic aortic valve through the LVOT and measure the velocity at which it exits the stenotic valve, then the equation can be rearranged to solve for the area of the stenotic valve (19) (Table 12.3).

One must first calculate the cross-sectional area of the LVOT. In the ME aortic valve long-axis view (120 degrees), the LVOT annular diameter is obtained by measuring the *inner* dimension (endocardium to endocardium) of the LVOT at the insertion point of the aortic valve leaflets in midsystole with the electronic calipers (Figure 12.4B). The diameter of the LVOT is generally approximately 2.0 ± 0.2 cm and varies somewhat with body surface area. Inaccuracies in measurement of the outflow tract can account for much of the error in this technique because the radius is squared in the continuity equation. The most common discrepancies occur during the imaging of elderly women, who often have a smaller outflow tract (and body surface area) than average, and large men, who often have a larger outflow tract (and body surface area). If we assume that the LVOT is a circle, one calculates its area as πr^2 (or $\pi [D/2]^2$).

The LVOT time-velocity integral (TVI) is then determined by either of two methods. Pulsed wave Doppler can be used, with the sample volume just proximal to the aortic valve cusps within the LVOT (Figure 12.5). The sample volume is gradually moved toward the aortic valve until a smooth LVOT velocity profile is obtained *at the level of the outflow tract where the annular dimension was obtained*. The internal calculation package available on all echocardiographic machines traces the LVOT velocity, allowing calculation of the LVOT TVI. Pulsed wave Doppler is essential for this flow measurement because it must be made at

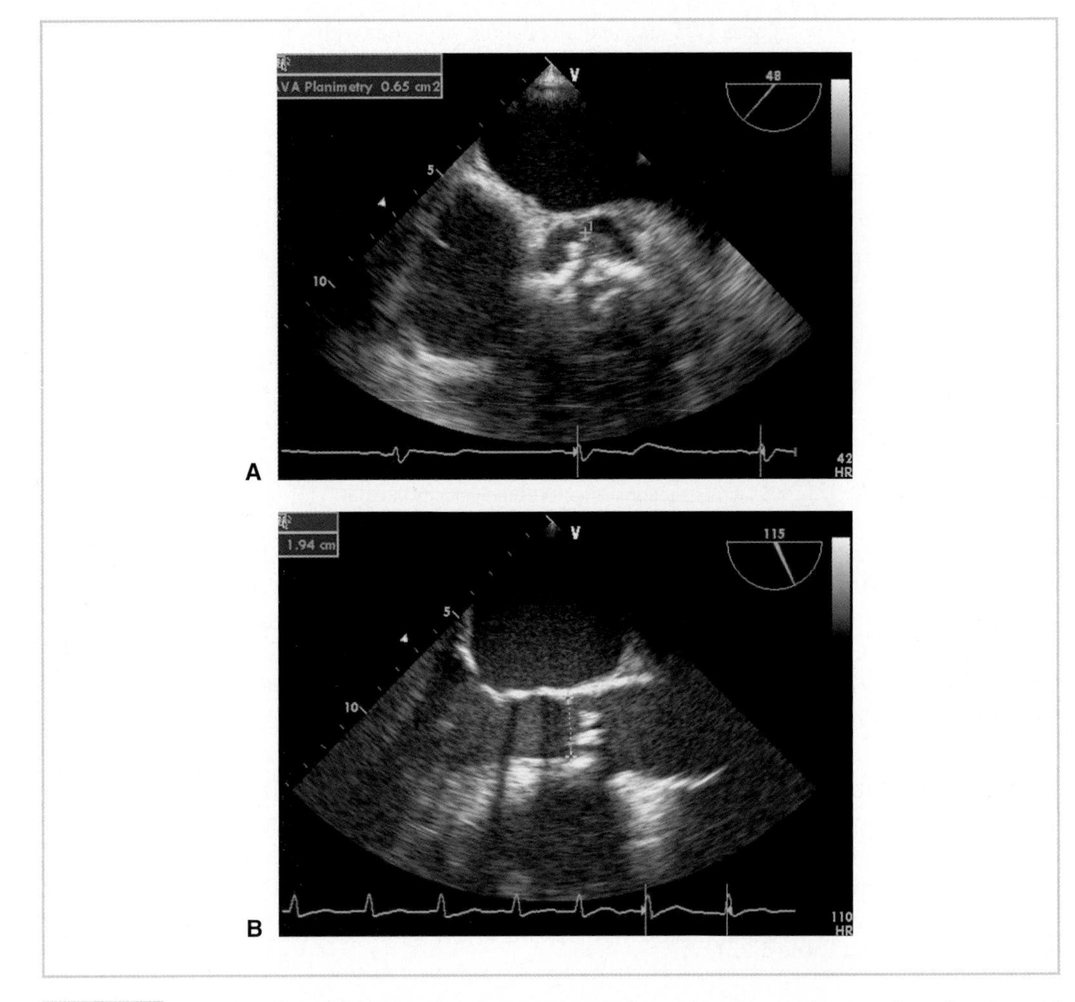

Figure 12.4. **A:** Midesophageal aortic valve short-axis view demonstrating aortic stenosis and a tricuspid aortic valve with heavy calcification. Aortic valve area by planimetry is 0.65 cm^2. **B:** Midesophageal aortic valve long-axis view in midsystole with measurement of the left ventricular outflow tract (LVOT) diameter (1.94 cm). The diameter is measured from the inner surfaces (endocardium to endocardium) of the LVOT at the insertion points of the aortic cusps. The continuity equation–derived aortic valve area is 0.70 cm^2. Continuous wave Doppler values are from Figure 12.2.

the level at which the outflow tract was measured to calculate the stroke volume through that area. An alternative method, which is less well validated, uses continuous wave Doppler interrogation through the aortic valve. If the alignment is correct, a more intense lower-velocity inner envelope representing the lower-velocity LVOT flow is imaged within the higher-velocity aortic jet envelope and can be traced as previously described to calculate the LVOT TVI (20) (Figure 12.2). However, this envelope peak can be erroneously high because the subaortic jet accelerates into the stenotic orifice to form a proximal isovelocity surface area as it narrows to fit into the orifice (Chapter 11). This can raise the apparent peak velocity to a level higher than it would be at the annular level and result in an overestimation of the valve area. The "envelope in envelope" configuration defines proper alignment with the jet and facilitates pulse wave confirmation of the velocity at the annular level.

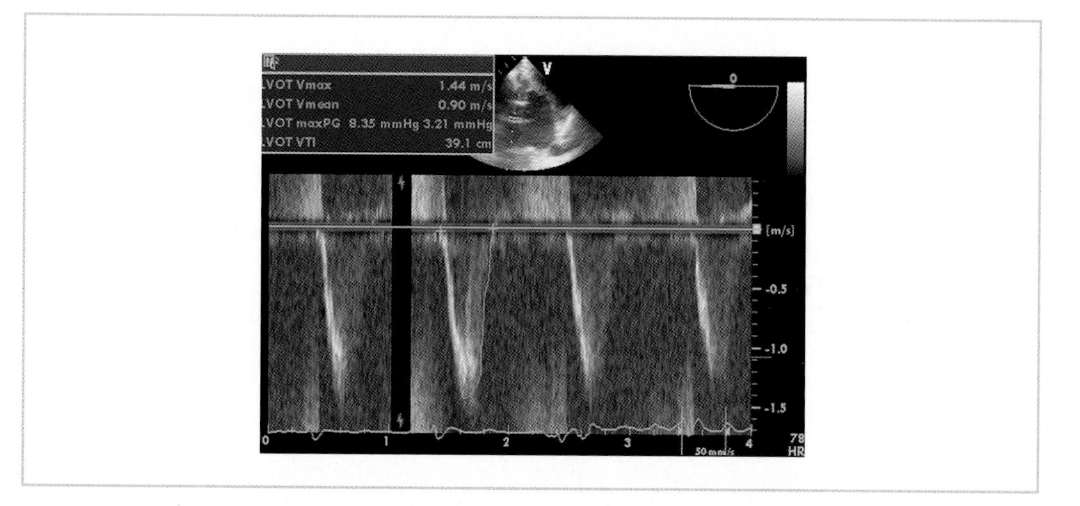

Figure 12.5. Deep transgastric view of the aortic valve with pulsed wave Doppler assessment of the left ventricular outflow tract (LVOT) flow velocity. The LVOT time-velocity integral is assessed to be 39.1 cm. Note correlation with inner envelope technique valve area of 33.1 cm (same patient as in Figure 12.2.)

Finally, the aortic valve TVI is traced from the larger envelope of the continuous wave Doppler profile (Figure 12.2). These measurements require that the Doppler probe be as close to parallel as possible to the direction of flow (usually from the deep TG long-axis view). The resulting values for the LVOT diameter, LVOT TVI, and aortic valve TVI are entered into the continuity equation to solve for the aortic valve area. Some clinicians use the peak velocity instead of the TVI in these analyses, although the TVI should correlate better from a theoretic standpoint.

Technical Considerations

AS is a technically challenging valvular lesion to assess by Doppler TTE, and the limitations imposed by the angle of incidence of the Doppler beam in TEE are even more of a challenge. Often, the orientation of the jet is such that the transducer cannot be aligned parallel to it. Acceptance of an inadequate jet as representative of the true jet is a significant source of error in estimating the severity of stenosis. Unless a clearly defined velocity envelope can be seen, no quantitative estimate of severity should be made.

The jet of mitral insufficiency can easily be mistaken for that of AS. Both jets have several features in common: they are negative, high-velocity jets when interrogated from the mid to low esophagus, tend to peak in midsystole, and may lie in the same path of interrogation because the Doppler beam often traverses both the anterior left atrium (LA) and the adjacent posterior aortic root. In the latter situation, anteriorly oriented mitral regurgitant (MR) jets and stenotic aortic jets can be interrogated. It is important to document visually that an MR jet is not traversed when color Doppler imaging is used. In cases in which this is difficult, it is useful to look at the time of onset of an MR jet during pulsed Doppler recording to determine the relationship of the onset of flow velocity to the electrocardiographic QRS complex for reference. MR jets start early (during isovolumic systole) because the LV pressure exceeds the LA pressure (normal, 0–12 mm Hg) almost as soon as LV contraction begins. AS jets start later in systole because flow begins when the LV pressure exceeds the central aortic diastolic pressure (60–90 mm Hg). This is generally in the mid or latter portion of the QRS complex. This determination is facilitated by recording the jets at a faster sweep speed (100 mm/s). It may be helpful to look at the aortic valve morphology to assess whether significant obstruction is suggested by the mobility of the valve on 2-D imaging. It should be borne in mind, however, that in a low-output state, aortic valve motion may be decreased by reduced CO rather than by significant stenosis.

SPECIAL CONSIDERATIONS

Assessment in the Presence of a Low Cardiac Output: The "Dimensionless" Index and Dobutamine Testing

As previously noted, *the gradient across a stenosis varies with the flow across the stenosis* (21,22). The gradient will increase during exercise or in a hyperadrenergic state (e.g., in the operating room) because it is directly proportional to the CO, but the valve area remains constant. This relationship is reflected in the Gorlin formula used to calculate valve areas, in which the CO is in the numerator and the gradient is in the denominator. In patients with a normal CO, significant and possibly critical stenosis usually results in a peak pressure gradient of greater than 50 mm Hg and often significantly higher. However, in patients with a low CO, a peak gradient in potentially critical stenosis may be in the range of 20 to 30 mm Hg. Gradients this low with a normal CO are generally minor and not hemodynamically important. Therefore, the CO is an important determinant of the significance of a given valve gradient. Accordingly, an echocardiographic assessment of LV function should routinely be performed before "small" gradients are reported as insignificant. Finding a significantly reduced ejection fraction should raise concerns about this issue.

DOBUTAMINE STRESS TESTING

The fact that patients with poor LV function may be unable to mount a significant gradient, has led to the use of dobutamine stress testing or stimulation to determine whether a low gradient is caused by intrinsic myocardial disease or valvular disease. A low dose of dobutamine (usually 5 to 10 μ/kg/min) is infused intravenously to increase the CO while the relevant Doppler parameters are monitored. An increase in CO and in gradient with a *constant valve area* suggests severe valvular disease. An *increase in valve area* with increase in CO suggests primary myocardial disease as an issue and would contraindicate valve replacement as sole definitive therapy (3). In general, but not invariably, the surgical outcome of these patients may be poorer than that of patients with high gradients and normal baseline function (23). However, AS is unique in being one of the few cardiovascular conditions where patients with a low ejection fraction preoperatively may normalize after valve replacement.

DIMENSIONLESS INDEX

In patients with a decreased LV ejection fraction, in addition to calculation of estimated aortic valve area, the echocardiographer can use the LVOT TVI/aortic valve TVI ratio or LVOT peak velocity/aortic valve peak velocity ratio to assess the degree of AS. This approach is a modification of the continuity equation (Table 12.3) but eliminates the aortic root area ($Area_{LVOT}$), which is a common source of measurement error (since the square of diameter is used in the formula), to provide a *dimensionless index*. The aortic root area is essentially a constant and therefore can be eliminated from the equation to provide this alternative index of severity. A ratio of 0.25 or less denotes critical disease. This approach is also helpful in determining whether an erroneous measurement of the aortic annular dimension may have resulted in an estimated aortic valve area that seems disproportionately high or low to the measured gradient across the valve. It is also a useful index for following patients with prosthetic aortic valves where measurement of an aortic annular dimension is often not clear.

Assessment of Aortic Stenosis Gradient in Aortic Regurgitation

As a result of the leak in aortic insufficiency the volume of blood that must be ejected from the ventricle during systole increases. The reason is that the forward stroke volume now equals the volume of blood returning from the lungs plus the volume leaking back from the aorta. The latter can exceed 50% of the forward stroke volume. This increased volume must be ejected through the LVOT, which has only a limited ability to dilate to accommodate it. Therefore, velocity in the LVOT increases because the area is relatively stenotic for the volume of blood traversing it. The increased velocity in the outflow tract is further exaggerated in the aorta by the acceleration resulting from the narrowing caused by the valvular stenosis. The modified Bernoulli equation must be used to calculate the true valve gradient accurately when the LVOT flow velocity is 1.5 m/s or more, whether from aortic regurgitation or from another hyperdynamic state (Table 12.3). The outflow tract velocity should be sampled using pulsed wave Doppler at the level at which the outflow tract diameter was measured.

Pre and Postoperative Subaortic Obstruction

The anterior MV leaflet and the intraventricular septum are relatively close to each other. In a small percentage of patients in whom the septum is hypertrophic as an adaptive response to AS, the septum bulges into the outflow tract and may appear to underlie most of the right coronary cusp in the ME 120-degree TEE long-axis view (mirrored in the parasternal long-axis TTE view preoperatively). The so-called sigmoid septum, seen in some older patients with or without hypertrophy, has a similar appearance (24). This situation is frequently encountered in elderly hypertensive women who have marked left ventricular hypertrophy and, frequently, small left ventricular cavities with significant mitral annular calcification. Occasionally systolic anterior motion (SAM) of the MV with true subaortic stenosis physiology is present. Replacement of the aortic valve, with the resultant decrease in afterload on the ventricle, may then cause subaortic stenosis (SAM) when it was not present or worsen it if it was present.

Valvular AS can also coexist with true idiopathic hypertrophic subaortic stenosis and SAM of the MV (25). In that situation the accelerated velocity to the subaortic stenosis can extend into the LVOT and make it impossible to calculate the transvalvular gradient. In this situation, the best approach to estimating the severity of the valvular stenosis is by planimetry of the short-axis view of the aortic orifice (see earlier text). Here too, valve replacement may bring the anterior mitral leaflet closer to the septum, and SAM may develop or worsen, causing a secondary subaortic stenosis physiologically identical to that of idiopathic hypertrophic subaortic stenosis. The classic finding is the so-called dagger-shaped (or late peaking) jet seen in dynamic subaortic obstruction, caused by an increase in the gradient late in systole as the MV moves closer to the septum when the ventricle becomes smaller (Figure 12.6). A similar phenomenon can occur with redundant, elongated mitral leaflets after a ''floppy'' MV is repaired (26,27). Occasionally, postoperative intracavitary gradients or midcavity obliteration occurs with the decrease in afterload after valve replacement in ventricles that are markedly hypertrophic in response to the stenotic valve.

The result of all of these phenomena is that weaning from bypass may be impossible unless the subvalvular obstruction is recognized as a cause of postoperative hypotension. In this situation, interrogation of the LVOT in the long-axis view demonstrates SAM of the MV. Color flow Doppler shows the mosaic appearance of high-velocity aliasing flow

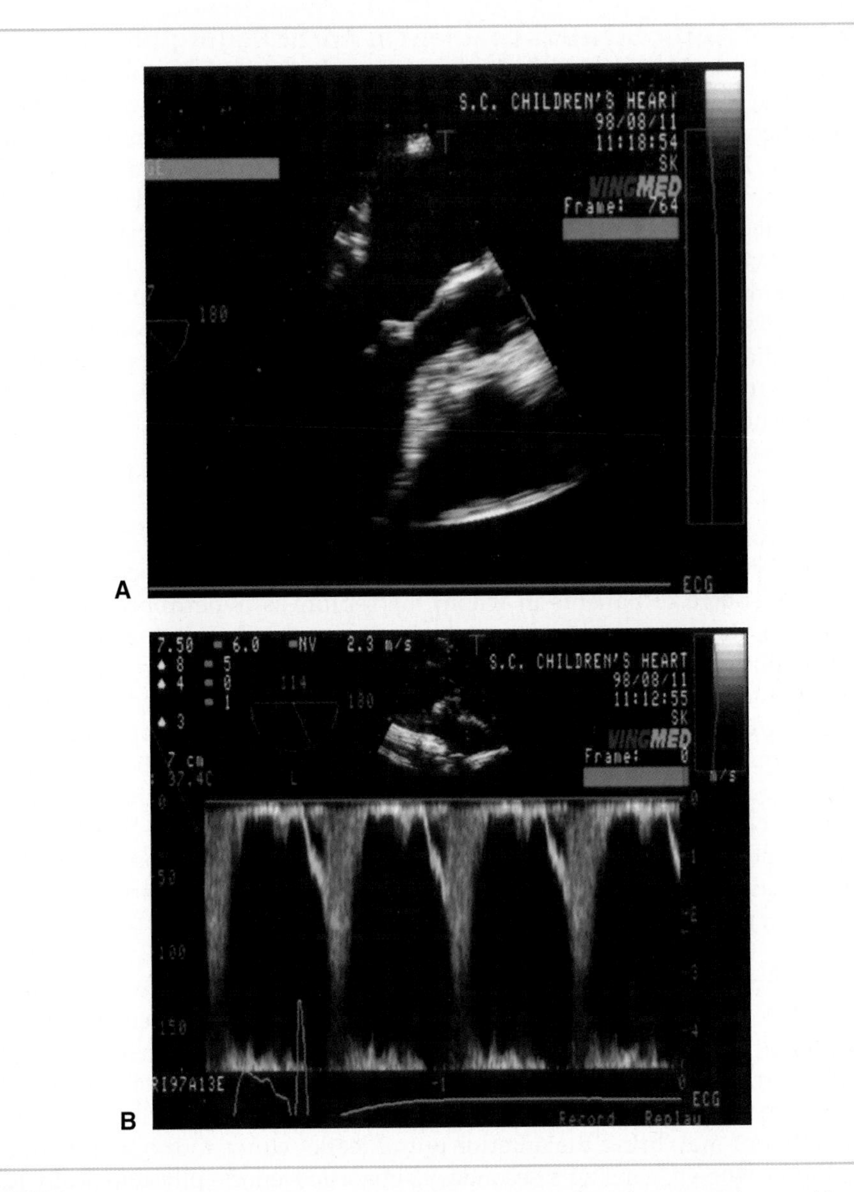

Figure 12.6. **A:** Midesophageal long-axis view demonstrating profound asymmetric septal hypertrophy involving the left ventricular outflow tract (LVOT). Note the acute narrowing of the LVOT at the proximal border of the area of septal hypertrophy. **B:** High pulse repetition frequency Doppler demonstrating the classic "dagger" flow velocity pattern of dynamic outflow obstruction.

caused by the resultant gradient across the LVOT (or within the cavity at an area of intracavitary narrowing). Interrogation by continuous wave Doppler demonstrates a high velocity proportional to the gradient caused by the obstruction that can be quantified with the modified Bernoulli equation. *The treatment for the resultant hypotension is counterintuitive; the patient requires volume loading to increase the LV volume and the negative inotropic effect of β-blocker therapy to decrease contractility and prolong the diastolic filling period by slowing the heart.* On rare occasions, the obstruction may be intractable, and septal myomectomy (28) or MV replacement with a low-profile prosthetic valve is required.

SUMMARY

Assessment of the stenotic aortic valve remains a challenge. Echocardiography provided valuable insights into the rate of progression by permitting serial noninvasive measurements for the first time. As is generally the case in echocardiography, the application of a variety of techniques allows a more reliable estimate of the severity of disease, particularly if the results support each other. In clinical practice, however, the integration of patient data is essential, and a good correlation of the clinical and echocardiographic findings remains essential. Accordingly, echocardiographers must be thoroughly familiar with the application of all these techniques for an optimal assessment of AS in the operating room.

REFERENCES

1 Roger VL, Tajik AJ. Progression of aortic stenosis in adults: new insights provided by Doppler echocardiography. *J Heart Valve Dis* 1993;2:114–118.
2 Rosenhek R, Binder T, Porenta G, et al. Predictors of outcome in severe, asymptomatic aortic stenosis. *N Engl J Med* 2000;343:611–617.
3 Bonow RO, Carabello BA, Kanu C, et al. ACC/AHA 2006 guidelines for the management of patients with valvular heart disease: a report of the American College of Cardiology/American Heart Association Task Force on Practice Guidelines. *Circulation* 2006;114:e84–231.
4 Godley RW, Green D, Dillion JC, et al. Reliability of two-dimensional echocardiography in assessing the severity of valvular aortic stenosis. *Chest* 1981;79:657–662.
5 Chin ML, Bernstein RF, Child JS, et al. Aortic valve systolic flutter as a screening test for severe aortic stenosis. *Am J Cardiol* 1983;51:981–985.
6 Okura H, Yoshida K, Hozumi T, et al. Planimetry and transthoracic two-dimensional echocardiography in noninvasive assessment of aortic valve area in patients with valvular aortic stenosis. *J Am Coll Cardiol* 1997;30:753–759.
7 Stoddard MF, Arce J, Liddell NE, et al. Two-dimensional transesophageal echocardiographic determination of aortic valve area in adults with aortic stenosis. *Am Heart J* 1991;122:1415–1422.
8 Hoffmann R, Flachskampf FA, Hanrath P. Planimetry of orifice area in aortic stenosis using multiplane transesophageal echocardiography. *J Am Coll Cardiol* 1993;22:529–534.
9 Kim KS, Maxted W, Nanda NC, et al. Comparison of multiplane and biplane transesophageal echocardiography in the assessment of aortic stenosis. *Am J Cardiol* 1997;79:436–441.
10 Tardif JC, Miller DS, Pandian NG, et al. Effects of variations in flow on aortic valve area in aortic stenosis based on *in vivo* planimetry of aortic valve area by multiplane transesophageal echocardiography. *Am J Cardiol* 1995;76:193–198.
11 De la Fuente Galan L, San Roman Calvar JA, Munoz San Jose JC, et al. Influence of the degree of aortic valve calcification on the estimate of valvular area using planimetry with transesophageal echocardiography [in Spanish]. *Rev Esp Cardiol* 1996;49:663–668.
12 Bernard Y, Meneveau N, Vuillemenot A, et al. Planimetry of aortic valve area using multiplane transoesophageal echocardiography is not a reliable method for assessing severity of aortic stenosis. *Heart* 1997;78:68.
13 Hatle L, Angelsen BA, Tromsdal A. Non-invasive assessment of aortic stenosis by Doppler ultrasound. *Br Heart J* 1980;43:284–292.
14 Owen AN, Simon P, Moidl R, et al. Measurement of aortic flow velocity during transesophageal echocardiography in the transgastric five-chamber view. *J Am Soc Echocardiogr* 1995;8:874–878.
15 Skjaerpe T, Hegrenaes L, Hatle L. Noninvasive estimation of valve area in patients with aortic stenosis by Doppler ultrasound and two-dimensional echocardiography. *Circulation* 1985;72:810–818.
16 Harris SN, Luther MA, Perrino AC. Multiplane transesophageal echocardiography acquisition of ascending aortic flow velocities: a comparison with established techniques. *J Am Soc Echocardiogr* 1999;12:754–760.
17 Cooper J, Pinheiro L, Fan P, et al. A practical approach to cardiovascular Doppler ultrasound. In: Nanda V, ed. *Doppler echocardiography*. Baltimore: Williams & Wilkins, 1993:59–68.
18 Laskey WK, Kussmaul WG. Pressure recovery in aortic valve stenosis. *Circulation* 1994;89:116–121.
19 Richards KL. Assessment of aortic and pulmonic stenosis by echocardiography. *Circulation* 1991;84:I182–I187.
20 Maslow AD, Mashikian J, Haering JM, et al. TEE evaluation of native aortic valve area: utility of the double envelope technique. *J Cardiothorac Vasc Anesth* 2001;15:293–299.

21 Burwash IG, Dickinson A, Teskey RJ, et al. Aortic valve area discrepancy by Gorlin equation and Doppler echocardiography continuity equation: relationship to flow in patients with valvular aortic stenosis. *Can J Cardiol* 2000;16:985–992.
22 Burwash IG, Pearlman AS, Kraft CD, et al. Flow dependence of measures of aortic stenosis severity during exercise. *J Am Coll Cardiol* 1994;24:1342–1350.
23 Brogan WC III, Grayburn PA, Lange RA, et al. Prognosis after valve replacement in patients with severe aortic stenosis and a low transvalvular pressure gradient. *J Am Coll Cardiol* 1993;21:1657–1660.
24 Maron BJ, Gottdiener JS, Roberts WC, et al. Nongenetically transmitted disproportionate ventricular septal thickening associated with left ventricular outflow obstruction. *Br Heart J* 1979;41:345–349.
25 Chung KJ, Manning JA, Gramiak R. Echocardiography in coexisting hypertrophic subaortic stenosis and fixed left ventricular outflow obstruction. *Circulation* 1974;49:673–677.
26 Kronzon I, Cohen ML, Winer HE, et al. Left ventricular outflow obstruction: a complication of mitral valvuloplasty. *J Am Coll Cardiol* 1984;4:825–828.
27 Mihaileanu S, Marino JP, Chauvaud S, et al. Left ventricular outflow obstruction after mitral valve repair (Carpentier's technique). Proposed mechanisms of disease. *Circulation* 1988;78:I78–I84.
28 Turina M. Asymmetric septal hypertrophy should be resected during aortic valve replacement. *Z Kardiol* 1986;75:198–200.

QUESTIONS

1. Use of the Gorlin equation in the catheterization suite has all of the following limitations except

a. In patients with aortic insufficiency, the aortic valve area may be falsely elevated.
b. The cardiac output (CO) of multiple beats must be averaged for patients in atrial fibrillation.
c. The peak-to-peak gradient is required.
d. The systolic ejection period must be calculated.

2. The following statements regarding the usefulness of planimetry in the evaluation of AS are true except

a. The midesophageal (ME) aortic valve short-axis view is preferred.
b. The results of planimetry correlate extremely well with catheterization-derived determinations of the aortic valve area.
c. An adequate planimetry-derived determination of the aortic valve area depends on an adequate CO.
d. Significant valvular calcification decreases the accuracy of planimetry-derived determinations of area.

3. All of the following statements regarding continuous wave Doppler evaluation of the aortic valve are true except

a. The preferred view is the deep transgastric (TG) long-axis view because of the parallel alignment of the Doppler beam with flow.
b. The deep TG long-axis view offers a correlation of more than 0.9 with transthoracic echocardiography (TTE)-derived aortic valve flow velocities.
c. If a mitral prosthetic valve is present, the TG long-axis view at 120 degrees can be used to obtain aortic valve flow velocities.
d. Accurate flow velocities can be obtained with the ME views by electronically steering (angle correction) the resulting signal.

4. A patient is determined to have the following Doppler parameters: left ventricular outflow tract (LVOT) velocity, 1.7 m/s; aortic valve velocity, 4.6 m/s. The pressure gradient across the aortic valve is

a. 84.64 mm Hg
b. 73.00 mm Hg
c. 33.64 mm Hg
d. 11.56 mm Hg

5. In regard to pressure gradients in the left ventricle (LV) and aortic valve, the following is/are true:

a. The Doppler-derived maximal instantaneous gradient approximates the catheterization-derived maximal instantaneous gradient.
b. The peak-to-peak gradient is usually the highest gradient recorded.
c. The Doppler-derived maximal instantaneous gradient is comparable with the peak-to-peak catheterization gradient.
d. All of the above.

6. A patient has an LV ejection fraction of 10%. Which measurements are preferred in determining the severity of the AS?

a. Peak aortic valve flow velocity
b. Aortic valve mean gradient
c. Planimetric aortic valve area

d. LVOT time-velocity integral (TVI)/aortic valve TVI ratio
e. **a** and **b**
f. **c** and **d**
g. All of the above

7. When the continuity equation is used, which of the following statements regarding measurement of the LVOT diameter is true?
a. The diameter is measured 1 cm proximal to the aortic valve.
b. The diameter is measured at the insertion point of the aortic valve leaflets.
c. The diameter is measured at the leaflet tips.
d. The chance of introducing error into this measurement is small.

8. A patient is found to have aortic sclerosis. What maneuvers will increase the gradient across the aortic valve?
a. Exercise
b. Aortic insufficiency
c. Acute myocardial ischemia
d. **a** and **b**
e. All of the above

9. All of the following statements regarding systolic anterior motion (SAM) of the mitral valve (MV) are true except
a. It commonly occurs following a noncircumferential ring annuloplasty.
b. It occurs in patients with redundant anterior MV leaflets.
c. The pathophysiology is similar to that of idiopathic hypertrophic subaortic stenosis.
d. It can develop after aortic valve replacement because of changes in LV geometry.

10. Treatment for SAM can include which of the following
a. MV replacement
b. Volume expansion
c. Reduction in inotropes
d. All of the above

Answers appear at the back of the book.

13 Prosthetic Valves

Albert T. Cheung

The first successful artificial heart valves were implanted in 1960. Starr implanted a Starr-Edwards caged-ball valve in a patient with rheumatic mitral stenosis and Harken implanted the Harken caged-ball prosthesis in the subcoronary aortic position in a patient with rheumatic aortic stenosis and regurgitation. Over the next 45 years prosthetic valves of various designs made by different manufacturers became available for clinical use. These developments have led to a large number of patients with many different kinds of prosthetic valves. This effort is ongoing and new types of valve prosthesis are continually being developed and are in various stages of clinical testing.

ROLE OF TRANSESOPHAGEAL ECHOCARDIOGRAPHY IN THE EVALUATION OF PROSTHETIC CARDIAC VALVES

Multiplane transesophageal echocardiography (TEE) is considered the diagnostic technique of choice for the identifying the type of prosthesis, assessing its function, and diagnosing prosthetic dysfunction (1–5). The ability of TEE to combine two-dimensional (2-D) with color flow Doppler and spectral Doppler imaging enables TEE to generate diagnostic information based on both the structure and hemodynamic function of the prosthetic valve. However, the evaluation of prosthetic heart valves using ultrasound imaging poses special problems because mechanical valves and components of bioprosthetic valves have poor acoustic properties making it difficult to image the valve and the surrounding soft tissues in detail. In addition, the small size of the valves and their mechanical components make detailed examination of the motion of the stent and occluder mechanisms challenging.

Despite incremental improvements in instrumentation, the imaging resolution that can be achieved using transthoracic echocardiography does not match that achieved by TEE. The improved imaging resolution provided by TEE with the ultrasound transducer close to the cardiac valve structures permits a detailed assessment of both prosthetic valve function and determining the etiology of prosthetic valve dysfunction. High-resolution 2-D imaging can distinguish between normal and abnormal motion of the valve leaflets and occluder mechanisms. Abnormal motion of the valve stent or dehiscence of the prosthetic valve annulus can be also detected. In addition, vegetations, calcifications, pannus, and thrombus formation on the prosthetic valve can be detected using 2-D imaging.

Color Doppler flow imaging can distinguish normal closure and leakage regurgitant jets from pathologic transvalvular or paravalvular regurgitant jets. Quantification of blood flow velocity using spectral Doppler techniques often permits the estimation of transvalvular pressure gradients and the effective orifice area (EOA) of the prosthetic valves (6–9).

Clinical indications for TEE include the evaluation of the native valve before valve replacement, evaluation of prosthetic valve function immediately after implantation, the diagnosis of prosthetic valve dysfunction, and assessment of patient-prosthetic mismatching (Table 13.1).

Table 13.1 Prosthetic heart valves and clinical indications for transesophageal echocardiography

TEE evaluation before valve replacement 1. Verify disease of native valve 2. Assess the extent of annular calcification 3. Estimate the annular diameter of the native valve; in aortic valve disease, a small annulus may dictate the type of valve to be implanted 4. Evaluate the feasibility of valve repair; considering the limitations of prosthetic valves, it is almost always preferable to repair a valve rather than replace it
TEE evaluation immediately after valve replacement 1. Verify that all leaflets or occluders move normally 2. Verify the absence of paravalvular regurgitation 3. Verify that no air remains in the cardiac chambers 4. Verify that there is no left ventricular outflow tract obstruction by struts or subvalvular apparatus
TEE diagnosis of prosthetic valve dysfunction 1. Identify prosthetic valve type 2. Detect and quantify transvalvular or paravalvular regurgitation 3. Detect annular dehiscence 4. Detect vegetations associated with endocarditis 5. Detect thrombosis or pannus formation on the valve 6. Detect and quantify valve stenosis 7. Detect structural valvular degeneration or calcification

TEE, transesophageal echocardiography.

TECHNICAL CONSIDERATIONS IN PERFORMING TRANSESOPHAGEAL ECHOCARDIOGRAPHY EXAMINATIONS OF PROSTHETIC VALVES

Many of the ultrasound imaging techniques used to evaluate native valve function can be applied to the evaluation of prosthetic heart valves, but certain special considerations are necessary. Ultrasound does not penetrate through the metallic and polymeric components of mechanical and biologic valves. These material components produce highly specular echoes and impair the imaging of distal structures because of shadowing. For these reasons, decreasing the transmit gain helps to decrease imaging artifacts and to resolve structural details in the vicinity of nonbiologic materials. To compensate for ultrasound shadowing, it is necessary to image the prosthetic valve from different transducer positions that generate imaging planes from both above and below the prosthetic valve. For example, the midesophageal aortic valve long-axis imaging plane will not reliably display the motion of the mechanical aortic prosthesis because of shadowing from the valve sewing ring (Figure 13.1). By advancing the TEE probe to the transgastric position, prosthetic aortic leaflet motion can be observed from the apical or mid-left ventricular transgastric long-axis view through the aortic valve without interference from the sewing ring (Figure 13.2). Similarly, imaging the ventricular side of mitral prosthetic valves using the transgastric midventricular or deep transgastric long-axis imaging planes provides detail that cannot be observed with the midesophageal views alone.

Doppler echocardiography can be used to estimate the transvalvular pressure gradient across bileaflet, tilting disc, and biologic valves that have a centrally directed, linear transvalvular flow. In contrast, for caged-ball or caged-disc valves where the occluder alters the direction of blood flow through the valve, the Bernoulli equation will not accurately estimate the transvalvular pressure gradient.

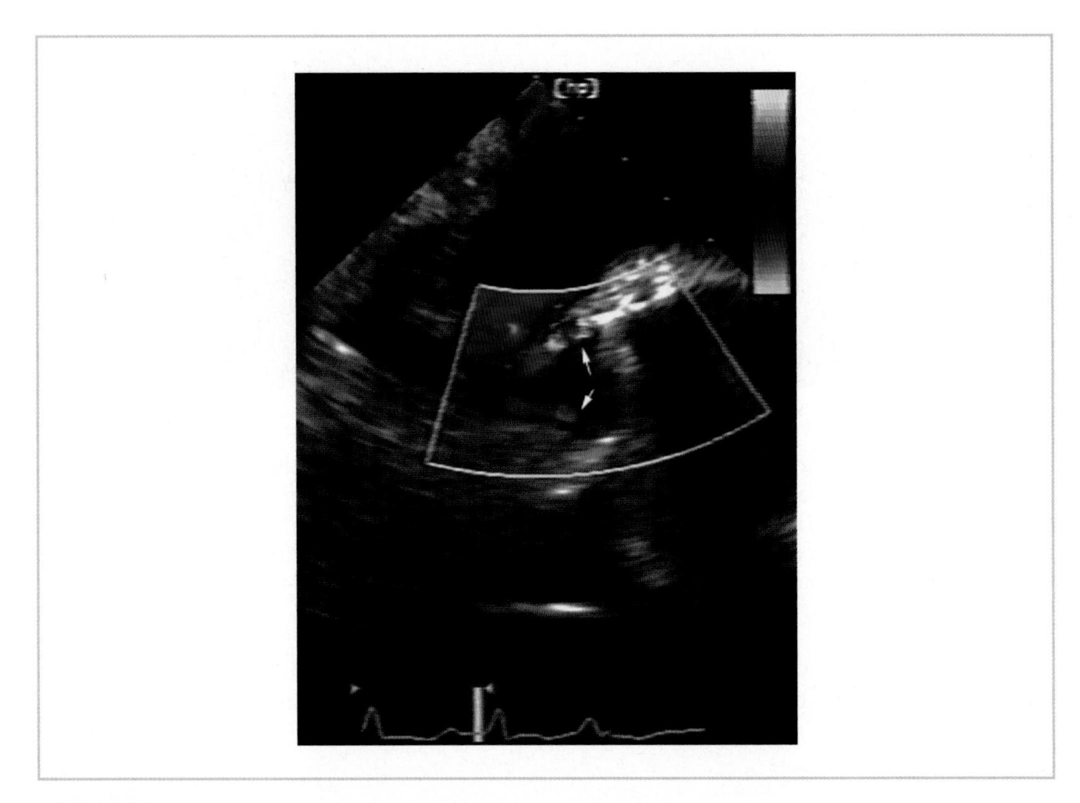

Figure 13.1. Bileaflet mechanical prosthesis in the aortic position. Transesophageal echocardiographic midesophageal aortic valve long-axis view at a multiplane angle of 135 degrees in a patient with a bileaflet mechanical prosthesis in the aortic position. Color Doppler flow imaging in diastole shows the normal appearance of the two leakage regurgitant jets that originate at the leaflet hinge points (*arrows*). Note that ultrasound shadowing caused by the annular stent makes it difficult to assess the motion of the leaflets from this imaging angle. The transgastric long-axis or the deep transgastric long-axis views through the aortic valve are necessary to evaluate the motion of the individual leaflets.

ECHOCARDIOGRAPHIC CHARACTERISTICS OF THE VARIOUS PROSTHETIC CARDIAC VALVE TYPES

Each type of prosthetic valve has distinct echocardiographic features and hemodynamic characteristics. The type, shape, and motion of the structural components of the valve allow it to be identified by the TEE examination. Knowing the published and manufacturers' specifications for the normal range of motion of the valve components, the average transvalvular pressure gradient, and average EOA is necessary to verify normal functioning of the prosthesis and to diagnose prosthetic dysfunction (7–9). In general, prosthetic valves are classified as mechanical or biological (Table 13.2).

Mechanical Heart Valves

Mechanical heart valves are more durable than biologic valves, but are thrombogenic and require systemic anticoagulation. For these reasons, mechanical valves are typically considered for younger patients who are more likely to experience structural failure after implantation of a biologic prosthetic as a consequence of their longer life expectancy. Mechanical prosthetics may also be preferred in patients who require anticoagulation

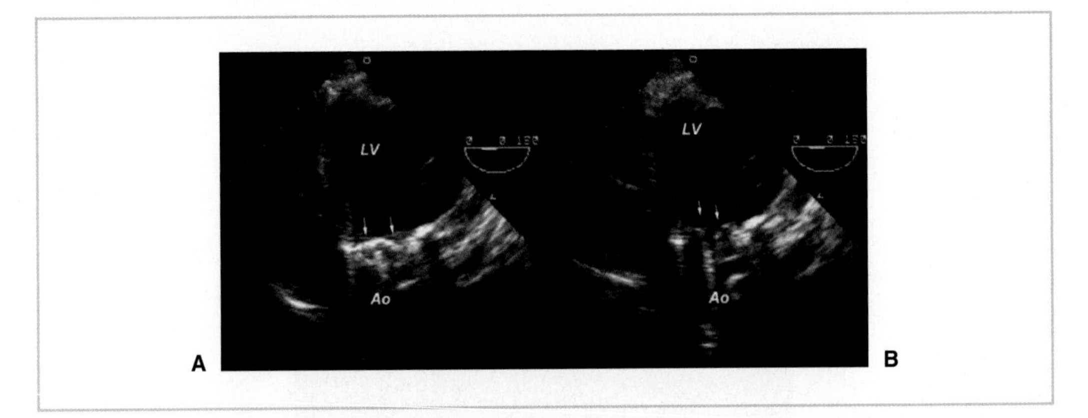

Figure 13.2. Bileaflet mechanical prosthesis in the aortic position. Transesophageal echocardiographic deep transgastric apical long-axis view at a multiplane angle of 0 degree permits imaging of prosthetic valve leaflets (arrows) and their motion. In diastole (panel **A**), both leaflets are in the fully closed position at an angle of 30 degrees in relation to the plane of the valve annulus. In systole (panel **B**), both leaflets are in the fully open position at an angle of 90 degrees in relation to the plane of the valve annulus. LV, left ventricle; Ao, aorta.

therapy for other reasons or in whom the risk of reoperation is unacceptable. The silastic, metal, and pyrolytic carbon components of mechanical valves are poor conductors of ultrasound and cause acoustic shadowing, reverberations, and strong specular signals.

BILEAFLET VALVES

The bileaflet mechanical valve prostheses are the most commonly implanted mechanical valves because of their outstanding record of durability and large valve orifice area in

Table 13.2 Prosthetic valve types

Valve	Description
Bioprosthetic	
Allograft	Indistinguishable from the native valve, used only in the aortic position (CryoLife aortic allograft)
Porcine bioprostheses	Porcine aortic valve on polypropylene mount with three support struts, (e.g. Hancock, Carpentier-Edwards, Medtronic Mosaic, St. Jude Bioimplant, Wessex)
Bovine pericardial	Trileaflet valve fashioned from bovine pericardium in dacron-covered support frame with three struts, (e.g. Bioflo pericardial, Carpentier-Edwards Pericardial, Carpentier-Edwards Perimount Magna, Labcor-Santiago pericardial, Mitroflow, Ionescu-Shiley, Sorin Pericarbon)
Stentless	Reinforced porcine aortic root, (Biocor stentless, CryoLife-O'Brien stentless, Edwards Prima stentless, Medtronic Freestyle, Toronto Stentless Porcine)
Mechanical	
Ball-in-cage	Circular sewing ring with two U-shaped arches containing a silastic ball, (e.g. Braunwald-Cutter, Harken, Starr-Edwards)
Caged-disc	Circular sewing ring with short cage containing a lightweight silastic centrally occluding disc, (e.g. Beall, Kay-Shiley, Kay Suzuki, Starr-Edwards Model 6520)
Tilting disc	Eccentrically hinged single tilting disc in circular ring opening to form two orifices, (e.g. Bjork-Shiley, Lillehei- Kaster, Medtronic Hall, Omnicarbon, Omniscience, Sorin Allcarbon monoleaflet, Wada-Cutter)
Bileaflet	Two semicircular hinged leaflets in a circular ring opening almost perpendicularly to form three orifices, (e.g. ATS, Carbomedics, Duromedics, Edwards MIRA, Jyros bileaflet, ON-X, St. Jude Medical, Sorin Allcarbon, Sorin Bicarbon)

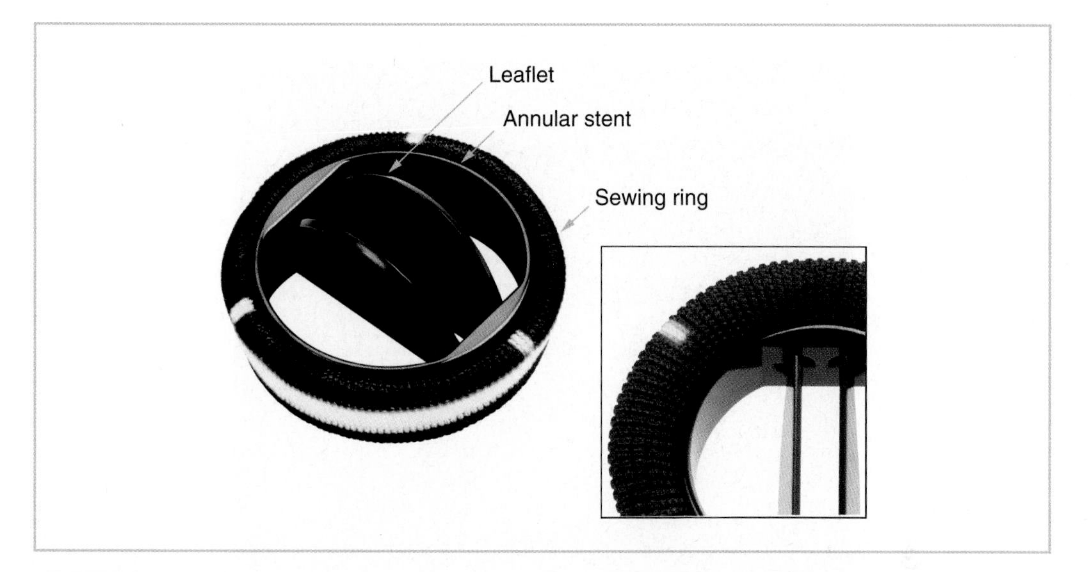

Figure 13.3. Photograph of a Carbomedics R-series mechanical bileaflet prosthetic aortic valve. The valve consists of two semicircular pyrolytic carbon leaflets supported within a pyrolytic carbon annular stent surrounded by the sewing ring. The inset shows a close-up of the hinge points of the leaflets. The valve is designed to permit a small amount of leakage backflow at the hinge points.

relation to sewing ring diameter. They can be implanted in the aortic, mitral, or tricuspid positions. The valves are constructed of two semicircular leaflets suspended from four hinge points in a circular annulus surrounded by a sewing ring (Figure 13.3). When the leaflets open, three separate orifices are formed within the valve annulus.

A systematic TEE examination of the prosthetic valve includes verification of normal leaflet motion, proper seating of the prosthesis within the native valve annulus, and normal blood flow pattern through the valve. In addition, the TEE examination should verify the absence of significant paravalvular regurgitation and abnormal transvalvular regurgitation. Finally, TEE can be used to estimate the transvalvular pressure gradient or calculate the EOA of the valve.

1. ***Confirm leaflet motion.*** 2-D imaging confirms the opening and closure of the two mechanical leaflets. In the short-axis imaging plane, the two leaflets in the open position produce two linear shadows within a circular annulus (Figure 13.4). For valves implanted in the mitral position, leaflet motion is best examined using the midesophageal long-axis views (Figure 13.5). Multiplane rotation through the valve to generate a cross-sectional imaging plane that is perpendicular to the two leaflets permits the motion of both leaflets to be observed simultaneously (Figure 13.5B). The two leaflets tilt open symmetrically to an angle of 85 to 90 degrees and close at an angle of 30 degrees in relation to the plane of the annulus. Leaflet motion of a valve implanted in the aortic position is more difficult to evaluate (Figure 13.1). Acoustic shadowing from the sewing ring and leaflets typically obscure leaflet motion in the midesophageal aortic valve long-axis view. Individual leaflet motion is better visualized in the transgastric long axis and deep transgastric long-axis views that provide unobstructed views of the aortic valve in the far field through the left ventricle and left ventricular outflow tract (LVOT) (Figure 13.2).

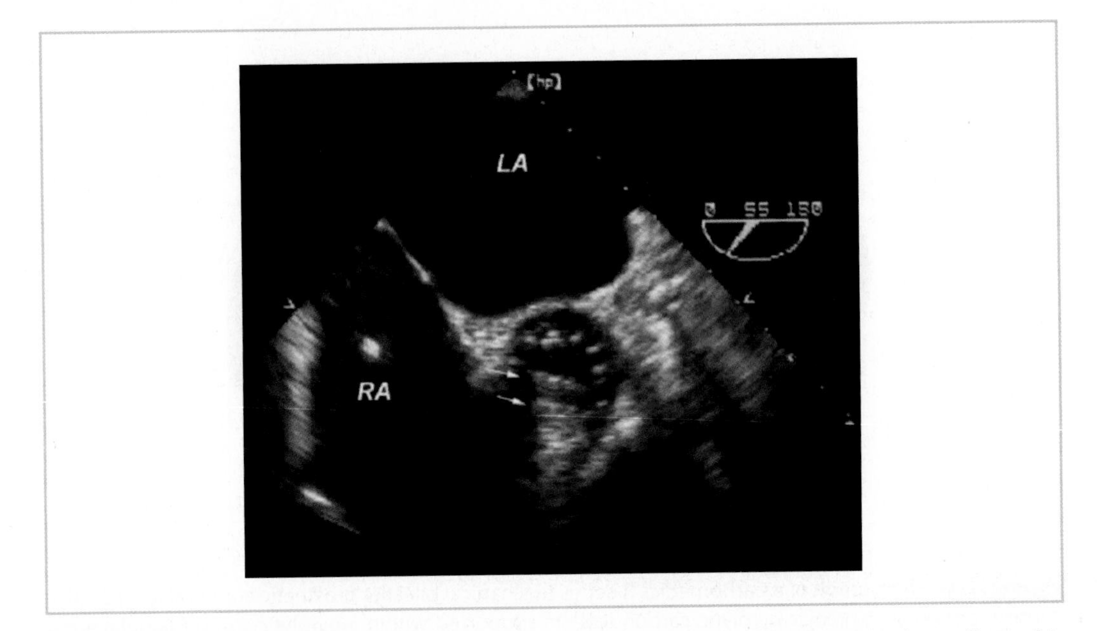

Figure 13.4. Bileaflet mechanical prosthesis in the aortic position. Transesophageal echocardiographic midesophageal short-axis image just above the plane of the valve annulus in systole provides permits cross-sectional imaging of the two parallel leaflets (*arrows*) of the mechanical valve in the open position. Note the acoustic shadowing caused by the mechanical leaflets in the far field making it difficult to resolve detail in the distal portion of the valve annulus. LA, left atrium; RA, right atrium.

2. ***Confirm proper valve seating.*** Incomplete fixation of the prosthetic sewing ring to the native annulus or dehiscence of the sewing ring will cause paravalvular regurgitation. Paravalvular regurgitation is defined as regurgitation originating outside of the prosthetic valve annulus or sewing ring. The most common cause for incomplete fixation immediately after prosthetic implantation is a severely calcified native valve annulus. Prosthetic endocarditis is the most common cause for late valve dehiscence and can produce a "rocking" motion of the entire valve apparatus on 2-D imaging. Proper seating of the prosthetic valve, paravalvular regurgitation, and dehiscence are best identified from the multiplane long-axis images of the valve.
3. ***Confirm normal blood flow patterns and the absence of pathologic transvalvular and paravalvular regurgitation.*** Color flow Doppler imaging will demonstrate central antegrade flow through the valve annulus when the leaflets open and small characteristic regurgitant jets during leaflet closure. A small amount of regurgitation is normal for bileaflet prosthetic valves and is caused by closure backflow and leakage backflow. Closure backflow is the reversal of flow required for closure of the leaflets. Leakage backflow occurs after closure of mechanical valves, originates from the four hinge points of the leaflets, and produces four centrally directed regurgitant jets (Figures 13.1 and 13.5). The leakage backflow jets originating from the hinge points are best visualized in the long-axis image through the prosthetic valve at a multiplane angle aligned parallel to the leaflets (Figure 13.5A). The bileaflet valves are designed to permit a small amount of regurgitation at the hinge points to prevent the formation of thrombus within the hinge mechanism. Sometimes, small leakage regurgitant jets originating along the edge of the leaflet where it meets the annulus during closure can also be imaged by color Doppler (Figure 13.5B). Normal physiologic regurgitant jets are small and short in

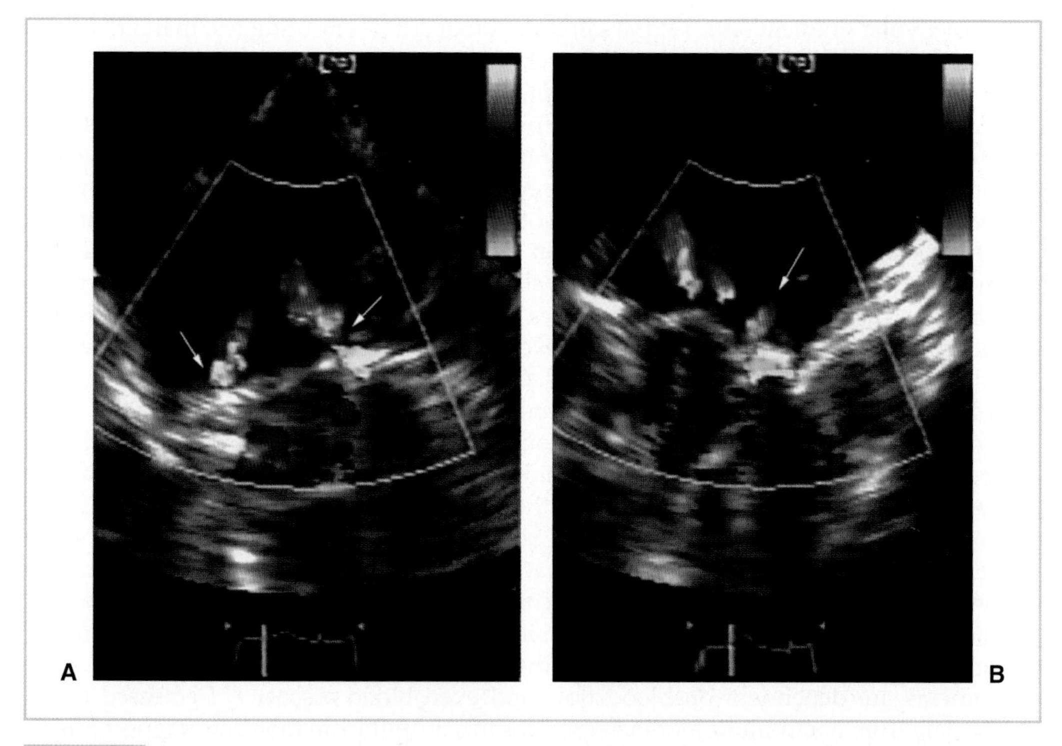

Figure 13.5. Bileaflet mechanical prosthesis, mitral position. Color Doppler flow transesophageal echocardiographic midesophageal mitral valve commissural view at a multiplane angle of 60 degrees (panel **A**) and long-axis view at a multiplane angle of 150 degrees (panel **B**) showing the normal appearance of leakage regurgitant jets that are characteristic of bileaflet valves. In panel **A**, individual leakage jets originate from the hinge points of the leaflets (*arrows*) and are directed toward the center of the valve. In panel **B**, a third leakage regurgitant jet (*arrow*) can be visualized originating at the point of contact between the leaflet and the valve stent.

duration and can be distinguished from pathologic transvalvular regurgitation based on their size, location, direction, and duration.

Pathologic regurgitation with a jet originating within the sewing ring is called *transvalvular regurgitation*. Pathologic transvalvular regurgitation immediately after valve implantation indicates malfunctioning of the valve leaflets. Intraoperative causes of leaflet malfunction causing transvalvular regurgitation include retained tissue preventing valve closure, a misplaced suture interfering with leaflet motion, or debris within the hinges causing trapping of the leaflet in a fixed position. Regurgitant jets originating outside of the sewing ring are always pathologic and called *paravalvular regurgitation*.

4. ***Calculate valve gradient and EOA.*** The hemodynamic performance of the prosthetic valve can be assessed using Doppler echocardiography. The interpretation of Doppler-derived prosthetic valve hemodynamic parameters is complicated because even normally functioning prosthetic valves are inherently obstructive to blood flow and blood flow velocity profiles across prosthetic valves are not uniform depending upon prosthetic valve type, model, and annular diameter. Because the blood flow velocity through the central rectangular orifice is greater than the blood flow velocity through the two semicircular orifices of the bileaflet valves, some studies suggest that Doppler-derived gradients based on the simplified Bernoulli equation may overestimate the true

transvalvular gradient (10). Yet the same and other studies also suggest that differences observed between Doppler- and catheter-derived gradients across prosthetic valves can be explained by localized gradients and pressure recovery downstream from the valve orifice (10,11). On the basis of this interpretation, differences between Doppler- and catheter-derived pressure gradients may not represent an overestimation of catheter-derived gradients, but instead represent inherent differences in measurement technique, line of interrogation, and precise location of pressure gradients relative to the prosthetic valve orifices. Furthermore, the equation used to estimate mitral valve area (MVA) based on pressure half-time ($MVA = 220/PHT$) may not apply to prosthetic valves that differ in structure and flow characteristics to the native valve. For clinical purposes of quantifying prosthetic valve function, several approaches can be applied for interpretation of Doppler-derived measurements. One approach is to report only actual values of Doppler transvalvular peak and mean flow velocities across the prosthetic valve and compare the values to established normal values for the specific type, model, and size of the prosthetic valve based on clinical reports or specifications published by the manufactures that can be obtained from their respective websites or the package insert accompanying the prosthetic valve (9). Similarly, Doppler-derived estimated orifice areas calculated using the continuity equation (Table 13.3) for a prosthetic valve can be compared to those observed for that specific prosthetic valve type, model, and size (9). Another aspect adding to the complication of interpreting Doppler-derived hemodynamic information in patients with prosthetic valves is that Doppler-derived pressure gradients are dependent on blood flow and even blood viscosity. Decreased blood viscosity from hemodilution or increased cardiac output from inotropic support immediately after prosthetic valve implantation may lead to overestimation of prosthetic valve gradients using the simplified Bernoulli equation. One approach to potentially overcome this problem for assessing aortic valve prosthetics is to index transvalvular Doppler blood flow velocity through the prosthetic valve relative to the blood flow velocity through the LVOT (12,13). For example, using a "double envelope" technique for assessing the function of a prosthetic valve in the aortic position, a peak blood flow velocity in the LVOT (V_{LVOT}) to peak transvalvular blood flow velocity (V_{AoV}) ratio less than 0.35 ($V_{LVOT}/V_{AoV} < 0.35$) may indicate prosthetic valve stenosis (12). Similarly, for assessing the function of a prosthetic valve in the mitral position, a transvalvular velocity time integral (VTI_{MV}) to LVOT velocity time integral (VTI_{LVOT}) ratio greater than 2.2 ($VTI_{MV}/VTI_{LVOT} > 2.2$) may indicate prosthetic valve stenosis (13).

CAGED BALL

Caged-ball valves were the first prosthetic valves implanted in humans. They consist of a silastic or metal ball occluder housed in a wire cage with three or four struts. The ball occluder casts a large acoustic shadow and its motion within the cage is best imaged in the long-axis plane of the valve (Figure 13.6A). In the short-axis imaging plane, the ball occluder can be imaged within the wire struts. Doppler color flow imaging in the short-axis plane of the valve demonstrates blood flow between the wire struts through the outside perimeter of the ball occluder (Figure 13.6B).

CAGED DISC

Caged-disc valves consist of a disc occluder housed within a wire cage. Motion of the disc occluder up and down within the wire cage is best imaged in the long-axis plane. Doppler color flow imaging should demonstrate flow through the central orifice in the plane of the stent then out the side of the wire cage between the stent and the disc occluder. The multidirectional blood flow through the valve precludes reliable Doppler-derived estimates of valve orifice area and transvalvular gradient.

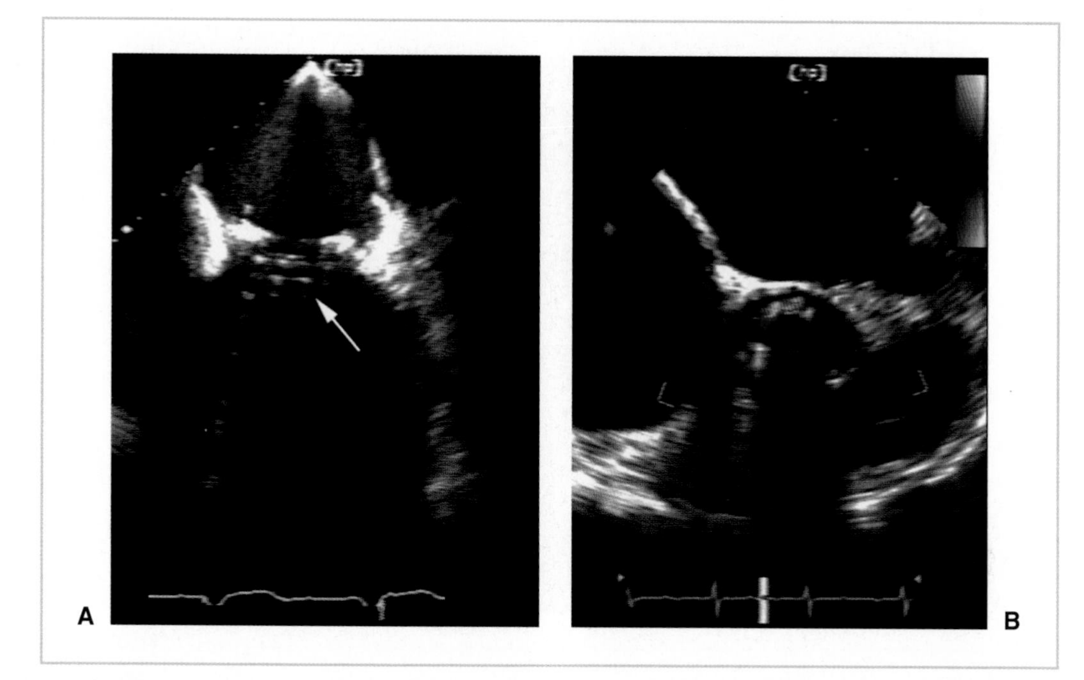

Figure 13.6. Starr-Edwards caged-ball mechanical valve. Panel **A** is a transesophageal echocardiographic midesophageal four-chamber view of a caged-ball valve prosthesis in the mitral position at end-diastole. Ultrasound shadowing caused by the silastic ball occluder (*arrow*) contained within the wire form cage makes it difficult to image the distal side of the valve. Panel **B** is a TEE midesophageal aortic valve short-axis view at a multiplane angle of 50 degrees during systole in a patient with a caged-ball valve in the aortic position. Note the three metal struts of the cage. Color Doppler flow imaging demonstrates blood flow through the valve at the perimeter of the silastic ball occluder. Again, the silastic ball occluder causes ultrasound shadowing.

TILTING DISC

Tilting disc valves are utilized in the aortic or mitral positions. They consist of a disc occluder supported by struts. The single disc occluder pivots open 60 to 80 degrees to form two orifices of different size and shape. They have a low profile and offer the advantage of providing a large orifice size in relation to its stent size.

Echocardiographic examination includes:

1. Confirm proper tilting action of the occluder in the long-axis imaging plane.
2. In the short-axis imaging plane, one edge of the disc occluder should move in and out of the imaging plane as the valve tilts opens.
3. Doppler color flow imaging showing small centrally directed leakage backflow regurgitant jet originating from the hinge point of the disc occluder or small jets originating at the site of contact between the disc and the annular stent are normal findings.
4. Abnormal findings: Strut fracture is a serious complication that can cause occluder malfunction and even disc embolization. Other complications such as thrombus or pannus formation on the valve can impair occluder motion resulting in stenosis or transvalvular regurgitation (Figure 13.7).

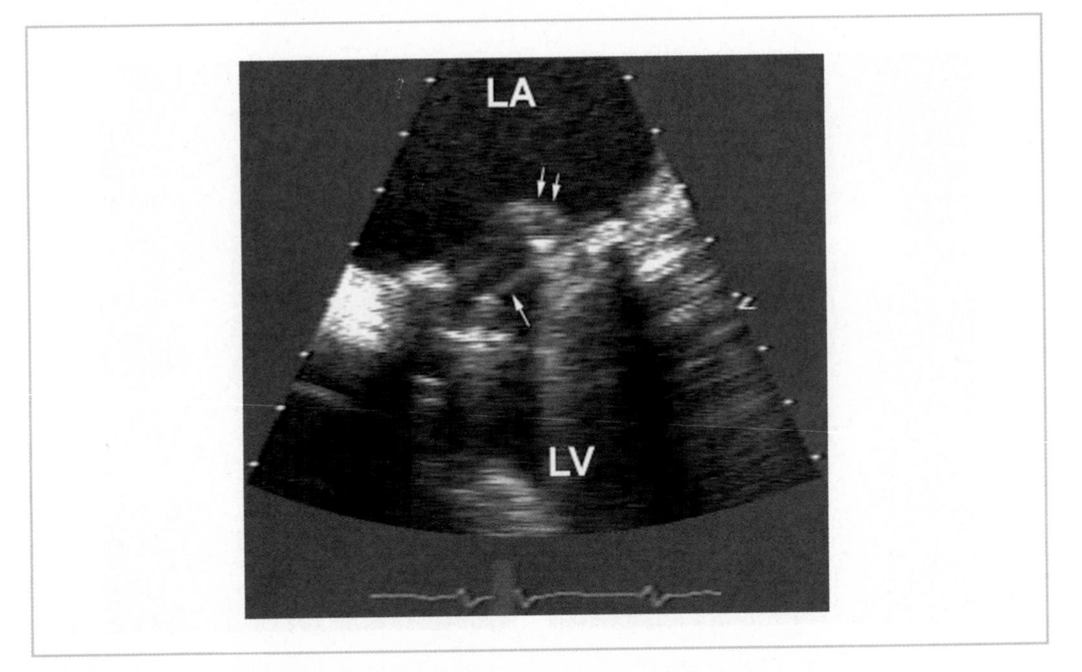

Figure 13.7. Pannus formation on Bjork-Shiley tilting disc mechanical prosthesis in the mitral position. Transesophageal echocardiographic midesophageal four-chamber view during systole in a patient with a tilting disc mechanical prosthesis in the mitral position. The single-disc occluder (single *arrow*) failed to close completely during systole and open completely during diastole (not shown). Pannus formation on the valve (double *arrows*) limited the motion of the disc occluder causing both prosthetic mitral stenosis and transvalvular mitral regurgitation. LA, left atrium; LV, left ventricle.

Biologic Valves or Tissue Valves

Biologic valves do not require systemic anticoagulation, but have an effective life span of only 12 to 15 years. The biologic components of bioprosthetic valves are susceptible to structural valvular deterioration such as leaflet calcification, tear, or perforation. Unstented bioprosthetic aortic valves are also susceptible to regurgitation from annular or aortic root dilatation. Bioprosthetic valves are typically preferred for elderly patients with a life expectancy less than 15 years or for patients who cannot tolerate anticoagulation therapy or in whom anticoagulation therapy is not feasible. The biologic components of bioprosthetic valves have favorable acoustic properties and permit imaging by ultrasound. In general, the same principles used to examine native cardiac valves can be applied to the TEE examination of biologic valve prostheses.

STENTED PORCINE HETEROGRAFTS

Stented porcine heterografts are constructed from a glutaraldehyde preserved porcine aortic xenograft mounted on a cloth-covered wire or polymer frame with an attached sewing ring (Figure 13.8). They can be implanted in the aortic, mitral, or tricuspid positions. In short axis, the three leaflets supported by struts open to form a central orifice in the shape of a bulging triangle. In long axis, the valve leaflets separate symmetrically when open and coapt at the center of the valve when closed. The stent struts that support the leaflets extend from the base of the annulus and point toward the downstream side of the valve. Doppler color flow imaging can sometimes detect a small closure or leakage backflow jet originating from the central coaptation point.

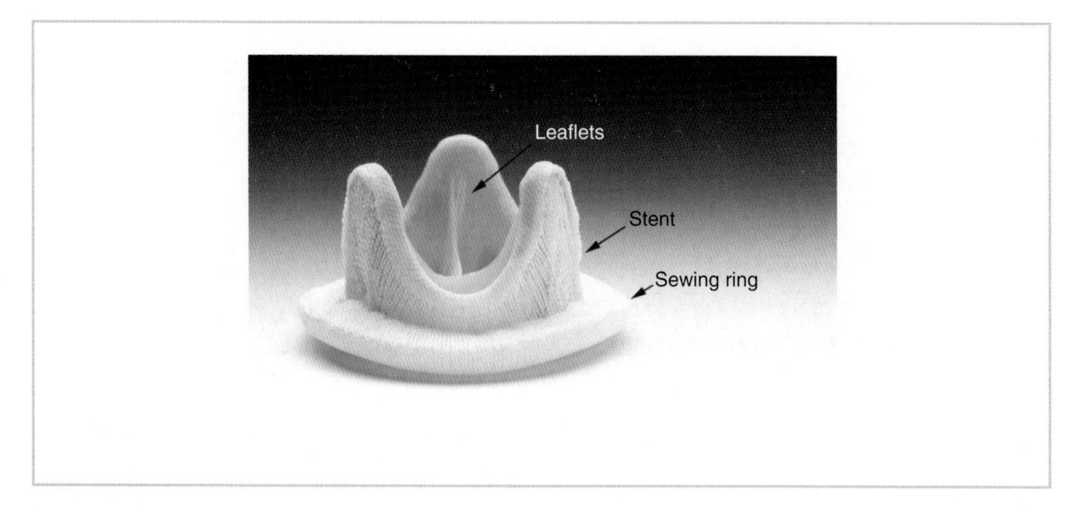

Figure 13.8. Photograph of a Carpentier-Edwards model 6625 porcine bioprosthetic mitral valve. The valve is constructed from a porcine aortic xenograft mounted on a wire form stent surrounded by a sewing ring.

STENTED BOVINE PERICARDIAL VALVES

Stented bovine pericardial valves are constructed from bovine pericardium fashioned into three leaflets supported by a wire frame with three struts attached to a sewing ring (Figure 13.9). The pericardial bioprosthetic valves have a lower profile compared to the stented porcine bioprosthetic valves, but the echocardiographic appearance of these valves is very similar to that of a stented porcine aortic heterograft. The pericardial bioprosthesis implanted in the mitral position sometimes exhibits mild central transvalvular regurgitation immediately after implantation that typically decreases over time (Figure 13.10A). Small transvalvular regurgitant leakage jets can sometimes be identified originating from the fabric-covered regions of the stent struts or from the region between the stent and

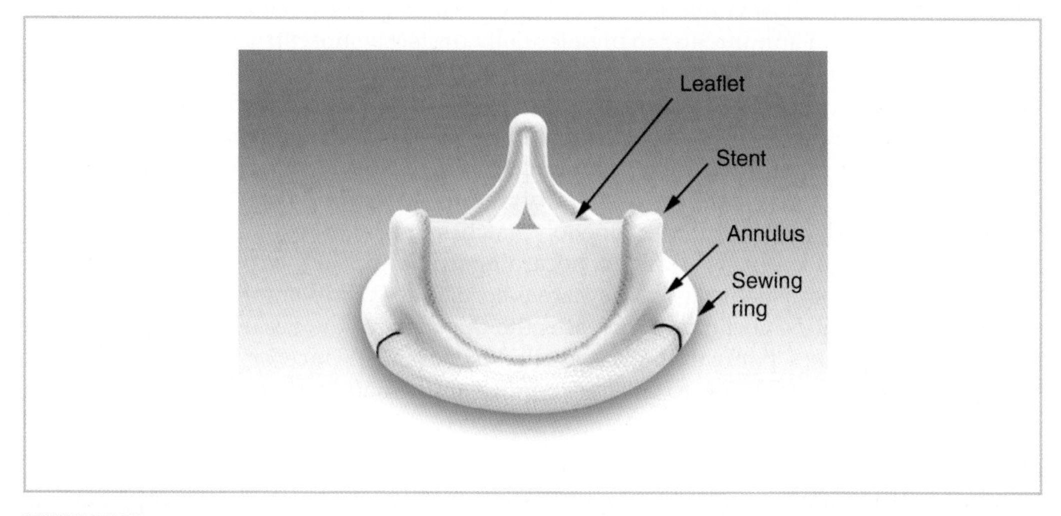

Figure 13.9. Photograph of a Carpentier-Edwards model 6900 bovine pericardial bioprosthetic mitral valve. The valve leaflets are constructed from bovine pericardium mounted on a wire form stent surrounded by a sewing ring.

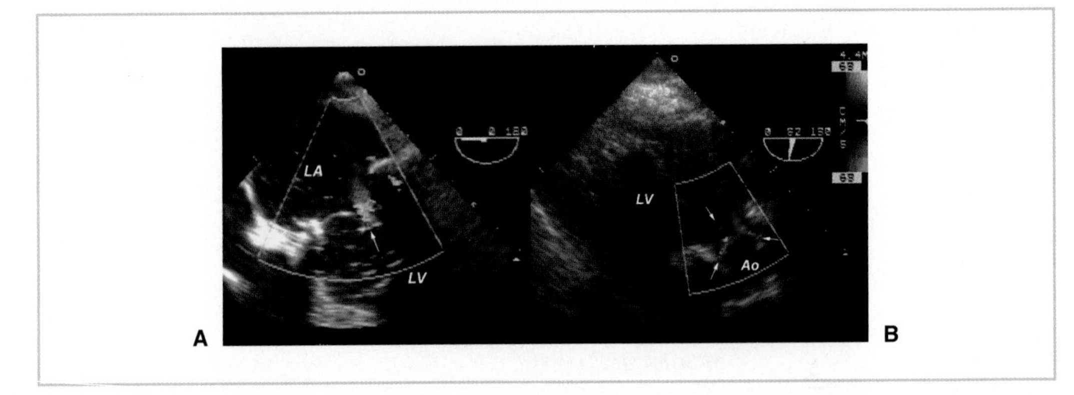

Figure 13.10. Mild transvalvular regurgitation can normally be detected immediately after implantation of bovine pericardial bioprosthetic valves. Midesophageal four-chamber view with color Doppler flow imaging demonstrated mild central regurgitation (*arrow*) through the leaflet commissures in a bovine pericardial bioprosthetic valve implanted in the mitral position (panel **A**). Transgastric mid-left ventricular long-axis view through the aortic valve with color Doppler flow imaging detected mild regurgitation through the fabric-covered stent struts (arrows) in a bovine pericardial bioprosthetic valves implanted in the aortic position (panel **B**). These transvalvular regurgitant jets typically decrease in severity over time. LA, left atrium; LV, left ventricle; Ao, aorta.

the sewing ring (Figure 13.10B). These regurgitant leakage jets through the fabric of the bioprosthetic valve typically resolve over time as the fabric becomes sealed with cellular elements or endothelium.

STENTLESS VALVES

Stentless bioprosthetic valves are fabric-reinforced glutaraldehyde preserved porcine aortic heterografts constructed without the wire form frame, stents, and sewing ring. They are designed for use in the aortic position or for replacement of the aortic root. Elimination of the stent and sewing ring increases the EOA that can be achieved after valve replacement, making them particularly useful in patients with a native aortic valve annulus less than 20 mm in diameter. Elimination of the stent also permits greater freedom of movement of the valve leaflets and annulus and may potentially protect against structural deterioration. However, the competency of the stentless aortic valve is contingent on the geometry of the aortic root. Mismatching of the annular size, malalignment of the leaflets in the annular plane, or dilatation of the aortic root will alter leaflet coaptation and cause regurgitation. For this reason, it is important for the intraoperative echocardiographic examination to accurately size the native annulus and verify that the ascending aorta is not dilated and that the diameter of the sinotubular junction matches or is within 10% the diameter of the stentless valve (Figure 13.11) (14). The echocardiographic appearance of the stentless valve is virtually indistinguishable from the native aortic valve. Implantation of the stentless valve within the native aortic root increases the thickness of the vessel wall at the region of overlap and makes paravalvular regurgitation possible. Trace or mild central aortic regurgitation is detectable up to 25% of the time immediately after implantation of the stentless bioprosthetic valve.

ALLOGRAFT VALVES

Cryopreserved human aortic root allografts are commercially available for implantation. They are sized according to the aortic valve annulus diameter in a range from 20 mm to 26 mm. Absence of a stent requires that the annular size of the allograft match the size of the native valve annulus to ensure valve competence. Implantation of an

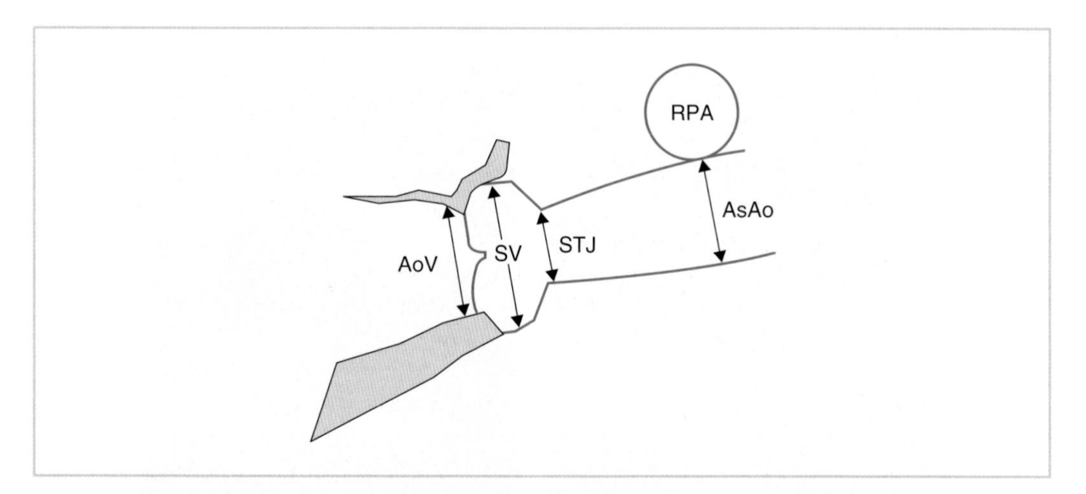

Figure 13.11. Schematic of the transesophageal echocardiographic midesophageal aortic valve long-axis imaging plane demonstrating the anatomic landmarks used to measure the diameter of the native aortic valve (AoV) annulus, sinus of Valsalva (SV), sinotubular junction (STJ), and ascending aorta (AsAo) at the level of the right pulmonary artery (RPA).

undersized or oversized allograft may result in aortic regurgitation. The echocardiographic appearance of the aortic allograft is indistinguishable from the native aortic valve and aortic root. Replacement of the aortic root and reimplantation of the coronary arteries with a human aortic root allograft, stentless porcine aortic root, or mechanical valved-conduit is performed for aortic valve endocarditis with aortic root abscess, bicuspid aortic valve with dilated aortic root, type A aortic dissection, or aneurysms involving the aortic root and ascending aorta.

CLINICAL CAVEATS TO ECHOCARDIOGRAPHIC DIAGNOSIS OF PROSTHETIC VALVE DYSFUNCTION

Prosthetic valve dysfunction can result in regurgitation, stenosis, or hemolysis. TEE is recognized as the diagnostic examination of choice for the diagnosis and evaluation of suspected prosthetic valve dysfunction.

1. ***Prosthetic valve regurgitation.*** When the Doppler examination reveals regurgitation in a prosthetic valve, it is important to distinguish physiologic regurgitation from pathologic regurgitation.
   a. A small amount of regurgitation is normally observed in all mechanical prosthetic valves and in approximately 10% of bioprosthetic valves. Closure backflow is the reversal of flow required for closure of the valve. In contrast, leakage backflow occurs after closure of mechanical valves and originates from the hinges and the regions of coaptation between the occluders and the valve ring (Figures 13.1, 13.5, and 13.10). Physiologic regurgitation jets are small and short in duration. The leakage backflow patterns for each valve type are unique and distinct from pathologic regurgitation. Mild transvalvular regurgitation can often be detected by TEE Doppler flow imaging in bioprosthetic valves immediately after implantation. Regurgitant jets that originate at the sites of leaflet coaptation are directed centrally. Regurgitant jets from leakage at the fabric-covered regions of the valve stent originate at the valve struts and are directed toward the center of the valve. Mild physiologic transvalvular regurgitation

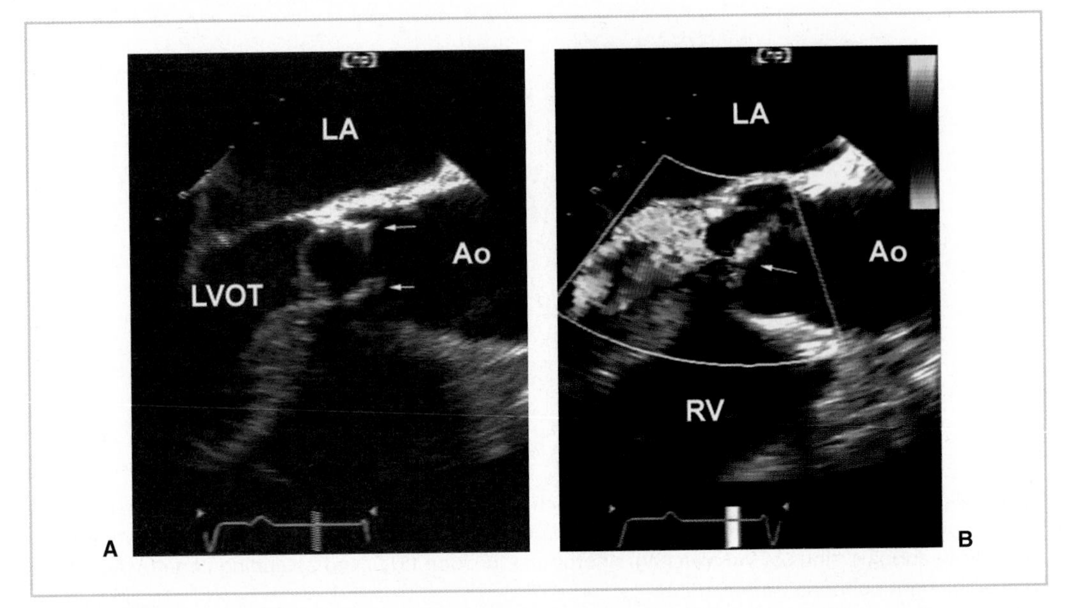

Figure 13.12. Transvalvular regurgitation, porcine bioprosthetic valve in the aortic position. Transesophageal echocardiographic midesophageal aortic valve long-axis image at a multiplane angle of 150 degrees in a patient with a porcine bioprosthetic valve in the aortic position. 2-D imaging (panel **A**) in diastole shows the appearance of the valve struts (*arrows*) that support the leaflets. The leaflets prolapse into the left ventricular outflow tract. Color Doppler flow imaging during diastole (panel **B**) shows the aortic regurgitant jet (*arrow*) originating between the valve struts indicating transvalvular regurgitation cause by structural degeneration of the bioprosthetic valve. LVOT, left ventricular outflow tract; LA, left atrium; RV, right ventricle; Ao, aorta.

in bioprosthetic valves detected by TEE immediately after implantation typically decrease or even disappear by the end of the surgery.

b. Pathologic transvalvular regurgitation in bioprosthetic valves is commonly associated with chronic degenerative changes including leaflet calcification, perforation, tears, or prolapse (Figure 13.12) or from leaflet destruction caused by endocarditis. In mechanical prosthetic valves, pathologic transvalvular regurgitation will result when the formation of pannus, thrombus, vegetations, or foreign material on valve components prevents complete closure of the occluder (Figure 13.13). 2-D imaging of leaflet or occluder motion in mechanical valves is useful for detecting transvalvular regurgitation caused by impingement of the occluder by pannus, thrombus, or vegetations. Grading systems based on Doppler measurements of regurgitant fraction, regurgitant jet area, jet length, and vena contracta or jet width also apply for assessing the clinical severity of prosthetic valve regurgitation.

c. Paravalvular regurgitation is always pathologic and is caused by incomplete fixation of the prosthetic sewing ring to the native annulus or dehiscence of the sewing ring. Incomplete fixation is typically caused by native annular calcification that increases the difficulty of prosthetic implantation. Paravalvular regurgitant jets imaged using color Doppler flow imaging originate from outside of the sewing ring, characteristically produce eccentric jets that track along the walls of the receiving chamber, and usually produce zones of flow acceleration adjacent to the site of regurgitation in the chamber proximal to the prosthetic valve (Figure 13.14). Evidence to support the best course of action in response to the TEE detection of paravalvular

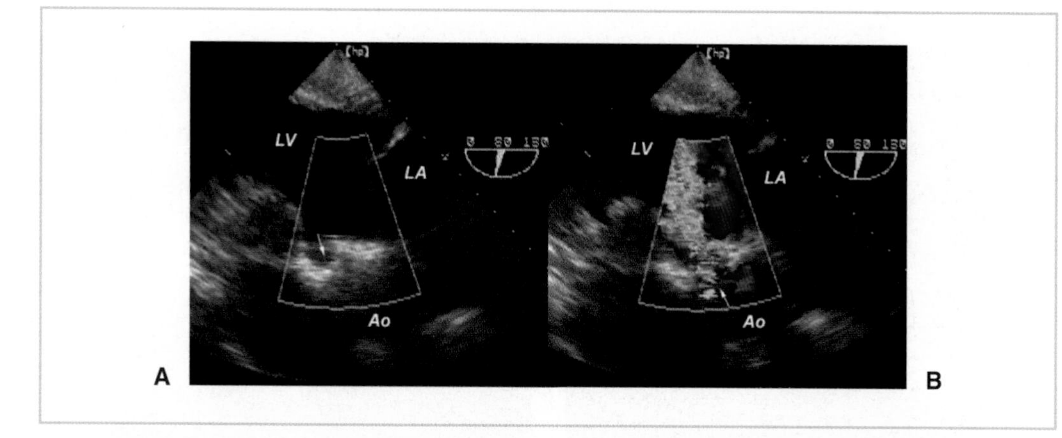

Figure 13.13. Severe transvalvular regurgitation caused by a leaflet trapped in the open position due to pannus in-growth. Transgastric mid-left ventricular long-axis view through the aortic valve in a patient with a bileaflet mechanical prosthetic valve in the aortic position. 2-D imaging (panel **A**) demonstrated one of the valve leaflets was immobile and trapped in the open position (*arrow*). Color Doppler flow imaging (panel **B**) demonstrated severe transvalvular regurgitation through the region of the prosthetic valve with the leaflet trapped in the open position (*arrow*). LA, left atrium; RV, right ventricle; Ao, aorta.

regurgitation immediately after prosthetic valve implantation is limited. Some clinical series suggested that intraoperative TEE was useful for detecting paravalvular regurgitation and prompted revision of the valve replacement (15). In a very small series, two out of six patients with mild paravalvular regurgitation and two out of two patients with moderate paravalvular regurgitation detected by TEE immediately

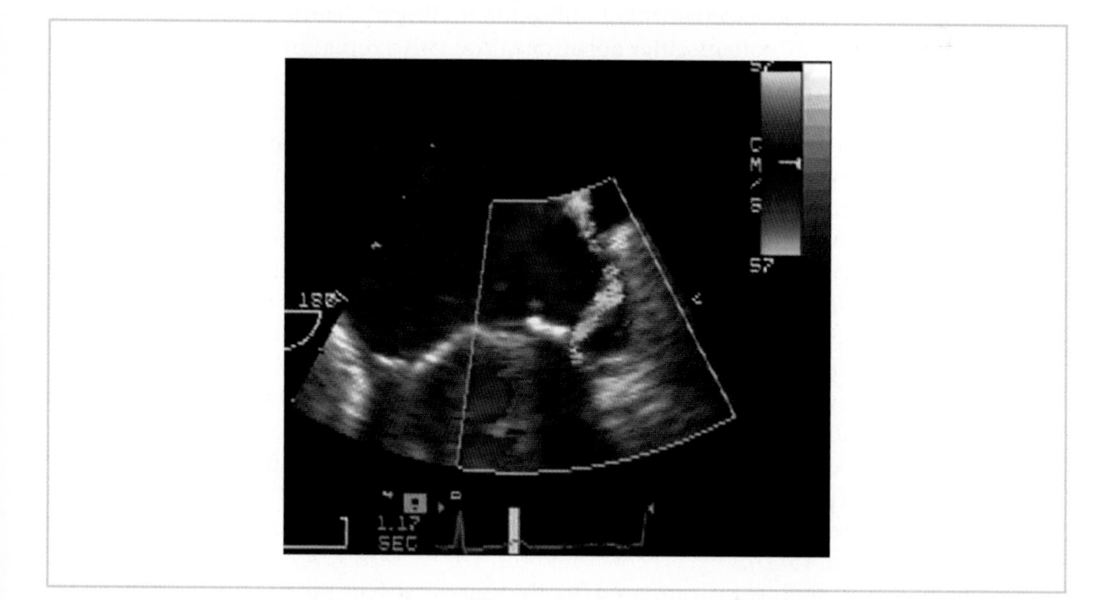

Figure 13.14. Paravalvular regurgitation, mechanical bileaflet valve in the mitral position. Transesophageal echocardiographic midesophageal long-axis view at a multiplane angle of 22 degrees of a mechanical bileaflet prosthesis in the mitral position demonstrating paravalvular regurgitation. Color Doppler flow imaging demonstrates an eccentric regurgitant jet originating outside of the prosthetic annulus.

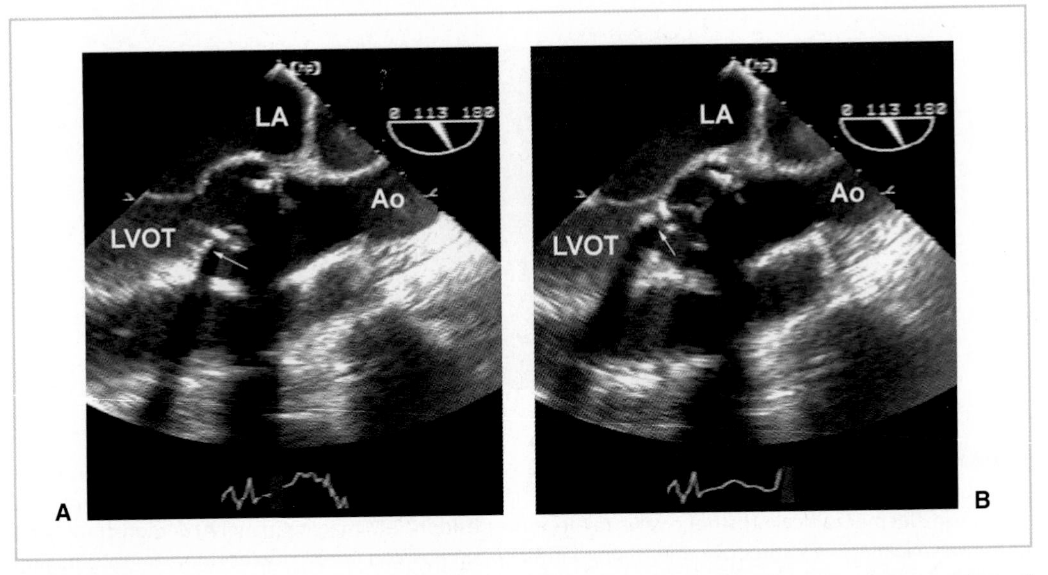

Figure 13.15. Dehiscence, bovine pericardial bioprosthesis in the aortic position. Transesophageal echocardiographic midesophageal aortic valve long-axis image at a multiplane angle of 113 degrees showing dehiscence of a pericardial bioprosthesis in the aortic position. In systole (panel **A**), the anterior region of the prosthetic stent (*arrow*) is displaced toward the left ventricular side of the native aortic valve annulus. In diastole (panel **B**) the anterior region of the prosthetic stent is completely detached from the aortic valve annulus (*arrow*). Dehiscence with partial annular detachment produced a "rocking" motion of the prosthetic valve and paravalvular regurgitation in the region of separation (*arrow*). LA, left atrium; LVOT, left ventricular outflow tract; Ao, aorta.

after mitral valve replacement had subsequent clinical deterioration (16). Another study examining 27 patients after aortic or mitral valve replacement found that small paravalvular regurgitant jets detected by TEE using Doppler color flow imaging were common after valve replacement, decreased in size and number after protamine administration, and were not associated with early postoperative morbidity (17). Finally, in a large series of 608 consecutive patients undergoing aortic or mitral valve replacement, trivial or mild paravalvular regurgitation defined as a regurgitant jet area less than 3.0 cm^2 by Doppler color flow imaging was detected by intraoperative TEE in 18.3% of patients (18). At early follow-up, paravalvular regurgitation had resolved in 50% of the patients. At late follow-up, only 4 out of the original 113 patients with mild paravalvular regurgitation had worsening of regurgitation. Precise characterization of the location and severity of paravalvular regurgitant jets detected by TEE after valve implantation may be useful for guiding decisions for surgical intervention. Dehiscence is a late complication after valve replacement and is often associated with endocarditis. Dehiscence of part of the sewing ring may destabilize the prosthetic valve producing a "rocking" motion of the entire prosthesis and a visible separation of the native and prosthetic valve annulus detected by 2-D imaging (Figure 13.15).

2. ***Prosthetic valve stenosis***. Compared to the native valve, all prosthetic valves are mildly stenotic depending upon the valve type, size, and the hemodynamic condition of the patient. The mean pressure gradient across prosthetic valves calculated using the simplified Bernoulli equation depends on the prosthetic valve type, its position, its size, and the cardiac output. For this reason, the package insert or published

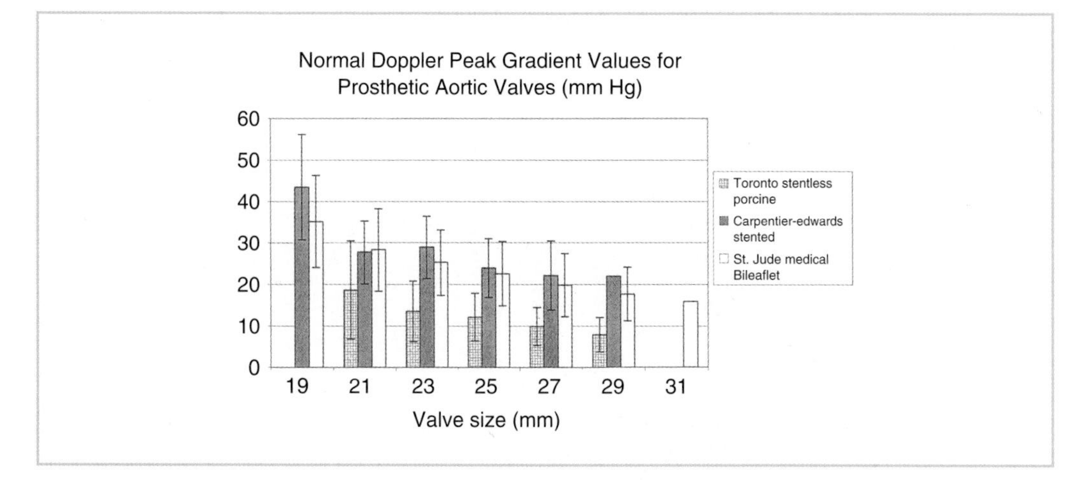

Figure 13.16. Pressure gradients across prosthetic aortic valves. Maximum transvalvular pressure gradients across aortic valve prostheses measured using Doppler echocardiography based on the simplified Bernoulli equation for representative prosthetic valve type and annular size in the aortic position. Values are the mean and the error bars indicate the standard deviations. (Values are the composite of published reports from Rosenhek R, Binder T, Maurer G, et al. Normal values for Doppler echocardiographic assessment of heart valve prostheses. *J Am Soc Echocardiogr* 2003;16:1116–1127.)

normal values that lists the hemodynamic specifications for the particular valve type according to annular size is often used as a reference when examining the hemodynamic performance of a prosthetic valve (7–9). The peak transvalvular gradient for valves in the mitral position ranges from 3 to 4 mm Hg and the peak transvalvular gradient for valves in the aortic position ranges from <10 to >30 mm Hg (Figure 13.16). The continuity method can also be used to estimate the EOA of prosthetic valves in the mitral or aortic positions (Table 13.3). This method uses Doppler to measure the velocity time integral (VTI) across the prosthetic valve in relation to the cross-sectional area and VTI through the LVOT. Average values for the EOA estimated by the continuity equation range from 1.4 to 3.0 cm^2 for valves in the mitral position and 1.0 to 2.5 cm^2 for valves in the aortic position (Figure 13.17). Stenosis of bioprosthetic valves is caused by chronic degenerative changes resulting in leaflet calcification, thickening, and rigidity restricting their ability to open completely. Degenerative changes and restricted leaflet mobility

Table 13.3 Determining the effective orifice area using the continuity method

$EOA = LVOT_{area} (VTI_{LVOT}/VTI_{transvalvular})$
Where:
EOA = effective orifice area of prosthetic valve
$LVOT_{area}$ = cross-sectional area of left ventricular outflow tract (LVOT)
$= \pi(\text{diameter of LVOT}/2)^2$
$VTI_{transvalvular}$ = velocity time integral of blood flow across valve
VTI_{LVOT} = velocity time integral of blood flow across LVOT

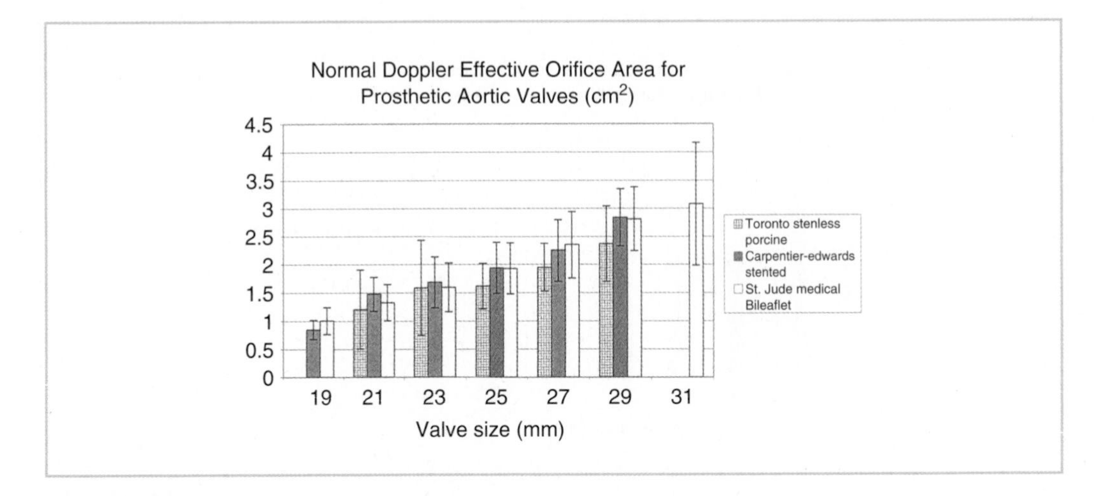

Figure 13.17. Effective orifice area for prosthetic aortic valves. Effective orifice area for aortic valve prostheses measured using Doppler echocardiography based on the continuity method for representative prosthetic valve types and prosthetic valve annular size in the aortic position. Values are the mean and the error bars indicate the standard deviations. (Values are the composite of published reports from Rosenhek R, Binder T, Maurer G, et al. Normal values for Doppler echocardiographic assessment of heart valve prostheses. *J Am Soc Echocardiogr* 2003;16:1116–1127.)

can be detected by the 2-D examination. In mechanical valves, stenosis can be caused by thrombus, pannus, vegetation, suture, or even retained subvalvular structures that trap the occluder mechanism in the closed position or impinge its ability to open completely (Figures 13.7 and 13.18).

3. ***Prosthesis-patient mismatch***. Prosthetic heart valves are inherently stenotic relative to native cardiac valves. Although still somewhat controversial, several clinical studies have provided evidence that implantation of a prosthetic valve that is sized too small for an individual patient has the potential to cause significant obstruction to flow (19–22). The hemodynamic consequences of flow obstruction caused by a normally functioning prosthetic valve increased the likelihood of mortality and cardiac complications after aortic valve replacement (20–22). Implantation of a stenotic prosthetic valve in the aortic position has also been shown to be associated with decreased ventricular mass regression after operation (23). This condition been called *prosthesis-patient mismatch* and may be particularly important in patients with decreased left ventricular function. Prosthesis-patient mismatching has been best described after aortic valve replacement because the diameter of the native aortic valve annulus limits the size of the prosthetic valve that can be implanted. However, several studies have also suggested that prosthesis-patient mismatching may occur after mitral valve replacement and was manifested by pulmonary hypertension (24). Intraoperative TEE provides an opportunity to measure the diameter of the native aortic valve annulus to determine the size of prosthetic valve that can be implanted, thereby helpful for predicting the risk of patient-prosthetic mismatch based on the indexed EOA ($EOA_i = EOA/BSA$, were EOA_i is the indexed effective orifice area, EOA is the effective orifice area of the prosthetic valve and BSA is the body surface area of the patient in m^2). Prosthesis-patient mismatch is considered severe after aortic valve replacement if the EOA_i less than or equal to 0.65 cm^2/m^2, moderate if the EOA_i is between 0.65 cm^2/m^2 and 0.85 cm^2/m^2, and not significant if the EOA_i is equal to or greater than 0.85 cm^2/m^2 (20). Prosthesis-patient mismatch is considered significant after mitral valve replacement if the EOA_i less than or equal to

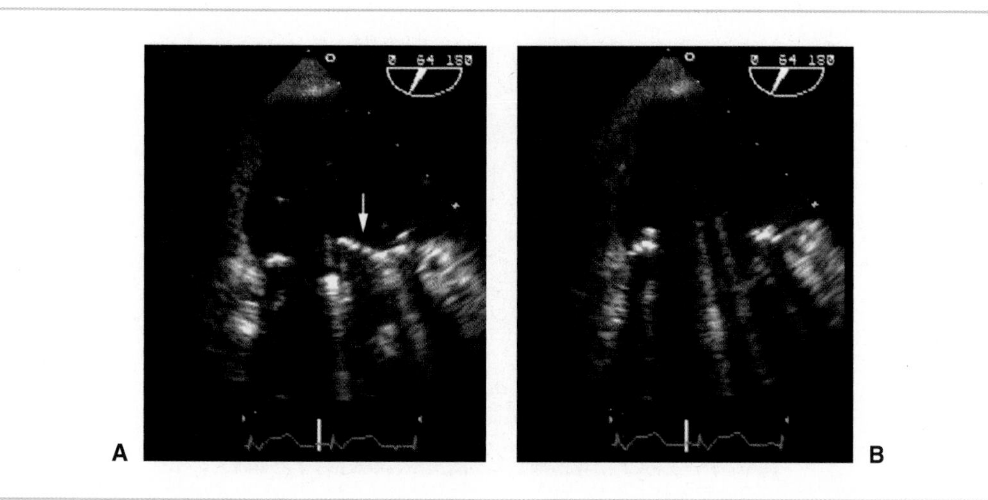

Figure 13.18. Trapped leaflet, mechanical bileaflet valve in the mitral position. Transesophageal echocardiographic midesophageal mitral valve commissural view at a multiplane angle of 64 degrees in mid-diastole provided a cross-section to demonstrate the motion of both leaflets in a patient with a mechanical bileaflet valve in the mitral position. Note that in panel **A**, the anterior leaflet of the prosthesis is trapped in the closed position (*arrow*). Panel **B** shows both leaflets opening completely after the trapped leaflet was freed surgically. Color Doppler flow imaging (not shown) demonstrated mitral inflow in diastole through the region of the valve with the open leaflet, but not across the region of the valve with the leaflet trapped in the closed position.

1.2 cm^2/m^2 (20). If intraoperative TEE measurements detect a small aortic valve annulus before aortic valve replacement, operative options to decrease the risk of patient-prosthetic mismatch include supra-annular implantation of the prosthetic valve, choose a prosthetic valve model with more a favorable hemodynamic flow profile in relation to its annular dimension, perform an aortic root enlargement to permit implantation of a larger prosthetic valve, or perform a root replacement.

4. ***Thrombosis and pannus.*** Acute thrombosis, usually as a result of inadequate anticoagulation can cause stenosis or regurgitation by obstructing blood flow through the valve or by interfering with leaflet opening and closure. Stenosis or regurgitation can also be caused by in-growth of pannus, a subacute condition. 2-D imaging may demonstrate abnormal masses attached to the prosthetic valve sometimes interfering with or limiting the range of motion of the occluder device (Figure 13.7). Pannus, with its fibrous composition, is echodense and firmly fixed to the valve apparatus. Thrombus tends to be more mobile, larger in size, and associated with spontaneous echocontrast indicating regions of low flow (25). Color Doppler imaging may demonstrate transvalvular regurgitation or an eccentric inflow pattern across the affected leaflet. Sometimes, the only evidence of pannus obstruction is the demonstration of an abnormally increased transvalvular pressure gradient by Doppler examination.
5. ***Hemolysis.*** Hemolysis is unusual with modern valve prostheses, but hemolysis can occur when blood is subjected to high peak shear stresses. These hydrodynamic conditions can occur when blood accelerates rapidly or decelerates rapidly upon collision or impingement with prosthetic material (26). Regurgitant jets associated with hemolysis often exhibit patterns of flow fragmentation, collision, or rapid acceleration by color Doppler flow imaging. Free regurgitant jets or jets that decelerate gradually are less likely to produce hemolysis.

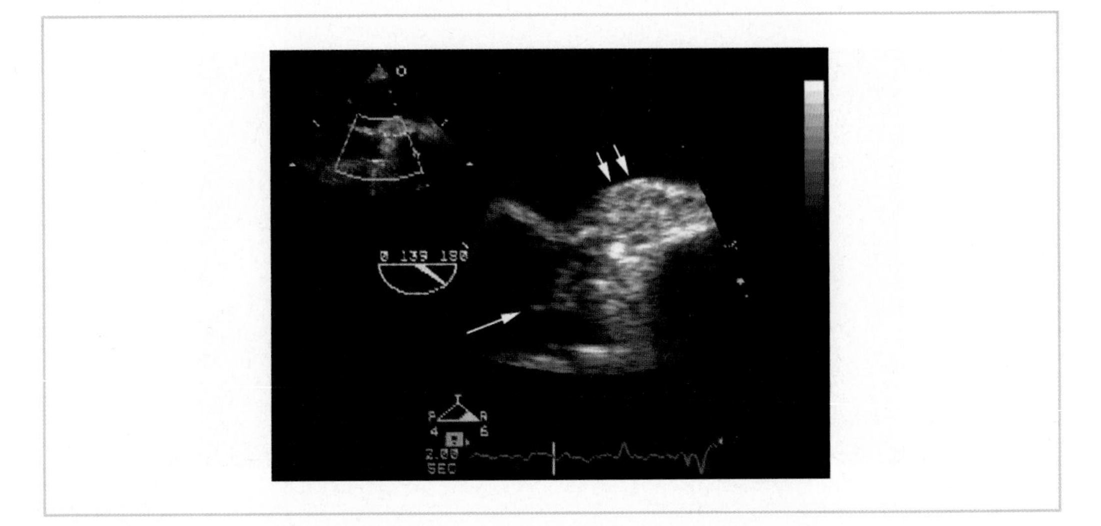

Figure 13.19. Endocarditis and aortic root abscess, mechanical bileaflet valve, aortic position. Transesophageal echocardiographic midesophageal aortic valve long-axis image at a multiplane angle of 139 degrees demonstrating prosthetic endocarditis in a patient with a mechanical bileaflet valve in the aortic position. A vegetation attached to the prosthetic valve was imaged in the left ventricular outflow tract during diastole (single *arrow*). Thickening of the posterior wall of the aortic root (double *arrows*) suggested aortic root abscess.

6. ***Endocarditis***. Prosthetic endocarditis occurs in approximately 3% to 6% of patients after valve replacement and has a mortality that ranges between 20% and 80% (2). TEE is currently the best diagnostic technique for detecting vegetations, dehiscence, or annular abscess for the diagnosis of prosthetic endocarditis (Figure 13.19) (27). Because imaging the distal side of the prosthetic valve is difficult due to shadowing of the ultrasound beam, it is important to use both midesophageal and transgastric imaging planes to examine both sides of the prosthesis for vegetations.
7. ***LVOT obstruction***. LVOT obstruction causing subvalvular aortic stenosis is an uncommon, but is a recognized complication of mitral valve replacement (28–30). After mitral valve replacement performed using the valve sparing or chordal sparing techniques, residual mitral valve leaflet or chordal apparatus remaining in the LVOT can cause LVOT obstruction. LVOT obstruction can also be caused by a porcine bioprosthesis in the mitral position with a strut impinging left ventricular outflow. The transgastric long-axis view provides a means to image the LVOT after mitral valve replacement and to estimate the LVOT pressure gradient using continuous wave Doppler.

CONCLUSION

The evaluation of prosthetic heart valves, the diagnosis of prosthetic valve dysfunction, and the detection of complications associated with valve replacement are important clinical applications of TEE.

REFERENCES

1 Seward JB, Labovitz AJ, Lewis JF, et al. ACC position statement. Transesophageal echocardiography. *J Am Coll Cardiol* 1992;20:506.

2 Vongpatanasin W, Hillis DL, Lange RA. Medical progress: prosthetic heart valves. *N Engl J Med* 1996;335:407–416.
3 Daniel WG, Mugge A, Grote J, et al. Comparison of transthoracic and transesophageal echocardiography for detection of abnormalities of prosthetic and bioprosthetic valves in the mitral and aortic positions. *Am J Cardiol* 1993;71:210–215.
4 Khandheria BK, Seward JB, Oh JK, et al. Value and limitations of transesophageal echocardiography in assessment of mitral valve prostheses. *Circulation* 1991;83:1956–1968.
5 Karalis DG, Chandrasekaran K, Ross JJ, et al. Single-plane transesophageal echocardiography for assessing function of mechanical or bioprosthetic valves in the aortic position. *Am J Cardiol* 1992;69: 1310–1315.
6 Chambers J, Fraser A, Lawford P, et al. Echocardiographic assessment of artificial heart valves: British Society of Echocardiography position paper. *Br Heart J* 1994;71(4 Suppl):6–14.
7 Panidis IP, Ross J, Mintz GS. Normal and abnormal prosthetic valve function as assessed by Doppler echocardiography. *J Am Coll Cardiol* 1986;8:317–326.
8 Reisner SA, Meltzer RS. Normal values of prosthetic valve Doppler echocardiographic parameters: a review. *J Am Soc Echocardiogr* 1988;1:201–210.
9 Rosenhek R, Binder T, Maurer G, et al. Normal values for Doppler echocardiographic assessment of heart valve prostheses. *J Am Soc Echocardiogr* 2003;16:1116–1127.
10 Baumgartner H, Khan S, DeRobertis M, et al. Discrepancies between Doppler and catheter gradients in aortic prosthetic valves *in vitro*. A manifestation of localized gradients and pressure recovery. *Circulation* 1990;82:1467–1475.
11 Bech-Hanssen O, Gjertsson P, Houltz E, et al. Net pressure gradients in aortic prosthetic valves can be estimated by Doppler. *J Am Soc Echocardiogr* 2003;16:858–866.
12 Maslow AD, Haering JM, Heindel S, et al. An evaluation of prosthetic aortic valves using transesophageal echocardiography: the double-envelope technique. *Anesth Analg* 2000;91:509–516.
13 Malouf JF, Ballo M, Connolly HM, et al. Doppler echocardiography of 119 normal-functioning St Jude Medical mitral valve prostheses: a comprehensive assessment including time-velocity integral ratio and prosthesis performance index. *J Am Soc Echocardiograph* 2005;18:252–256.
14 Guarracino F, Zussa C, Polesel E, et al. Influence of transesophageal echocardiography on intraoperative decision making for Toronto stentless prosthetic valve implantation. *J Heart Valve Dis* 2001;10: 31–34.
15 Shapira Y, Vaturi M, Weisenberg DE, et al. Impact of intraoperative transesophageal echocardiography in patients undergoing valve replacement. *Ann Thorac Surg* 2004;78:579–583.
16 Movsowitz HD, Shah SI, Ioli A, et al. Long-term follow-up of mitral paraprosthetic regurgitation by transesophageal echocardiography. *J Am Soc Echocardiogr* 1994;7:488–492.
17 Morehead AJ, Firstenberg MS, Shiota T, et al. Intraoperative echocardiographic detection of regurgitant jets after valve replacement. *Ann Thorac Surg* 2000;69:135–139.
18 O'Rourke DJ, Palac RT, Malenka DJ, et al. Outcome of mild periprosthetic regurgitation detected by intraoperative transesophageal echocardiography. *J Am Coll Cardiol* 2001;38:163–166.
19 Koch CG, Khandwala F, Estafanous FG, et al. Impact of prosthesis-patient size on functional recovery after aortic valve replacement. *Circulation* 2005;111:3221–3229.
20 Blais C, Dumesnil JG, Baillot R, et al. Impact of valve prosthesis-patient mismatch on short-term mortality after aortic valve replacement. *Circulation* 2003;108:983–988.
21 Tasca G, Mhagna Z, Perotti S, et al. Impact of prosthesis-patient mismatch on cardiac events and midterm mortality after aortic valve replacement in patients with pure aortic stenosis. *Circulation* 2006;113: 570–576.
22 Mohty-Echahidi D, Malouf JF, Girard SE, et al. Jr Impact of prosthesis-patient mismatch on long-term survival in patients with small St Jude Medical mechanical prostheses in the aortic position. *Circulation* 2006;113:420–426.
23 Tasca G, Brunelli F, Cirillo M, et al. Impact of valve prosthesis-patient mismatch on left ventricular mass regression following aortic valve replacement. *Ann Thorac Surg* 2005;79:505–510.
24 Li M, Dumesnil JG, Mathieu P, et al. Impact of valve prosthesis-patient mismatch on pulmonary arterial pressure after mitral valve replacement. *J Am Coll Cardiol* 2005;45:1034–1040.
25 Barbetseas J, Nagueh SF, Pitsavos C, et al. Differentiating thrombus from pannus formation in obstructed mechanical prosthetic valves: an evaluation of clinical, transthoracic, and transesophageal echocardiographic parameters. *J Am Coll Cardiol* 1998;32:1410–1417.
26 Garcia MJ, Vandervoort P, Stewart WJ, et al. Mechanisms of hemolysis with mitral prosthetic regurgitation. Study using transesophageal echocardiography and fluid dynamic simulation. *J Am Coll Cardiol* 1996;27:399–406.
27 Piper C, Korfer R, Horstkotte D. Prosthetic valve endocarditis. *Heart* 2001;85:590–593.

28 Jett GK, Jett MD, Banhart GR, et al. Left ventricular outflow tract obstruction with mitral valve replacement in small ventricular cavities. *Ann Thorac Surg* 1986;41:70–74.
29 Come PC, Riley MF, Weintraub RM, et al. Dynamic left ventricular outflow tract obstruction when the anterior leaflet is retained at prosthetic mitral valve replacement. *Ann Thorac Surg* 1987;43:561–563.
30 Gallet B, Berrebi A, Grinda JM, et al. Severe intermittent intraprosthetic regurgitation after mitral valve replacement with subvalvular preservation. *J Am Soc Echocardiogr* 2001;14:314–316.

QUESTIONS

1. The first clinically successful prosthetic valve type was a
   a. Porcine bioprosthesis
   b. Caged-ball mechanical prosthesis
   c. Tilting-disc mechanical prosthesis
   d. Pericardial bioprosthesis

2. An important limitation of ultrasound imaging for the evaluation of prosthetic heart valves is
   a. Limited cross-sectional imaging planes
   b. Inability to quantify the severity of valve stenosis
   c. Acoustic shadowing
   d. Poor imaging resolution of structural details

3. Doppler echocardiography using the continuity method can estimate the effective orifice area of
   a. A bileaflet mechanical valve in the aortic position
   b. A caged-disc mechanical prosthesis in the mitral position
   c. A caged-ball mechanical prosthesis in the aortic position
   d. A caged-ball mechanical prosthesis in the mitral position

4. A Doppler echocardiographic characteristic of a pathologic regurgitant jet is
   a. Regurgitant jet originating from the hinge points of a mechanical valve
   b. Small regurgitant jet at the central coaptation point of a biologic valve
   c. Regurgitant jets of short duration early in the cardiac cycle during valve closure
   d. Eccentric regurgitant jets that tract along the wall of the receiving chamber

5. Prosthesis-patient mismatch is a term used to describe the following condition
   a. Native aortic valve annular diameter small relative to prosthetic valve diameter
   b. Native aortic valve annular diameter large relative to prosthetic valve diameter
   c. Prosthetic valve effective orifice area small relative to native aortic valve annulus diameter
   d. Prosthetic valve effective orifice area small relative to body surface area

6. Left ventricular outflow tract obstruction can occur after implantation of a
   a. Stented porcine valve in the mitral position
   b. Aortic root allograft
   c. Stentless aortic valve
   d. Mechanical bileaflet valve in the aortic position

7. Prosthetic valve dehiscence produces the following echocardiographic finding
   a. Increased effective orifice area
   b. Vegetations
   c. "Rocking" of the valve prosthesis
   d. Transvalvular regurgitation

8. The best transesophageal echocardiography (TEE) view for assessing valve leaflet motion in a patient with a mechanical bileaflet prosthesis in the aortic position is the
   a. Transgastric long axis
   b. Midesophageal aortic valve long axis
   c. Midesophageal long axis
   d. Midesophageal aortic valve short axis

9. A characteristic feature of regurgitant jets causing hemolysis in patients with prosthetic heart valves is

a. Low velocity, wide-based regurgitant jet
b. High velocity jet that collides with the valve prosthesis
c. Free regurgitant jet
d. Regurgitant jets originating from the hinge points of the occluder mechanism

10. An echocardiographic criteria for the diagnosis of prosthetic endocarditis is

a. Vegetations on the prosthetic valve
b. Leaflet calcification
c. Valve stenosis
d. Thrombosis of the valve

Answers appear at the back of the book.

14 Right Ventricle, Right Atrium, Tricuspid Valve, and Pulmonic Valve

Rebecca A. Schroeder, Gautam M. Sreeram, and Jonathan B. Mark

Right ventricular (RV) dysfunction is a common concern in the perioperative period. Inadequate myocardial protection, increases in pulmonary vascular resistance, air embolism to the RV coronary supply, and acute valvular dysfunction can compromise RV performance. This chapter surveys the echocardiographic approaches for evaluating the right side of the heart and its associated valves.

RIGHT VENTRICLE

Anatomy

Echocardiographic evaluation of the RV is complicated by the nongeometric, asymmetric, crescent shape of this chamber. The RV consists of a free wall and a septum that it shares with the left ventricle (LV). The RV free wall can be divided into basal, mid, and apical segments corresponding to the adjacent LV segments seen in the midesophageal (ME) four-chamber view. The RV can also be described in terms of its inflow and outflow tracts, which reflect the separate embryologic origins of these portions of the RV. An encircling muscular band separates the inflow and outflow portions of the RV. Its most apical portion, the moderator band, is often seen with transesophageal echocardiography (TEE). Present in most normal individuals, the moderator band is a muscular trabeculation extending from the lower interventricular septum to the anterior RV wall (Figure 14.1).

Transesophageal Echocardiographic Views

1. ***ME four-chamber view.*** This long-axis view of the RV allows assessment of the apical, mid, and basal segments of the RV. In the four-chamber view, the RV appears triangular in comparison with the elliptic LV, and its length is only two thirds the length of the LV (see Chapter 2 and Appendices).
2. ***ME RV inflow-outflow view.*** This view is often termed the *wraparound view*, owing to the fact that the right atrium (RA), RV, and pulmonary artery (PA) appear to "wrap around" the aortic valve and left atrium, describing a 270-degree arc (see Chapter 2 and Appendices).
3. ***Transgastric (TG) midpapillary short-axis view.*** In addition to allowing monitoring of LV function, this view serves to assess the RV free wall and interventricular septum. (Figure 14.2).
4. ***TG RV inflow view.*** This is a long-axis view of the RV similar to the TG two-chamber view of the LV. To acquire this view, one begins with the TG short-axis view of the RV (described earlier) and advances the multiplane angle to approximately 90 degrees, or until the RA and RV are seen in long axis, with the RV inflow and tricuspid valve (TV) centered in the image. Alternatively, one develops the TG two-chamber view of the left atrium and ventricle and then rotates the probe clockwise (rightward) until the two right-sided chambers are displayed. Both techniques should result in the same image of the RV inflow tract and the long axis of the RA and RV (Figure 14.3).

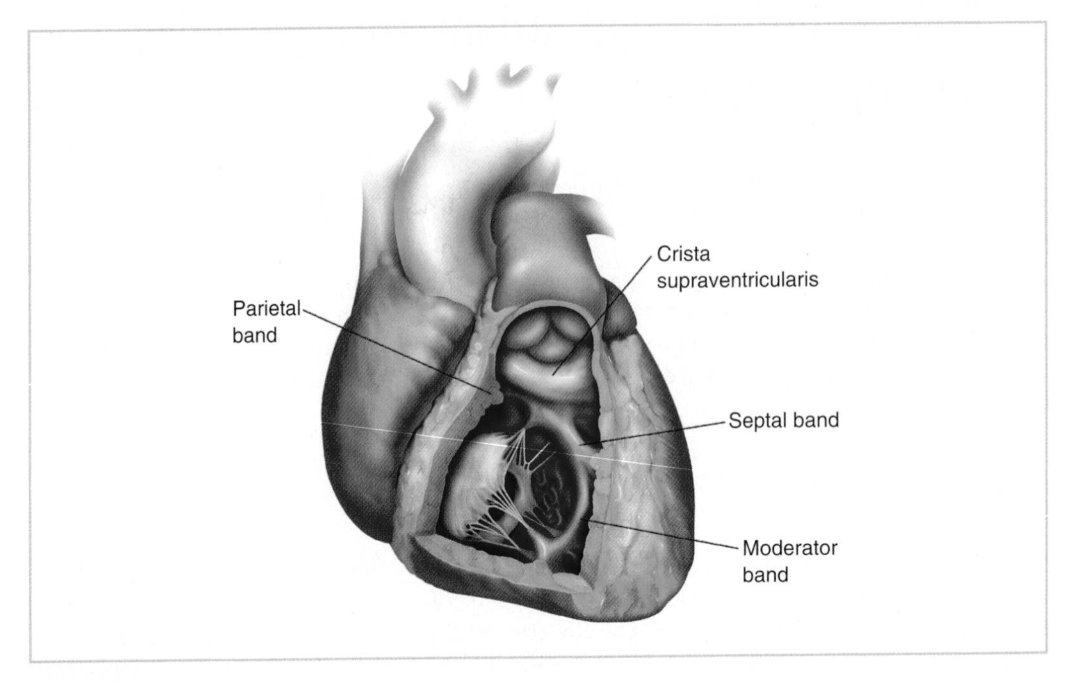

Figure 14.1. Schematic drawing of anatomic structures in the right ventricle.

Assessment of Global Right Ventricular Function

HYPERTROPHY

The normal thickness of the RV free wall is less than half that of the LV and measures less than 5 mm at end-diastole (1). RV hypertrophy is present when the RV free wall thickness exceeds 5 mm and may indicate elevated PA pressure or pulmonic stenosis (PS) (2). For example, in patients with chronic cor pulmonale, the RV wall thickness may exceed 10 mm

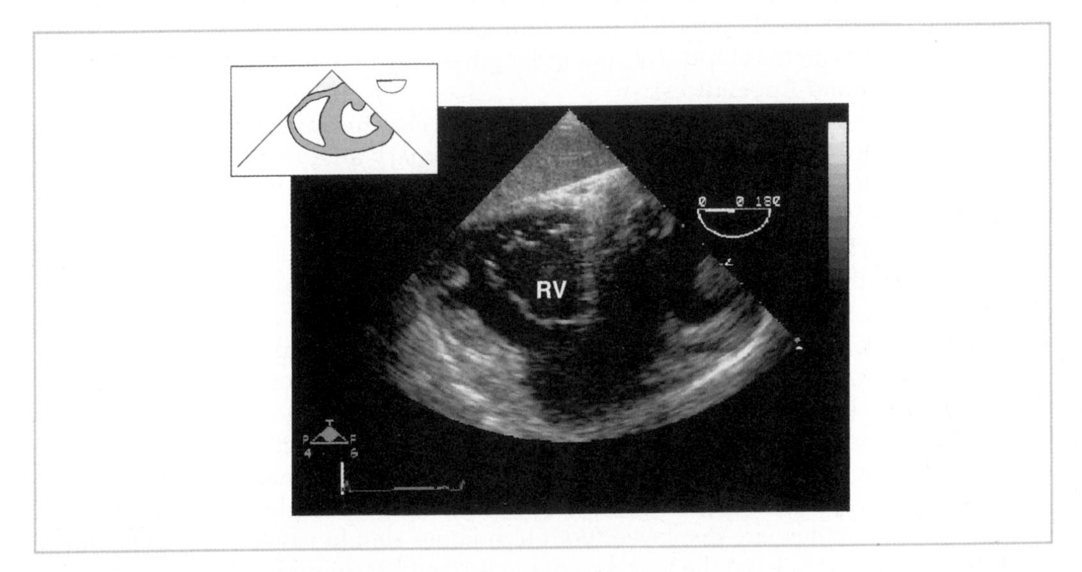

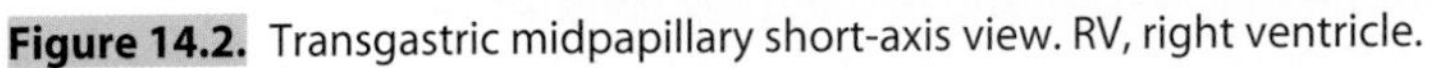
Figure 14.2. Transgastric midpapillary short-axis view. RV, right ventricle.

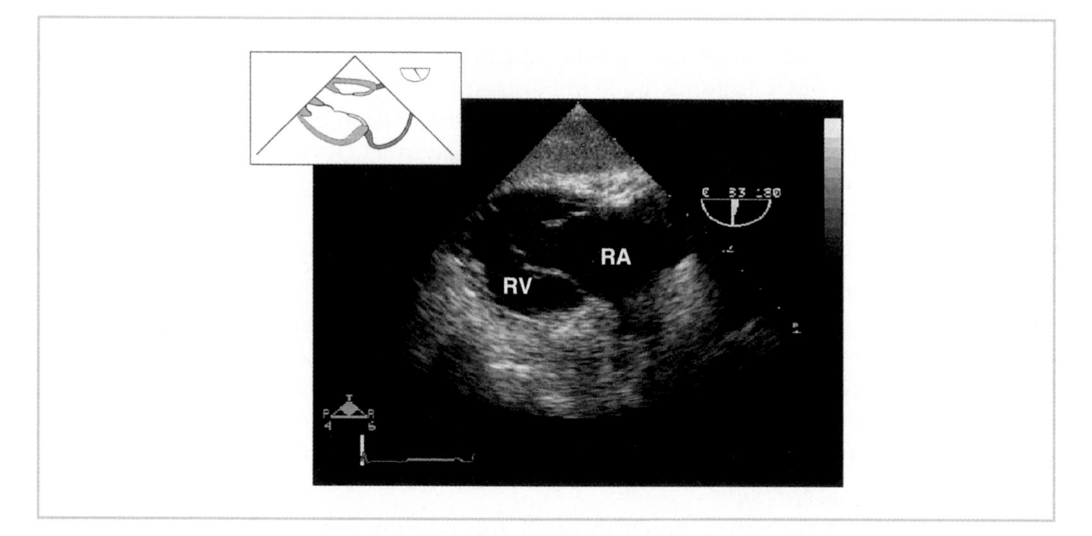

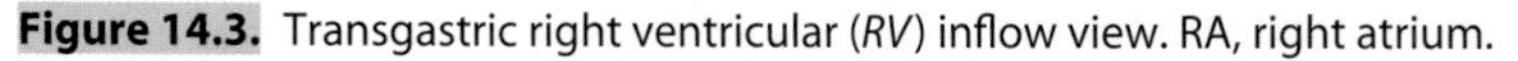

Figure 14.3. Transgastric right ventricular (*RV*) inflow view. RA, right atrium.

when severe pulmonary hypertension raises PA pressures to systemic levels. Additionally, the intracavitary trabecular pattern is more prominent, particularly at the apex in patients with RV hypertrophy.

DILATION

RV dilation may be seen with RV volume overload or chronic RV pressure overload. Normally, the RV end-diastolic cross-sectional area is approximately 60% of the area of the LV. As the RV dilates, its shape changes from triangular to round. An additional clue to the presence of RV dilation may be found through examination of the cardiac apex, which is formed by the apex of the LV in the ME four-chamber view. *When the RV forms part of the cardiac apex, then RV dilation is present.* With mild RV dilation, the RV area is 60% to 100% of the LV area. With moderate RV dilation, the RV area may equal the LV area, and with severe RV enlargement, the RV area often exceeds the LV area (2) (Figure 14.4).

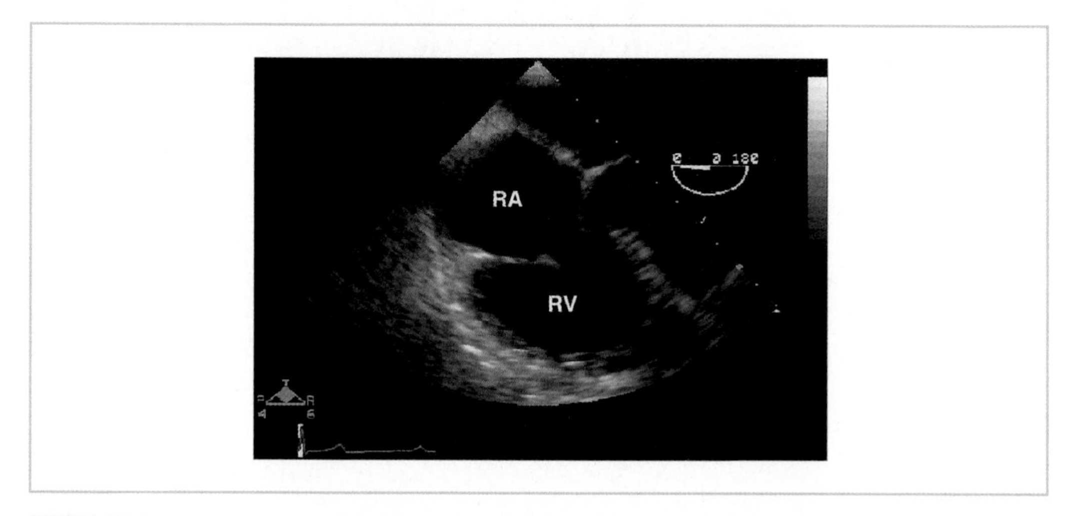

Figure 14.4. Right ventricular (*RV*) dilation. Note the change in shape of the dilated right ventricle from triangular to round. RA, right atrium.

SYSTOLIC FUNCTION

The quantitative assessment of RV systolic function is limited by the unique geometry of the RV. Furthermore, variations in chamber shape may occur readily with changes in volume. RV ejection is produced primarily by inward motion of the RV free wall, with lesser contributions from the right ventricular outflow tract (RVOT) and descent of the cardiac base (1). Signs of RV dysfunction include severe hypokinesis or akinesis of the RV free wall, RV enlargement, change in shape of the RV from crescent to round, and flattening or bulging of the interventricular septum from right to left.

TRICUSPID ANNULAR PLANE SYSTOLIC EXCURSION

Long-axis systolic excursion of the lateral aspect of the tricuspid annulus may be used as an indicator of RV systolic function. The normal tricuspid annular plane systolic excursion is 20 to 25 mm toward the cardiac apex, slightly greater than the normal mitral annular plane excursion (3). The tricuspid annulus tilts toward the apex, whereas the mitral annulus moves more symmetrically toward the apex, somewhat like a piston (3).

HEPATIC VENOUS FLOW PATTERNS

Blood from the hepatic veins flows through the inferior vena cava toward the RA. Examination of the patterns of flow velocity during the different phases of the cardiac cycle with pulsed wave Doppler can reveal important clues about RV function. Normal hepatic venous flow patterns have four phasic components (Figures 14.5 and 14.6). The initial forward flow toward the RA occurs during systole and is caused by the fall in atrial pressure resulting from atrial relaxation and apical movement of the TV during RV systole. This corresponds to the x-descent in atrial pressure. Forward flow in diastole is caused by a fall in atrial pressure during early ventricular filling and corresponds to the y-descent in atrial pressure. Two small retrograde waves may be observed, one corresponding to atrial contraction at end-diastole and one appearing at end-systole, before the y-descent in atrial pressure. When RV systolic function is impaired, the systolic inflow wave of hepatic venous flow is attenuated.

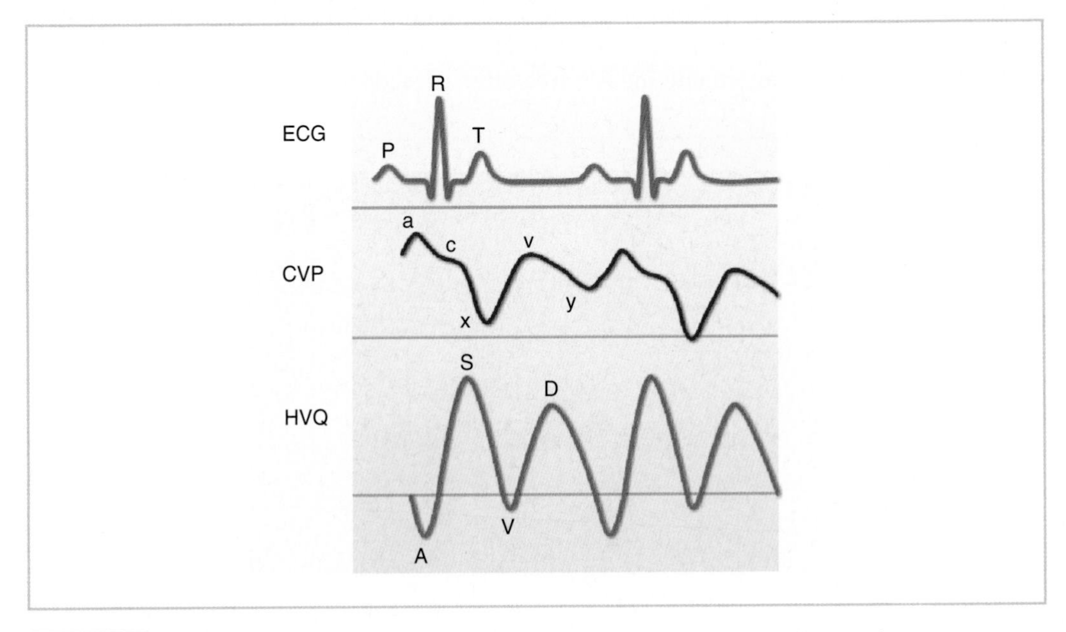

Figure 14.5. Schematic diagram of the correlation of hepatic vein flow (HVQ) with central venous pressure (CVP) and electrocardiogram (ECG).

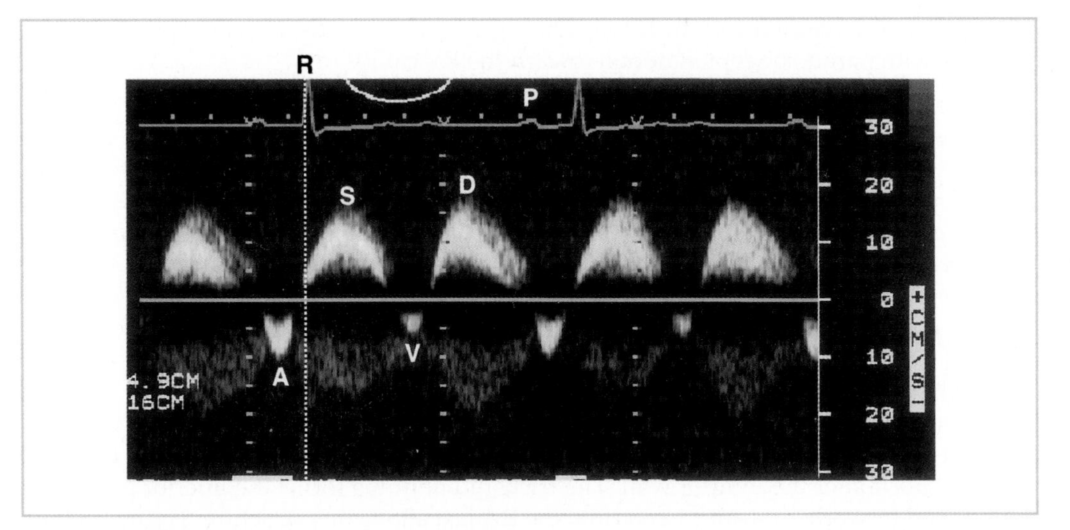

Figure 14.6. Pulsed wave Doppler image of normal hepatic venous flow with forward flow in systole and diastole and two small retrograde waves (A and V).

Assessment of Regional Right Ventricular Function

RV perfusion is supplied primarily by the right coronary artery, although a small portion of the anterior free wall may be supplied by the conus branch of the left anterior descending artery (4). Regional RV ischemia is difficult to detect with TEE, in part because RV wall motion is more dependent on afterload than that of the LV. Because the thin-walled RV is a volume-pumping chamber, its ejection fraction is extremely sensitive to acute increases in PA pressure. In contrast, the thick-walled LV is a pressure-pumping chamber, and its ejection fraction, although influenced by the systemic arterial pressure, is generally preserved despite marked increases in systemic arterial pressure. Furthermore, the irregularity and asymmetry of the RV make the detection of mild changes in contractility difficult. Akinesis or dyskinesis of the RV is more readily identified and is a very sensitive indicator of RV infarction (5). Less common findings in RV infarction include RV dilation, papillary muscle dysfunction, tricuspid regurgitation (TR), and paradoxic interventricular septal motion (6,7).

Interventricular Septum

Examination of interventricular septal motion can help distinguish RV volume overload from RV pressure overload.

RIGHT VENTRICULAR VOLUME OVERLOAD

RV volume overload may be seen with atrial or ventricular septal defects, TR, and pulmonic regurgitation (PR). Although features of RV volume and RV pressure overload may overlap, *RV volume overload more consistently produces dilation of the RV*. Examination of the interventricular septum may yield additional clues to the etiology of RV overload. Normally, the interventricular septum functions as part of the LV and maintains a convex curvature toward the RV throughout the cardiac cycle because its motion is controlled by the center of cardiac muscle mass located in the LV cavity. As the RV dilates or becomes hypertrophic and the RV mass increases to equal that of the LV, the septum flattens, and when RV mass exceeds LV mass, paradoxic septal motion appears. With RV volume overload, septal distortion is maximal at end-diastole, corresponding to the time of peak diastolic overfilling of the RV (8). During systole, the end-diastolic septal flattening reverses, with paradoxic septal motion toward the RV cavity.

RIGHT VENTRICULAR PRESSURE OVERLOAD

RV pressure overload may be seen with pulmonary hypertension or PS. RV pressure overload is characterized primarily by hypertrophy of the RV free wall and, if chronic, hypertrophy of the interventricular septum. *In contrast to RV volume overload, RV pressure overload produces maximal septal distortion at end-systole and early diastole, corresponding to the time of peak systolic afterloading of the RV* (9).

RIGHT ATRIUM

Anatomy

The RA is a thin-walled structure with an irregular shape. The superior vena cava enters the right anterior portion of the superior wall, and the inferior vena cava enters the right posterior portion of the inferior wall. The tricuspid annulus forms the inferior portion of the RA, and the coronary sinus opens into the RA just above this structure. The eustachian valve and Chiari network are two structures associated with the orifice of the inferior vena cava. Failure of regression of the right or inferior valve of the sinus venosus during gestation may result in a persistent eustachian valve. The Chiari network is a fenestrated, strand-like structure within the RA cavity. Although it most often arises from the orifice of the inferior vena cava, the Chiari network may have a primary origin of attachment to the RA free wall, coronary sinus, or interatrial septum.

Transesophageal Echocardiographic Views

TEE evaluation of the RA may be performed from the standard ME four-chamber view and the ME RV inflow-outflow view. The ME bicaval view is also very useful (see Chapter 2 and Appendices), particularly for evaluation of the RA free wall and interatrial septum. The superior-inferior dimension of the RA at end-systole is 4.2 ± 0.4 cm, and the medial-lateral dimension is 3.7 ± 0.4 cm (10).

TRICUSPID VALVE

Anatomy

The TV consists of the valve leaflets, chordae tendineae, papillary muscles, annular ring, and RV myocardium. The TV is trileaflet, with anterior, septal, and posterior leaflets of unequal size (Figure 14.7). Likewise, there are three papillary muscles; the anterior papillary muscle is the largest and originates from the moderator band as it courses toward the RV free wall. The chordae tendineae connect the papillary muscles to the tricuspid leaflets. The TV annulus is larger and located in a slightly more apical position than the mitral valve annulus. This normal apical displacement of the TV is not present in patients with endocardial cushion defects or primum atrial septal defects and is exaggerated in patients with Ebstein anomaly of the TV.

Transesophageal Echocardiographic Views

TEE evaluation of the TV focuses on the same standard views as those used to evaluate the RV.

1. ***ME four-chamber view.*** From the standard ME four-chamber view, slight rightward (clockwise) rotation of the probe moves the TV to the center of the scan plane;

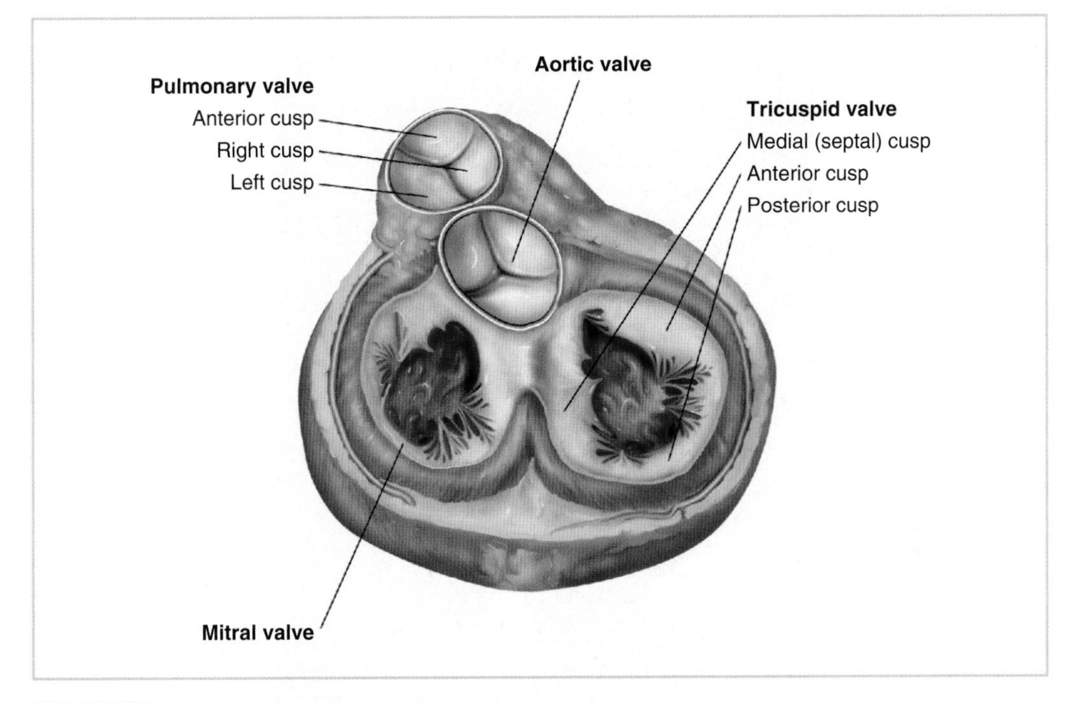

Figure 14.7. Schematic drawing of tricuspid valve anatomy.

advancing and withdrawing the transducer then allows imaging of the entire TV. This view demonstrates the anterior and septal leaflets.

2. *ME RV inflow-outflow view.* This view provides an additional, nearly orthogonal view of the TV. In this scan plane, the plane of the TV orifice is more nearly parallel to the ultrasound beam, so that quantitative measurement of TV flow velocities with continuous wave Doppler is optimized.
3. *TG views.* The TG views used to evaluate the RV also provide useful windows for imaging the TV. Rightward (clockwise) rotation of the TEE transducer from the TG mid short-axis view of the LV provides a good view of the TV in short axis, allowing identification of its septal, anterior, and posterior leaflets. The TG RV inflow view provides the best image of the chordae tendineae and RV papillary muscles supporting the TV.

Tricuspid Regurgitation

TR is the most common right-sided valvular lesion in adults. *It is most commonly caused by tricuspid annular dilation secondary to RV enlargement or pulmonary hypertension.*

TWO-DIMENSIONAL ECHOCARDIOGRAPHY

Features of TR may include dilation of the RA, RV, and tricuspid annulus, causing incomplete TV closure. TV prolapse may be seen when the valve leaflets are displaced beyond the tricuspid annulus into the RA.

Doppler echocardiography

COLOR FLOW DOPPLER

The degree of regurgitation is usually assessed with color flow Doppler; severe regurgitation is represented by a large color flow disturbance that fills more than half of the RA.

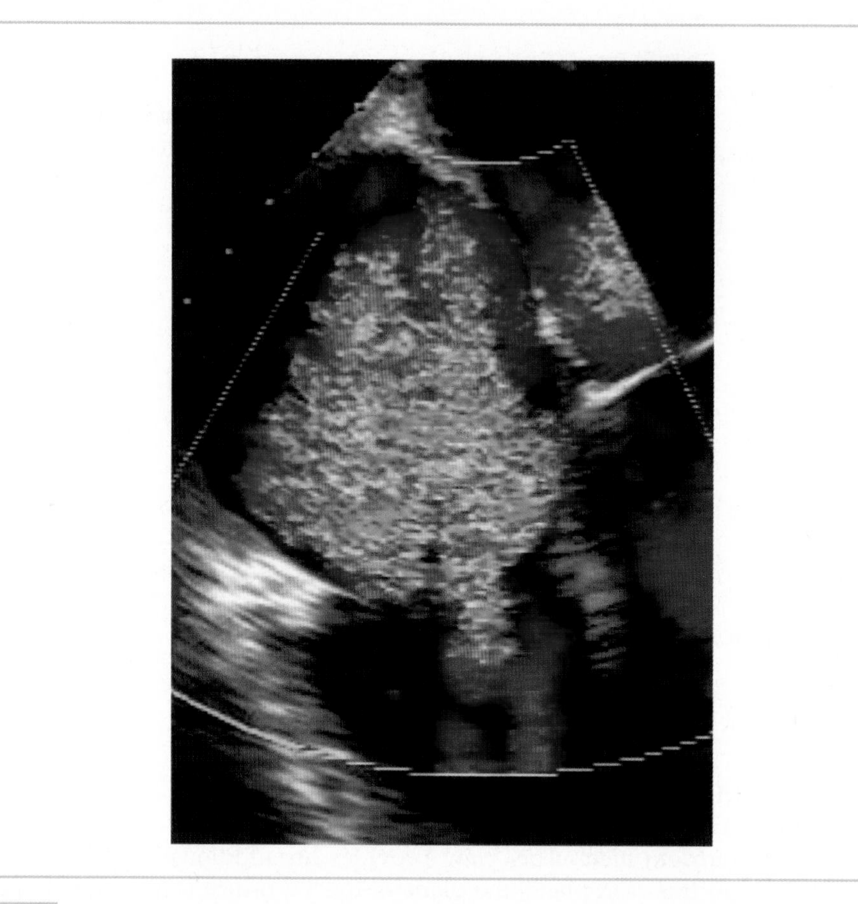

Figure 14.8. Color flow Doppler image demonstrating severe tricuspid regurgitation.

When the regurgitant jet is directed toward the atrial septum, it must be distinguished from normal caval inflow or an atrial septal defect (Figure 14.8).

PULSED WAVE DOPPLER

Assessment of caval or hepatic vein flow by pulsed wave Doppler may reveal abnormal reversed (retrograde) flow in systole, which represents severe TR (Figure 14.9).

USE OF CONTINUOUS WAVE DOPPLER TO DETERMINE THE PULMONARY ARTERY SYSTOLIC PRESSURE

The jet of TR can also be interrogated with continuous wave Doppler to measure the peak velocity of the regurgitant jet. With the simplified Bernoulli equation, the systolic transvalvular pressure gradient (ΔP) is calculated as $\Delta P = 4v^2$, where v is the peak velocity of the TR jet. RV systolic pressure is calculated by adding the tricuspid transvalvular gradient to an estimate of the RA pressure. In the absence of obstruction to RV outflow, this calculated RV systolic pressure provides a good estimate of the PA systolic pressure. Because the vast majority of patients with elevated PA pressure have some degree of TR, even in the absence of clinical signs, this measurement is widely applicable. However, when the calculation is performed, considerable care must be taken to align the ultrasound beam with the regurgitant jet to avoid an underestimation of the pressures (Figure 14.10).

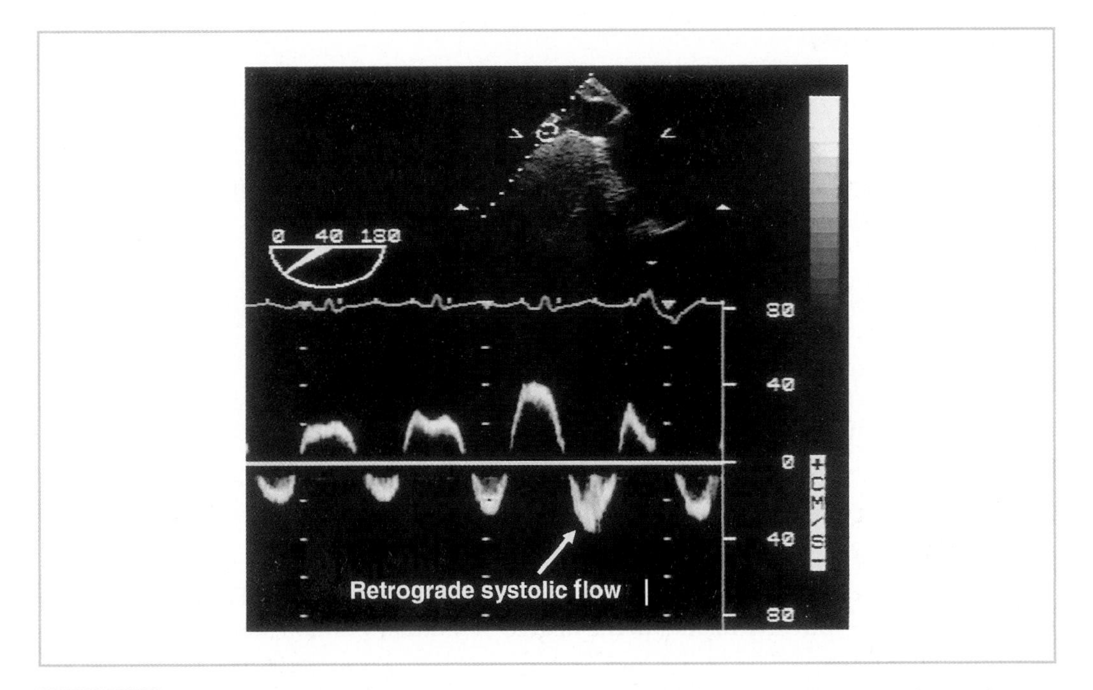

Figure 14.9. Pulsed wave Doppler image of hepatic venous flow with retrograde systolic flow, indicating severe tricuspid regurgitation.

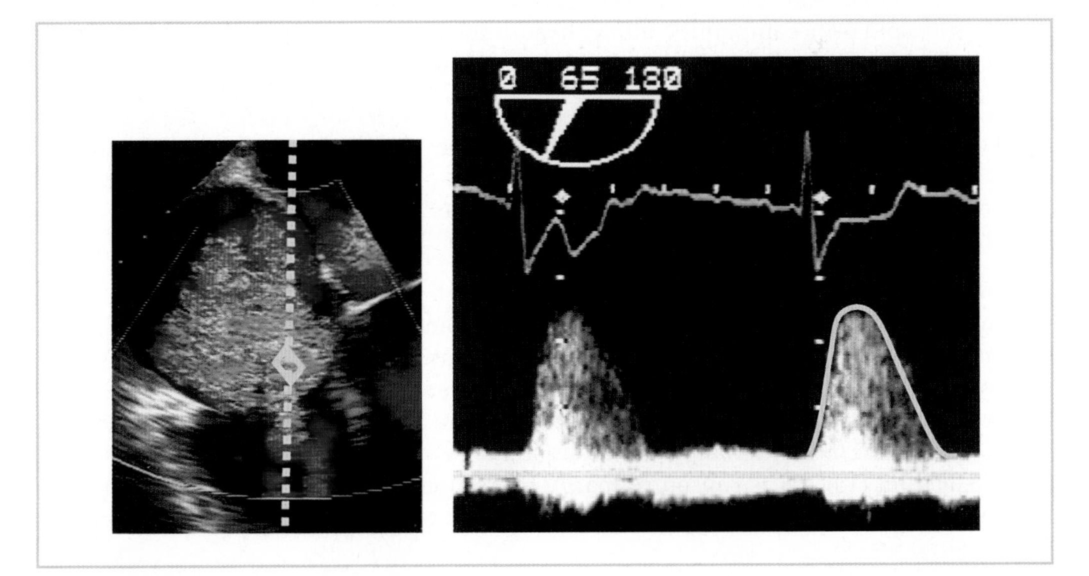

Figure 14.10. Continuous wave Doppler image of tricuspid regurgitation. A sample calculation of the pulmonary artery systolic pressure follows: $\Delta P = 4(2.6)^2$; systolic pulmonary artery pressure = 27 + right atrial pressure; systolic pulmonary artery pressure = 42 mm Hg. (Maslow A, Communale ME, Haering JM, et al. Pulsed wave Doppler measurements of cardiac output from the right ventricular outflow tract. *Anesth Analg* 1996;83:466–471.)

Tricuspid Stenosis

Tricuspid stenosis (TS) is diagnosed by the structural abnormalities of the leaflets and quantified by continuous wave Doppler examination of the transtricuspid flow.

TWO-DIMENSIONAL ECHOCARDIOGRAPHY

Characteristic features of TS include increased echo density of the thickened leaflets, diastolic leaflet doming, and decreased size of the TV orifice.

DOPPLER ECHOCARDIOGRAPHY

Because the tricuspid is the largest of the four cardiac valves, flow velocities are the lowest across this valve, typically less than 0.7 m/s (11). Although normal prosthetic valves in the tricuspid position may demonstrate peak velocities nearly twice normal, velocities greater than 1.5 m/s suggest significant TS, which may be confirmed by noting a deterioration in the effective valve orifice area (12).

Etiology of Tricuspid Valve Disease

ANNULAR DILATION

Annular dilation results in decreased leaflet coaptation, which leads to TR. The severity of the regurgitation is directly related to the degree of annular dilation, and the patient may require annuloplasty.

RHEUMATIC DISEASE

Rheumatic disease is the most common cause of acquired TS and results in fibrosis and scarring of the valve leaflets, leaflet doming, and commissural fusion. Reduced leaflet mobility and a smaller tricuspid orifice impair RV filling. In addition to TS, rheumatic tricuspid disease is characterized by TR, and the mitral valve is almost always involved.

ENDOCARDITIS

TV vegetations appear as oscillating, echo-dense masses attached to the leaflets or annulus. Typically, TV vegetations involve the atrial surface of affected leaflets and are larger than left-sided vegetations. Endocarditis may cause leaflet destruction that results in a flail leaflet and TR.

CARCINOID SYNDROME

Carcinoid tumors typically originate in the ileum and release serotonin, bradykinins, histamine, and prostaglandins. These vasoactive substances can damage the TV and pulmonic valve (PV), but they typically do not affect the left-sided heart valves as a consequence of inactivation of the tumor secretions in the lungs by monoamine oxidase. *Typical features include thickening and fibrosis of the TV and PV with moderate to severe TR, mild TS, and PS* (13). TR is caused primarily by restricted leaflet mobility. In contrast to rheumatic heart disease, carcinoid syndrome does not result in tricuspid leaflet doming or commissural fusion.

EBSTEIN ANOMALY

Ebstein anomaly is a congenital condition in which a malformed TV is displaced into the RV cavity. Typically, the anterior leaflet is the least affected, with the septal and posterior leaflets either rudimentary or absent. Ebstein anomaly should be suspected when the long-axis separation between the mitral and tricuspid annular planes exceeds 8 mm/m^2. This marked apical displacement of the TV causes a portion of the morphologic RV to become atrialized (14). Associated features may include impaired RV function, conduction abnormalities, and TR.

PULMONIC VALVE

Anatomy

The PV is a trileaflet valve with anterior, right, and left posterior semilunar cusps. The PV leaflets are thinner than the aortic valve leaflets and are directly connected to the musculature of the RV.

Transesophageal Echocardiographic Views

Because of its anterior position, detailed images of the PV are difficult to obtain with TEE. In fact, complete ultrasound assessment of the PV often requires a transthoracic echocardiographic (TTE) examination. The anteriorly located structures of the right side of the heart are more accessible to TTE imaging, and TTE also provides a greater number of acoustic windows and a greater ability to angulate the ultrasound probe, thereby improving the alignment of the Doppler beam.

1. ***ME RV inflow-outflow view.*** The most reliable TEE scan plan for imaging the PV is the ME RV inflow-outflow view. In this imaging plane, the aortic valve provides a useful anatomic guide. The PV can be identified in its normal location adjacent to the commissure separating the right and left coronary cusps of the aortic valve. Because the PV is oriented roughly at a right angle to the aortic valve, it is typically seen in its long axis when the aortic valve is seen in short axis.
2. ***ME aortic valve short-axis view.*** In the ME aortic valve short-axis view, the PV may be seen again in long axis adjacent to the aortic valve. Further gradual withdrawal of the probe will display the main PA above the PV and its bifurcation into left and right branches. With the probe at this position high in the esophagus, advancement of the transducer angle to 90 degrees reveals the upper esophageal aortic arch short-axis view. In many patients, the main PA, the PV, and the distal RVOT can be seen beneath the aortic arch. This may be a particularly useful view for detecting PR or quantifying PS with continuous wave Doppler because of the advantageous parallel alignment with blood flow (Figure 14.11).

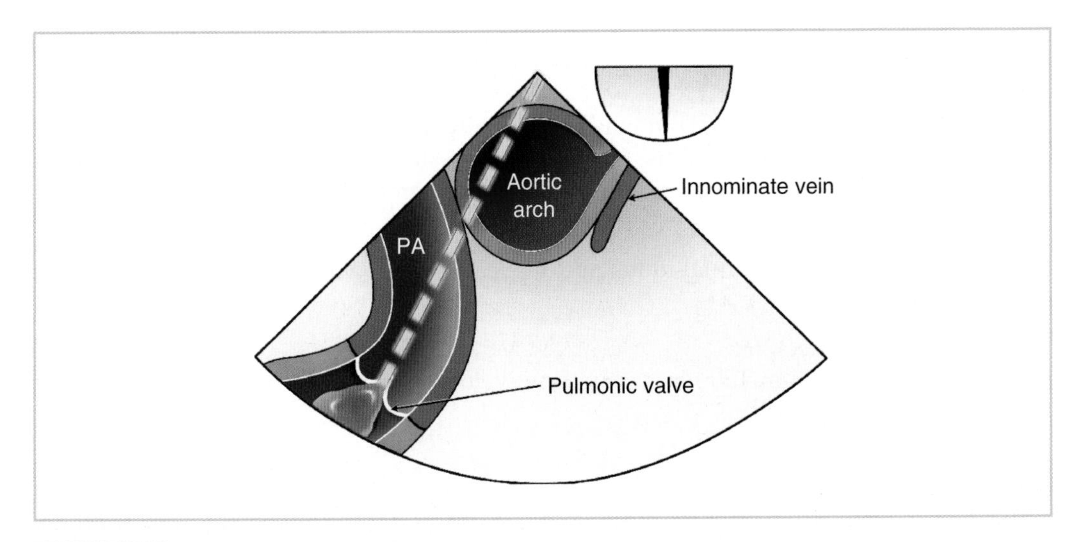

Figure 14.11. Schematic diagram of image used to evaluate the severity of pulmonic regurgitation or stenosis. PA, pulmonary artery.

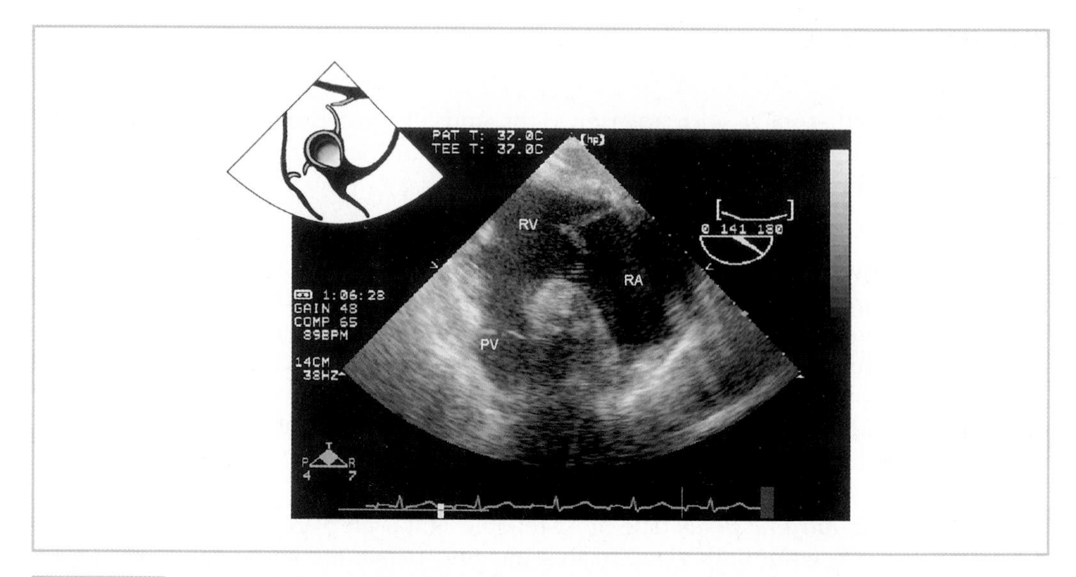

Figure 14.12. Transesophageal echocardiographic image of the transgastric pulmonic valve view. RV, right ventricle; RA, right atrium; PV, pulmonic valve.

3. ***TG PV view.*** From the TG LV midpapillary short-axis view, the probe is rotated to examine the structures of the right side of the heart. The transducer is then rotated to 110 to 140 degrees to obtain a view of the RVOT and PV (Figure 14.12). This view is useful for obtaining Doppler measurements of cardiac output from the RVOT (15).

Pulmonic Regurgitation

Congenital PR may result from abnormal cusp number or development. Acquired PR often results from pulmonary hypertension and subsequent annular dilation and structural distortion. Evaluation of the severity of PR is primarily through the qualitative examination of color flow Doppler mapping. *PA catheters have a minimal effect on the severity of PR or TR* (16).

Pulmonic Stenosis

PS is most commonly congenital but may occasionally result from rheumatic heart disease, carcinoid, or infective endocarditis. The severity of stenosis can be evaluated through qualitative assessments of leaflet motion or Doppler examination.

TWO-DIMENSIONAL ECHOCARDIOGRAPHY

Features of PS include abnormal initial systolic leaflet motion and subsequent doming of stenotic leaflets into the PA.

DOPPLER ECHOCARDIOGRAPHY

Doppler features of PS include increased flow velocities through the stenotic valve and turbulence beyond the orifice.

Ross Procedure

In 1967, Donald Ross first described the replacement of a diseased aortic valve with the patient's own PV (i.e., a pulmonary autograft). The TEE examination plays an important role in determining the suitability of candidates for this procedure. The examination should include an assessment for PR and measurement of the annular dimensions of both the pulmonic and aortic valves. *Significant PR or a mismatch in semilunar valve annular dimensions of more than 2 mm is considered a contraindication to this procedure* (17). *Following the Ross procedure, the patient should be evaluated for aortic insufficiency because this is a primary indication of autograft failure.* Additionally, an assessment of LV wall motion may reveal a new septal LV regional wall motion abnormality, which can result from the unintentional ligation of a septal coronary artery branch during dissection and excision of the PV.

SUMMARY

This chapter has explained how TEE provides an extensive evaluation of the right side of the heart and its associated valves. By using the standard TEE views, the echocardiographer can learn to evaluate the right side of the heart as efficiently as the left.

REFERENCES

1 Weyman AE. *Principles and practices of echocardiography*. Philadelphia: Lea & Febiger, 1994:914–915.
2 Otto CM. *Textbook of clinical echocardiography*. Philadelphia: WB Saunders, 2000:120–122.
3 Hammerstrom E, Wranne B, Pinto FJ, et al. Tricuspid annular motion. *J Am Soc Echocardiogr* 1991;14:131–139.
4 Wilson BC, Cohn JN. Right ventricular infarction complicating left ventricular infarction secondary to coronary heart disease. *Am J Cardiol* 1978;42:885–894.
5 D'Arcy B, Nanda NC. Two-dimensional echocardiographic features of right ventricular infarction. *Circulation* 1982;65:1967–1973.
6 Sharkey SW, Shelley W, Carlyle PF, et al. M-mode and two-dimensional echocardiographic analysis of the septum in experimental RV infarction: correlation with hemodynamic alterations. *Am Heart J* 1985;110:1210–1218.
7 Judgutt BI, Sussex BA, Sivaram CA, et al. Right ventricular infarction: two-dimensional echocardiographic evaluation. *Am Heart J* 1984;107:505–515.
8 Louie EK, Rich S, Levitsky S, et al. Doppler echocardiographic demonstration of the differential effects of right ventricular pressure and volume overload on left ventricular geometry and filling. *J Am Coll Cardiol* 1992;19:84–90.
9 Jardin F, Dubourg O, Bourdarias J-P. Echocardiographic pattern of acute cor pulmonale. *Chest* 1997; 111:209–217.
10 Triulizi MO, Gillam LD, Gentile F, et al. Normal adult cross-section echo values: linear dimensions and chamber areas. *Echocardiography* 1984;1:403–426.
11 Perez JE, Ludbrook PA, Ahumada GG. Usefulness of Doppler echocardiography in detecting tricuspid valve stenosis. *Am J Cardiol* 1985;55:601–603.
12 Feigenbaum H. *Echocardiography*, 5th ed. Philadelphia: Lea & Febiger, 1994:302–307.
13 Pellikka PA, Tajik AJ, Khandheria BK, et al. Carcinoid heart disease: clinical and echocardiographic spectrum in 74 patients. *Circulation* 1993;87:1188–1196.
14 Shiina A, Seward JB, Edwards WD, et al. Two-dimensional echocardiographic spectrum of Ebstein's anomaly: detailed anatomic assessment. *J Am Coll Cardiol* 1984;3:356–370.
15 Maslow A, Communale ME, Haering JM, et al. Pulsed wave Doppler measurements of cardiac output from the right ventricular outflow tract. *Anesth Analg* 1996;83:466–471.
16 Goldman ME, Guarino T, Fuster V, et al. The necessity for tricuspid valve repair can be determined intraoperatively by two-dimensional echocardiography. *J Thorac Cardiovasc Surg* 1987;94:542–550.
17 Albertucci M, Karp RB. Aortic valvular allografts and pulmonary autografts. In: Edmunds LH, ed. *Cardiac surgery in the adult*. New York: McGraw-Hill, 1997:911–937.

QUESTIONS

1. **Which of the following standard transesophageal echocardiography (TEE) scan planes allows an assessment of ventricular septal motion?**
   a. Midesophageal (ME) bicaval
   b. ME right ventricular (RV) inflow-outflow
   c. ME two-chamber
   d. Transgastric (TG) midpapillary short-axis
   e. TG RV inflow

2. **In patients with RV volume overload, ventricular septal displacement toward the left ventricle (LV) is maximal at which point in the cardiac cycle?**
   a. End-diastole
   b. End-systole
   c. Mid-diastole
   d. Mid-systole

3. **Which of the following structures is located in the RV?**
   a. Chiari network
   b. Crista terminalis
   c. Eustachian valve
   d. Moderator band

4. **In patients with RV dysfunction resulting from severe tricuspid regurgitation (TR), the cardiac apex**
   a. Is akinetic
   b. Is formed by the RV
   c. Is displaced toward the base of the heart
   d. Moves paradoxically outward during systole

5. **Which of the following standard TEE scan planes allows assessment of tricuspid stenosis (TS) with continuous wave Doppler?**
   a. ME bicaval
   b. ME RV inflow-outflow
   c. TG midpapillary short-axis
   d. TG RV inflow

6. **Which of the following features distinguishes Ebstein anomaly from endocardial cushion defects?**
   a. Conduction abnormalities
   b. Long-axis position of the TV
   c. Pulmonary stenosis (PS)
   d. TR

7. **In the schematic diagram of normal hepatic venous flow shown, which of the following waves is indicated by the asterisk?**
   a. A wave
   b. D wave
   c. S wave
   d. V wave

8. Which of the following diagnoses is suggested by the observation of a 5-mm tricuspid annular plane systolic excursion?

a. RV hypertrophy
b. RV hypokinesia
c. TR
d. TS

9. Compared with the aortic valve, the PV

a. Has a more rigid annular ring
b. Has thinner leaflets
c. Is adjacent to the noncoronary cusp
d. Is oriented in a parallel scan plane

10. Following a pulmonary autograft (Ross) procedure, which of the following must be sought/evaluated echocardiographically to detect the complications associated with this operation?

a. Aortic valve stenosis
b. Mitral valve regurgitation
c. TS
d. Ventricular septal function

Answers appear at the back of the book.

IV Clinical Challenges

15 Transesophageal Echocardiography for Coronary Revascularization

Stuart J. Weiss and John G. Augoustides

Transesophageal echocardiography (TEE) has evolved to become a critical element in the advanced care of the cardiac surgical patient. Its importance for valvular surgery is widely accepted, but its role for coronary artery bypass grafting (CABG) is still evolving. TEE is a powerful and versatile tool that can be used to diagnose the cause of (a) ischemia, (b) acute hemodynamic decompensation, or the presence of (c) occult pathology, (d) to facilitate the conduct and management of bypass, and (e) to initiate and titrate pharmacologic therapies. Echocardiography can also be used as a hemodynamic monitor to determine cardiac output (CO), stroke volume, pulmonary artery (PA) and right ventricular (RV) systolic pressures. At the current time, it is doubtful that TEE will supplant the PA catheter for hemodynamic monitoring. TEE and the PA catheter have complementary roles in the perioperative setting; the choice depends on factors such as clinician preference, cost, and resource availability. The PA catheter permits continuous measurement of intracardiac pressures and CO, particularly in the postoperative setting, when TEE is often not readily available. Although the PA catheter detects cardiac dysfunction, it often does not diagnose the cause. The forte of TEE is the rapid diagnosis of cardiac dysfunction and analysis that immediately affects both surgical and hemodynamic management, even in the setting of PA catheterization.

INDICATIONS AND APPLICATIONS OF TRANSESOPHAGEAL ECHOCARDIOGRAPHY

TEE is particularly useful during CABG to assess the clinical significance of dynamic valvular dysfunction, diagnose the cause of ischemia and acute hemodynamic instability, and assist in the conduct of circulatory management and surgery. TEE is the approach most commonly used because the examination does not interfere with the progress of surgery. A number of studies support an important role of TEE in improving outcome, especially in high-risk patients undergoing coronary revascularization (1). In comparison with historical matched controls, patients evaluated with TEE show decreased rates of mortality and infarction. Savage et al. observed that in 33% of high-risk patients undergoing CABG, at least one major surgical management alteration was initiated on the basis of TEE and that 51% of patients had at least one major anesthetic or hemodynamic change initiated by a TEE finding. However, the importance of TEE for routine CABG surgery in patients with preserved function is less clear.

The value of perioperative echocardiography was evaluated in 1996 by the American Society of Anesthesiologists and the Society of Cardiovascular Anesthesiologists (2) and again by the American Heart Association and American College of Cardiology in 2003 (3). The application of TEE for CABG was assessed to be a class II indication; "conditions for which there is conflicting evidence and/or a divergence of opinion about the usefulness/efficacy of a procedure or treatment." Patients at increased risk of myocardial ischemia, infarction, or hemodynamic disturbance were categorized as a class IIa indication (weight of evidence/opinion is in favor of usefulness/efficacy). The role of intraoperative

Table 15.1 Uses of transesophageal echocardiography in patients undergoing coronary artery bypass grafting

To supplement an incomplete cardiac workup
Confirm diagnosis and evaluate cardiac function for patients undergoing emergent surgery
Provide an updated examination of cardiac and valvular function
Evaluate potential target sites of coronary revascularization by administration of contrast agents (evaluate coronary perfusion) or dobutamine (stress test to evaluate viability)
To assist the surgeon in the conduct of circulatory management
Positioning/placement of:
Aortic cross-clamp
Coronary sinus catheter
Intra-aortic balloon pump
Femoral venous cannula
Ventricular assist device cannula
MIDCAB (endoaortic catheter, venous cannula, pulmonary artery drainage catheter, coronary sinus catheter)
To diagnose cause of acute cardiovascular compromise
To diagnose impact of previously unrecognized pathology on surgical procedure
Valvular pathology:
Aortic insufficiency distension of the ventricle during cardiopulmonary bypass
Mitral regurgitation (MR): dynamic MR, ischemic MR
Patent foramen ovale/atrial septal defect
Emboli, thrombus, or mass
Persistent left superior vena cava
Onset of regional wall motion abnormalities
Aortic dissection
Atherosclerotic disease
To facilitate the conduct of circulatory management or surgical procedure
Redo sternotomy
Conduct of bypass: assess left ventricle chamber size for distension
Plan management strategies for separation from cardiopulmonary bypass for patients with poor cardiac function
Separation from cardiopulmonary bypass (titration of volume and pharmacologic support)

TEE for the evaluation of regional myocardial function, coronary anatomy, or graft patency was deemed less apparent, class IIb (usefulness/efficacy is less well established by evidence/opinion). However, these guidelines were based on limited clinical data and need to be periodically reevaluated in light of advances in technology, improvements in surgical and anesthetic techniques, and an expanding base of literature.

In our current health care environment, a significant number of patients arrive in the operating room for surgery with an incomplete preoperative evaluation. TEE can serve an important function in the evaluation of patients who are undergoing emergent surgery with an inadequate cardiac evaluation and the potential for undiagnosed cardiac pathology that would affect perioperative management. TEE can assist the surgeon, cardiologist, and anesthesiologist at each stage of CABG surgery (Table 15.1).

CONTRAINDICATIONS AND COMPLICATIONS OF TRANSESOPHAGEAL ECHOCARDIOGRAPHY

The risk for complications associated with insertion of the TEE probe and performance of the examination is low. In a case series of 7,200 cardiac surgical patients studied at a single institution, the reported incidence of morbidity was 0.2% (severe odynophagia, 0.1%; displacement of the endotracheal tube, 0.3%; upper gastrointestinal hemorrhage,

0.03%; dental injury, 0.03%; esophageal perforation, 0.01%) (4). Although esophageal trauma leading to mediastinitis is rare, it has a significant mortality of approximately 10% (5). Therefore, esophageal pathology (e.g., web, stricture, diverticulum, cancer) and prior esophageal surgery are contraindications to insertion of the TEE probe. In such cases, surface scanning with a hand-held probe should be considered.

SURFACE SCANNING: EPICARDIAL AND EPIAORTIC SCANNING

The alternative to TEE is surface scanning with a hand-held probe from a standard echocardiography machine or a less expensive surface ultrasound device that is used to image the internal jugular vein for cannulation (6). Surface scanning of the heart (epicardial imaging) and aorta (epiaortic imaging) is the procedure of choice when TEE is contraindicated or the acoustic window for TEE is inadequate. *Because the air-filled trachea is interposed, TEE provides only limited imaging of the ascending aorta. Epiaortic scanning is being increasingly used to detect severe atheromatous disease, a significant risk factor for poor neurologic outcome.*

Surface scanning with a hand-held probe requires considerable patience and experience if optimal results are to be obtained (Figure 15.1). The ultrasound probe is inserted in a sterile sheath filled with saline solution and positioned such that a column of fluid acts as a "standoff" between the structure of interest and the ultrasound crystal. This standoff enhances the imaging of structures in the near field (i.e., the anterior surface of the ascending aorta). Alternatively, a standoff device can be purchased or made to improve visualization of the near field. The probes typically feature 5- to 10-MHz transducers with two-dimensional and Doppler capability. Although surface scanning is suitable for most applications that require TEE, *the major applications of surface scanning include assessing the severity of aortic atherosclerotic disease, confirming the patency of coronary grafts (7,8), elucidating the anatomy of intramyocardial coronary vessels, and diagnosing acute aortic dissections.*

BASIC APPROACH TO THE TRANSESOPHAGEAL ECHOCARDIOGRAPHIC EXAMINATION

The indication for the study should determine the direction and focus of the perioperative TEE examination. Regardless of the indication, each study should proceed in a routine and organized manner in which each structure of the heart and great vessels is examined in several imaging planes (9). The initial examination before cardiopulmonary bypass (CPB) is usually a more thorough standardized approach, whereas the post-CPB, "postintervention" examination is commonly focused on a full assessment of the intervention and possible complications thereof. Digital cine loops of pre-CPB cardiac function should be recorded for readily available review and comparison with the post-CPB examination findings. Excessive focus of the pre-CPB examination on one aspect may jeopardize patient care as a consequence of missed or incorrect diagnoses. Unexpected findings are not uncommon and may have a significant impact on perioperative management. For example, the diagnosis of persistent left superior vena cava is a contraindication to retrograde cardioplegia, and the finding of previously unrecognized dynamic mitral valvular insufficiency might alter surgical management (10). The strategy of progressing through a standardized protocol will decrease the chances of missing important findings (Table 15.1). A complete TEE examination should include a written report for the medical record and a review of the findings with the cardiac surgeon. The process of writing a report provides a mechanism for critically reviewing the recorded study and making sure that all relevant images and measurements have been acquired.

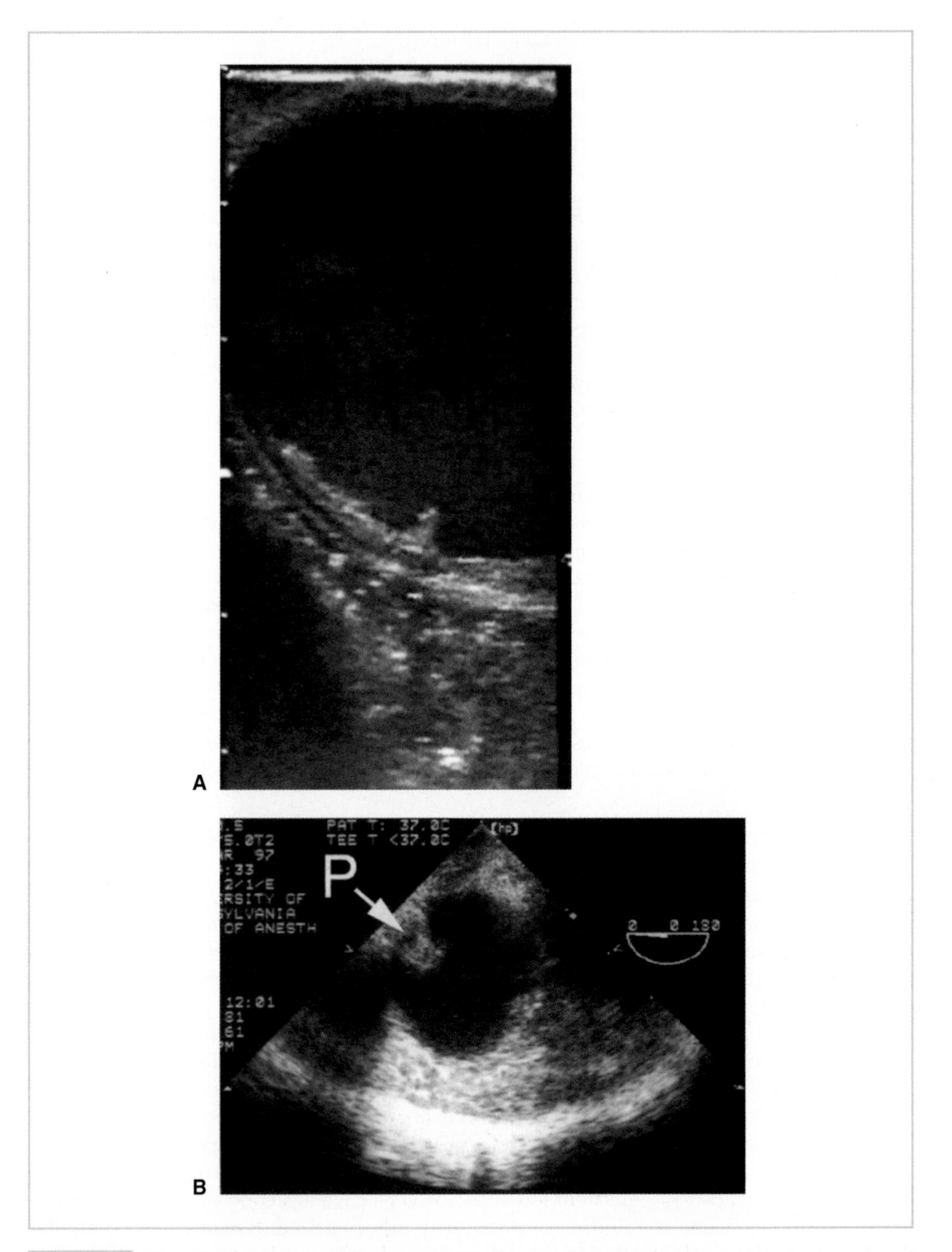

Figure 15.1. Ultrasound imaging of the aorta is useful for detecting and assessing the severity of atherosclerotic disease. **A:** A high-frequency ultrasound probe that is placed in a sterile sheath is used to examine the ascending aorta before aortic cannulation and cross-clamping. A mobile plaque can be visualized in the posterior aspect of the aorta. **B:** A transesophageal echocardiographic probe can be used to evaluate the severity of disease in the descending thoracic aorta. A large plaque (*P*) is visualized just distal to the left subclavian artery.

Table 15.2 Assessment of cardiac function by transesophageal echocardiography

Preload
LV end-diastolic area
LV end-diastolic pressure (estimated from AI jet)
LA pressure (estimated from pulmonary vein flow)
Contractility
Fractional area change (calculated)
Ejection fraction (visual estimate)
Segmental wall motion
Fractional shortening
Tissue Doppler
Quantitative hemodynamics
Stroke volume/cardiac output
Systemic vascular resistance
RV systolic pressure
Diastolic function
Mitral inflow velocities
Pulmonary vein blood flow velocities

LV, left ventricle; AI, aortic insufficiency; LA, left atrium; RV, right ventricle.

TRANSESOPHAGEAL ECHOCARDIOGRAPHIC ASSESSMENT OF VENTRICULAR FUNCTION

Two-Dimensional Measurements of Ventricular Size

TEE is a versatile monitor of cardiac function in that it can provide either a rapid qualitative assessment of chamber size and function or quantitative measures of chamber size, intracardiac pressures, and hemodynamic indices, such as stroke volume and CO (Table 15.2). Quantitative assessment of chamber size and ventricular function is a common task that provides prognostic value regarding cardiac function postbypass and the need for pharmacologic support. For example, significant LV dilation would predict difficulty in separating from bypass or the presence of ventricular hypertrophy would support the need for increased perfusion pressure and diagnosis of diastolic dysfunction. A good resource for the normative (reference) values that describe both normal and the severity of pathology is the consensus paper proposed by the American Society of Echocardiography (11).

Left ventricular (LV) function is first evaluated from the midesophageal (ME) four-chamber long-axis and two-chamber views; the TEE probe should then be advanced into the stomach to obtain a series of transgastric (TG) short-axis views. The ME views permit rapid qualitative evaluation of all four cardiac chambers but are used less commonly for quantitative planimetry because of apical foreshortening. The TG short-axis ventricular views are most commonly used to monitor global and regional function because the image planes are relatively easy to maintain (Figure 15.2). Experienced echocardiographers use these views to quantify global ventricular function, the ejection fraction, and the adequacy of the LV preload. In a study by Cheung et al. (12), TEE was highly sensitive for detecting changes in LV function and preload following controlled decreases in the circulating blood volume. The changes in the LV end-diastolic area (EDA) accurately reflected the decrement in LV preload and PA pressures. This application is perhaps the best method for assessing the effects volume or inotropic administration during separation from CPB or periods of bleeding.

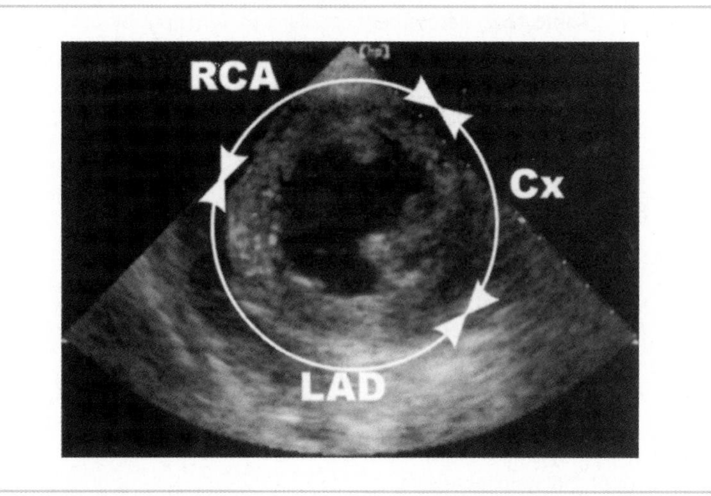

Figure 15.2. The transgastric short-axis view is routinely used intraoperatively to assess left ventricular function and diagnose myocardial ischemia. Myocardial function at the midpapillary level reflects the vascular distribution of the three major coronary arteries: the left anterior descending (*LAD*), circumflex (*Cx*), and right coronary (*RCA*) arteries.

Planimetry can quantify changes in LV area (LV EDA and end-systolic area [ESA]). The fractional area change (FAC) is then calculated as follows: FAC = 100 × (EDA − ESA)/EDA. The TEE-derived changes in LV area are accurate and reproducible but may not directly correlate with changes in LV volume. Assumptions based on LV areas measured in one plane may not reliably reflect LV volume, particularly in patients with regional wall motion abnormalities (RWMAs) and LV aneurysms. Geometric algorithms can be used to calculate LV volume; they typically require multiple measurements in several imaging planes. The correlation of end-diastolic and end-systolic volumes with the ejection fraction is clinically acceptable but consistently underestimates the true changes in ventricular volume because of foreshortening of LV length in the four-chamber view. *Because performing planimetry and the aforementioned calculations is time consuming, their application is usually limited to off-line analysis.*

Until recently, TEE was limited in regard to the continuous processing and reporting of reliable quantitative numeric parameters. The development of continuous automated border detection uses proprietary algorithms to discriminate the endocardial interface. Tracking of the continuous changes in chamber area, FAC, are calculated on-line by measuring the difference between the LV end-diastolic and the LV ESAs (see Figure 3.5). Perrino et al. (13) demonstrated good correlation between automated measurement of ventricular dimensions and off-line manual measurements, but acceptance of this proprietary automated border detection technology of has not gained wide clinical popularity. However, the promise of on-line three-dimensional TEE may prove more useful for quantitative assessment of both global and regional ventricular function.

Quantitative Assessment of Left Ventricular Function: Cardiac Output

Two-dimensional and Doppler echocardiography are used to evaluate stroke volume and CO. This is accomplished by measuring the transit of blood through an area of known size (e.g., the mitral valve, LV outflow tract, or PA). Although the transmitral inflow velocity is easy to obtain, its agreement with measurements obtained by thermodilution is unacceptable because of inaccuracy in measuring the area of the mitral valve orifice (14). Savino et al. (15) describe a better correlation with the use of the transpulmonic flow. This approach may be limited by the difficulty of consistently interrogating the transpulmonic blood flow and measuring the dimensions of the proximal PA. The alternative method is to measure the transit of blood through the LV outflow tract or aortic valve in the TG long-axis and deep TG long-axis views (16) (see Figure 6.3). Combining the TEE-derived CO with the mean arterial pressure and the mean central venous pressure can yield the systemic vascular resistance. These measures of stroke volume, CO, and systemic vascular resistance are particularly useful when PA catheter measurements are not available.

Assessment of Intracardiac Pressures

TEE measures important intracardiac pressures by quantifying the pressure gradient across a regurgitant valve (Table 15.2). The flow velocity of the regurgitant jet (v) is measured with Doppler echocardiography. The pressure gradient (ΔP) across the regurgitant valve is then calculated with the simplified Bernoulli equation: $\Delta P = 4v^2$. The accuracy of the measurements depends on the presence of valvular insufficiency and correct alignment of the regurgitant jet. Like the TEE measurements of CO, these measurements are laborious and not automated. Consequently, the PA catheter is currently still preferred over TEE for the on-line measurement of intracardiac pressures.

MONITORING OF ISCHEMIA

Predictive Value of Regional Wall Motion Abnormalities for Myocardial Infarction

The clinical application of TEE to detect and monitor myocardial ischemia gained considerable attention in the early 1980s (17). TEE can diagnose and characterize myocardial ischemia by a more sensitive method than either the electrocardiogram or PA catheter. Canine studies documented that the reduction in coronary blood flow occurs in rapid association with the decrease in regional myocardial function and precedes any ischemic changes on the electrocardiogram (18,19). The TG short-axis view is the one most commonly used to monitor and diagnose ischemia because it reflects the distribution of all three major coronary vessels (Figure 15.2).

In two classic studies by Roizen et al. (20) and Smith et al. (17), the occurrence of postoperative myocardial infarction was increased in patients who exhibited new RWMAs during CABG or aortic vascular surgery. The incidence of postoperative infarction was more strongly associated with the new RWMAs than with new electrocardiographic changes. *Although TEE may be sensitive in diagnosing ischemia, a new RWMA does not always predict myocardial infarction.* In the study of Leung et al. (21), a myocardial infarction was subsequently diagnosed in only one of eight patients in whom a new, persistent RWMA had developed. This apparent discrepancy is consistent with the concept of "myocardial stunning," in which an acute episode of myocardial ischemia can result in wall motion abnormalities that later resolve without any permanent injury. Alternatively, new RWMAs may be related to loading conditions of the ventricle, electrolyte abnormalities, blood viscosity, level of inotropic support, hypothermia, off-pump CABG stabilizing devices, cardiac pacing, and bundle branch conduction abnormalities. *Any apparent dyskinesis that is attributable to conduction abnormalities can be differentiated from ischemia by closely evaluating the area in question for the presence of myocardial thickening.*

Table 15.3 Strategy for management of a new regional wall motion abnormality after separation from cardiopulmonary bypass

Increase the coronary perfusion pressure
Restore normal conduction pathways (sinus rhythm, A-pace)
Normalize electrolytes and arterial blood gases
Inspect coronary grafts
Visual inspection and stripping
Doppler flow examination
Echo contrast examination
Return to cardiopulmonary bypass

Strategy for the Management of a New Regional Wall Motion Abnormality after Cardiopulmonary Bypass

The appearance of new RWMAs after bypass is common, but the interpretation is complicated by factors such as infusion of inotropic drugs, inadequate recovery from cardioplegia, conduction abnormalities, and transient ischemia resulting from the distal coronary embolization of air or debris. Although some investigators have suggested that the detection of new RWMAs warrants further surgical intervention, no prospective study is available to support such an aggressive approach. The additional morbidity/mortality associated with the resumption of bypass to place another graft would likely outweigh the potential benefit in most cases. A more rational, conservative approach may include the following: increasing the coronary perfusion pressure to flush any emboli or residual cardioplegic agents, restoring normal conduction pathways, normalizing the arterial blood gases and electrolytes, and inspecting the coronary grafts to confirm patency (Table 15.3). New RWMAs, such as ventricular septal wall motion abnormalities, are often related to conduction disturbances caused by ventricular pacing or bundle branch block. Atrial pacing commonly restores the normal ventricular conduction pathway and contractile synchrony of the ventricular septum. If atrial pacing is not possible, the most common bundle branch conduction abnormalities usually resolve within the first postoperative day. In addition, the surgeon can assess graft patency and flow by visual inspection to confirm the absence of graft kinking or torsion, by stripping the vein graft to confirm refill, by palpation, and by use of a Doppler flow probe. Decreased flow in an arterial conduit can result from poor distal runoff, a compromised anastomosis, or vasospasm that can be effectively treated by infusing a calcium channel antagonist such as nicardipine. Differentiation between poor perfusion and stunned myocardium is more difficult. Possible strategies include epicardial scanning and the administration of a contrast agent to determine coronary flow patterns. If the area demonstrates flow of the contrast agent, the RWMA may resolve with time. The absence of contrast agent suggests a technical problem at the anastomosis or distal obstruction in the native coronary. Such information can help guide any possible surgical intervention. The technique of contrast perfusion can also be performed before bypass. If a specific area is likely to be infarcted, as demonstrated by the absence of contrast flow and significant wall thinning, surgical interventions are not likely to be of value. This technique is uncommonly applied in routine operative practice, and its impact remains to be determined.

ACUTE CARDIAC DYSFUNCTION: ASSESSMENT AND MANAGEMENT

Cardiac dysfunction may develop at any time during the perioperative period. *The prompt, accurate diagnosis of the cause of hemodynamic instability is one of the major applications, if not the forte, of TEE.* Ultrasound examination of the heart and great vessels can provide a quick

Table 15.4 Echocardiographic findings in hypotension and cardiac dysfunction

	LVEDA	LVESA	FAC	CO
Decreased LV preload	↓	↓	0	↓
Decreased LV afterload	0	↓↓	↑↑	↑
Increased LV afterload	↑	↑	↓	↓
LV dysfunction	↑	↑↑	↓↓	↓
RV dysfunction	↓	↓	↓/0	↓
Acute mitral regurgitation LV distension	↑↑	0/↑	↓	↓

LVEDA, left ventricular end-diastolic diameter; LVESA, left ventricular end-systolic diameter; FAC, fractional area change; CO, cardiac output; LV, left ventricle; RV, right ventricle; ↑, increased; ↓, decreased; 0, unchanged.

assessment of the primary factors related to hypotension: preload, afterload, myocardial contractility, valvular function, and integrity of the aorta. TEE can significantly affect the surgical and anesthetic management, especially in high-risk patients or in patients with acute hemodynamic collapse. The reader is reminded that post-CPB cardiac function must be interpreted in the context of the prebypass examination findings and the occurrence of any significant bypass events.

The echocardiographic examination quickly provides data that guides pharmacologic therapy and volume resuscitation. In several studies, echocardiography significantly modified both surgical and hemodynamic decision making during the perioperative period (22,23). The echocardiographic findings associated with common causes of hypotension and cardiac dysfunction are presented in Table 15.4.

Hypovolemia

Hypovolemia, a common cause of perioperative hypotension, is often related to the obstruction of venous inflow as a consequence of prebypass cannula placement, volume re-equilibration after separation from bypass, and bleeding. Hypovolemia can be differentiated from low systemic vascular resistance by assessing the LV chamber size and contractility. The assessment of LV chamber size by TEE has been shown to be a sensitive measure of LV preload. In the study of Cheung et al. (12), the quantitative analysis of changes in the TG short-axis area could reliably detect even a 2.5% decrease in intravascular volume.

Dynamic Mitral Regurgitation

The development of mitral regurgitation may be associated with hypotension, increased pulmonary pressures, RV failure, and decreased CO. Excessive volume resuscitation or increased afterload can result in LV distension with incomplete coaptation of the mitral leaflets and a central jet of regurgitation. Alternatively, ischemia or LV dysfunction can lead to papillary muscle dysfunction or LV distension. Significant mitral regurgitation may require mitral valve surgery or hemodynamic management, such as adjusting the systemic vascular resistance, administering inotropic agents, or decreasing the LV preload.

Right Ventricular Dysfunction

RV dysfunction is another common cause of perioperative hypotension. The ME four-chamber view allows a rapid assessment of ventricular chamber size and function. RV dysfunction is associated with RV dilation, tricuspid regurgitation, abnormal septal wall

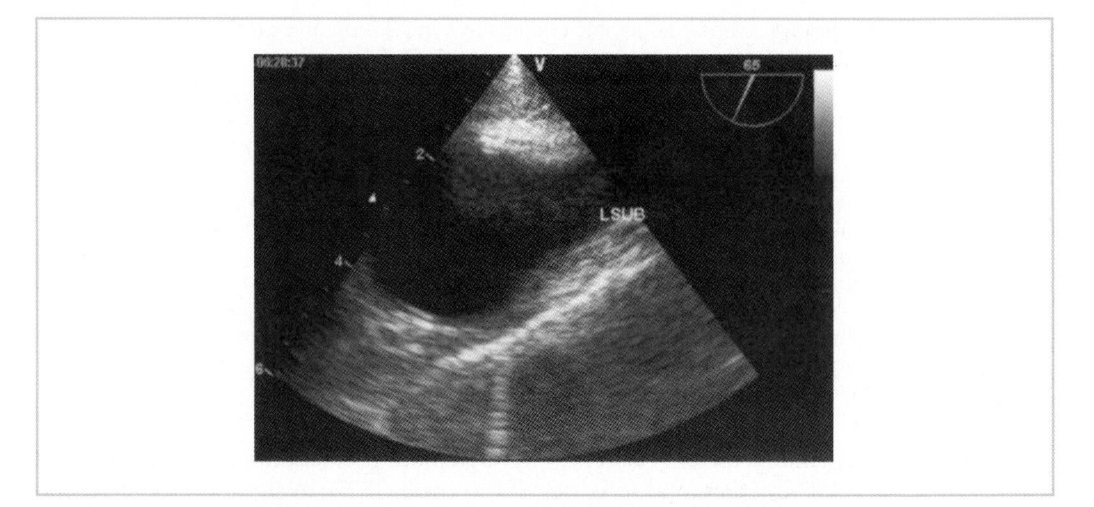

Figure 15.3. The descending aorta short-axis view demonstrating the takeoff of the left subclavian artery (*LSUB*). An intra-aortic balloon pump should not be visualized in this view but 2 cm distally for optimal placement.

motion, and decreased LV chamber size. The management of RV dysfunction includes checking for ischemia in the distribution of the right coronary artery, hyperventilation to decrease pulmonary vascular resistance, administration of inotropic agents that also decrease pulmonary vascular resistance (e.g., milrinone, dobutamine), and titration of pulmonary vasodilators (nitric oxide, prostaglandin E_1, or nitroglycerin).

Intra-aortic Balloon Counterpulsation

Severe global LV dysfunction may require more aggressive management, including the institution of intra-aortic balloon counterpulsation (IABP). TEE is often used to confirm proper location of the guidewire and positioning of the IABP. The cross section of the descending thoracic aorta can be visualized by positioning the TEE probe at the ME level and rotating it counterclockwise. The image depth is then decreased to approximately 6 cm, and the probe is slowly withdrawn until the origin of the left subclavian artery and distal aortic arch are visualized (Figure 15.3). The pulsatile hyperrefractile IABP is advanced to a location 1 to 2 cm distal to the origin of the left subclavian artery. If the cardiac dysfunction is refractory to such interventions, TEE can also be used to assist the surgeon in placing a mechanical ventricular assist device.

TRANSESOPHAGEAL ECHOCARDIOGRAPHY FOR PREVENTING LEFT VENTRICULAR DISTENSION

Distension of the LV during bypass results in increased chamber pressure that decreases coronary perfusion and stretches myocardial fibers. If unrecognized or untreated, LV distension can result in severe cardiac dysfunction that complicates attempts at separation from CPB. LV distension may be caused by excessive return from the bronchial and thebesian veins or by unsuspected aortic regurgitation during the administration of antegrade cardioplegia.

Distension of the RV is usually obvious to the observer because of its anterior location. In contrast, LV distension may not be visually appreciated in the surgical field because it is located posteriorly.

TEE can be used to evaluate the chamber size serially by imaging the LV in the TG short-axis and ME four-chamber views. If LV distension or a gradual increase in the pulmonary pressures is noted, the conduct of bypass is altered by placing a drainage cannula in the PA or superior pulmonary vein to aspirate blood and decompress the ventricle. TEE provides a direct assessment of LV size whereas monitoring of PA pressure is indirect. For example, a malpositioned pulmonary vein vent cannula that failed to cross the mitral valve would result in LV distension despite the low PA pressure values.

ROLE OF TRANSESOPHAGEAL ECHOCARDIOGRAPHY IN VASCULAR CANNULATION

Imaging the Ascending Aorta

Atherosclerotic disease of the ascending aorta is a significant risk factor for stroke and a poor neurologic outcome after CABG (24–26). Assessment of the aorta is feasible with both TEE and epiaortic imaging. Palpation by the surgeon is not sensitive in detecting atherosclerotic disease except for hard calcific plaques (27). TEE is an excellent modality with which to examine the descending thoracic aorta and aortic arch, but the acoustic window of the mid and distal ascending aorta is inadequate. *TEE fails to image 42% of the ascending aorta because visualization is obstructed by the air-filled trachea and left main bronchus* (27). In comparison, epiaortic scanning provides excellent imaging of these areas and is significantly more sensitive than TEE in detecting clinically significant atherosclerotic disease in the ascending aorta. In a study of 81 cardiac surgical patients, epicardial imaging detected 14 of 15 patients with significant atherosclerotic disease, whereas TEE identified only 5 of 15 patients (28).

The ascending aorta is best imaged by epicardial scanning, with the transducer placed in a sterile sheath filled with saline solution (Figure 15.1). The surgeon usually performs the manipulation with the assistance of the echocardiographer (29). The examination should proceed in the following manner:

1. The scanning depth is set to approximately 5 cm, and the probe is positioned at the level of the aortic valve to produce a cross-sectional image.
2. The probe is then slowly advanced distally to the arch, with care taken to identify atheroma on the anterior surface at the sites of cannulation and cross-clamping.
3. The longitudinal image can be obtained by manually rotating the transducer approximately 90 degrees until the long axis of the aorta is visualized, after which the probe is again slowly advanced along the aorta.

The epiaortic examination should determine the plaque thickness in millimeters and its mobility and location. The presence of mobile plaque or a plaque thickness greater than 5 mm indicates severe atheromatous disease and is a risk factor for poor outcome.

Management Strategy for Aortic Atheromatous Disease

The detection of significant pathology warrants consideration of modifying the aortic cannulation to reduce the risk for cerebral atheroembolism. The possible modifications of surgical technique include the following: avoiding bypass with off-pump CABG, alternating the aortic cannulation and cross-clamp sites, using endoaortic balloon occlusion, avoiding a side-biting aortic clamp by performing both distal and proximal coronary anastomoses within a single ischemic period, and performing coronary revascularization under hypothermic circulatory arrest (30–34). In the presence of severe aortic pathology, the surgeon may consider elective aortic atherectomy or replacement of the ascending aorta and arch. *We recommend that epiaortic scanning of the aorta be performed in patients who are considered at increased risk for neurologic complications.* The patients most likely to benefit are those with a history of stroke or prior CABG surgery, an age past 70 years, diabetes mellitus, hypertension, peripheral vascular disease, or a diagnosis of significant atheromatous disease by TEE examination or surgical palpation (24–26). The main objection to the use of this technology is the additional training, equipment, and time required to perform an examination adequately. Such concerns should diminish as individual surgeons gain more experience and the technology enters the mainstream of clinical practice.

Administration of Antegrade Cardioplegia

Antegrade cardioplegia is the most common method of cardiac preservation during bypass. It is usually administered by cannulating the ascending aorta. The delivery of cardioplegia depends on a competent aortic valve to pressurize the aortic root and drive the agent into the coronary vessels. *The presence of aortic valvular regurgitation not only compromises myocardial preservation but can result in LV distension, an important cause of post-CPB LV dysfunction.* It may be difficult for the surgeon to diagnose significant aortic regurgitation clinically because the LV is located posteriorly and therefore not easily visible. The prompt diagnosis of significant aortic regurgitation by TEE can alter the conduct of surgery as follows: administration of antegrade cardioplegia using a hand-held cannula after aortotomy, use of retrograde cardioplegia, decompression of the LV, or replacement of the aortic valve. Aortic regurgitation is best detected and characterized by using the ME long-axis view of the aortic valve. The severity of regurgitation is determined by comparing the diameter of the regurgitant jet with the diameter of the outflow tract (see Chapter 11). The diagnosis of anything more than mild aortic regurgitation should prompt the aforementioned considerations.

Administration of Retrograde Cardioplegia

Retrograde cardioplegia is routinely performed during CABG surgery as an adjunct to antegrade cardioplegia. This technique is often used in the presence of severe LV hypertrophy, severe proximal coronary artery disease, aortic regurgitation, or pathology within the aortic root that may compromise the delivery of antegrade cardioplegia. An incision is made in the right atrium, and the coronary sinus cannula is directed into the ostium of the coronary sinus, which lies inferiorly and medially in the right atrium adjacent to the tricuspid valve. Placement is commonly confirmed by palpating the catheter in the coronary sinus as it courses along the atrioventricular groove. Catheter malposition, which can be difficult to detect, puts the patient at risk for myocardial ischemia during bypass. Positioning the catheter may be difficult because of variations in the anatomy, such as eustachian valves, a thickened Chiari network, or thebesian valves. Another anatomic variant that complicates the administration of retrograde cardioplegia is the presence of a persistent left superior vena cava that empties the left central venous circulation into the coronary sinus instead of the superior vena cava through the innominate vein. Although the incidence of this congenital variant is low, timely detection is important to prevent the misdirection of cardioplegia into the left arm away from the heart. In addition, misdirection of the cannula through the tricuspid valve into the RV or insufficient advancement of the cannula negates the benefit of cardioplegia.

Echocardiography is useful to assist the surgeon in positioning the catheter. The stippled appearance of the balloon at the tip of the retrograde catheter can be easily identified

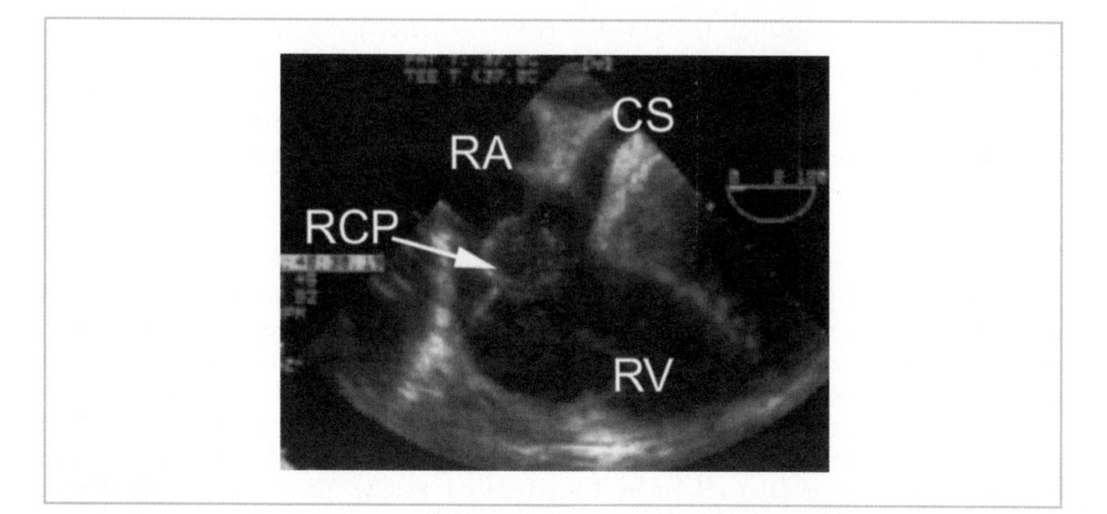

Figure 15.4. A modified midesophageal four-chamber view can be used to visualize the coronary sinus. Transesophageal echocardiography can be used to assist the surgeon in positioning the retrograde cardioplegia cannula in the coronary sinus (*CS*). The *arrow* points to the balloon of the retrograde cannula (*RCP*), right atrium (*RA*), and right ventricle (*RV*). The ostium of the coronary sinus is best viewed by slightly retroflexing the probe in the midesophageal four-chamber view.

because it is engaged in the ostium of the coronary sinus. The ostium of the coronary sinus is best viewed by slight retroflexion of the probe in the ME four-chamber view. The final position of the catheter can be confirmed by the presence of the thin hollow cannula within the lumen of the coronary sinus (Figure 15.4).

Femoral Venous Cannulation

The surgical placement of a femoral venous cannula can be facilitated with the use of TEE, first to confirm the location of the guidewire in the right atrium and later to verify adequate positioning of the cannula tip at the junction of the atrium and superior vena cava. The best view to visualize the cannula is the ME bicaval imaging plane. Slight rotation of the probe or readjustment of the angle should enable visualization of the echogenic cannula wall. Obstruction of the venous drainage can often be corrected by slightly advancing or withdrawing the catheter, which often abuts the venous wall or interatrial septum.

Femoral Arterial Cannulation

Femoral arterial cannulation is often used in cases of previous sternotomy, aortic dissection, or MIDCAB (endoaortic catheter, venous cannula, PA drainage catheter, coronary sinus catheter) surgery. The presence of severe athermanous disease with mobile debri raises concerns regarding increased risk embolization and retrograde aortic dissection. After the surgeon has accessed the femoral artery, a guidewire is threaded proximally into the descending aorta. Because it is very echogenic, the wire can easily be seen in the thoracic aorta. It is important to confirm the absence of an aortic dissection and correct placement of the cannula by visualizing the bypass blood flow with color flow Doppler.

TRANSESOPHAGEAL ECHOCARDIOGRAPHY IN PORT ACCESS SURGERY

In an effort to avoid median sternotomy and minimize invasiveness, a limited thoracotomy exposure is now being used for coronary revascularization. In this approach, the percutaneous cannulation for CPB and coronary artery anastomoses are performed through a series of small ports in the chest wall. The catheter-based Port Access system (Heartport, Redwood City, California) is based on a modified extracorporeal circulation and a combination of five intravascular cannulas (coronary sinus catheter, PA drainage catheter, intra-aortic occlusive balloon, venous drainage catheter, and arterial drainage catheter).

Coronary Sinus and Pulmonary Catheters

The coronary sinus and pulmonary catheters are inserted percutaneously by the anesthesiologist using the right jugular venous approach. TEE or fluoroscopy can be used as a complementary technique to assist in positioning these cannulas. The PA drainage catheter decompresses the heart by aspirating blood from the PA. This catheter is inserted through a 9F introducer and advanced to a position distal to the pulmonic valve. Correct placement is confirmed by visualizing the catheter in the PA with TEE and by detecting a change in the pressure wave form as it is advanced distally. The PA is best visualized by slightly anteflexing and withdrawing the probe in the ME view. Adequate drainage with this catheter is confirmed by using TEE to evaluate distension of the cardiac chambers. This is best achieved by monitoring the TG LV short-axis and ME four-chamber views.

Endoaortic Clamp

The endoaortic clamp is a triple-lumen balloon-tipped catheter that is introduced through the femoral arterial cannula and advanced into the ascending aorta. TEE is used to guide placement of the balloon catheter centrally in a position just distal to the sinuses of Valsalva. The ME long-axis view of the aortic valve is the best view for endoclamp positioning and monitoring during balloon inflation. The anesthesiologist must not only confirm correct initial positioning but also monitor to detect balloon migration. Migration of the balloon proximally can damage the aortic valve and distally can occlude blood flow to the arch vessels, resulting in cerebral ischemia. TEE is also used to monitor the delivery of antegrade cardioplegia through the lumen within the cannula and to detect LV distension.

TRANSESOPHAGEAL ECHOCARDIOGRAPHY FOR THE DIAGNOSIS OF OCCULT DISEASE

The detection of anatomic variants or incidental findings is fairly common (Table 15.5). No prospective outcome studies have addressed the issue of altering surgery based on unanticipated echocardiographic findings. Some findings, such as a pleural effusion, do not affect the progress of the intended surgery, whereas others markedly alter surgical management. The implications of significant atheromatous disease in the ascending aorta and persistent left vena cava have already been discussed.

Thrombus

The detection of intracardiac thrombus by TEE is infrequent but may alter the surgical management. Thrombus in the left atrial appendage can be managed by minimizing manipulation of the heart or plication of the appendage. Mobile fresh thrombus, especially in the left side of the heart, merits surgical extraction. Thrombus can increase the risk for postoperative complications, and its detection is likely to alter postoperative management with the initiation of long-term anticoagulation.

Table 15.5 Transesophageal echocardiography for the diagnosis of incidental disease

Incidental findings	Clinical considerations
Patent foramen ovale	Shunting, risk for paradoxical embolism
Persistent left superior vena cava	Contraindication for retrograde cardioplegia
Atherosclerotic disease	Modify cannulation/cross-clamping of aorta
Aortic regurgitation	Inadequate antegrade cardioplegia, distension of left ventricle
Valvular disease	Valve repair or replacement
Intracardiac thrombus	Risk for embolism, alter surgical management
Pleural effusion	Drainage of effusion

Patent Foramen Ovale

The management of an unsuspected patent foramen ovale, which has an incidence of 20% to 25% in adult cardiac surgical patients, can affect the anticipated surgical plan and long-term neurologic prognosis (35). Closure of an incidental patent foramen ovale should be considered in a patient with a history of stroke or when an open chamber procedure is performed in conjunction with CABG surgery. A patent foramen ovale is most reliably detected when the interatrial septum is interrogated with both color flow Doppler and imaging after contrast injection in the ME four-chamber and bicaval views (36,37). The contrast agent is made by agitating 10 mL of saline that is forcefully injected back and forth through a three-way stopcock into another syringe. The excess air is then removed and the solution injected as the interatrial septum is interrogated by TEE. The passage of contrast bubbles in the left atrium within five cardiac cycles confirms the diagnosis patent foramen ovale.

Pleural Effusions

Pleural effusions are often present in patients undergoing CABG surgery as a result of decompensated coronary artery disease, coexisting valvular disease, or other pathology. Large effusions that cause significant atelectasis result in decreased ventilatory capacity and increased alveolar-to-arterial oxygen gradients. The left pleural space is best imaged by counterclockwise rotation of the TEE probe to image the short axis of the descending thoracic aorta. An effusion surrounds the aorta, displacing normal parenchyma of the lung.

Aortic Stenosis

The natural history of aortic stenosis in the adult begins with a prolonged asymptomatic period associated with minimal mortality. In patients having either mild or severe disease, the decision is apparent. In addition, the finding of a congenital bicuspid aortic valve which predisposes to progressive aortic stenosis and aneurysmal dilation of the root may also be more aggressively pursued. However, the decisions regarding valve replacement for moderate aortic valve disease in the setting of otherwise routine CABG surgery is complicated by the variability in the natural progression of the disease. The pathogenesis of aortic stenosis is not a random degenerative process, but an active progressive disease associated with hypercholesterolemia, inflammation, and osteoblast activity. Factors to consider when deciding to replace the aortic valve include age (life expectancy), peak pressure gradient, valve area, and rate of progression of the aortic stenosis. Several investigators have examined this controversial scenario (38–40). Recent data suggests that a combined procedure does not increase operative mortality but may confer a survival benefit in those with moderate and severe aortic stenosis but not mild stenosis.

Mitral Regurgitation

The presence of significant mitral regurgitation may merit surgical intervention. However, there is no consensus regarding the specifics of any pharmacologic or volume challenge that should be used to induce valvular insufficiency. It is important to assess the severity and dynamic nature of mitral valvular disease under conditions that best mimic the preoperative state and to consider the patient's preoperative symptoms and cardiac function. Coronary revascularization alone may significantly decrease mitral regurgitation as a consequence of improved coronary perfusion and ventricular function. The surgical plan should be modified by the surgeon and cardiologist with input from the echocardiographer.

TRANSESOPHAGEAL ECHOCARDIOGRAPHY IN OFF-PUMP CORONARY ARTERY BYPASS GRAFTING

Off-pump coronary artery bypass grafting (OPCAB) surgery has gained popularity because some practitioners believe that it avoids the morbidity of CPB. During the critical time when the heart is surgically positioned for distal coronary anastomosis, hemodynamic instability and coronary ischemia can develop. One of the factors critical to the success of this procedure is that the anesthesiologist remains vigilant and communicates with the cardiac surgeon. Effective communication and gradual positioning of the heart greatly facilitate the maintenance of stable hemodynamics. Because this surgical procedure is relatively new, the national consensus in regard to monitoring with TEE is still emerging. The application of TEE in OPCAB surgery may vary within an institution and is generally physician-specific.

Hemodynamic Compromise during Off-Pump Coronary Artery Bypass

Hemodynamic compromise during OPCAB can be caused by hypovolemia (bleeding, manual compression of the heart, chamber distortion during positioning), ischemia (coronary air or debris), valvular dysfunction, or arrhythmias (secondary to ischemia or mechanical perturbation). Echocardiography can serve a valuable role in discriminating between these etiologies and monitoring the effectiveness of any subsequent intervention.

Regional Wall Motion Abnormalities in Off-Pump Coronary Artery Bypass

New RWMAs are common but may not indicate ongoing ischemia. As discussed previously, these can be attributed to altered volume status, positioning, and stabilization devices that distort the anatomy to reduce the excursion of affected myocardium. Positioning the heart to enable the anastomosis of distal left coronary grafts may cause torsion and compression of the right atria and ventricle, impeding venous return. This problem can be alleviated in part by administering fluid, placing the patient in a slight Trendelenburg position, opening the pericardium to the right side of the chest, and using a positioning device that is affixed to the apex of the heart and shifts the heart into a less compromising position.

Mitral Regurgitation in Off-Pump Coronary Artery Bypass

Distortion of the heart during anastomosis of the right or posterior coronary arteries can also exacerbate mitral regurgitation. The mechanism is most likely distortion of the mitral valve annulus and supportive structures that interferes with leaflet coaptation. In some cases, the mitral regurgitation may cause sufficient hemodynamic compromise that conversion to circulatory bypass is required.

Patent Foramen Ovale in Off-Pump Coronary Artery Bypass

The presence of a patent foramen ovale, which has an incidence of approximately 20%, has the potential to influence operative management. Positioning the heart during OPCAB can also be associated with profound hypoxemia that results from right-to-left intracardiac shunting through a patent foramen ovale (41). The patent foramen ovale may be unmasked by an acute increase in pressure in the right side of the heart that occurs during positioning. Repositioning the heart should permit closure of the shunt and resolution of the hypoxia. However, in the case of refractory hypoxia, it may be necessary to perform the surgery with CPB and also close the patent foramen ovale (41). In a small retrospective case series of 11 patients having this pathology, no patients who had a preexisting shunt or one induced by lifting of the heart had clinically relevant desaturation due to right to left shunting through the foramen ovale (42).

Deciding whether to Use Transesophageal Echocardiography during Coronary Artery Bypass Surgery

The use of TEE for routine CABG is somewhat controversial and reflects factors including perceived utility and availability of equipment and trained personnel. Whereas the value of this technology for valvular surgery is widely acknowledged, its application for CABG surgery is less clear. This view is reflected by the lack of reimbursement for performing TEE for routine CABG surgeries. Although its usefulness as a monitoring device for CABG surgery is acknowledged, many payers consider TEE as part of the anesthetic care plan and is therefore poorly reimbursed, if at all.

Most clinicians attest to the potential value of TEE to help manage administration and titration of pharmacologic therapy and volume resuscitation, a category II indication according to recent consensus papers (2,3). However, its documented role in significantly altering surgical management or the conduct of circulatory support ranged from 5% to 17% (23,42–44). The notable exception is its application in patients having substantial cardiac dysfunction for high-risk cases, where TEE has been shown to significantly influence intraoperative clinical management (1). However its necessity in patients having preserved function is debatable. The absence of prospective randomized controlled studies that demonstrate the benefit of TEE for routine CABG surgery has precluded a national consensus that affirms its benefit. At present, the rationale for its use relies on anecdotal reports and individual clinical experiences. The critical importance of TEE for CABG surgery in altering hemodynamic management in patients having preserved ventricular function is relatively low; it generally serves as an adjunct to supplement the practitioner's clinical acumen and the use of routine invasive monitors. As discussed previously, cardiac pacing or distortion of the heart, which is often associated with the application of stabilizing devices, complicate interpretation by producing nonischemic RWMAs and valvular insufficiency. Perhaps the strongest impetus for performing TEE in routine CABG surgery may lie in its capacity to detect occult, subclinical disease that would impact the conduct of circulatory management or the surgical procedure. Although relatively uncommon, its incidence of such findings may increase as economic pressures limit preoperative evaluation and profile of "healthy" patient coming for isolated CABG become less frequent. Early intervention to correct aortic valvular stenosis or mitral regurgitation may produce a positive benefit by reducing the need for redo sternotomy or progressive deterioration in cardiac function.

The decision to use this technology for CABG surgery is often institutional and individual specific. At the author's institution, patients having preserved cardiac function and no history of cardiac valvular abnormalities are less likely to have an intraoperative TEE examination. However, this segment of the population is becoming increasing rare. Patients having significant cardiac and valvular dysfunction will often benefit from its use.

SUMMARY

The major role of echocardiography in patients undergoing coronary revascularization is as a versatile diagnostic device that can dramatically alter the conduct and management of a surgical procedure. It is unlikely that echocardiography will supplant the traditional PA catheter because the PA catheter offers the advantage of providing continuous quantitative assessment of overall cardiac function and loading conditions throughout the perioperative period. However, advances in echocardiography have markedly expanded its applications and importance in cardiac surgery. As explained in this chapter, the potential indications for this technology include both monitoring and diagnosis. The multiple modalities (two-dimensional imaging, color flow mapping, spectral Doppler imaging, and use of contrast agents) provide for both the qualitative and quantitative assessment of cardiac function and pathophysiology. In the future, the increased availability of equipment, trained personnel, and technologic advances will foster an expanded role of echocardiography in selected groups of cardiac surgical patients.

REFERENCES

1 Savage RM, Lytle BW, Aronson S, et al. Intraoperative echocardiography is indicated in high-risk coronary artery bypass grafting. *Ann Thorac Surg* 1997;64(2):368–373.
2 American Society of Anesthesiologists. Practice guidelines for perioperative transesophageal echocardiography. A report by the American Society of Anesthesiologists and the Society of Cardiovascular Anesthesiologists Task Force on Transesophageal Echocardiography. *Anesthesiology* 1996;84(4):986–1006.
3 Cheitlin MD, Armstrong WF, Aurigemma GP, et al. ACC/AHA/ASE 2003 guideline update for the clinical application of echocardiography–summary article: a report of the American College of Cardiology/American Heart Association Task Force on Practice Guidelines (ACC/AHA/ASE Committee to Update the 1997. Guidelines for the Clinical Application of Echocardiography). *J Am Coll Cardiol* 2003;42(5):954–970.
4 Kallmeyer IJ, Collard CD, Fox JA, et al. The safety of intraoperative transesophageal echocardiography: a case series of 7200 cardiac surgical patients. *Anesth Analg* 2001;92(5):1126–1130.
5 Cheung EH, Craver JM, Jones EL, et al. Mediastinitis after cardiac valve operations. Impact upon survival. *J Thorac Cardiovasc Surg* 1985;90(4):517–522.
6 Staples JR, Tanaka KA, Shanewise JS, et al. The use of the SonoSite ultrasound device for intraoperative evaluation of the aorta. *J Cardiothorac Vasc Anesth* 2004;18(6):715–718.
7 Schellenberg AG, Marshall MB, Salgo IS. Intraoperative ultrasound for localization of patent left internal mammary artery grafts in repeat cardiothoracic surgery. *J Cardiothorac Vasc Anesth* 2001;15(2):228–230.
8 Arruda AM, Dearani JA, Click RL, et al. Intraoperative application of power Doppler imaging: visualization of myocardial perfusion after anastomosis of left internal thoracic artery to left anterior descending coronary artery. *J Am Soc Echocardiogr* 1999;12(8):650–654.
9 Shanewise JS, Cheung AT, Aronson S, et al. ASE/SCA guidelines for performing a comprehensive intraoperative multiplane transesophageal echocardiography examination: recommendations of the American Society of Echocardiography Council for Intraoperative Echocardiography and the Society of Cardiovascular Anesthesiologists Task Force for Certification in Perioperative Transesophageal Echocardiography. *Anesth Analg* 1999;89(4):870–884.
10 Weiss SJ, Savino JS. Decision-making and perioperative transesophageal echocardiogarphy. In: Kaplan JA, Reich DL, Konstadt SN, eds. *Cardiac anesthesia*. Philadelphia: WB Saunders, 2006.
11 Lang RM, Bierig M, Devereux RB, et al. Recommendations for chamber quantification: a report from the American Society of Echocardiography's Guidelines and Standards Committee and the Chamber Quantification Writing Group, developed in conjunction with the European Association of Echocardiography, a branch of the European Society of Cardiology. *J Am Soc Echocardiogr* 2005;18(12):1440–1463.

12 Cheung AT, Savino JS, Weiss SJ, et al. Echocardiographic and hemodynamic indexes of left ventricular preload in patients with normal and abnormal ventricular function. *Anesthesiology* 1994;81(2):376–387.
13 Perrino AC Jr, Luther MA, O'Connor TZ, et al. Automated echocardiographic analysis. Examination of serial intraoperative measurements. *Anesthesiology* 1995;83(2):285–292.
14 Muhiudeen IA, Kuecherer HF, Lee E, et al. Intraoperative estimation of cardiac output by transesophageal pulsed Doppler echocardiography. *Anesthesiology* 1991;74(1):9–14.
15 Savino JS, Troianos CA, Aukburg S, et al. Measurement of pulmonary blood flow with transesophageal two- dimensional and Doppler echocardiography. *Anesthesiology* 1991;75(3):445–451.
16 Darmon PL, Hillel Z, Mogtader A, et al. Cardiac output by transesophageal echocardiography using continuous- wave Doppler across the aortic valve. *Anesthesiology* 1994;80(4):796–805.
17 Smith JS, Cahalan MK, Benefiel DJ, et al. Intraoperative detection of myocardial ischemia in high-risk patients: electrocardiography versus two-dimensional transesophageal echocardiography. *Circulation* 1985;72(5):1015–1021.
18 Battler A, Froelicher VF, Gallagher KP, et al. Dissociation between regional myocardial dysfunction and ECG changes during ischemia in the conscious dog. *Circulation* 1980;62(4):735–744.
19 Gallagher KP, Kumada T, Koziol JA, et al. Significance of regional wall thickening abnormalities relative to transmural myocardial perfusion in anesthetized dogs. *Circulation* 1980;62(6):1266–1274.
20 Roizen MF, Beaupre PN, Alpert RA, et al. Monitoring with two-dimensional transesophageal echocardiography. Comparison of myocardial function in patients undergoing supraceliac, suprarenal-infraceliac, or infrarenal aortic occlusion. *J Vasc Surg* 1984;1(2):300–305.
21 Leung JM, O'Kelly B, Browner WS, et al. Prognostic importance of postbypass regional wall-motion abnormalities in patients undergoing coronary artery bypass graft surgery. SPI Research Group. *Anesthesiology* 1989;71(1):16–25.
22 Deutsch HJ, Curtius JM, Leischik R, et al. Diagnostic value of transesophageal echocardiography in cardiac surgery. *Thorac Cardiovasc Surg* 1991;39(4):199–204.
23 Bergquist BD, Bellows WH, Leung JM. Transesophageal echocardiography in myocardial revascularization: II. Influence on intraoperative decision making. *Anesth Analg* 1996;82(6):1139–1145.
24 Gardner TJ, Horneffer PJ, Manolio TA, et al. Stroke following coronary artery bypass grafting: a ten-year study. *Ann Thorac Surg* 1985;40(6):574–581.
25 Newman MF, Kirchner JL, Phillips-Bute B, et al. Longitudinal assessment of neurocognitive function after coronary-artery bypass surgery. *N Engl J Med* 2001;344(6):395–402.
26 Roach GW, Kanchuger M, Mangano CM, et al. Adverse cerebral outcomes after coronary bypass surgery. Multicenter Study of Perioperative Ischemia Research Group and the Ischemia Research and Education Foundation Investigators. *N Engl J Med* 1996;335(25):1857–1863.
27 Konstadt SN, Reich DL, Quintana C, et al. The ascending aorta: how much does transesophageal echocardiography see? *Anesth Analg* 1994;78(2):240–244.
28 Konstadt SN, Reich DL, Kahn R, et al. Transesophageal echocardiography can be used to screen for ascending aortic atherosclerosis. *Anesth Analg* 1995;81(2):225–228.
29 Eltzschig HK, Kallmeyer IJ, Mihaljevic T, et al. A practical approach to a comprehensive epicardial and epiaortic echocardiographic examination. *J Cardiothorac Vasc Anesth* 2003;17(4):422–429.
30 Byrne JG, Aranki SF, Cohn LH. Aortic valve operations under deep hypothermic circulatory arrest for the porcelain aorta: "no-touch" technique. *Ann Thorac Surg* 1998;65(5):1313–1315.
31 Cohn LH, Rizzo RJ, Adams DH, et al. Reduced mortality and morbidity for ascending aortic aneurysm resection regardless of cause. *Ann Thorac Surg* 1996;62(2):463–468.
32 Grossi EA, Kanchuger MS, Schwartz DS, et al. Effect of cannula length on aortic arch flow: protection of the atheromatous aortic arch. *Ann Thorac Surg* 1995;59(3):710–712.
33 Kouchoukos NT, Wareing TH, Daily BB, et al. Management of the severely atherosclerotic aorta during cardiac operations. *J Card Surg* 1994;9(5):490–494.
34 Paul D, Hartman GS. Foley balloon occlusion of the atheromatous ascending aorta: the role of transesophageal echocardiography. *J Cardiothorac Vasc Anesth* 1998;12(1):61–64.
35 Louie EK, Konstadt SN, Rao TL, et al. Transesophageal echocardiographic diagnosis of right to left shunting across the foramen ovale in adults without prior stroke. *J Am Coll Cardiol* 1993;21(5):1231–1237.
36 Konstadt SN, Louie EK, Black S, et al. Intraoperative detection of patent foramen ovale by transesophageal echocardiography. *Anesthesiology* 1991;74(2):212–216.
37 Augoustides JG, Weiss SJ, Weiner J, et al. Diagnosis of patent foramen ovale with multiplane transesophageal echocardiography in adult cardiac surgical patients. *J Cardiothorac Vasc Anesth* 2004;18(6):725–730.
38 Gillinov AM, Garcia MJ. When is concomitant aortic valve replacement indicated in patients with mild to moderate stenosis undergoing coronary revascularization? *Curr Cardiol Rep* 2005;7(2):101–104.
39 Rahimtoola SH. "Prophylactic" valve replacement for mild aortic valve disease at time of surgery for other cardiovascular disease? . . . No. *J Am Coll Cardiol* 1999;33(7):2009–2015.

40 Smith WT, Ferguson TB Jr, Ryan T, et al. Should coronary artery bypass graft surgery patients with mild or moderate aortic stenosis undergo concomitant aortic valve replacement? A decision analysis approach to the surgical dilemma. *J Am Coll Cardiol* 2004;44(6):1241–1247.
41 Akhter M, Lajos TZ. Pitfalls of undetected patent foramen ovale in off-pump cases. *Ann Thorac Surg* 1999;67(2):546–548.
42 Sukernik MR, Mets B, Kachulis B, et al. The impact of newly diagnosed patent foramen ovale in patients undergoing off-pump coronary artery bypass grafting: case series of eleven patients. *Anesth Analg* 2002;95(5):1142–1146; table.
43 Couture P, Denault AY, McKenty S, et al. Impact of routine use of intraoperative transesophageal echocardiography during cardiac surgery. *Can J Anaesth* 2000;47(1):20–26.
44 Michel-Cherqui M, Ceddaha A, Liu N, et al. Assessment of systematic use of intraoperative transesophageal echocardiography during cardiac surgery in adults: a prospective study of 203 patients. *J Cardiothorac Vasc Anesth* 2000;14(1):45–50.

QUESTIONS

1. **All of the following statements regarding transesophageal echocardiography (TEE) for coronary artery bypass grafting (CABG) surgery are true except**
   a. TEE is more sensitive than electrocardiography (ECG) for the detection of ischemia.
   b. TEE can play an important role during cardiac surgery by influencing circulatory and surgical management.
   c. The morbidity associated with TEE is low.
   d. TEE completely images the ascending and descending thoracic aorta.

2. **Epiaortic imaging in CABG surgery**
   a. Does not offer any significant benefit beyond that of TEE
   b. Images the ascending aorta better than TEE
   c. Is contraindicated in the case of a friable or atherosclerotic aorta
   d. Always requires the use of a "standoff" to improve resolution in the far field

3. **The TEE examination for CABG surgery**
   a. Should focus only on the specific surgical indication of ischemia detection
   b. Is classified as a "group 1 indication" according to the guidelines of the American Society of Anesthesiologists/Society of Cardiovascular Anesthesiologists
   c. Should be reviewed with the attending cardiac surgeon
   d. Has been shown to significantly improve the clinical outcome of off-pump surgery

4. **TEE assessment of ventricular function**
   a. Requires only the "classic" transgastric (TG) short-axis view
   b. Is independent of afterload
   c. Uses the volumetric determination of fractional area change (FAC)
   d. Is dependent on ventricular preload

5. **The TEE measurement of cardiac output (CO)**
   a. Cannot be performed in cases of high blood flow velocity
   b. Is most commonly achieved by interrogating blood flow through the mitral valve
   c. Shows good agreement with measurements determined by thermodilution
   d. Is dependent on the absence of valvular stenosis

6. **Which of the following statements is the most accurate?**
   a. TEE provides for the continuous on-line measurement of intracardiac pressures.
   b. The TEE-derived measurement of CO is often inaccurate because of left ventricular (LV) foreshortening.
   c. A change in pulmonary artery (PA) pressure is a more sensitive diagnostic indicator of cardiac ischemia than a new regional wall motion abnormality (RWMA).
   d. TEE and PA catheterization function as complementary technologies during CABG surgery.

7. **New RWMAs that develop after separation from bypass during CABG surgery**
   a. May respond to the administration of calcium channel antagonist
   b. Are diagnostic of myocardial ischemia
   c. Support the further intervention of returning to bypass and performing another coronary anastomosis
   d. Result in myocardial infarction

8. Which of the following is the most appropriate statement?

a. TEE often inaccurately assesses LV preload because of LV foreshortening.

b. An increase in FAC should not be equated with an increase in contractility.

c. With TEE, it is difficult to distinguish a low systemic vascular resistance syndrome from a pulmonary embolism.

d. The septal wall motion abnormality that is observed after bypass is most commonly related to transient ischemia.

9. TEE is used for all the following except

a. Confirming the absence of significant aortic valvular insufficiency

b. Diagnosing LV distension

c. Guiding arterial cannulation of the ascending aorta

d. Assisting in placement of a coronary sinus catheter

10. Which of the following is the most appropriate statement?

a. The diagnosis of a patent foramen ovale has more important implications for CABG surgery that uses cardiopulmonary bypass (CPB) than for off-pump surgery.

b. TEE assists with positioning the endoaortic clamp during port access procedures.

c. Incidental findings of the intraoperative TEE examination have no effect on cardioplegia techniques.

d. The presence of bubbles emerging from the coronary sinus following an injection of contrast in a peripheral vein is of minimal importance in conducting bypass surgery.

Answers appear at the back of the book.

16 Transesophageal Echocardiography of the Thoracic Aorta

Kim J. Payne, John S. Ikonomidis, and Scott T. Reeves

In few diseases is an accurate and timely diagnosis more important than in those of the thoracic aorta. This chapter guides the reader through the classification systems used for thoracic aortic aneurysms and dissections, their echocardiographic manifestations, and the surgical decision-making process. Emphasis is placed on obtaining a quick and accurate examination, with particular attention given to the echocardiographic findings diagnostic of aortic disease. The chapter concludes with a discussion of associated thoracic disease states, including intramural hematoma and atheroma.

CLASSIFICATION SYSTEMS

Diseases of the thoracic aorta include aortic aneurysms, aortic dissections, intramural hematomas, giant penetrating ulcers, and significant atherosclerosis that can present problems at the time of cardiac surgery.

Aortic Aneurysms

Aortic aneurysms can be classified according to their location in the ascending aorta, aortic arch, descending thoracic aorta, or any combination thereof. Any patient with a thoracic aortic aneurysm larger than 5 cm in diameter should be considered for operative repair because of the considerable risks for rupture. A further corollary is that any patient with an aneurysmal segment of the aorta that attains a luminal diameter more than two times that of a normal aortic segment, which can usually be estimated in an unaffected area at the level of the aortic arch or the abdominal aortic vessels, should be considered for surgery. Patients with connective tissue disease, such as Marfan syndrome or Ehlers-Danlos syndrome, may be considered for surgery at an earlier time.

The Crawford classification delineates four types of thoracoabdominal aneurysms (1) (Figure 16.1). Type I originates in the proximal descending thoracic aorta and ends above the renal arteries. Type II begins in the proximal descending thoracic aorta and terminates below the renal arteries. Type III originates in the distal descending aorta, conveniently identified as being below the level of the thoracic incision in the sixth intercostal space. Type IV involves most of the abdominal aorta. Figure 16.2 illustrates the distribution, frequency, and morphology of thoracic aortic aneurysms.

Aortic Dissections

Thoracic aortic dissections are classified by either of two schemes. The Stanford classification (2) separates aortic dissections into type A, in which the dissection involves the ascending aorta, and type B, in which the dissection is confined to the descending thoracic aorta. The DeBakey system (3) classifies dissections as type I, in which the dissection starts in the ascending aorta and involves variable portions of the descending aorta; type II, in which the dissection is confined to the ascending aorta; and type III, in which the dissection originates distal to the left subclavian artery and either involves only the descending

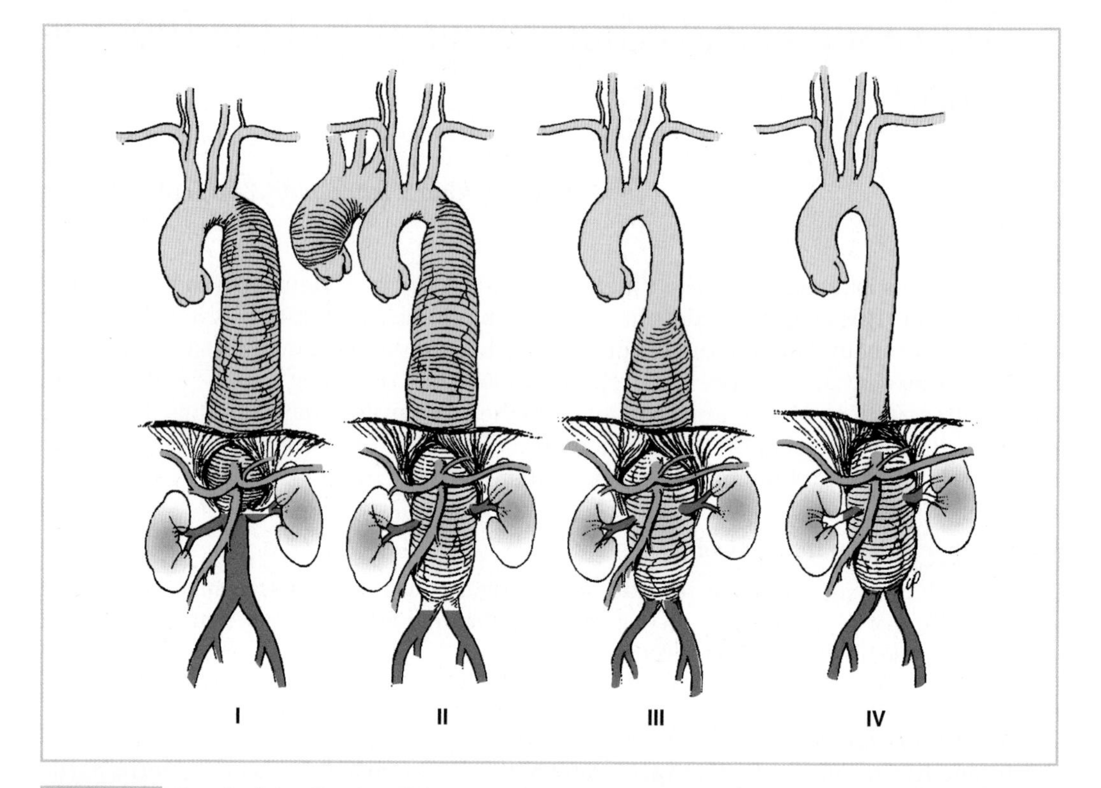

Figure 16.1. Crawford classification of thoracoabdominal aortic aneurysms according to extent of involvement of the thoracoabdominal aorta. Crawford type *I*, most or all of the descending thoracic aorta and the suprarenal abdominal aorta; type *II*, most or all of the descending thoracic aorta and most or all of the abdominal aorta; type *III*, distal descending thoracic aorta and varying segments of the abdominal aorta, including the renal and visceral arteries; type *IV*, most or all of the abdominal aorta. (From Crawford ES, Svensson LG, Hess HE, et al. A prospective randomized study of cerebrospinal fluid drainage to prevent paraplegia after high-risk surgery on the thoracoabdominal aorta. *J Vasc Surg* 1991;13:37, with permission.)

thoracic aorta (III-A) or extends into the abdominal segment of the descending aorta (III-B) (Figure 16.3).

Intramural Hematomas

Intramural hematomas of the thoracic aorta are classified the same way as thoracic aortic dissections.

Giant Penetrating Ulcers

Giant penetrating ulcer disease of the thoracic aorta is still a relatively poorly defined condition that is generally classified in relation to the anatomic location of the lesion (i.e., ascending aorta, arch, or descending thoracic aorta).

DIAGNOSTIC MODALITIES FOR AORTIC DISSECTION

The mortality rate for acute aortic dissection can be as high a 1% per hour among untreated patients during the first 48 hours (4) and has a mortality of 80% at 2 weeks. Death is caused by acute aortic insufficiency, major branch vessel obstruction, or aortic rupture. A quick and accurate diagnosis is imperative if one is to improve survival

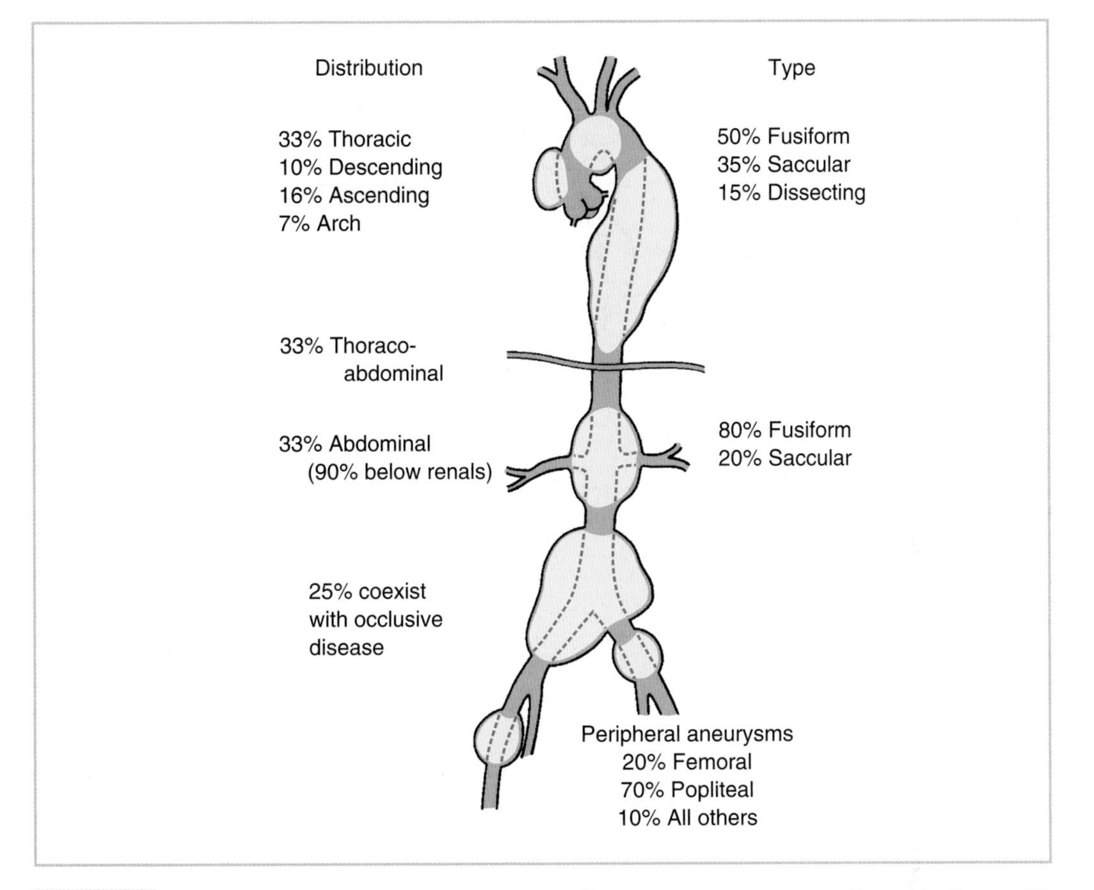

Figure 16.2. Distribution frequency and morphology of type A aortic aneurysms. (From Estafanous FG, Barash PG, Reves JG, eds. *Cardiac anesthesia principles and clinical practice,* second ed. Philadelphia: Lippincott Williams & Wilkins, 2001:785, with permission.)

and initiate the appropriate surgical or medical therapy. Until recently, aortography was the gold standard for evaluating patients with suspected aortic dissection (5). Currently, multiple imaging modalities, including computed tomography (CT) (6–8), transesophageal echocardiography (TEE) (5–12), and magnetic resonance imaging (MRI) (6–9), have been shown to be useful. The relative advantages of each modality are presented in Table 16.1. One must consider availability, time required to perform the study, safety, and cost when considering the four different modalities.

Aortography

Aortography requires the visualization of a double lumen or intimal flap to be completely diagnostic. Indirect signs that suggest acute dissection include thickening of the aortic wall, aortic insufficiency, ulcer-like projections along the aortic wall, abnormalities of branch vessels, an abnormal position of a catheter in the aorta, and compression of a true aortic lumen by a false lumen (5). As Table 16.1 shows, aortography may be the least sensitive of the modalities currently available (7). Furthermore, it is difficult to perform on an emergent basis because adequate personnel must be available in the hospital, the patient must be transferred to the interventional suite, and intravenous contrast, which can be detrimental in patients with renal insufficiency, must be used.

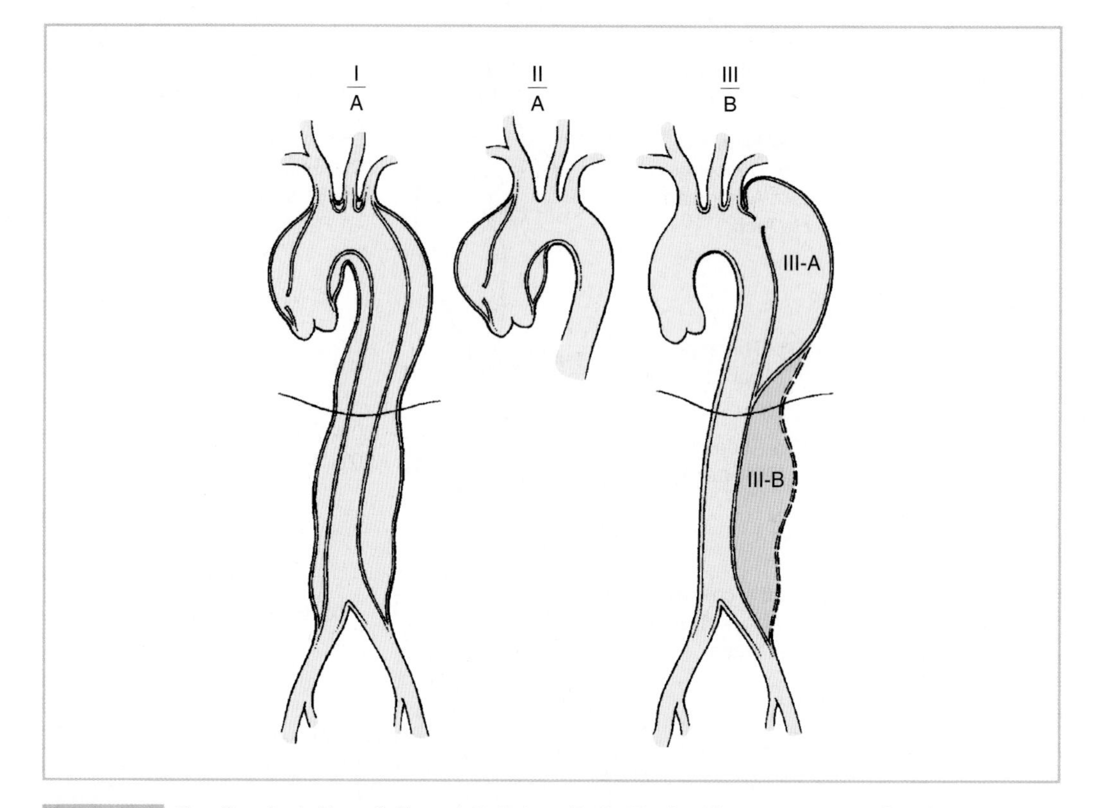

Figure 16.3. The Stanford (*A* and *B*) and DeBakey (*I*, *II*, *III*) classification systems for thoracic aorta dissections. (From Crawford ES, Crawford JL. *Diseases of the aorta.* Baltimore: Williams & Wilkins, 1984:174, with permission.)

Table 16.1 Diagnostic performance of imaging modalities in the evaluation of suspected dissection

Diagnostic performance	Angiography	CT	MRI	TEE
Sensitivity	++	++	+++	+++
Specificity	+++	+++	+++	++/+++
Site of intimal tear	++	+	+++	++
Presence of thrombus	+++	++	+++	+
Presence of aortic insufficiency	+++	—	+	+++
Pericardial effusion	—	++	+++	+++
Branch vessel involvement	+++	+	++	+
Coronary artery involvement	++	—	—	++

CT, computed tomography; MRI, magnetic resonance imaging; TEE, transesophageal echocardiography; +++, excellent; ++, good; +, fair; —, not detected. Modified from Cigarro JE, Isselbacher EM, DeSanctis RW, et al. Diagnostic imaging in the evaluation of suspected aortic dissection: old standards and new directions. *N Engl J Med* 1993;328:35, with permission.

Computed Tomography

CT requires the identification of two distinct lumina with a visible intimal flap. CT is more sensitive than aortography but is still less sensitive than MRI and TEE. CT rarely identifies the intimal flap entry site. CT also cannot reliably identify aortic insufficiency or coronary artery involvement (6–8).

Magnetic Resonance Imaging

MRI is the most sensitive and specific methodology currently available for evaluating aortic dissection. Unfortunately, an MRI examination is contraindicated for the many patients with pacemakers, certain types of aneurysm clips, or orthopedic hardware. Patients with acute aortic dissection are often hemodynamically unstable, require intravenous antihypertensive agents, and are intubated, so that proper management in the MRI scanner is further complicated (6–9).

Transesophageal Echocardiography

TEE is becoming the standard modality for the acute evaluation of a suspected acute aortic dissection. It is widely available, noninvasive, and cost effective, and it can be performed quickly at the bedside. *One must demonstrate an undulating intimal flap in the aorta in two different views to make the diagnosis.* The skill of the reader is paramount in making an accurate diagnosis with TEE. The study usually requires only 5 to 20 minutes to complete. The distal ascending aorta and proximal aortic arch may be poorly visualized with TEE because of the juxtaposition of the air-filled trachea and left main bronchus, which can lead to false-negative results. Visualization of this area has improved with the use of newer technologies, such as multiplane probes. TEE is also extremely helpful in detecting aortic insufficiency, pericardial effusion, and coronary artery involvement. In addition, other information, such as the left ventricular (LV) ejection fraction and parameters of valvular function, can easily be obtained (5–12).

Because it is safe, quick, accurate, and convenient and can be performed at the bedside, even in an unstable patient, we feel that TEE should be considered first when a patient is being evaluated for possible acute aortic dissection. For patients with chronic dissection and those requiring postoperative evaluation, MRI appears to be the test of choice (6–9).

EXAMINATION TECHNIQUES

Because of the close proximity of the thoracic aorta to the esophagus, TEE is the preferred echocardiographic approach. Figure 16.4 illustrates the changing relationship of the thoracic aorta to the esophagus along its course from the upper thorax to the diaphragm. At the level of the distal arch, the aorta is anterior to the esophagus, whereas at the level of the diaphragm, the aorta is posterior to the esophagus. This changing anatomic relationship makes it difficult for the echocardiographer to designate the anterior and posterior and the left and right orientation of the descending thoracic aorta. *To communicate the location of a lesion to the surgeon, we find it useful to relate its location to known anatomic landmarks. We measure the distance of lesions in the ascending aorta from the aortic valve, and the distance of those in the descending aorta from the left subclavian artery.* It is also useful to record the distance of a lesion from the incisors to guide follow-up examinations in the echocardiography suite; however, the usefulness of this measurement in directing the surgeon to lesions within the aorta is limited.

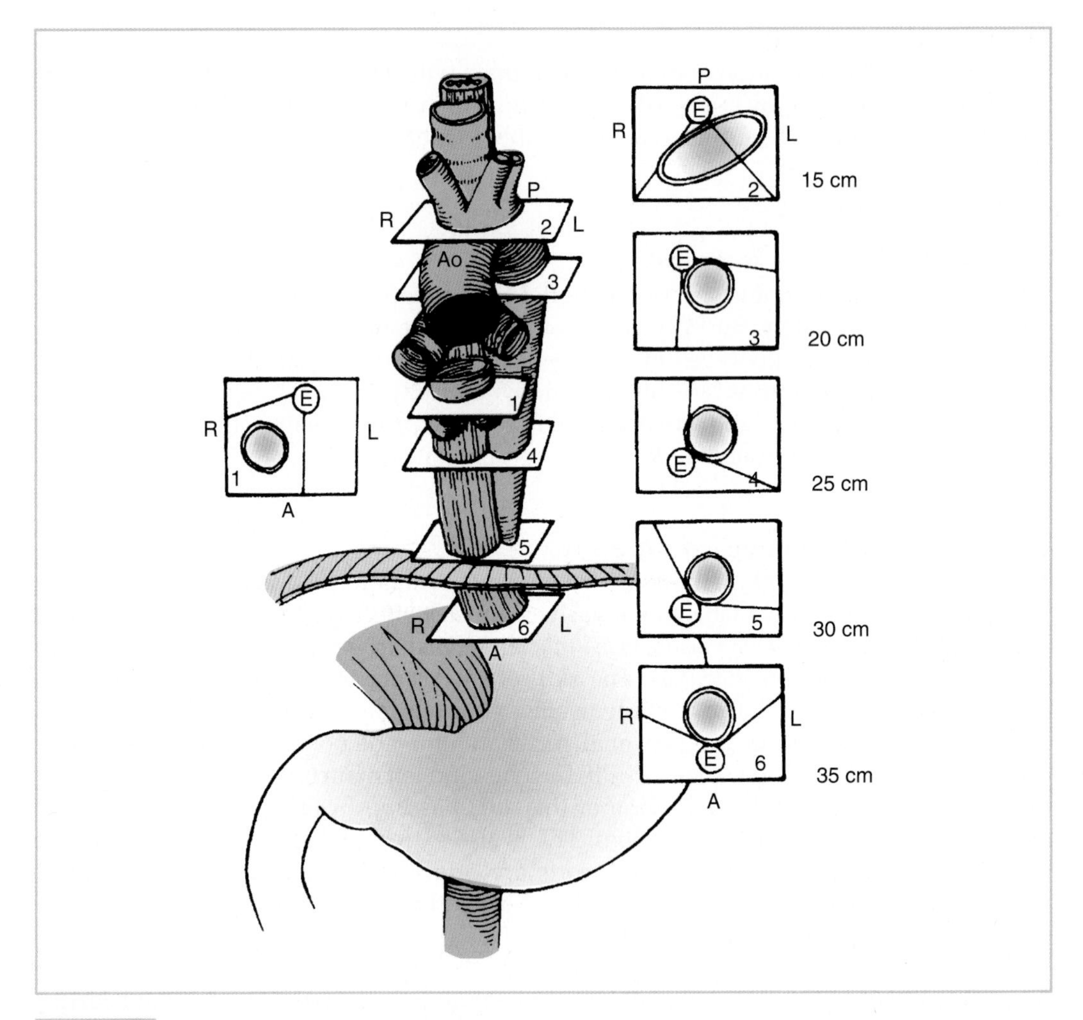

Figure 16.4. Relationship between the esophagus and aorta at different levels of the thoracic esophagus. (From Estafanous FG, Barash PG, Reves JG, eds. *Cardiac anesthesia principles and clinical practice,* second ed. Philadelphia: Lippincott Williams & Wilkins, 2001:785, with permission.)

As is discussed later, two areas are of primary concern in acute aortic dissection. These are the area just distal to the aortic valve in the region of the sinotubular junction, where acute ascending aortic dissections tend to occur, and the area just distal to the left subclavian artery, where descending dissections originate. A complete thoracic aortic examination is necessary to delineate both the aneurysm and the acute dissection pathology. These two high-risk areas must be carefully examined. One must remember also that the air-filled trachea is interposed between the esophagus and the distal ascending aorta and proximal aortic arch. *The distal ascending aorta may not be visualized clearly, even with multiplane TEE technology* (13).

Examination of the Ascending Thoracic Aorta

The examination technique that follows focuses on rapidly determining whether an aortic dissection is present. The examination of the thoracic aorta is begun at a probe depth of 30 to 35 cm from the incisors. At 0 degree, the midesophageal (ME) five-chamber view is identified. The angle is rotated first to 40 to 60 degrees for the ME aortic valve short-axis view and then to 90 to 120 degrees to identify the ME aortic valve long-axis view. The long-axis view allows interrogation of the proximal ascending aorta and measurement of the diameter of the sinus of Valsalva and sinotubular junction. To optimize this view, one generally rotates the handle toward the patient's right side. By gradually withdrawing the probe from the ME aortic valve long-axis view, one can frequently visualize an additional 2 to 3 cm of the ascending aorta. It is paramount that this view be carefully examined to detect proximal ascending aortic dissections. *Extreme care must be taken if a Swan-Ganz catheter is in place because it frequently appears as an artifact within the ascending aorta at this level* (Figure 16.5). If a question arises regarding the diagnosis of an intimal flap verses an artifact, our motto is *"when in doubt, pull the Swan out!"* The angle is now gradually decreased to 60 degrees and then 0 degree as the probe is gradually withdrawn from the patient's mouth. This demonstrates the ME ascending aorta short-axis view, in which the ascending aorta lies adjacent to the pulmonary artery and its right main branch.

Examination of the Descending Thoracic Aorta

Attention is now turned to the descending thoracic aorta. Again, one starts with the ME four- or five-chamber view, and the probe is manually rotated to the left until the circular short-axis image of the descending thoracic aorta is located in the center of the near field. This view is called the descending aorta short-axis view. It can be more easily seen by adjusting the depth settings on the machine to 6 to 8 cm thereby increasing the size of the aorta on the display screen. By advancing and withdrawing the probe within the esophagus, one can evaluate the entire descending thoracic aorta and a portion of the upper abdominal aorta from this position. The probe is advanced within the esophagus starting at the level of the distal arch and is gradually rotated farther to the left to keep the descending aorta in view. Once the stomach is entered, the ability to evaluate the descending abdominal aorta is lost. At this level, one gradually withdraws the probe

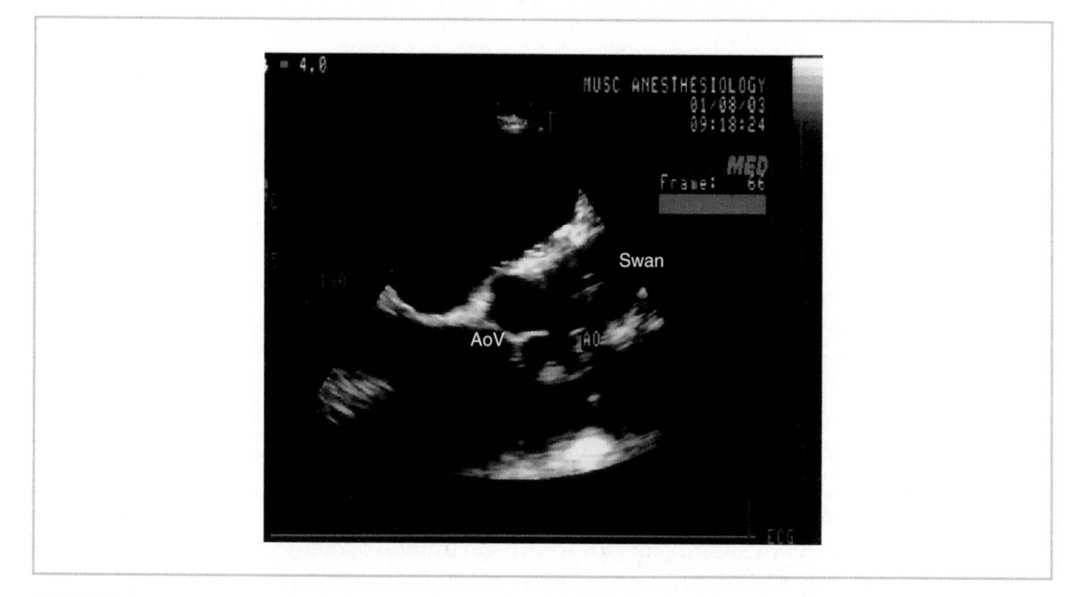

Figure 16.5. Transesophageal echocardiographic image demonstrating a linear streak in the middle of the proximal ascending aorta, representing an image artifact caused by a Swan-Ganz catheter. AoV, aortic valve; Ao, aorta.

while watching the descending aorta until the left subclavian artery is reached. Further withdrawal demonstrates the upper esophageal aortic arch long-axis view. One then rotates the probe 90 degrees to obtain the upper esophageal aortic arch short-axis view.

The probe is again advanced into the stomach until the descending aorta short-axis view is visualized. The transducer is then rotated 90 degrees and the descending aortic long-axis view is demonstrated. The probe is withdrawn until the left subclavian artery is again identified.

With careful inspection of the aorta in at least two planes and the use of color Doppler, most pathology of the ascending and descending aorta can be identified by this technique. Once the examination of the thoracic aorta is complete, attention can be turned to other matters of concern, such as pericardial effusion, aortic insufficiency, and LV function.

TRANSESOPHAGEAL ECHOCARDIOGRAPHIC EVALUATION OF AORTIC DISSECTION

Surgeons' Questions (What They Need to Know)

The goals of intraoperative TEE for the evaluation of aortic dissection include the following:

1. Confirmation of the preoperative diagnosis.
2. Determination of the dissection entry site, including differentiation of true and false lumina.
3. Intraoperative monitoring of the patient's volume status by assessing the LV chamber area and ventricular wall motion during the operative procedure and by determining whether aortic insufficiency is present. In cases of circulatory arrest, it is critical to know whether aortic insufficiency is present to detect ventricular distension if an aortic cross-clamp is not planned. Also, short-axis monitoring for LV distension when fibrillation occurs allows early chamber decompression through vent insertion, either through the LV apex or a pulmonary vein.
4. Examination to detect complications.
5. Confirmation of the integrity of the surgical repair.

Characteristics of Aortic Dissection

In aortic dissection, an accumulation of blood dissects the intima from the media. On TEE examination, most cases are associated with an intimal flap, seen as a mobile linear echo within the vascular lumen (4,14–17) (Figure 16.6). The intimal flap is the most important evidence of an aortic dissection (15,18). An intimal flap and flow within the true and false lumina on either side of the flap are highly sensitive features of aortic dissection (14,17,18) (Figure 16.6 and Figure 16.7). Additional TEE findings consistent with aortic dissection include the following: (a) complete thrombosis of the false lumen, (b) central displacement of intimal calcification with bright echogenic densities within the aorta, and (c) separation of the intimal layers from the thrombus (14,17,19).

Location and Entry Sites

TEE is a valuable tool for evaluating the location of an intimal tear entry site. The entry site of an intimal tear is defined as a disruption in the continuity of the flap, often identified by color flow Doppler (20) (Figure 16.8). With color Doppler, small intimal tears can be identified that may not be visualized by two-dimensional echocardiography. A turbulent jet of bright mosaic color can be seen flowing from the true to the false lumen (7,21,22) (Figure 16.8).

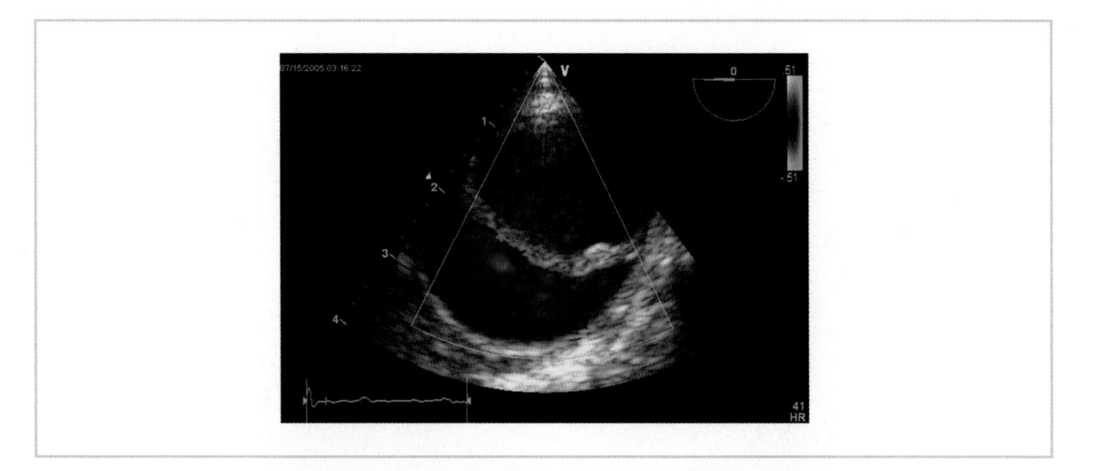

Figure 16.6. The true and false lumen of a type B aortic dissection are noted. Note the spontaneous echo contrast within the false lumen. Color Doppler demonstrates early systolic flow within the true lumen. Note proximity of the timing tracer to the QRS complex indicating early systole.

The intimal tear occurs in the ascending aorta 1 to 3 cm above the right or left sinus of Valsalva in approximately 70% of cases. (Figure 16.9) In the remaining 20% to 30% of cases, the intimal flap is located at the site of the ligamentum arteriosum in the descending thoracic aorta (4,7,21). The exact location of a tear can be estimated by the depth of probe insertion in relation to a major anatomic landmark, such as the sinus of Valsalva or the left subclavian artery. In some cases, the primary tear cannot be accurately identified because multiple tears are present or TEE visualization of the distal ascending aorta "blind spot" is poor. In a study by Adachi et al. (23), the entry site was identified in 88% patients with acute dissection. Type B dissection entry sites were identified in 90% of cases, and type A dissections in 83% of cases.

The dissection of the medial layer may be localized or split longitudinally. In the ascending aorta and arch, the plane of dissection usually courses along the greater curvature, whereas

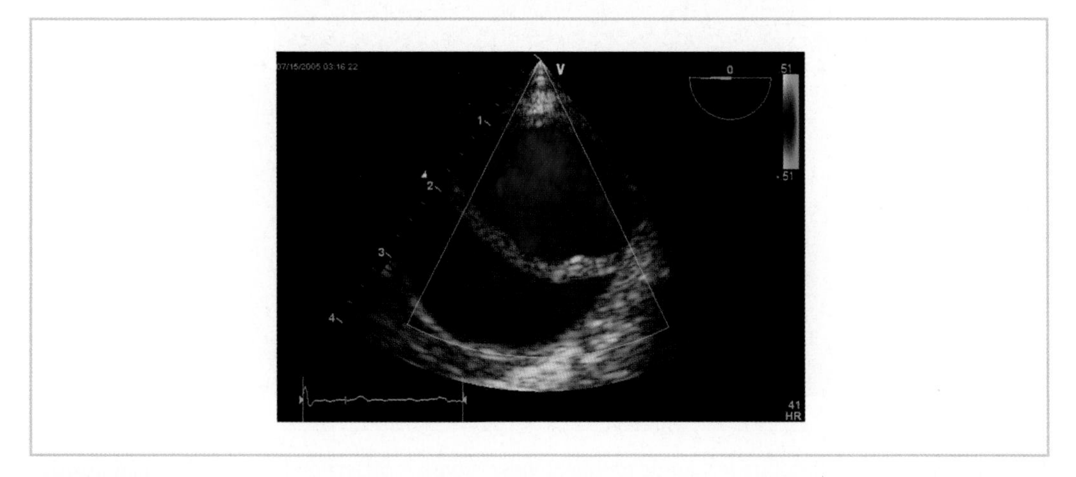

Figure 16.7. A color Doppler image demonstrating late systolic flow within the false lumen. Note the timing tracer is later in systole than that of Figure 16.6.

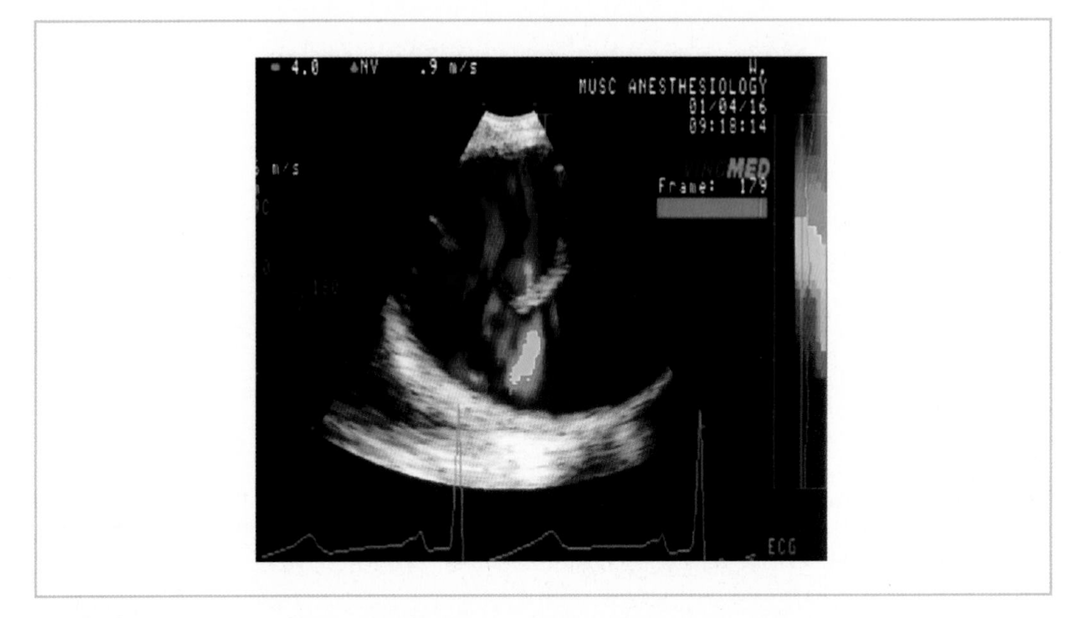

Figure 16.8. The image demonstrates the entry site of an intimal tear within the descending thoracic aorta. Note flow from the true lumen to the false lumen through the entry site.

in the descending thoracic aorta, the dissection plane is usually localized lateral to the true lumen, although it may spiral along the longitudinal axis (21).

As previously noted, the location and extent of the dissection flap are used to determine the type of aortic dissection. Identification and localization of the primary tear are important to the success of the surgical repair (24). Surgical resection of the primary entry site may decrease the incidence of late reoperation and complications (25).

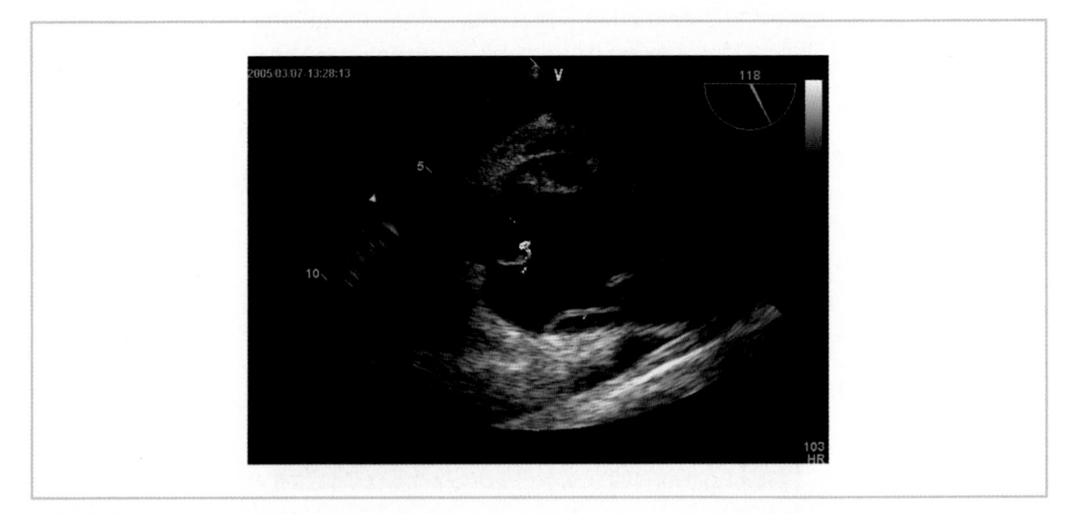

Figure 16.9. In this midesophageal aortic long-axis view, a type A dissection is evident with an obvious dissection flap. This dissection flap involves the sinuses of Valsalva with the potential for coronary artery involvement.

False versus True Lumen

Identification of the true and false lumina by TEE is critical to the assessment of aortic dissection (17,20). It may be difficult to differentiate the true from the false lumen, especially when the dissection involves the entire aorta and the intimal flap separates the lumen into halves (17).

Multiple indirect findings differentiate true from false lumina on TEE (17,19,20,26,27). The true lumen usually expands during systole and is compressed during diastole (15). A motion mode (M-mode) cursor placed through the dissection timed early in systole may identify expansion of the true lumen. (Figures 16.10 and 16.11) The true lumen has a thin, less echogenic inner layer, whereas the false lumen has a bright echogenic layer adjacent to the aortic lumen. Spontaneous echo contrast and variable amounts of thrombus are frequently present in the false lumen as a consequence of the stagnant flow. The false lumen is usually larger than the true lumen, especially in chronic dissections (17,19,20,26,27) (Figure 16.10).

Color flow Doppler imaging provides additional information regarding aortic flow patterns in dissection. The true lumen is identified by forward systolic flow, whereas flow in the false lumen is complicated and variable. With large, proximal entry tears, flow in the nearby segments of the false lumen may be the same in direction and timing as flow in the true lumen (27). With small distal tears, flow in the false lumen less closely resembles flow in the true lumen; it may be in the opposite direction and peak later in the cardiac cycle because of the delay of flow into the false lumen (15).

Multiple communications between the true and false lumina can frequently be identified by pulsed wave and color flow Doppler. Some communications represent entry sites with flow from the true toward the false lumen during systole, whereas others represent exit sites with bidirectional flow (20,22,27–29).

Thrombosis of the False Lumen

Thrombosis of the false lumen is an indirect finding of aortic dissection and requires further evaluation by TEE (15,20,22,26) (Figure 16.12). A thrombus can be identified as a mass

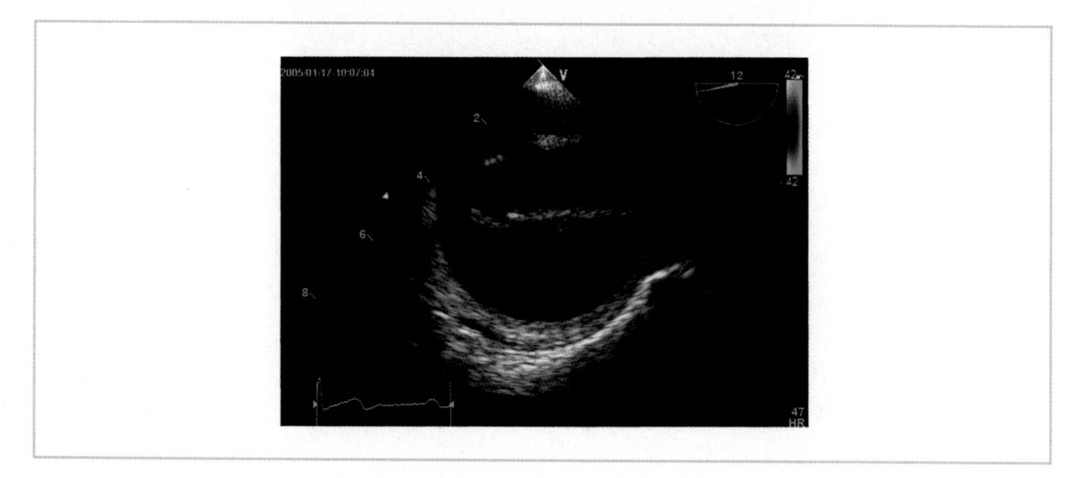

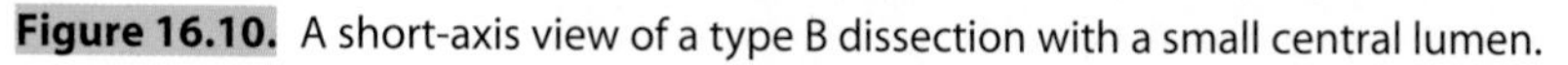

Figure 16.10. A short-axis view of a type B dissection with a small central lumen.

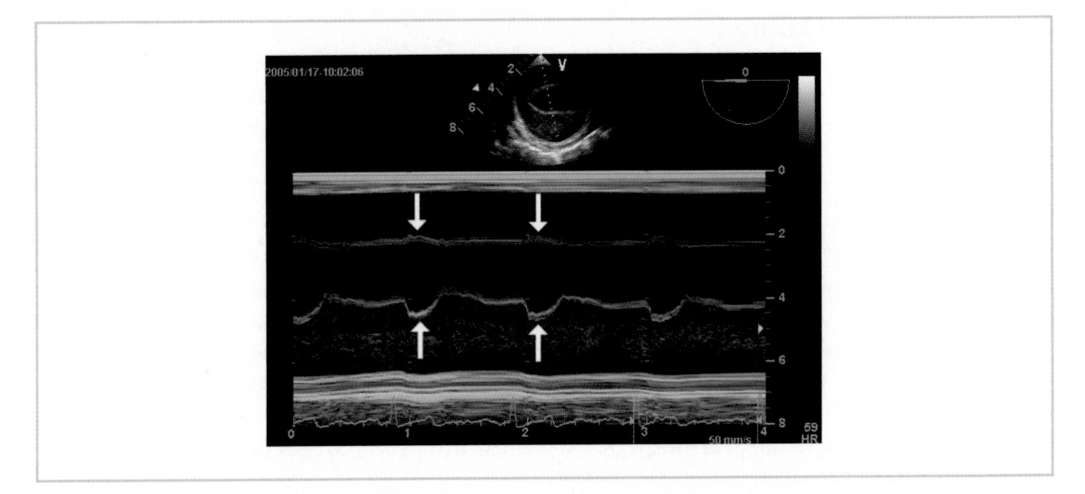

Figure 16.11. Motion mode (M-mode) examination reveals expansion of the true lumen during early systole with the intimal flaps moving towards the false lumens, arrows. Note the spontaneous echo contrast within the false lumen.

within the vascular true or false lumen that is separate from the intimal flap and aortic wall (29). A thickening of the aortic wall in excess of 15 mm has been considered a sign of dissection, suggesting thrombosis of a false channel, and can make the intimal flap difficult to identify (15). Many areas of the false lumen may show spontaneous echo contrast with stagnant flow and often exhibit partial thrombosis. These thrombosed segments tend to develop in areas remote from high-velocity large entry or exit sites.

The differentiation of a descending thoracic aortic aneurysm with laminated clot from a completely thrombosed false lumen is an important function of TEE. In a patient with a thrombosed false lumen, persistent small and limited areas with a sluggish, swirling flow pattern are typically seen, consistent with a false lumen rather than intraluminal clot. The

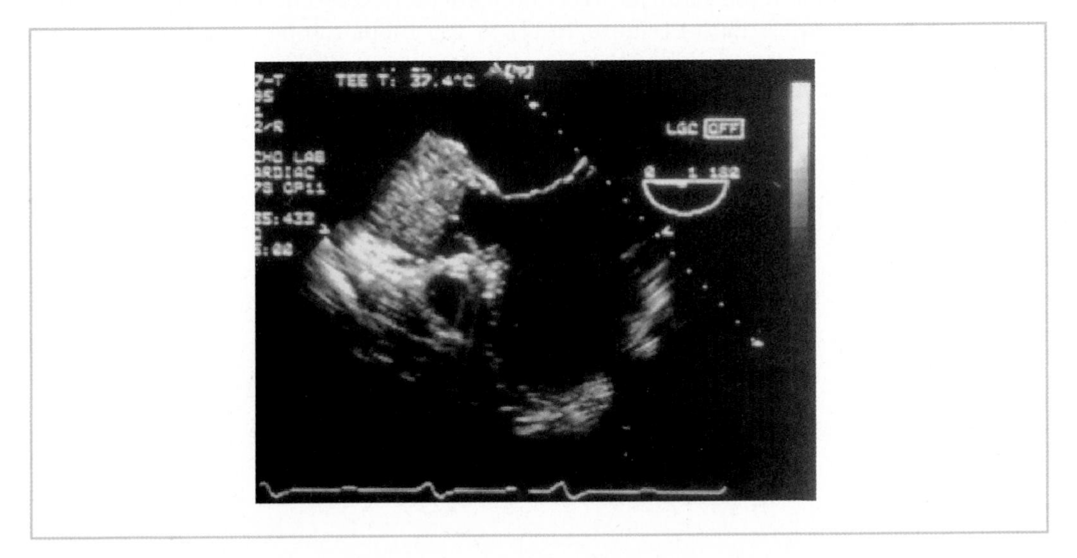

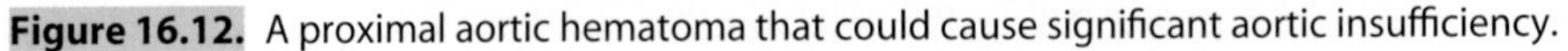

Figure 16.12. A proximal aortic hematoma that could cause significant aortic insufficiency.

presence of thrombus in the ascending aorta suggests thrombosis of the false lumen of an aortic dissection.

Aortic Insufficiency

A TEE evaluation of aortic valve structure and function is integral in the assessment of aortic dissection; aortic insufficiency is associated with 50% to 70% of proximal dissections and 10% of descending thoracic aortic dissections, and its presence carries important surgical implications (30). TEE is more sensitive than aortography in detecting mild aortic insufficiency (31). Aortic insufficiency is diagnosed with color flow Doppler (see Chapter 11). We have found that the ratio of the regurgitant jet height to the LV outflow tract width is the most useful method for grading aortic insufficiency as mild (1%–24%), moderate (25%–46%), moderate-severe (47%–64%), or severe (>65%) (28).

TEE can also demonstrate the causes of aortic insufficiency, thereby facilitating surgical decision making. The mechanisms of aortic insufficiency in the face of aortic dissection include the following: (a) dilation of the aortic root with widening of the aortic annulus and disturbance of aortic valve cusp coaptation (Figure 16.13); (b) disturbance of cusp closure by hematoma at the annulus (Figure 16.12); (c) destruction of annular support of the cusps with subsequent cusp prolapse; and (d) prolapse of the dissection flap into the aortic valve orifice and LV outflow tract with interference of aortic cusp motion (20,32) (Figure 16.14).

Aortic insufficiency has a negative effect on outcome in aortic dissection and may dictate the surgical approach. Preservation of the native aortic valve with repair and resuspension is possible in 86% of type A dissections, especially if the aortic valve leaflets appear normal (33). Specific involvement of the aortic annulus by Marfan syndrome or annuloaortic ectasia may dictate aortic valve replacement because of the limited long-term durability of

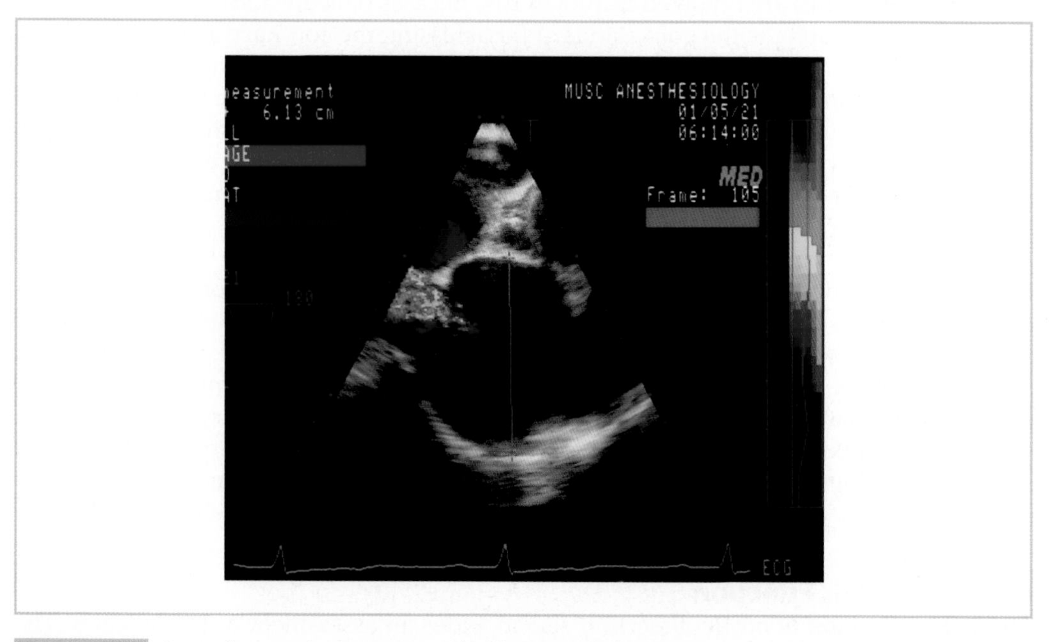

Figure 16.13. Ascending aortic aneurysm with dilation in the proximal ascending aorta resulting in poor coaptation of the aorta valve leaflets and a central jet of aortic regurgitation.

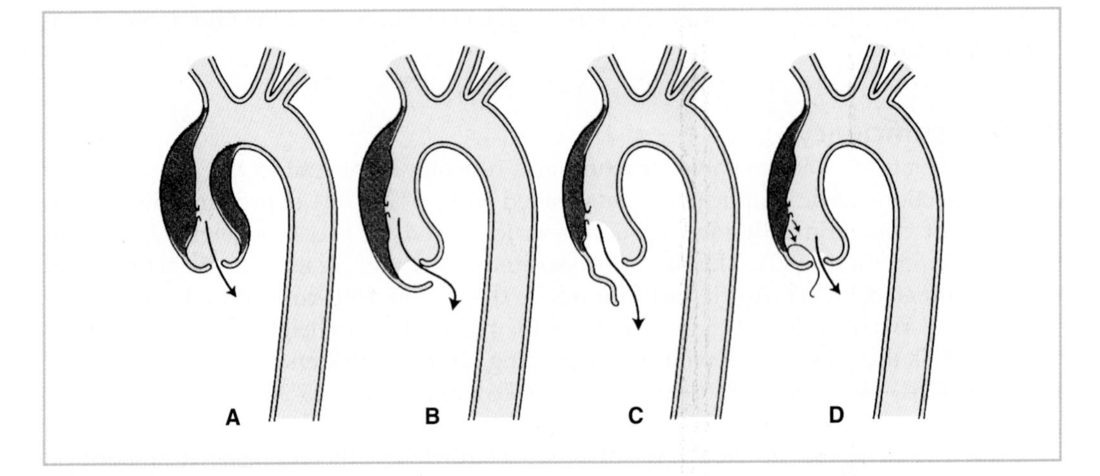

Figure 16.14. Mechanism of aortic regurgitation in proximal aortic dissection. **A:** An extensive or circumferential tear dilates the aortic root and annulus, causing failure of coaptation of the aortic valve leaflets. **B:** With asymmetric dissection, pressure from the false lumen depresses one aortic leaflet below the coaptation line of the other leaflets. **C:** The annular support is disrupted, resulting in a flail aortic leaflet. **D:** Prolapse of a mobile intimal flap through the aortic valve during diastole, which prevents leaflet coaptation. (From Braunwald E, ed. *Heart disease: a textbook of cardiovascular medicine,* fifth ed, Vol. 2. Philadelphia: WB Saunders, 1997:1557, with permission.)

aortic valve reconstruction. As previously noted, the presence of aortic insufficiency necessitates the use of either ostial or retrograde cardioplegia during cardiopulmonary bypass.

Involvement of the Coronary Arteries

The coronary arteries are involved in 10% to 20% of cases of acute aortic dissection (4,32). Although angiography is the gold standard for assessing the coronary anatomy, TEE has been shown to be a reliable tool for evaluating the proximal coronary anatomy, especially in the critical setting of aortic dissection (32). The coronary arteries can be visualized as two parallel lines originating from the aortic lumen in the ME aortic valve short-axis view (7). The relationship of the dissection flap to the proximal left and right coronary arteries, the extent of dissection into the coronary arteries, and the degree of coronary blood flow obstruction caused by the flap should be evaluated by TEE.

Ballard et al. (32) detected coronary artery involvement with TEE in six of seven surgically documented cases of coronary artery dissection. Adequate views of the ostia and proximal vessels were obtained in 88% of the left main coronary arteries and 50% of the right coronary arteries. Although no studies have shown that coronary artery bypass grafting affects the ultimate outcome in patients with aortic dissection, coronary involvement in patients with proximal aortic dissection is an indication for urgent surgery (34). *TEE, which enables a rapid diagnosis and a relative sensitive assessment of the proximal coronary anatomy, is the test of choice for defining the coronary anatomy in the setting of aortic dissection* (24,32,34).

Left Ventricular Function

The TEE evaluation of aortic dissection also includes an assessment of LV function. The heart represents an end organ that may experience significant ischemia during aortic dissection and subsequent coronary dissection. Global dysfunction may be secondary to diffuse ischemia with dissection of both coronary arteries or to aortic insufficiency–related LV decompensation. Left ventricular regional wall motion abnormalities are seen in 10% to 15% of patients with aortic dissection due to compression of a coronary artery by expansion of the false lumen, extension of the dissection into a coronary artery, or hypotension. The right coronary artery is more commonly affected (35–37).

Pericardial and Pleural Effusion

In an aortic dissection, the aortic wall may rupture through the adventitia at the site of the dissection. Proximal extension of the dissection with rupture at the aortic root may result in cardiac tamponade as blood enters the pericardium. In most cases of aortic dissection, pericardial effusion is not secondary to rupture or leak, but rather it is due to transudation of fluid into the pericardial cavity through the intact wall of the false lumen (35,38). (Figure 16.15) From the descending thoracic aorta, blood will enter the left pleural space, leading to hemothorax. Uncontained rupture into the mediastinum or pleural space causes sudden death, whereas ruptures contained by the aortic adventitia result in pseudoaneurysm formation or hematoma. Echo-free spaces around the aorta are a sign of penetration and periaortic hematoma. Mediastinal hematomas are identified when the distance from the esophagus to the left atrium or aorta increases and a pleural effusion develops (29).

Intraoperative Assessment of Aortic Graft Repair

After surgical repair, TEE assessment of the integrity of the aortic graft and detection of a residual flow signal in the false lumen provide vital information to the surgical team. The absence of a false luminal blood flow signal after repair indicates successful closure of the communication between the true and false lumina. This may reduce the risk for subsequent dissection and rupture, thereby improving the long-term prognosis (19,32).

Limitations of Transesophageal Echocardiography

Although the TEE evaluation of aortic dissection is sensitive and specific, it has notable limitations. Whereas the proximal ascending aorta and descending thoracic aorta are easily

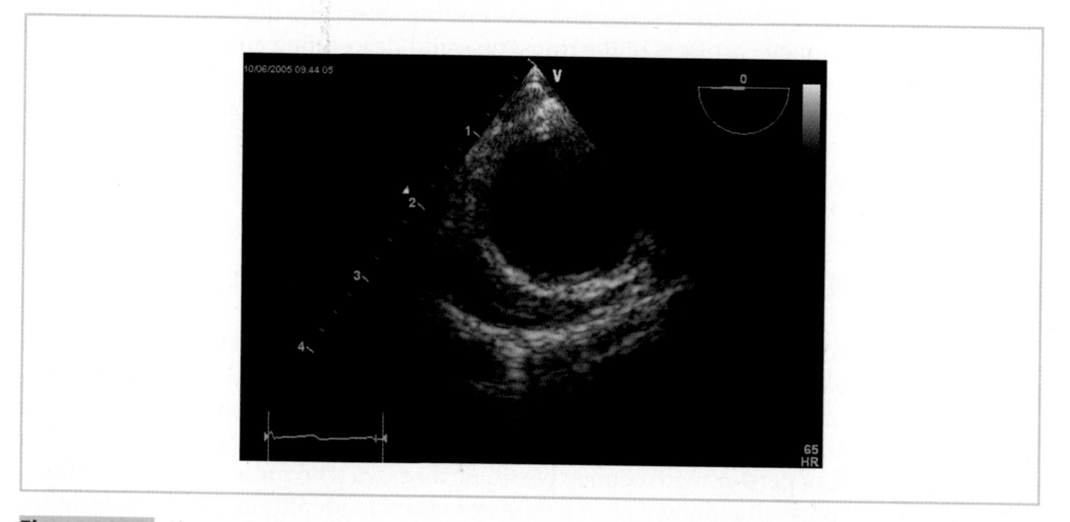

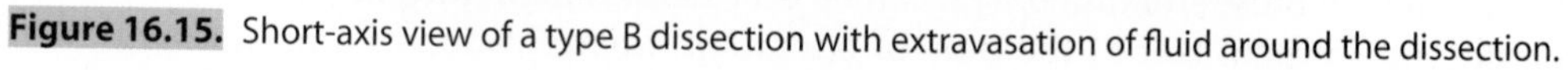

Figure 16.15. Short-axis view of a type B dissection with extravasation of fluid around the dissection.

visualized by TEE, the distal ascending aorta may be inadequately visualized because of the interposed air-filled trachea. Longitudinal plane imaging has significantly improved imaging of the distal ascending aorta; however, in a study by Konstadt (39), a variable portion of the distal ascending aorta (4.5–10.7 cm) could not be visualized.

Side branch involvement of the brachiocephalic arch vessels and thoracoabdominal aortic branches is not visualized by TEE (24). To obtain supplementary information regarding these arteries, angiography may be required.

Transesophageal Echocardiographic Artifacts

All ultrasound imaging techniques can produce artifacts when ultrasound is reflected back and forth between strongly reflective surfaces. These multiple-path artifacts introduce apparent boundaries and structures into an image when no structures actually exist. A multitude of tissue–fluid and tissue–air interfaces produce an ideal setting for imaging artifacts during a TEE examination of the heart and aorta (24).

Artifacts involving the ascending aorta are an important clinical problem in the evaluation of aortic dissection because whether or not the ascending aorta is involved determines the need for surgery. In a study by Appelbe et al. (40), linear artifacts were detected in the ascending aorta in 44% of the cases, leading to false-positive results and a decreased specificity of TEE. Linear artifacts in the ascending aorta are caused by reverberation of the aortic wall in the presence of arteriosclerosis, a sclerotic aortic root, or calcific aortic disease, and they produce echo images that resemble an intimal flap (7,20). Linear artifacts are also commonly encountered at the level of the left atrium in the presence of a dilated aorta. Side lobe artifacts from the aortic valve can also simulate an intimal flap. A linear artifact of the ascending aorta can be distinguished from an intimal flap by (a) indistinct borders of the artifact, (b) lack of the rapid oscillatory movement associated with an intimal flap, (c) extension of the artifact through the aortic wall as a straight line, and (d) the ability to extrapolate the linear artifact to the starting point of the transducer (40,41). In the presence of an artifact, color Doppler imaging will demonstrate homogeneous color on both sides of the linear echo, without any transverse or communicating jets.

Artifacts also occur in the transverse and descending aorta. In the study of Appelbe et al. (40), "mirror image" artifacts of the transverse and descending aorta were present in more than 80% of patients. These artifacts appear as a reduplication of the aortic lumen. The mirror image is caused by a highly reflective aorta–lung interface and is easy to distinguish from a true anatomic structure. The mirror image occurs at a predictable distance related to the width of the aorta, and the double-lumen appearance of the aorta disappears where the lung is not adjacent to the aorta.

SPECIAL CONSIDERATIONS IN THE EVALUATION OF TYPE III (STANFORD B) DISSECTIONS

The approach to a descending thoracic aortic dissection depends on the location of the primary intimal tear and the status of the patient. Surgery is considered for those patients who present with complications of the dissection, such as impending rupture, intractable pain, expanding size of the aorta, and signs of poor visceral or limb perfusion; it is also considered for young persons with connective tissue diseases who present with dissections at an early age. In these situations, TEE can be very helpful in identifying the exact location of the primary intimal tear at the time of operation. Identification of a normal proximal segment of aorta indicates that the patient can be safely cross-clamped. Currently, however, patients who have type B aortic dissections with primary intimal tears close to the left subclavian artery or extension of the dissection to the left subclavian artery or distal aortic arch should be treated with circulatory arrest. Under these circumstances, TEE is useful for identifying pathology and also for careful monitoring of the LV diameter in the short-axis view. During cooling for circulatory arrest, when the ventricle fibrillates, it is important to monitor for dilation of the LV secondary to aortic insufficiency. If this is identified, it is necessary to place an LV vent through the apex of the LV or across the mitral valve through a pulmonary vein. Currently, it is felt that avoidance of cross-clamping of the dissected aorta facilitates visualization for a proximal anastomosis and may reduce the incidence of residual aortic dissection and pseudoaneurysm formation at the anastomotic site following surgery.

INTRAMURAL HEMATOMA

Intramural hematoma is felt to be a noncommunicating aortic dissection that does not fall within the traditional DeBakey classification system. Intramural hematomas most often involve the ascending or descending aorta and are characterized by a thickened aortic wall without an intimal flap or dissection entry site. The false lumen is felt to be secondary to rupture of the vasa vasorum that results in massive hemorrhage into the vessel wall. The natural history of this disease is such that 60% of patients progress to either rupture or dissection within 1 year (42–44). Aortic rupture usually occurs within several days in patients who have ascending aortic involvement; therefore, rapid diagnosis and surgical treatment are imperative. In patients with a descending thoracic aorta intramural hematoma, the decision between surgical therapy and medical management with a strict antihypertensive regimen and frequent imaging follow-up remains controversial.

The initial TEE classification of intramural hematoma was described by Mohr-Kahaly (45). Intramural hematoma is characterized by circular or crescentic thickening of the aortic wall of more than 7 mm (Figure 16.16), central displacement of intimal calcification, a longitudinal extent of 1 to 20 cm, a layered appearance, and the absence of an intimal tear or dissection membrane. The thickness is measured from the internal border of the intima

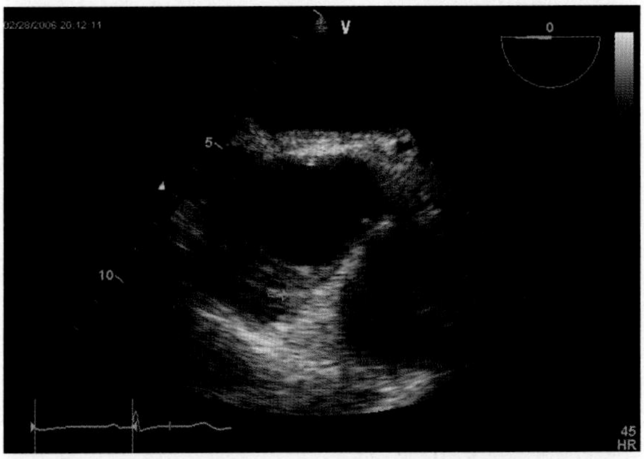

Figure 16.16. Short-axis view of the ascending aorta demonstrating a crescent-shaped intramural hematoma, arrow.

to the outer edge of the adventitia. Harris (43) further clarified the TEE findings by noting that an intramural hematoma involving the ascending aorta typically measures 7 ± 2 mm, whereas a hematoma in the descending aorta is much thicker, measuring 15 ± 6 mm. Most of the patients had a crescent-shaped intramural hematoma involving one wall predominantly that compressed the aortic lumen. Compression of the normal circular lumen of the aorta resulted in a major–minor axis ratio of the aortic lumen of 1.3% ± 0.2% (43).

GIANT PENETRATING ULCER

Giant penetrating atherosclerotic ulcer disease usually occurs in elderly patients who have hypertension, hyperlipidemia, and atherosclerosis (35,46). This disease typically occurs in the descending thoracic aorta and is characterized by a discrete ulcer with a thickened underlying aortic wall. Progressive penetration into the aortic wall may result in an intramural hematoma with aortic wall weakening and resultant aneurysm formation (35,47).

THORACIC AORTIC PLAQUE

Stroke continues to be a serious complication of cardiac surgery, occurring in approximately 1% to 5% of patients. The ability to detect atheroma within the thoracic aorta and alter the surgical approach is an important part of most strategies for stroke prevention (48). Royse (49) proposed dividing the thoracic aorta into six zones corresponding to sites of surgical manipulation. Zones 1 through 3 are the proximal, mid, and distal ascending aorta. Zones 1 and 2 are the sites of incision for aortic valve replacement. Figure 16.17 shows a zone 1 atheroma. Zone 2 is also the site for proximal coronary artery bypass graft anastomosis and can be used for antegrade cardioplegia cannulation. Zone 3 is where the aortic cross-clamp is usually placed. Zone 4 includes the proximal arch and is typically the site where the aortic cannula is manipulated. Zone 5, which includes the distal arch, and zone 6, which includes the proximal descending aorta, are not typically manipulated during cardiac surgery (49). However, in these areas, atheroma can be dislodged by the

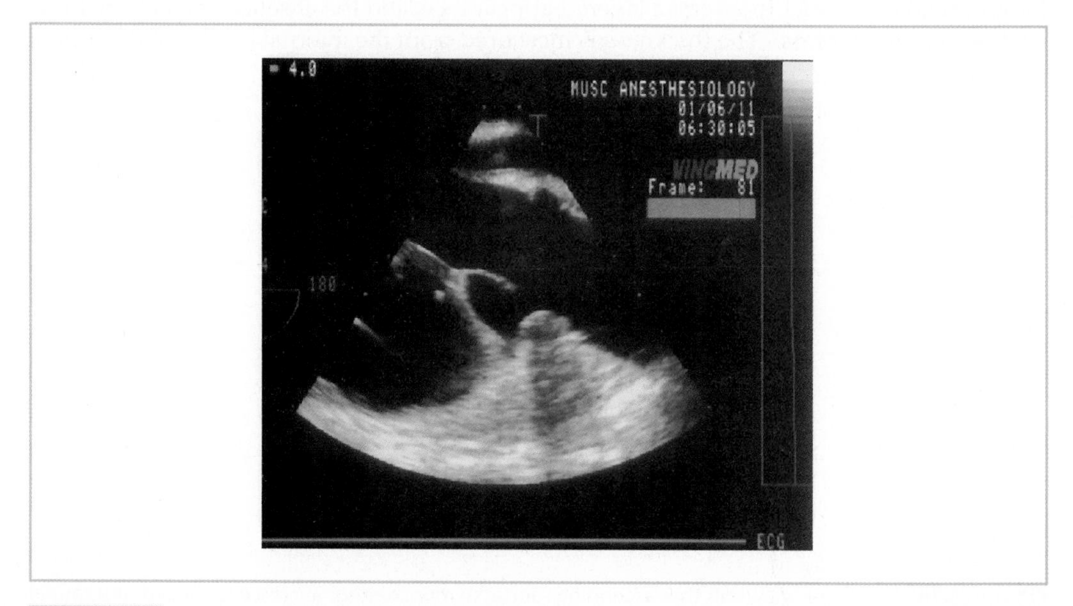

Figure 16.17. A grade 3 anterior atheroma in zone 1.

Table 16.2 Grading of thoracic aorta atheroma

Grade	Description
1	Normal aorta
2	Extensive intimal thickening
3	Protrudes <5 mm into aortic lumen
4	Protrudes >5 mm into aortic lumen
5	Mobile atheroma

aortic cannula or an endoluminal device, such as an intraaortic balloon pump. In the study of Royse (49), adequate imaging by TEE was obtained in zone 3 in only 58% of patients, and in zone 4 in 42% of patients. These findings are consistent with the work of Konstadt (39,50), who showed that as much as 42% of the length of the ascending aorta is not adequately visualized with TEE. Manual surgical palpation detects only 50% of important atheromas identified by epiaortic ultrasonography (49).

TEE has been proposed as an intraoperative screening tool to identify patients who should undergo epiaortic scanning before cannulation for cardiopulmonary bypass. When moderate to severe atheroma is identified in zones 5 and 6 by TEE, the incidence of moderate to severe atheroma in zones 1 through 4 is high. Therefore, epiaortic scanning should be performed. If all visualized zones (1, 2, 5, and 6) are negative for atheroma, epiaortic scanning of zones 3 and 4, the TEE potential blind spots, is not necessary.

In 1992, Katz (51) published a five-point grading system for aortic atheroma (Table 16.2). Figure 16.18 shows a grade 4 atheroma. Patients with a mobile (grade 5) atheroma had a 25% incidence of stroke, whereas stroke occurred in only 2% of patients without a mobile

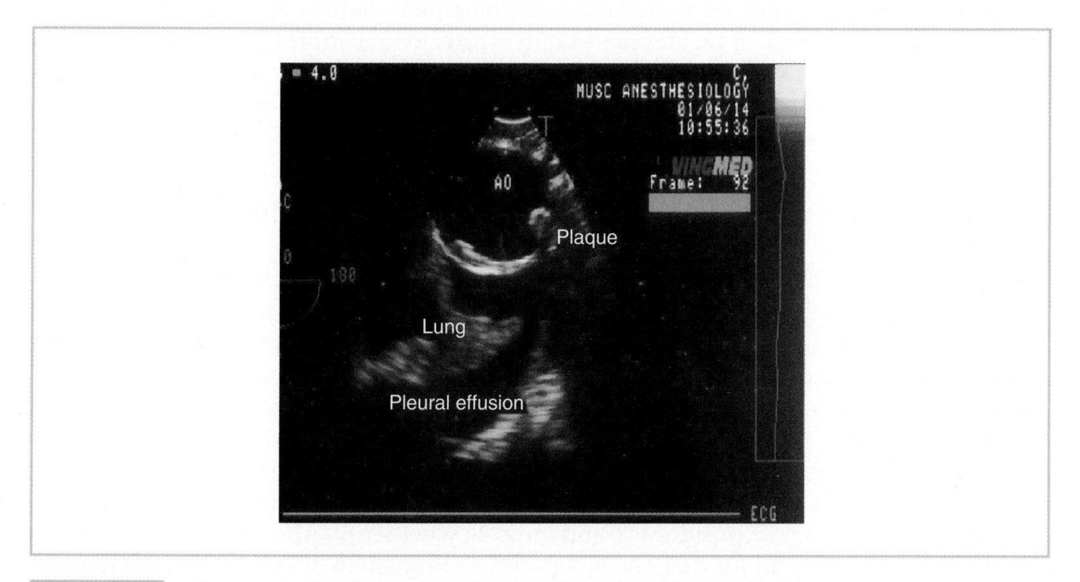

Figure 16.18. Atheroma in the descending thoracic aorta. Note the consolidated lung with a significant pleural effusion.

atheroma. In another study, the presence of aortic atheromas of 5 mm or larger increased the perioperative stroke rate by six fold and more than doubled the in-hospital mortality. It is therefore important to consider alternative surgical approaches for patients who have a significant protruding atheroma and especially patients with mobile components (51).

Severe ascending aortic calcification or atherosclerosis makes aortic cannulation and cardiopulmonary bypass dangerous and makes it difficult to construct aortic graft anastomoses. This problem has two potential solutions. One involves circulatory arrest with deep hypothermia, which usually requires replacement of a portion of the aorta. A second solution is a less complex operation that avoids cardiopulmonary bypass. Patients who are considered for coronary artery bypass grafting exclusively who present with a calcified ascending aorta can be managed with an off-pump approach. Through a median sternotomy, both the left internal and right internal mammary arteries can be used as conduits. Saphenous vein grafts or radial artery grafts can be taken off either of these conduits or separately anastomosed proximally to side branches of the aortic arch, such as the innominate artery.

The detection of atherosclerotic lesions in the aorta by TEE is a marker of diffuse atherosclerotic disease (52,53). A strong association between the presence and severity of aortic plaque imaged by TEE and the presence and extent of coronary artery disease has been identified (54,55). Complex plaques, which are defined as protuberant plaques greater than 4 mm in size or plaques with a mobile component detected on TEE, are associated with a high risk for cardiac death and coronary event (54,56). In a 2005 study by Weisenberg (57), a strong association between the presence of severe aortic stenosis and the presence and severity of aortic atheromas was identified with the suggestion that aortic stenosis may also be a manifestation of the atherosclerotic process.

Systemic Embolization of Aortic Plaque and Thrombus

TEE of the thoracic aorta may also aid in the identification of sources of arterial embolization. It is recognized that aortic atheromatous plaques are a potential source of embolization, especially if greater than 4 mm in size. Plaque morphology is important to consider, because ulcerated hypoechoic plaques with debris are at higher risk of embolization (58). The development of an overlying aortic thrombus is a rare, but potentially underestimated source of systemic embolization (59,60).

Transesophageal Echocardiographic Assessment of Endovascular Repair of Thoracic Aortic Aneurysms

Since its introduction in 1990, endovascular repair of the aorta (EVAR) has gained popularity as an alternative to open surgical repair of aortic aneurysms (61). The success of EVAR is dependent on satisfactory graft deployment as evidenced by proper positioning and the absence of a perigraft endoleak which has been routinely confirmed by aortography (62). TEE has also been found to be a valuable intraoperative tool for (a) identification of aortic pathology, (b) confirmation of placement of the guidewire within the aortic lumen, (c) aiding stent graft positioning, (d) supplementing angiography for detecting endoleaks, and (e) evaluating cardiac function (62–64). The TEE information can lead to modifications in endograft positioning and indicate whether EVAR is a feasible treatment option. TEE maybe useful for diagnosing endoleaks immediately after endograft deployment, because the TEE is able to image the space between the endograft and the aortic wall (63–66). Endoleaks are defined as persistent blood flow outside the endograft and within the aneurysm sac and they may occur in 20% of EVAR. The advantage of detecting an endoleak in the operating room is that an intervention to reposition the endograft or deploy a second prosthesis at the site of the leak can be undertaken (66).

SUMMARY

TEE plays an important role in the management of aortic pathology. Its ability to diagnose aortic aneurysm, dissection, and aortic atheroma rapidly and reliably has improved patient outcomes.

REFERENCES

1 Svensson LG, Crawford ES. Aortic dissection and aortic aneurysm surgery: clinical observations, experimental investigations, and statistical analyses. Part II *Curr Probl Surg* 1992;29:915–1057.
2 DeBakey ME, Henly WS, Cooley DA, et al. Surgical management of dissecting aneurysms of the aorta. *J Thorac Cardiovasc Surg* 1965;49:130–149.
3 Daily PO, Trueblood HW, Stinson EB, et al. Management of acute aortic dissections. *Ann Thorac Surg* 1970;10:237–247.
4 Hirst AE Jr, Johns VJ, Jr, Kime SW Jr. Dissecting aneurysm of the aorta: a review of 585 cases. *Medicine (Baltimore)* 1985;37:217–279.
5 Chirillo F, Cavillini C, Longhini C, et al. Comparative diagnostic valve of transesophageal echocardiography and retrograde aortography in the evaluation of thoracic aortic dissection. *Am J Cardiol* 1994;74:590–595.
6 Sommer T, Fehske W, Holzknecht N, et al. Aortic dissection: a comparative study of diagnosis with spiral CT, multiplanar transesophageal echocardiography, and MR imaging. *Radiology* 1996;199:347–352.
7 Cigarroa JE, Isselbacher EM, DeSanctis RW, et al. Diagnostic imaging in the evaluation of suspected aortic dissection. *N Engl J Med* 1993;328:35–43.
8 Barbant SD, Eisenberg MJ, Schiller NB. The diagnostic value of imaging techniques for aortic dissection. *Am Heart J* 1992;124:541–543.
9 Masani ND, Banning AP, Jones RA, et al. Follow-up of chronic thoracic aortic dissection. Comparison of transesophageal echocardiography and magnetic resonance imaging *Am Heart J* 1996;131:1156–1163.
10 Willens HJ, Kessler KM. Transesophageal echocardiography in the diagnosis of diseases of the thoracic aorta. *Chest* 1999;116:1172–1179.
11 Adachi H, Omoto R, Kyo S, et al. Emergency surgical intervention of acute aortic dissection with the rapid diagnosis by transesophageal echocardiography. *Circulation* 1991;84(Suppl III):III–14–III–19.
12 Keren A, Kim CB, Hu BS, et al. Accuracy of biplane and multiplane transesophageal echocardiography in diagnosis of typical acute aortic dissection and intramural hematoma. *J Am Coll Cardiol* 1996;28:627–636.
13 Shanewise JS, Cheung AT, Aronson S, et al. ASE/SCA guidelines for performing a comprehensive intraoperative multiplane transesophageal echocardiography examination: recommendations of the American Society of Echocardiography Council for Intraoperative Echocardiography and the Society of Cardiovascular Anesthesiologists Task Force for Certification in Perioperative Transesophageal Echocardiography. *Anesth Analg* 1999;89:870–884.
14 Erbel R, Engberding R, Daniel W, et al. Echocardiography in diagnosis of aortic dissection. *Lancet* 1989;1(8636):
457–461.
15 Iliceto S, Nanda NC, Rizzon P, et al. Color Doppler evaluation of aortic dissection. *Circulation* 1987;75:748–755.
16 Matthew T, Nanda NC. Two-dimensional and Doppler echocardiographic evaluation of aortic aneurysm and dissection. *Am J Cardiol* 1984;54:379–385.
17 Erbel R, Mohr-Kahaly S, Oelert H, et al. Diagnostic strategies in suspected aortic dissection: comparison of computed tomography, aortography, and transesophageal echocardiography. *Am J Card Imaging* 1990;4:157–172.
18 Erbel R, Borner N, Steller D, et al. Detection of aortic dissection by transesophageal echocardiography. *Br Heart J* 1987;58:45–51.
19 Mohr-Kahaly S, Erbel R, Rennollet H, et al. Ambulatory follow-up of aortic dissection by transesophageal two-dimensional and color-coded Doppler echocardiography. *Circulation* 1989;80:24–33.
20 Hashimoto S, Kumada T, Osakada G, et al. Assessment of transesophageal Doppler echocardiography in dissecting aortic aneurysm. *J Am Coll Cardiol* 1989;14:1253–1261.

21 Erbel K, Mohr-Kahaly S, Rennullet H, et al. Diagnosis of aortic dissection: the value of transesophageal echocardiography. *Thorac Cardiovasc Surg* 1987;35(1):126–133.
22 Dagli SV, Nanda NC, Roitman D, et al. Evaluation of aortic dissection by Doppler color flow mapping. *Am J Cardiol* 1985;56:497–498.
23 Adachi H, Kyo S, Takamoto S, et al. Early diagnosis and surgical intervention of acute aortic dissection by transesophageal color flow mapping. *Circulation* 1990;82(Suppl IV):IV–19–IV–23.
24 Taams MH, Gussenhoven WJ, Schippers LA, et al. The value of transesophageal echocardiography for diagnosis of thoracic aortic pathology. *Eur Heart J* 1988;9:1308–1316.
25 Heinemann M, Laas J, Karck M, et al. Thoracic aortic aneurysms after acute type A aortic dissection: necessity for follow-up. *Ann Thorac Surg* 1990;49:580–584.
26 Bansal RC, Shah PM. Transesophageal echocardiography. *Curr Probl Cardiol* 1990;15:643–720.
27 Erbel R, Mohr-Kahaly S, Rennollet H, et al. Diagnosis of aortic dissection: the value of transesophageal echocardiography. *Thorac Cardiovasc Surg* 1987;35:126–133.
28 Perry GJ, Helmcke F, Nanda NC, et al. Evaluation of aortic insufficiency by Doppler color flow mapping. *J Am Coll Cardiol* 1987;9:952–959.
29 Erbel R, Oelert H, Meyer J, et al. Effect of medical and surgical therapy on aortic dissection evaluated by transesophageal echocardiography. *Circulation* 1993;87:1604–1615.
30 Slater EE, DeSanctis RW. The clinical recognition of dissecting aortic aneurysm. *Am J Med* 1976;60:625–633.
31 Hunt D, Baxley WA, Kennedy JW, et al. Quantitative evaluation of cine aortography in the assessment of aortic regurgitation. *Am J Cardiol* 1973;31:696–700.
32 Ballard RS, Nanda NC, Gatewood R, et al. Usefulness of transesophageal echocardiography in assessment of aortic dissection. *Circulation* 1991;84:1903–1914.
33 Mazzucotelli JP, Deleuze PH, Baufreton C, et al. Preservation of the aortic valve in acute aortic dissection: long-term echocardiographic assessment and clinical outcome. *Ann Thorac Surg* 1993;55:1513–1517.
34 DeBakey ME, McCollum CH, Crawford ES, et al. Dissection and dissecting aneurysm of the aorta: twenty-year follow-up of five hundred twenty-seven patients treated surgically. *Surgery* 1982;92:1118–1134.
35 Khan IA, Nair CK. Clinical, diagnostic, and management perspectives of aortic dissection. *Chest* 2002;122:311–328.
36 Eisenberg MJ, Rice SA, et al. The clinical spectrum of patients with aneurysms of the ascending aorta. *Am Heart J* 1993;125:1380–1385.
37 Hennessy TG, Smith D, McCann HA, et al. Thoracic aortic dissection or aneurysm: clinical presentation, diagnostic imaging, and initial management in a tertiary referral center. *Ir J Med Sci* 1996;165:259–262.
38 Armstrong WF, Bach DS, Carey L, et al. Spectrum of acute aortic dissection of the ascending aorta: a transesophageal study. *J Am Soc Echocardiogr* 1996;9:646–656.
39 Konstadt SN, Reich DL, Kahn R, et al. Transesophageal echocardiography can be used to screen for ascending aortic atherosclerosis. *Anesth Analg* 1995;81:225–228.
40 Appelbe AF, Walker PG, Yeoh JK, et al. Clinical significance and origin of artifacts in transesophageal endocardiography of the thoracic aorta. *J Am Coll Cardiol* 1993;21:754–760.
41 Nienaber CA, Spielman RP, Von Kodolitsch Y, et al. Diagnosis of thoracic aortic dissection: magnetic resonance imagery versus transesophageal echocardiography. *Circulation* 1992;85:434–447.
42 Robbins RC, McManus RP, Mitchell RS, et al. Management of patients with intramural hematoma of the thoracic aorta. *Circulation* 1993;88:1–10.
43 Harris KM, Braverman AC, Gutierrez FR, et al. Transesophageal echocardiography and clinical features of aortic intramural hematoma. *J Thorac Cardiovasc Surg* 1997;114:619–626.
44 Kang DH, Song JK, Song MG, et al. Clinical and echocardiographic outcomes of aortic intramural hemorrhage compared with acute aortic dissection. *Am J Cardiol* 1998;81:202–206.
45 Mohr-Kahaly S, Erbel R, Kearney P, et al. Aortic intramural hemorrhage visualized by transesophageal echocardiography: findings and prognostic implications. *J Am Coll Cardiol* 1994;23:658–664.
46 Harris JA, Bis KG, Glover JL, et al. Penetrating atherosclerotic ulcers of the aorta. *J Vasc Surg* 1992;19:90–98.
47 Cooke JP, Kazmier FJ, Orszulak TA. The penetrating aortic ulcer: pathologic manifestations, diagnosis, and management. *Mayo Clin Proc* 1998;63:718–725.
48 Ribakove GH, Katz ES, Galloway AC, et al. Surgical implications of transesophageal echocardiography to grade the atheromatous aortic arch. *Ann Thorac Surg* 1992;53:758–763.
49 Royse C, Royse A, Blake D, et al. Screening the thoracic aorta for atheroma: a comparison of manual palpation, transesophageal and epiaortic ultrasonography. *Ann Thorac Cardiovasc Surg* 1998;4:347–350.
50 Konstadt SN, Reich DL, Quintana C, et al. The ascending aorta: how much does transesophageal echocardiography see? *Anesth Analg* 1994;78:240–244.
51 Katz ES, Tunick PA, Rusinek H, et al. Protruding aortic atheromas predict stroke in elderly patients undergoing cardiopulmonary bypass: experience with intraoperative transesophageal echocardiography. *J Am Coll Cardiol* 1992;20:70–77.

52 Witteman JC, Kannel WB, Wolf PA, et al. Aortic calcified plaques and cardiovascular disease (the Framingham Study). *Am J Cardiol* 1990;66:1060–1064.
53 Nihoyannopoulos P, Joshu J, Athanasopoulos G, et al. Detection of atherosclerotic lesions in the aorta by transesophageal echocardiography. *Am J Cardiol* 1993;71:1208–1212.
54 Rohani M, Jogestrand T, Ekberg M, et al. Interrelation between the extent of atherosclerosis in the thoracic aorta, carotid intima-media thickness, and the extent of coronary artery disease. *Atherosclerosis* 2005;179:311–316.
55 Fazio GP, Redberg RF, Winslow T, et al. Transesophageal echocardiography detected atherosclerotic plaque is a marker for coronary artery disease. *J Am Coll Cardiol* 1993;21:144–150.
56 Amanullah AM, Artel BJ, Grossman LB, et al. Usefulness of complex atherosclerotic plaque in the ascending aorta and arch for predicting cardiovascular events. *Am J Cardiol* 2002;89:1423–1426.
57 Weisenberg D, Sahar Y, Sahar G, et al. Atherosclerosis of the aorta is common in patients with severe aortic stenosis: an intraoperative transesophageal study. *J Thorac Cardiovasc Surg* 2005;130:29–32.
58 Bernard Y. Value of transesophageal echocardiography for the diagnosis of embolic lesions from the thoracic aorta. *J Neuroradiol* 2005;32:266–272.
59 Mirza IH, Mitchell ARJ, Timperley J. Transesophageal echocardiography for identification of a giant aortic thrombus. *Heart* 2005;91:778.
60 Aldrich HR, Girardi L, Bush HJ, et al. Recurrent systemic embolization caused by aortic thrombi. *Ann Thorac Surg* 1994;57:466–468.
61 Parodi JC, Palmaz JC, Barone HD. Transfemoral intraluminal graft implantation for abdominal aortic aneurysms. *Ann Vasc Surg* 1991;5:491–499.
62 Swaminathan M, Linebarger C, McCann R, et al. The importance of intraoperative transesophageal echocardiography in endovascular repair of thoracic aortic aneurysms. *Anesth Analg* 2003;97:1566–1572.
63 Rapezzi C, Rocchi G, Fattori R, et al. Usefulness of transesophageal echocardiography monitoring to improve the outcome of stent-graft treatment of thoracic aortic aneurysms. *Am J Cardiol* 2001;87:315–319.
64 Gonzalez-Fajardo JA, Gutierrez V, San Roman JA, et al. Utility of intraoperative transesophageal echocardioigraphy during endovascular stent-graft repair of acute thoracic aortic dissection. *Ann Vasc Surg* 2002;16:297–303.
65 van Marrewijk C, Buth J, Harris P, et al. Significance of endoleaks after endovascular repair of abdominal aortic aneurysms: the EUROSTAR experience. *J Vasc Surg* 2002;35:461–473.
66 Fattori R, Calderera J, Rapezzi C, et al. Primary endoleakage in endovascular treatment of the thoracic aorta: importance of intraoperative transesophageal echocardiography. *J Thorac Cardiovasc Surg* 2000;120:490–449.

QUESTIONS

1. **The Crawford classification of thoracoabdominal aneurysms includes all of the following definitions except**
   a. Type II aneurysms begin in the proximal descending thoracic aorta and terminate below the renal arteries.
   b. Type IV aneurysms involve the proximal descending thoracic aorta and the entire abdominal aorta.
   c. Type III aneurysms originate in the distal descending aorta.
   d. Type I aneurysms originate in the proximal descending thoracic aorta and end above the renal arteries.

2. **Which of the following is the most important evidence for an aortic dissection?**
   a. Separation of the intimal layers from the thrombus.
   b. Central displacement of intimal calcification with bright echogenic densities within the aorta.
   c. An intimal flap seen as a mobile line or echo within the vascular lumen.
   d. Complete thrombosis of the false lumen.

3. **Which of the following statements regarding aortic dissection is true?**
   a. In the majority of cases, the intimal flap is located at the site of the ligamentum arteriosum in the descending thoracic aorta.
   b. The intimal tear occurs in the ascending aorta 1 to 3 cm above the right or left sinus of Valsalva in 40% of cases.
   c. The entry site of a dissection can be identified in less than 60% of cases by transesophageal echocardiography (TEE) due to the "blind spot."
   d. Surgical resection of the primary entry site may decrease the incidence of late reoperation and complications.

4. **Which of the following statements regarding identification of the true and false lumen by TEE is false?**
   a. The false lumen has a thin, less echogenic layer.
   b. Spontaneous echo contrast and thrombus are frequently present in the false lumen.
   c. The true lumen usually expands during systole and is compressed during diastole.
   d. The false lumen is usually larger than the true in chronic dissections.
   e. The true lumen is identified by forward systolic flow.

5. **Which of the following statements regarding aortic dissection and aortic insufficiency is true?**
   a. TEE is less sensitive than aortography in detecting mild aortic insufficiency.
   b. Aortic insufficiency is diagnosed with pulse wave Doppler.
   c. Aortic insufficiency is associated with 50% to 70% of proximal dissections.
   d. Preservation of the aortic valve with repair and resuspension is rarely possible in type A dissections.

6. **Which of the following statements is true regarding aortic dissection and the coronary arteries.**
   a. The coronary arteries are involved in 10% to 20% of cases of acute aortic dissection.
   b. Coronary artery involvement in patients with proximal aortic dissections is an indication for urgent surgery.
   c. TEE can identify the relationship of the flap to the coronary arteries.

d. The extent of the dissection into the coronary arteries and the degree of blood flow obstruction can be evaluated by TEE.
e. All of the above.

7. Which of the following statements is true?
a. Left ventricular regional wall motion abnormalities are seen in 50% of patients with aortic dissection due to compression of a coronary artery by expansion of the false lumen.
b. The left coronary artery is more commonly affected by aortic dissection.
c. The majority of pericardial effusions associated with aortic dissection are secondary to leak or rupture of the aorta.
d. Echo-free spaces around the aorta are a sign of penetration and periaortic hematoma.

8. A linear artifact of the ascending aorta can be distinguished from an intimal flap by all of the following except
a. Lack of the rapid oscillatory movement associated with an intimal flap.
b. Extension of the artifact through the aortic wall as a straight line.
c. Distinct borders of the artifact.
d. The linear artifact can be extrapolated back to the starting point of the transducer.
e. Color Doppler will demonstrate homogenous color on both sides of the linear echo.

9. Which of the following statements regarding intramural hematoma is true?
a. Intramural hematomas only involve the descending thoracic aorta.
b. The false lumen is secondary to rupture of the vaso vasorum with hemorrhage into the vessel wall.
c. All intramural hematomas require surgical treatment.
d. Ten percent of patients progress to rupture or dissection within 1 year.
e. A dissection entry site and an intimal flap can be identified.

10. Which of the following statements regarding thoracic aortic plaque and atheroma is false?
a. Grade 4 disease is defined as the presence of mobile atheroma.
b. As much as 42% of the ascending aorta is not visualized by TEE.
c. Surgical palpation detects 50% of important atheromas.
d. Ulcerated hypoechoic plaques are at high risk of embolization.
e. Aortic atheromas greater than 5 mm increase the risk of perioperative stroke by six times.

11. Figure 16.19 shows a descending aorta long-axis view of an atheroma. This plaque is consistent with grade
a. 1
b. 2
c. 3
d. 4
e. 5

12. The appropriate response for the patient in Question 11 is
a. Doing nothing
b. Surgical manual palpation of the ascending aorta in the area of the aortic cross-clamp

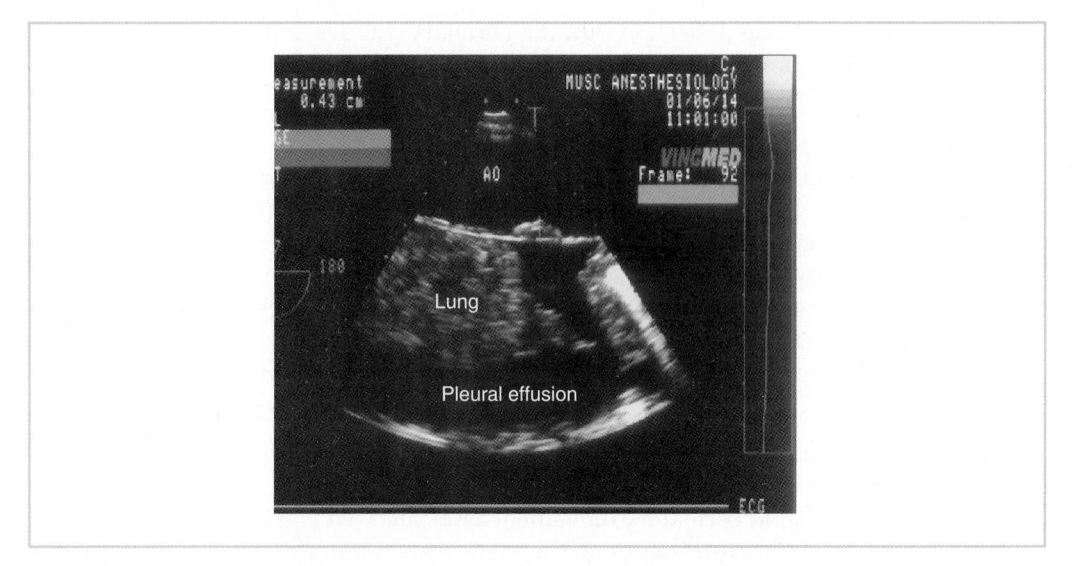

Figure 16.19.

c. Completely evaluating zones 1, 2, 5, and 6, and if no lesions above grade 3 are identified, proceeding with aortic cannulation in the normal manner
d. Completely examining zones 1, 2, 5, and 6, and if an atheroma of grade 4 or 5 is found, then performing epiaortic ultrasonography of zones 3 and 4

13. The following characteristics indicate an intramural hematoma except
a. A circular or crescentic thickening in the aortic wall larger than 7 mm
b. Central displacement of intimal calcification
c. A layered appearance
d. Longitudinal extent of 1 to 20 cm
e. A very fine intimal tear

14. Which statement most closely explains the relationship between TEE and the ascending distal aorta and proximal arch?
a. Multiplane TEE can clearly visualize the entire ascending aorta and proximal arch.
b. A blind spot is caused by the trachea overlying the ascending aorta.
c. A blind spot is caused by the trachea and left main bronchus overlying the ascending aorta and proximal arch.
d. A blind spot is caused by the trachea, left main bronchus, and right main bronchus overlying the ascending aorta and proximal arch.

15. Causes of aortic insufficiency secondary to aortic dissection include all of the following except
a. An extensive or circumferential tear dilates the aortic root and annulus, causing failure of coaptation of the aortic valve leaflets.
b. With asymmetric dissection, pressure from the false lumen depresses one aortic leaflet below the coaptation line of the other leaflets.
c. The annular support is disrupted, resulting in a flail aortic leaflet.
d. Prolapse of a mobile intimal flap through the aortic valve during systole prevents leaflet coaptation.
e. All of the above.

16. All of the following statements about the diagnostic performance of imaging modalities in the evaluation of suspected aortic dissections are true except

a. TEE is as sensitive as angiography, computed tomography (CT), and magnetic resonance imaging (MRI).
b. TEE is the most sensitive modality for detecting a thrombus within an aortic dissection.
c. TEE is extremely sensitive in detecting aortic insufficiency.
d. Angiography is not useful in determining whether a patient has a pericardial effusion.

17. Which of the following statements about the DeBakey and Stanford classification criteria for aortic dissections is false?

a. The DeBakey classification comprises three types.
b. Stanford type A includes both DeBakey type I and DeBakey type III.
c. The Stanford criteria were developed to determine whether a patient requires medical or surgical management.
d. A DeBakey type III-B dissection is a type III dissection that extends below the diaphragm.

18. The surgical goals of intraoperative TEE in the evaluation of aortic dissection include which of the following?

a. Confirmation of the preoperative diagnosis
b. Determination of the dissection entry site, including the differentiation of true from false lumina
c. Evaluation of ventricular distension and aortic insufficiency if planning for circulatory arrest
d. Assessment of the surgical repair
e. All of the above

19. Which of the following is/are TEE manifestations of acute aortic dissection?

a. Intimal flap
b. Complete thrombus of the false lumen
c. Central displacement of intimal calcification, evidenced as a bright echogenic area within the aorta
d. Separation of intimal layers secondary to thrombus
e. All of the above

20. Which of the following statements is false?

a. Aortic insufficiency is present in up to 70% of patients with a proximal dissection.
b. Aortic insufficiency is present in 10% of patients with a dissection of the descending thoracic aorta.
c. Preservation of the native aortic valve with repair and resuspension is possible in more 80% of patients with a type A dissection.
d. Coronary artery involvement by acute aortic dissection is rare, occurring in fewer than 5% of patients.

Answers appear at the back of the book.

17 Transesophageal Echocardiography in the Intensive Care Unit

Emilio B. Lobato and Jochen D. Muehlschlegel

Bedside ultrasonography has become an indispensable tool for the management of the critically ill patient. Of all modalities, the use of transesophageal echocardiography (TEE) continues to occupy a predominant role in the evaluation of hemodynamically unstable patients in the intensive care unit (ICU). In addition, the diagnostic impact of TEE in conditions such as unexplained hypoxemia or suspicion of endocarditis is well established. This chapter will examine the unique advantages of TEE and discuss its use in many of the common diagnostic dilemmas confronting the intensivist.

COMPARISON OF TRANSESOPHAGEAL ECHOCARDIOGRAPHY WITH OTHER DIAGNOSTIC AND MONITORING MODALITIES

Transesophageal Echocardiography versus Transthoracic Echocardiography

Echocardiography in intensive care settings is well described (1). Transthoracic echocardiography (TTE) is the easiest and least invasive way to image cardiac structures. However, in many critically ill patients, low-quality images are obtained because the acoustic windows are suboptimal. Despite advances in ultrasound technology which have improved the diagnostic accuracy of TEE, the examination is estimated to be inadequate in approximately 50% of patients on mechanical ventilation and in 60% of all ICU patients (2). Acoustic windows are frequently suboptimal in patients who are morbidly obese, have multiple chest tubes or extensive dressings, or are receiving mechanical ventilation (Table 17.1). TEE, although more invasive, often provides images of better quality and resolution than TTE because the acoustic windows from the esophagus to the heart and great vessels are unobstructed. In addition, the TEE probe can be left in place for many hours for the continuous monitoring of cardiac function, and its position can be readily reproduced to provide repeated comparisons. At present, only oral probes are available, which are poorly

Table 17.1 Challenges to transesophageal echocardiographic images in critical care

Obesity
Mediastinal drainage tubes
Chest dressings
Inability to position patient on left side
Chronic obstructive pulmonary disease
Positive end-expiratory pressure
Ribs, calcified rib cartilages

Table 17.2 Situations in which transesophageal is superior to transthoracic echocardiography

Mechanical ventilation
Cardiac tamponade
Diagnosis of vegetations and complications of endocarditis
Central pulmonary emboli
Exclusion of a cardiac source of embolism
Evaluation of a mediastinal hematoma
Diagnosis of ascending or descending thoracic aortic dissection
Structural and functional evaluation of native valves, including postoperative assessment of mitral repair
Acute hemodynamic instability

tolerated for continuous monitoring. However, newer, smaller probes placed transnasally for long-term use are currently being evaluated.

Conditions in which TEE is superior to TTE are listed in Table 17.2. TEE is by far more sensitive for the detection of left atrial thrombi, small vegetations, paraprosthetic valvular insufficiency, aortic dissection, and central pulmonary emboli. In patients receiving mechanical ventilation and positive end-expiratory pressure (PEEP), LV function is more easily and more accurately assessed with TEE. This diagnostic superiority is particularly important when mechanical ventilation is applied in patients with hemodynamic instability. *TEE provides unexpected diagnoses that are missed by TTE in up to 40% of cases* (3,4). The clinical impact of TEE on therapeutic decision making is substantial, frequently leading to changes in medical or surgical management.

Transesophageal Echocardiography versus Pulmonary Artery Catheterization

Pulmonary artery (PA) catheterization is often utilized in critically ill patients. The evaluation of left ventricular (LV) preload and function, and the measurement of cardiac output (CO) are considered essential for appropriate hemodynamic management. The PA occlusion pressure remains the most commonly used variable to assess LV preload; however, the values can be misleading. In the ICU setting, factors such as PEEP and changes in ventricular compliance can be associated with elevation of the PA occlusion pressure independently of LV volume. Similarly, LV function is evaluated indirectly based on the relationship of the PA occlusion pressure to the CO. As was noted previously, TEE rapidly visualizes the LV, providing direct estimates of ventricular dimensions and function. *Data obtained with TEE frequently differ significantly from PA catheterization assessments of the LV preload and systolic function and can lead to a change in therapy 40% to 60% of patients when utilized* (5,6). In patients with preexisting myocardial dysfunction and cardiomegaly, changes in the LV end-diastolic area and concomitant measurements of the PA occlusion pressure may serve to determine the optimal LV preload and provide a better titration of inotropic agents.

In addition, TEE measurement of the CO in critically ill patients, with Doppler analysis of the LV outflow, has been found to correlate well with bolus thermodilution (7). The ability to provide continuous CO measurements is compromised because minimal movement of the probe will significantly alter results.

PROBE INSERTION

Although relatively safe in experienced hands, TEE is a semi-invasive procedure that is not without risk. Critically ill patients represent a heterogeneous population, and an individualized approach to the TEE examination is required. The use of mechanical ventilation and the patient's hemodynamic and respiratory status and level of consciousness are important factors that must be considered. Placement of a TEE probe in an uncooperative patient can be associated with esophageal trauma, increased cardiovascular stress, hypoxia, and dysrhythmias. Emesis and aspiration are real concerns, particularly in nonfasting patients without an endotracheal tube.

Preparation

1. ***Fasting***. If possible, the patient should be fasting for at least 4 hours before the procedure.
2. ***History***. A history of esophageal/gastric pathology or dysphagia should be evaluated.
3. ***Monitoring***. Electrocardiography (ECG), pulse oximeter, and blood pressure monitors should be placed.
4. ***Sedation***. Passage of the TEE transducer tip through the oropharynx is not infrequently cumbersome; an adequate level of sedation ensures better patient cooperation. The choice of sedatives must be tailored to the patient's respiratory and hemodynamic status to decrease the likelihood of hypoxemia or hypotension. Small intravenous doses of benzodiazepines or opiates are commonly used, and pharmacologic reversal (naloxone, flumazenil) can be instituted if necessary. *Excessive sedation resulting in a lack of patient cooperation is problematic because swallowing on command facilitates probe insertion.*
5. ***Prevention of the gag reflex***. Topical anesthesia of the oropharynx effectively decreases the gag reflex. Lidocaine or benzocaine spray is applied to the posterior pharynx, or the patient is instructed to gargle with viscous lidocaine. A drying agent such as glycopyrrolate may decrease the possibility of salivary aspiration; however, it can be associated with tachyarrhythmias.
6. ***Tracheal intubation***. Sedation, paralysis, and tracheal intubation may be necessary in patients with severe respiratory distress or cardiovascular collapse in whom TEE must be performed urgently or emergently.
7. ***Nasogastric suction***. If a nasogastric tube is present, the stomach contents should be suctioned before the examination. *Nasogastric tubes usually do not interfere with insertion of the transducer or the quality of the images;* however, on occasion, they must be removed.
8. ***Patient positioning***. Patients are commonly placed in a semirecumbent, left lateral decubitus position with the head slightly flexed to facilitate probe placement and drainage of secretions. Supine positioning is most commonly used for intubated patients.

Technique

1. Place a mouth guard to protect the TEE probe unless the patient is edentulous.
2. Thoroughly lubricate the tip of the transducer with ultrasonic gel.
3. Check for free movement of the tip and *maintain in the unlocked position.*
4. With the patient's mouth open, gently depress the tongue with the index finger, place the transducer over the finger in the midline, and gently advance it posteriorly toward the esophagus.

5. Instruct the patient to swallow.
6. Advance the transducer into the esophagus. As you advance, slight resistance from the cricoid sphincter may have to be overcome before the probe enters the esophagus. However, significant resistance to advancement typically signifies that the probe has deviated from the midline and rests within the pyriform sinus. Withdraw the probe and make adjustments in the patient's position and flexion of the probe to advance it into the esophagus.
7. Intubated patients frequently require sedation and muscle relaxants. *On occasion, direct laryngoscopy, deflation of the endotracheal tube cuff, or both are necessary to facilitate passage of the transducer.*
8. Once the probe is advanced to approximately 30 cm from the incisors, the examination can begin.

CONTRAINDICATIONS AND COMPLICATIONS TO TRANSESOPHAGEAL ECHOCARDIOGRAPHY

Contraindications to TEE include significant esophageal or gastric pathology (e.g., tumors, strictures). Esophageal varices are not an absolute contraindication, especially when TEE is urgently indicated. However, bleeding can occur, particularly in the presence of coagulation abnormalities. In patients with cervical spinal disease or injury, manipulation of the neck must be avoided to prevent disastrous consequences.

Overall, complications associated with TEE are rare, averaging 0.5% in the general population (8,9). Table 17.3 lists the types and incidence of the complications most often encountered during TEE. A multicenter study of more than 10,000 TEE examinations

Table 17.3 Complications in 15,381 transesophageal examinations

Complication	Percentage (%)
Hypoxia	0.6
Hypotension	0.5
Hypertension	0.2
PSVT	0.2
NSVT	<0.1
Hematemesis	0.1
Laryngospasm	0.1
Esophageal tear	<0.02
Death	<0.02

PSVT, paroxysmal supraventricular tachycardia; NSVT, nonsustained ventricular tachycardia.
Modified from Oh JK, Seward JB, Tajik AJ. Transesophageal echocardiography. In: Oh JK, Seward JB, Tajik AJ, eds. *The echo manual,* second ed. Philadelphia: Lippincott Williams & Wilkins, 1999:23–36.

reported a procedural mortality of 0.01%. Cardiac, pulmonary, and bleeding events requiring interruption of the procedure occurred in 0.18% of cases (9).

It is logical to assume that in critically ill patients, TEE-associated complications may be more frequent as a consequence of their severe illness and unstable state. However, the incidence of complications remains low, albeit slightly higher than in patients who are not critically ill. A review of 943 TEE examinations performed in several ICUs reported a complication rate of 1.7%, with arrhythmias and hypotension occurring most frequently (7). Serious complications developed in only two patients (0.2%). Difficulties with probe insertion have been reported in only 1.4% of patients (7). Therefore, with appropriate monitoring, TEE is a safe technique, even in patients who are most compromised.

DISADVANTAGES AND LIMITATIONS

Transducer Size

The adult TEE probe is a modified gastroesophageal endoscope measuring approximately 100 cm in length and 1 cm in width. The transducer, located at the tip, measures between 10 and 16 mm. Because of its size, it can create significant discomfort. Occasionally, attempts at probe insertion are unsuccessful, and one should desist insertion or risk esophageal perforation. Although the probe can be safely left in place to provide continuous monitoring, many of these patients require high levels of sedation, so that its usefulness as a monitoring tool is limited. New, miniaturized TEE probes can be inserted transnasally and left in place for prolonged periods of time. They are currently being tested for image quality and patient acceptance, and it is hoped that they will be available in the near future.

Limited Acoustic Windows

The TEE views of some anatomic structures are limited. These limited acoustic windows include the following:

1. Superior portion of the ascending aorta (because of interference from the left main bronchus): frequent
2. Left branch of the pulmonary artery: frequent
3. LV apex: occasional.

In addition, proper alignment of the LV outflow tract and ascending aorta during Doppler spectral analysis to measure the CO or the aortic valve area can be technically demanding.

Time-Consuming Analysis

1. Off-line quantitative measurements of LV function (preload, afterload, and fraction of area of change) require meticulous interpretation and considerable time.
2. Real-time assessment with automatic border detection techniques may be limited by the inability to visualize the entire endocardium.

COMMON INDICATIONS FOR TRANSESOPHAGEAL ECHOCARDIOGRAPHY IN CRITICAL CARE

The indications for TEE examinations are varied and continue to increase (Table 17.4). Not surprisingly, the use of TEE varies according to the type of ICU. In medical ICUs, most patients were examined by TEE to rule out endocarditis; in coronary and surgical

Table 17.4 Indications for transesophageal echocardiography in the intensive care unit

Assessment of left ventricular function	Complications of myocardial infarction
Hemodynamic instability	Pericardial effusion
Assessment of valvular function	Evaluation of heart transplant donors
Suspected endocarditis	Hemodynamic management
Determination of source of systemic embolism	Evaluation of chest trauma
Pulmonary emboli	

ICUs, aortic dissection and valvular assessment were the primary indications; and in neurosurgical ICUs, a cardiac source of embolism was the principal indication (10).

Hemodynamic Instability

The evaluation of hemodynamic instability is one of the most common and important indications for TEE in the ICU. Because the patient is usually hypotensive, an accurate diagnosis expedites therapy and helps prevent an adverse event or death. Frequently, the physical examination findings are limited; placement of a PA catheter is time consuming, and the information obtained is often ambiguous and incomplete. TEE is a fast and accurate method to ascertain whether the hemodynamic instability is cardiac or noncardiac in origin. The lack of a blood pressure response to a fluid challenge leaves the clinician in doubt about whether to repeat the fluid challenge or obtain further diagnostic information. TEE can provide the necessary information less invasively and faster than a PA catheter. Furthermore, in patients with hemodynamic instability, TEE information is associated with higher interobserver agreement, when compared with PA catheter derived hemodynamic monitoring (11–13).

ASSESSMENT OF VENTRICULAR FUNCTION

Knowledge of the cardiac volume status and pump function is the major priority in the ICU. By providing rapid visualization of the left and right ventricles, TEE can aid both in the diagnosis and in monitoring the response to therapy. A recommended rapid examination to assess ventricular function follows.

Assessment of the left ventricular end-diastolic area

One starts at the transgastric (TG) mid short-axis view to evaluate the LV preload and global systolic function. Determination of the LV preload is of primary importance in critically ill patients. The LV end-diastolic area, obtained from this view, allows the rapid identification of LV volume depletion or overload. It provides a better estimate of LV preload than the PA occlusion pressure (14,15). The range of normal values for the LV end-diastolic area is wide; therefore, determination of the optimal preload may require a fluid challenge to assess changes.

Estimation of the left ventricular ejection fraction

A visual estimation of LV global systolic function (LV ejection fraction) is performed in the same view.

Assessment of regional wall motion abnormalities

An analysis of segmental wall motion in multiple views (TG mid short-axis, midesophageal [ME] four-chamber, ME two-chamber, and ME long-axis views) completes the assessment of LV function.

Assessment of right ventricular function

Right ventricular (RV) function is evaluated with the ME views. A visual assessment of ventricular dilation and systolic function provides a qualitative impression of RV function. The PA systolic pressure can be estimated by Doppler analysis of a tricuspid regurgitant jet if present.

Additional evaluation

The above sequence often allows an initial diagnosis and treatment. A more comprehensive TEE examination can be completed as therapy continues.

EVALUATION OF VALVULAR FUNCTION

TEE is invaluable in the assessment of valvular function. It can detect significant mitral regurgitation and unsuspected severe aortic valve disease in patients with unexplained heart failure (16). Besides providing a diagnosis and establishing the severity of disease, TEE can provide clues to its cause by detecting abnormal ventricular function, ruptured chordae, valvular perforation, abnormal masses, and vegetations (17).

Following prosthetic valve replacement, TEE can identify paravalvular regurgitation, especially in the mitral position. Paravalvular leaks from the aortic valve are not as easily detected because of acoustic shadowing of the LV outflow tract. Jets of paravalvular regurgitation must be differentiated from the normal cleansing regurgitation present in mechanical prostheses. TEE can also detect mitral and aortic bioprosthetic dysfunction secondary to degeneration and rupture of the cusps as the predominant mechanism of heart failure.

The echocardiographic evaluation of valve function is discussed in detail in Part III of this book.

EVALUATION OF HYPOTENSION

Table 17.5 summarizes the causes of hypotension and lists the associated TEE findings. Figure 17.1 shows a large hemopericardium with compression of the right atrium and ventricle.

Endocarditis

INDICATIONS FOR TRANSESOPHAGEAL ECHOCARDIOGRAPHY

Suspected infective endocarditis is a rather common indication for a TEE examination in the ICU. Critically ill patients are at high risk for bacteremia caused by indwelling catheters or colonized endotracheal tubes. TEE is cost-effective in ICU patients in comparison with other modalities when the probability of endocarditis exceeds 2% (7,18). *Because critically ill patients often present with nonspecific signs and symptoms, the threshold for performing TEE should be low.*

CLINICAL IMPLICATIONS OF THE TRANSESOPHAGEAL ECHOCARDIOGRAPHIC FINDINGS

The hallmark lesions are vegetations, which are generally attached to valves (Figure 17.2) but can also adhere to a wall in areas of denuded endocardium. The appearance is that of an echo-dense, often pedunculated mass exhibiting a variable range of motion. Multiplane TEE is credited with a 90% to 100% sensitivity in detecting left-sided vegetations, and a special benefit in detecting small vegetations in patients with a prosthetic valve (19). For right-sided vegetations, it may not offer a substantial benefit in comparison with TTE. *However, TEE is the procedure of choice to identify complications such as abscesses, perforation, mycotic aneurysms, and fistulae.* In addition, it offers important prognostic information. The

Table 17.5 Conditions associated with hypotension

Condition	Useful views	TEE findings
Pericardial tamponade	ME four-chamber view, transgastric short- and long-axis	Effusion Diastolic collapse of the atrium Exaggerated variation on E- or S-wave velocities with inspiration
Aortic dissection	ME five-chamber view, aortic valve and ascending and descending aorta	Intimal flap No flow on false lumen (color Doppler) Aortic regurgitation Pericardial effusion
Pulmonary embolus	ME four-chamber pulmonary artery and RVOT views	Echogenic density in pulmonary artery Dilated RA and RV Small LA and LV TR and PR jets Flow through PFO
Hypovolemia	Transgastric short-axis Transgastric long-axis	↓EDA ↑FAC "Kissing" papillary muscles
Decreased systolic function	Transgastric short-axis Transgastric long-axis	↑EDA ↑ESA ↓FAC
Severe valvular regurgitation or stenosis	Appropriate valvular plane	Doppler methods Planimetry
Vasodilation	Transgastric short-axis	Normal EDA ↑FAC Absence of severe valvular regurgitation

RVOT, right ventricular outflow tract; RA, right atrium; RV, right ventricle; LA, left atrium; LV, left ventricle; TR, tricuspid regurgitation; PR, pulmonary regurgitation; PFO, patent foramen ovale; EDA, end-diastolic area; FAC, fractional area of change; ESA, end-systolic area.

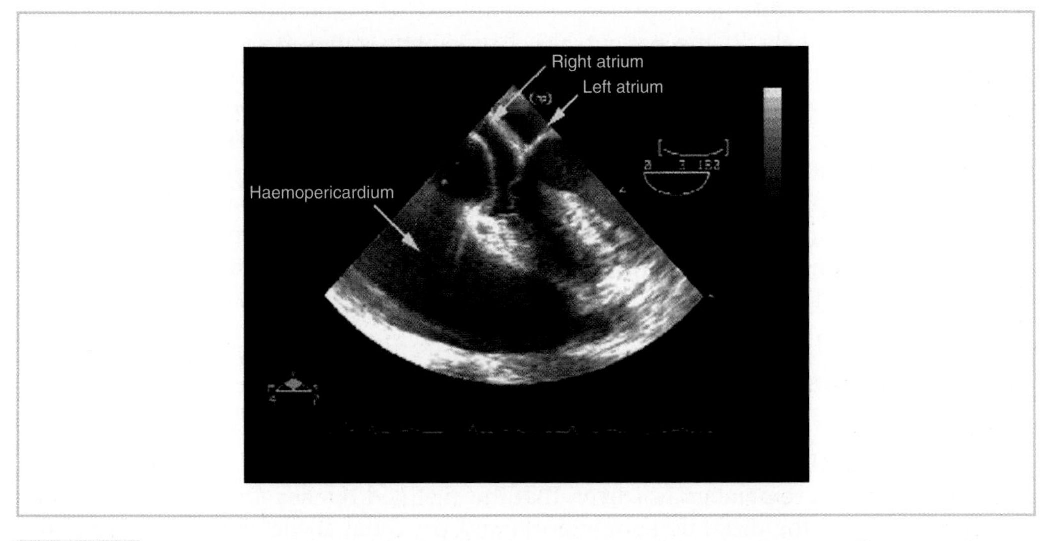

Figure 17.1. Midesophageal four-chamber view showing pericardial tamponade. The effusion is collapsing the right atrium and the right ventricle.

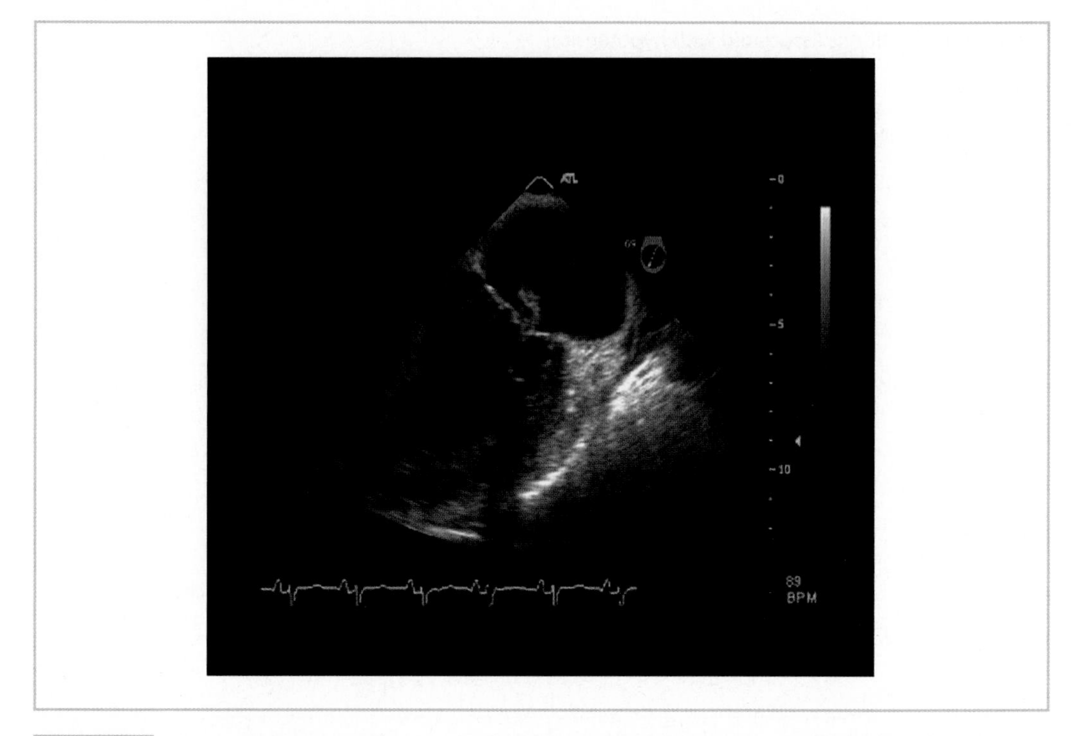

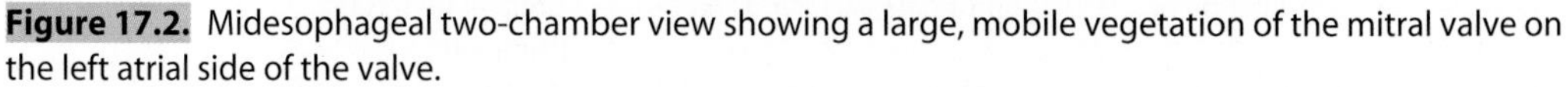

Figure 17.2. Midesophageal two-chamber view showing a large, mobile vegetation of the mitral valve on the left atrial side of the valve.

size of vegetations, location (mitral versus aortic), mobility, and number of valves affected are all related to the likelihood of complications (systemic embolization, congestive heart failure, failure to respond to treatment, death) (20). TEE may also assist in the decision to perform surgery, particularly when a prosthetic valve is involved.

When native endocarditis is suspected, a negative TEE examination result makes this diagnosis very unlikely. If the patient has a prosthetic valve, it is wise to repeat the examination when the clinical picture remains consistent with the presumptive diagnosis. Other echocardiographic findings, including myxomatous changes, Lambl excrescences in the aortic valve (small oscillating masses on the aortic side of the valve cusps), thrombus formation, and suture material, can be confused with infective endocarditis. Degenerative changes of the bioprosthesis are usually seen as prolapsing masses and can also be confused with vegetations. Finally, it must be remembered that vegetations may occur in the absence of infection, such as those associated with marantic endocarditis, systemic lupus erythematosus, and tumors.

Aortic Dissection

IMAGING CAVEATS

TEE is ideal for evaluating the thoracic aorta because of the proximity of the esophagus to the aorta. One must remember, however, that the air-filled trachea is interposed between the esophagus and the distal ascending aorta and proximal aortic arch. This area is not clearly visualized, even with multiplane technology. Fortunately, an isolated dissection in this area is rare. Multiplane TEE is a useful diagnostic modality in patients with suspected aortic dissection, having 99% sensitivity and better than 90% specificity (17). TEE should be the procedure of choice for an ICU patient because it can be performed safely and rapidly at the bedside.

TRANSESOPHAGEAL ECHOCARDIOGRAPHIC EXAMINATION

The goals of perioperative TEE in the evaluation of aortic dissection include the following: (a) establishing the diagnosis, (b) localizing primary and secondary entry sites, (c) differentiating the true from the false lumen, (d) evaluating the aortic valve for insufficiency, (e) establishing involvement of the coronary arteries, and (f) ruling out associated conditions such as pericardial infusions and tamponade.

Localization of the intimal flap

The diagnosis is established by identifying an intimal flap (a mobile linear echo within the vascular lumen) in at least two planes. Figure 17.3 demonstrates an intimal flap within the descending aorta with true and false lumina. Color flow Doppler can identify flow within the true and false lumina on either side of an intimal flap and is also highly sensitive for detecting aortic dissection. We find it most useful to begin in the stomach with the descending aortic short-axis view. Typically, the depth setting is reduced to enlarge the size of the aorta on the display monitor. The transducer is gradually withdrawn while an intimal flap is sought until the ME ascending aortic short-axis view is obtained. Special care must be taken in evaluating the aorta near the left subclavian artery (ligamentum arteriosum area) because approximately 30% of acute dissections originate at this location. The transducer is then rotated to approximately 90 degrees to obtain the ME ascending aortic long-axis view, and the probe is gradually advanced to achieve the descending aortic long-axis view, with careful observation throughout its path to detect an intimal flap.

Once the descending aorta has been evaluated, the ME aortic valve long-axis view is obtained to interrogate the proximal ascending aorta. *More than 70% of dissections exhibit an intimal tear originating in the ascending aorta 1 to 3 cm distal to the right or left sinus of*

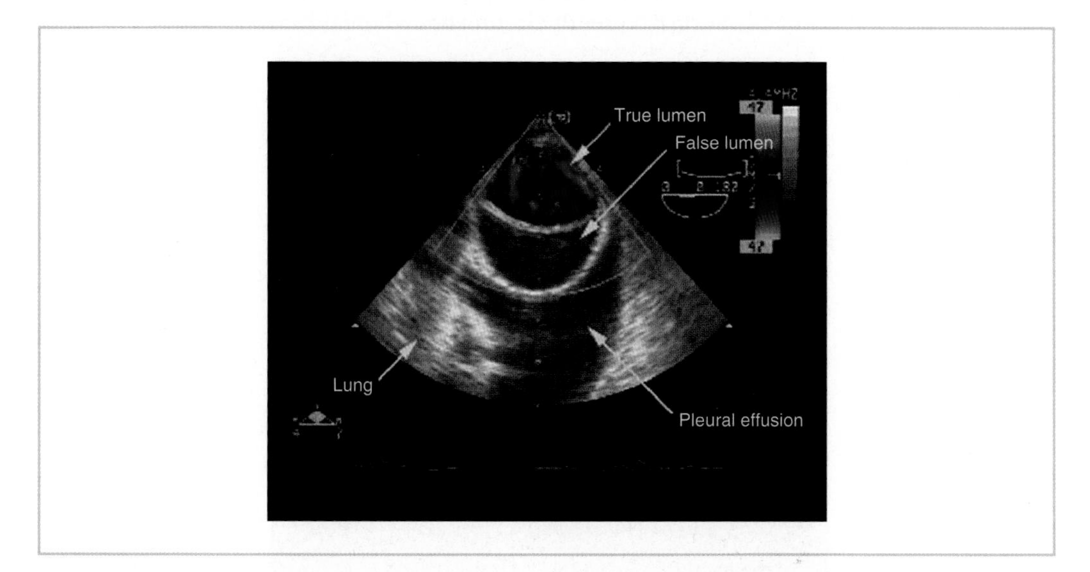

Figure 17.3. Descending aortic short-axis view. Aortic dissection showing the true and false lumina. The true lumen shows color Doppler flow and bulging of the wall toward the false lumen in systole. Also notable is a pleural effusion.

Valsalva. The surgeon will need to know the location of the entrance site. We use anatomic landmarks to assist in the surgical identification. In the ascending aorta, we use the distance (in centimeters) from the aortic valve. Within the descending aorta, we use the distance from the left subclavian artery.

Identification of true and false lumina

The true lumen can be identified by expansion during systole and by compression during diastole. M-mode is extremely helpful in identifying and timing these events (21). Thrombus or spontaneous echo contrast may be present in the false lumen as a consequence of stagnant flow. In chronic dissections, the false lumen is typically much larger (22–24). Small secondary tears and any exit sites must be identified to facilitate repair.

Evaluation of coronary artery involvement

Coronary artery involvement is evaluated by observing acute regional wall motion abnormalities.

Evaluation of cardiac tamponade

Cardiac tamponade is suspected and evaluated when a pericardial effusion is present. The echocardiographic manifestations of cardiac tamponade are discussed in Chapter 7 and later in this chapter.

Unexplained Hypoxemia

In some ICU patients, the degree of hypoxemia appears disproportionate to the severity of their illness. In patients with elevated right atrial pressure, TEE may diagnose an intracardiac shunt through a patent foramen ovale (Figure17.4) or an atrial septal defect. Right-to-left intracardiac shunting can be demonstrated by means of color flow Doppler or contrast echocardiography with agitated saline solution as a contrast agent or a commercially available agent. When right-to-left intracardiac shunting occurs through a patent foramen ovale, left atrial contrast is observed within three cardiac cycles, and the density does not match that of the right side (7). On the contrary, in intrapulmonary shunting, right-sided opacification frequently diminishes whereas the intensity of left-sided

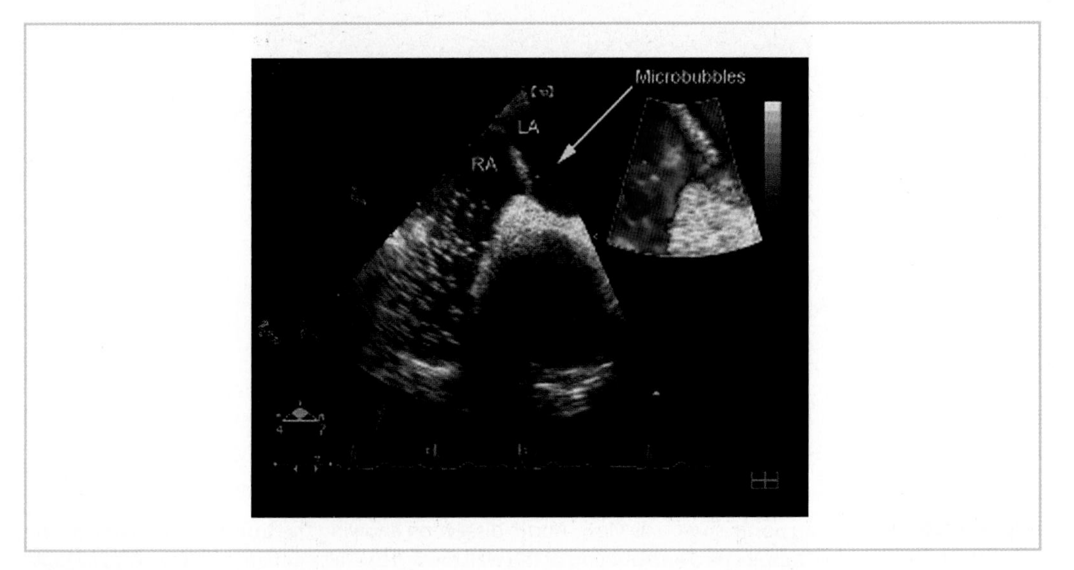

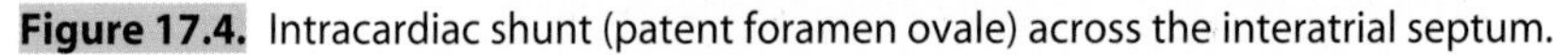
Figure 17.4. Intracardiac shunt (patent foramen ovale) across the interatrial septum.

contrast continues to increase (25). In intrapulmonary shunting, contrast is frequently seen entering the left atrium through the pulmonary veins. A diagnosis of intracardiac shunting leads to changes in management, such as the elimination of PEEP or the placement of catheter-based septal closure devices.

Embolism

PULMONARY EMBOLISM

Acute pulmonary embolism carries a high mortality. In the ICU, it remains difficult to diagnose, so that one must have a high index of suspicion. Successful imaging of acute pulmonary emboli within the main or right pulmonary artery has been extensively described (26–28) (Figure 17.5). The left pulmonary artery, however, is rarely seen beyond a few centimeters because of interposition of the left main bronchus. Pruszczyk et al. (28) have delineated the following echo manifestations of thrombus in an effort to minimize false-positive diagnoses of pulmonary embolism.

1. An unequivocal thrombus should have distinct borders and an echo density different from that of blood in the adjacent vascular walls.
2. The thrombus may protrude into the arterial lumen and thereby alter the blood flow by Doppler imaging.
3. The thrombus must be imaged in more than one plane.
4. The thrombus may have a distinct movement separate from that of the vascular wall and blood flow.

Although TTE is routinely used to screen patients with suspected pulmonary embolism, TEE is indicated if TTE is nondiagnostic, hemodynamic instability is present, or RV overload is identified (to confirm central pulmonary or intracardiac thromboemboli). Central thromboemboli are frequently demonstrated in patients with associated hemodynamic compromise. In these cases, TEE has a sensitivity of 80% and a specificity of approximately

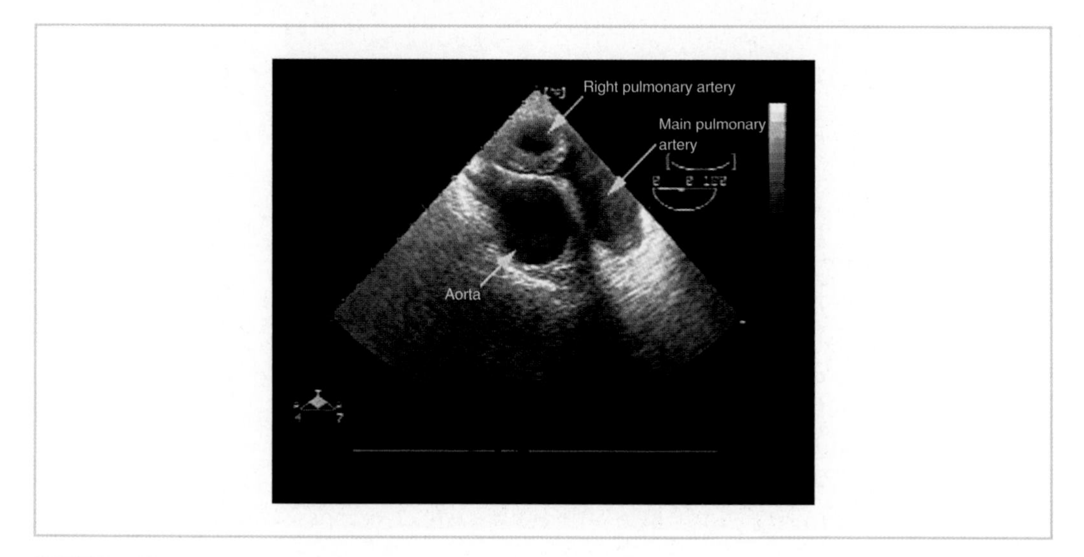

Figure 17.5. Upper esophageal ascending aortic short-axis view showing the aorta with the main pulmonary artery branching into the right pulmonary artery containing a large, obstructing, echo-dense structure (thrombus).

100% (28). Although a negative finding on TEE examination cannot rule out pulmonary embolism, positive TEE findings confirm the decision to institute either thrombolytic or surgical therapy.

SYSTEMIC EMBOLISM

TEE is useful in determining the source of emboli in patients with stroke, transient ischemic attack, or emboli in the extremities or viscera (29). Findings include atrial and ventricular thrombi, vegetations, tumors, and atrial septal aneurysms. Spontaneous echo contrast (''smoke'') in the atrium, particularly in patients with atrial fibrillation, indicates a low-flow state that may lead to thrombus formation (see Figure 10.10). In ICU patients with atrial fibrillation TEE is often necessary to rule out the presence of thrombi before cardioversion, when a long period of anticoagulation is not possible.

Mobile atheromatous plaques in the aorta are a frequent source of emboli that are readily identified by TEE (30). TEE can assess plaque mobility and overall load. Arteriosclerosis of the aorta is a marker of diffuse disease and is commonly associated with carotid and peripheral vascular disease. Hence, a thorough workup (e.g., carotid ultrasound) should be performed to evaluate the common sites of embolism and ensure that appropriate treatment is instituted.

Myocardial Infarction

In patients with myocardial infarction, particularly patients in cardiogenic shock, TEE can provide useful information regarding the extent of myocardial involvement and suspected complications (16). Acute mitral valve insufficiency (Figure 17.6), secondary to

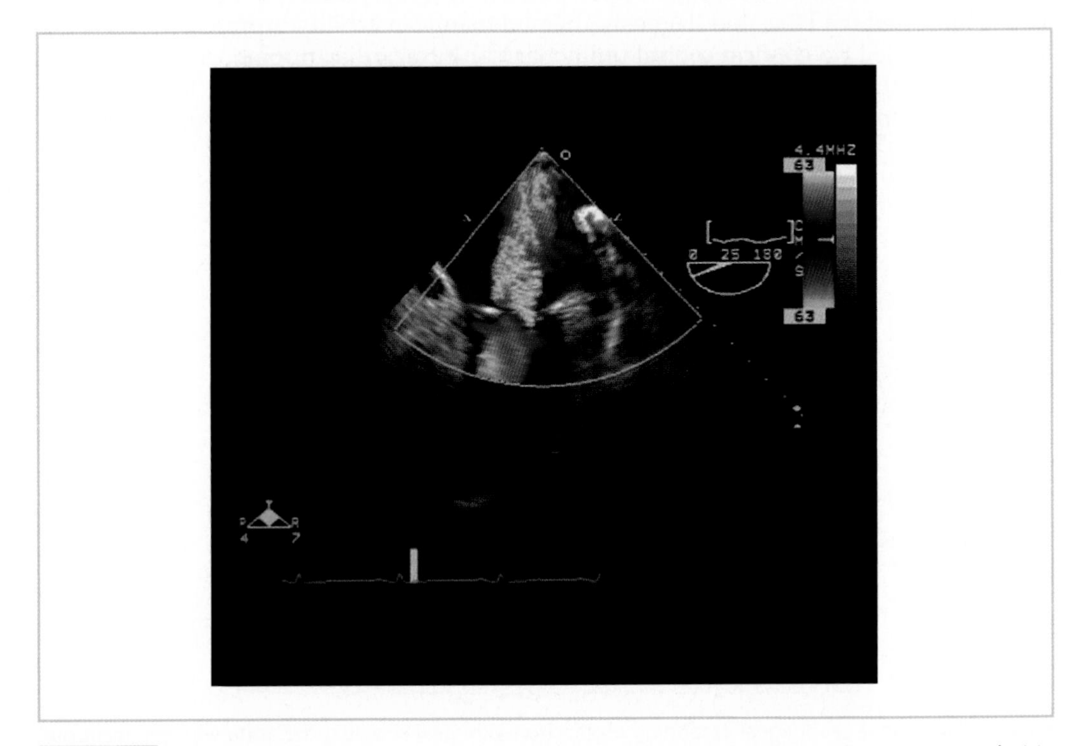

Figure 17.6. Color Doppler revealing new onset mitral regurgitation in a patient with hypotension during an acute myocardial infarction.

either chordal or papillary muscle rupture and the presence of mural thrombi, is best evaluated with TEE. Other mechanical complications, such as ventricular septal defect and ventricular pseudoaneurysm, are readily diagnosed with TEE. The latter condition is also associated with characteristic color flow Doppler findings of antegrade flow into the pseudoaneurysm during early systole and retrograde flow in early diastole. This flow pattern is helpful in differentiating a pseudoaneurysm from a true aneurysm or a loculated pericardial effusion (16).

One limitation of TEE is that the ventricular apex is sometimes poorly visualized, and therefore infarction, aneurysms, or thrombi in that location may not be obvious. In these situations, apical views with TTE may be required.

Blunt Chest Trauma

INJURY PATTERNS

In patients with severe chest wall injury, a complete assessment of cardiac structures and function may not be possible with TTE, as previously discussed. The most common abnormality following blunt chest trauma is myocardial contusion. The RV wall, because of its proximity to the sternum, is the most vulnerable structure and is involved in approximately 25% of patients. The LV is also involved in more than 15% of patients. Findings on TEE include ventricular dilation and poor systolic function (31).

Assessment of valvular function is also important because occasionally lacerations of the valvular annuli or ruptured chordae can be seen. Because of higher pressures on the left side of the heart, the aortic and mitral valves are at greater risk for damage.

Cardiac tamponade and pericardial effusion

Pericardial effusion resulting from hemopericardium and cardiac tamponade can easily be diagnosed with TEE. The most sensitive two-dimensional manifestation of cardiac tamponade is RV collapse during diastole in a patient with a pericardial effusion. Right atrial collapse frequently occurs in late diastole. Left atrial and ventricular collapse can occur, especially if LV pressures are low. This phenomenon is frequently encountered following cardiac surgery when a loculated pericardial effusion or thrombus impedes left atrial or ventricular filling.

The Doppler manifestations of cardiac tamponade consist of a significant increase in the early diastolic E-wave velocity across the tricuspid valve during inspiration in a spontaneously breathing patient. Because the patient's heart can be considered to be encased in a concrete box, the resulting increase in RV inflow creates a reciprocal decrease in LV inflow and therefore a fall in the early diastolic E-wave velocity across the mitral valve during inspiration. The opposite occurs in the tricuspid and mitral E-wave velocities during expiration. Diastolic pulmonary venous forward flow decreases during inspiration and increases during expiration. Finally, during expiration, hepatic venous flow is reduced in both diastole and systole (32,33).

SUMMARY

TEE is easily performed in the ICU setting with a wide margin of safety. In the ICU, TEE is frequently superior to TTE, particularly in mechanically ventilated patients. It also provides a better assessment of heart function than the PA catheter. TEE is most useful in patients with hemodynamic instability when accurate information must be obtained rapidly. Because of its ability to provide high-resolution images and a superior diagnostic yield, TEE has become indispensable in the ICU.

REFERENCES

1 Beaulieu Y, Marik PE. Bedside ultrasonography in the ICU. *Chest* 2005;128:881–895.
2 Vignon P, Mentec H, Terre S, et al. Diagnostic accuracy and therapeutic impact of transthoracic and transesophageal echocardiography in mechanically ventilated patients in the ICU. *Chest* 1994;106:1829–1834.
3 Pearson AC, Castello R, Labovitz AJ. Safety and utility of transesophageal echocardiography in the critically ill patient. *Am Heart J* 1990;119:1083–1089.
4 Hwang JJ, Shyu KG, Chen JJ, et al. Usefulness of transesophageal echocardiography in the critical care unit. *Chest* 1993;104:861–866.
5 Benjamin E, Griffin K, Leibowitz AB, et al. Goal-directed transesophageal echocardiography performed by intensivists to assess LV function: comparison with pulmonary artery catheterization. *J Cardiothorac Vasc Anesth* 1998;12:10–15.
6 Bouchard MJ, Denault A, Couture P, et al. Poor correlation between hemodynamic and echocardiographic indexes of left ventricular performance in the operating room and intensive care unit. *Crit Care Med* 2004;32:644–648.
7 Heidenreich PA. Transesophageal echocardiography in the critical care patient. *Cardiol Clin* 2000;18:789–805.
8 Seward JB, Khandheria BK, Oh JK, et al. Transesophageal echocardiography: technique, anatomic correlations, implementation, and clinical applications. *Mayo Clin Proc* 1988;63:649–680.
9 Daniel WG, Erbel R, Kasper W, et al. Safety of transesophageal echocardiography. A multicenter study of 10,419 examinations. *Circulation* 1991;83:817–821.
10 Alam M. Transesophageal echocardiography in critical care units: Henry Ford Hospital experience and review of the literature. *Prog Cardiovasc Dis* 1996;38:315–328.
11 Oh JK, Seward JB, Khandheria BK, et al. Transesophageal echocardiography in critically ill patients. *Am J Cardiol* 1990;66:1492–1495.
12 Slama MA, Novara A, Van de Putte P, et al. Diagnostic and therapeutic implications of transesophageal echocardiography in medical ICU patients with unexplained shock, hypoxemia, or suspected endocarditis. *Intensive Care Med* 1996;22:916–922.
13 Costachescu T, Denault A, Guimond JG, et al. The hemodnamically unstable patient in the intensive care unit: hemodynamic vs transesophageal echocardiographic monitoring. *Crit Care Med* 2002;30:1214–1223.
14 Greim CA, Roewer N, Apfel G, et al. Relation of echocardiographic preload indices to stroke volume in critically ill patients with normal and low cardiac index. *Intensive Care Med* 1997;23:411–416.
15 Vignon P. Hemodynamic assessment of critically ill patients using echocardiography Doppler. *Curr Opin Crit Care* 2005;11:227–234.
16 Foster E, Schiller NB. Transesophageal echocardiography in the critical care patient. *Cardiol Clin* 1993;11:489–503.
17 Keren A, Kim CB, Hu BS, et al. Accuracy of biplane and multiplane transesophageal echocardiography in diagnosis of typical acute aortic dissection and intramural hematoma. *J Am Coll Cardiol* 1996;28:627–636.
18 Heidenreich PA, Masoudi FA, Maini B, et al. Echocardiography patients with suspected endocarditis: a cost-effectiveness analysis. *Am J Med* 1999;107:198–208.
19 Shanewise JS, Martin RP. Assessment of endocarditis and associated complications with transesophageal echocardiography. *Crit Care Clin* 1996;12:411–427.
20 Sanfilippo AJ, Picard MH, Newell JB, et al. Echocardiographic assessment of patients with infectious endocarditis: prediction of risk for complications. *J Am Coll Cardiol* 1991;18:1191–1199.
21 Iliceto S, Nanda NC, Rizzon P, et al. Color Doppler evaluation of aortic dissection. *Circulation* 1987;75:748–755.
22 Erbel R, Engberding R, Daniel W, et al. Echocardiography in diagnosis of aortic dissection. *Lancet* 1989;1:457–460.
23 Erbel R, Mohr-Kahaly S, Oelert H, et al. Diagnostic strategies in suspected aortic dissection: comparison of computed tomography, aortography, and transesophageal echocardiography. *Am J Card Imaging* 1990;4:157–172.
24 Mohr-Kahaly S, Erbel R, Rennollet H, et al. Ambulatory follow-up of aortic dissection by transesophageal two-dimensional and color-coded Doppler echocardiography. *Circulation* 1989;80:24–33.
25 Dansky HM, Schwinger ME, Cohen MV. Using contrast material-enhanced echocardiography to identify abnormal pulmonary arteriovenous connection in patients with hypoxemia. *Chest* 1992;102:1690–1692.

26 Lengyel M. Should transesophageal echocardiography become a routine test in patients with suspected pulmonary thromboembolism? *Echocardiography* 1998;15:779–785.
27 Steiner P, Lund GK, Debatin JF, et al. Acute pulmonary embolism: value of transthoracic and transesophageal echocardiography in comparison with helical CT. *AJR Am J Roentgenol* 1996;167:931–936.
28 Pruszczyk P, Torbicki A, Pacho R, et al. Noninvasive diagnosis of suspected severe pulmonary embolism: transesophageal echocardiography versus spiral CT. *Chest* 1997;112:722–728.
29 Mariano MC, Gutierrez CJ, Alexander J, et al. The utility of transesophageal echocardiography in determining the source of arterial embolization. *Am Surg* 2000;66:901–904.
30 Montgomery DH, Ververis JJ, McGorisk G, et al. Natural history of severe atheromatous disease of the thoracic aorta. A transesophageal echocardiographic study. *J Am Coll Cardiol* 1996;27:95–101.
31 Garcia-Fernandez MA, Lopez-Perez JM, Perez-Castellano N, et al. Role of transesophageal echocardiography in the assessment of patients with blunt chest trauma: correlation of echocardiographic findings with the electrocardiogram and creatine kinase monoclonal antibody measurements. *Am Heart J* 1998;135:476–481.
32 Tsang TSM, Oh JK, Seward JM. Diagnosis and management of cardiac tamponade in the era of echocardiography. *Clin Cardiol* 1999;22:446–452.
33 Merce J, Sagrista-Sauleda J, Permanyer-Miralda G, et al. Imaging/diagnostic testing. Correlation between clinical and Doppler echocardiographic findings in patients with moderate and large pericardial effusion: implications for the diagnosis of cardiac tamponade. *Am Heart J* 1999;138:759–764.

QUESTIONS

1. **Limitations of transesophageal echocardiography (TEE) in the intensive care unit (ICU) include all of the following except**
   a. Poor visualization of the aortic arch
   b. Patient discomfort
   c. Foreshortening of the left ventricular (LV) apex
   d. Inability to evaluate the right ventricle (RV)

2. **Current indications for TEE in a critically ill patient are**
   a. Evaluation of the LV preload
   b. Assessment of the severity of aortic stenosis
   c. Unexplained heart failure
   d. All of the above

3. **In patients with suspected infective endocarditis, TEE**
   a. Is cost-effective in comparison with transthoracic echocardiography (TTE)
   b. Can detect small pedunculated masses of the mitral valve
   c. Allows identification of the organism
   d. Always detects tricuspid valve vegetations
   e. **a** and **b**

4. **TEE findings in acute pulmonary embolus include all of the following except**
   a. Dilated right atrium
   b. Echogenic mass in the right PA
   c. Tricuspid regurgitation
   d. Pulmonary filling defect

5. **In patients with an unexplained cerebrovascular accident, TEE can reveal all the following except**
   a. Patent foramen ovale
   b. Mural thrombus
   c. Carotid atheroma
   d. Spontaneous echo contrast in the left atrium

6. **The PA catheter is superior to TEE in the measurement of**
   a. LV preload
   b. LV contractility
   c. Mixed venous oxygen level
   d. Intermittent cardiac output (CO)

7. **In a patient with unexplained hypotension after cardiac surgery, common TEE findings include**
   a. Decreased LV end-diastolic area
   b. Compression of the right cardiac chambers
   c. New regional wall motion abnormalities
   d. All of the above

8. **Common reasons why TTE is often nondiagnostic in critically ill patients are**
   a. Mechanical ventilation with positive end-expiratory pressure
   b. Chest dressings
   c. Inability to lie on the left side
   d. All of the above

9. The following hemodynamic measurements are possible with TEE except
   a. Pulmonary artery (PA) systolic pressure
   b. CO
   c. Oxygen extraction ratio
   d. Systemic vascular resistance

10. Complications associated with TEE include all of the following except
   a. PA perforation
   b. Hypertension
   c. Supraventricular tachycardia
   d. Hematemesis

Answers appear at the back of the book.

18 Transesophageal Echocardiography for Congenital Heart Disease in the Adult

Kathryn Rouine-Rapp and Wanda C. Miller-Hance

The spectrum of congenital cardiovascular pathology seen in the adult varies widely. Malformations range from defects frequently found in isolation to complex lesions characterized by the presence of multiple coexistent defects. Echocardiography is the primary imaging modality for diagnostic assessment of congenital heart disease (CHD) in all age-groups. The transesophageal approach has further expanded the applications of echocardiography in patients with CHD by permitting the acquisition of anatomic information not obtainable by transthoracic imaging, particularly in the adult, with suboptimal precordial windows. As such, transesophageal echocardiography (TEE) enhances the characterization of structural defects, the estimation of hemodynamics, and evaluation of ventricular function. Additional major contributions of TEE in CHD include the intraoperative assessment of the adequacy of the surgical procedure and detection of residual pathology. The role of TEE has also been documented during monitoring of therapeutic catheter interventions in congenital pathology. This chapter addresses the applications of TEE in CHD patients with a focus on the intraoperative setting and as an adjunct during interventions in the cardiac catheterization laboratory.

CONGENITAL HEART DISEASE IN ADULTS: INCIDENCE, PREVALENCE, AND SURVIVAL

The incidence of CHD in the United States is estimated to be 6.2 per 1,000 live births. At birth, the most common CHD lesion is a ventricular septal defect (VSD). Other common CHD lesions include atrial septal defects (ASDs), patent ductus arteriosus (PDA), pulmonary stenosis (PS), aortic stenosis, coarctation of the aorta (CoA), atrioventricular-septal defects (AVSDs), tetralogy of Fallot (TOF), and transposition of the great arteries. Of infants born with CHD, the overall rate of survival to adulthood is 85%. Not surprisingly, the highest survival rate occurs among infants with simple lesions; however, survival of infants with complex lesions has improved dramatically since 1940.

Multiple factors, including prenatal diagnosis, definitive surgical repair at an earlier age, and improvements in the postoperative care of patients with complex defects, are expected to lead to continued increases in survival. Consequently, adults with CHD will soon exceed the numbers of children with CHD.

Normal Embryologic Development of the Heart

A study of normal cardiac embryology can enhance understanding of abnormal cardiac formation and resultant lesions of CHD. By the middle of the third week, clusters of angiogenic cells form and give rise to vascular structures in the human embryo. Over time, these cells form two endothelial heart tubes that fuse completely to form a single heart tube. This single heart tube differentiates into components that include the sinus venosus, atrium, primitive ventricle, and bulbus cordis (Figure 18.1A). Initially a short and straight structure, the single heart tube undergoes rapid growth within the pericardial sac that necessitates bending or looping such that the atria migrate in a cephalad direction

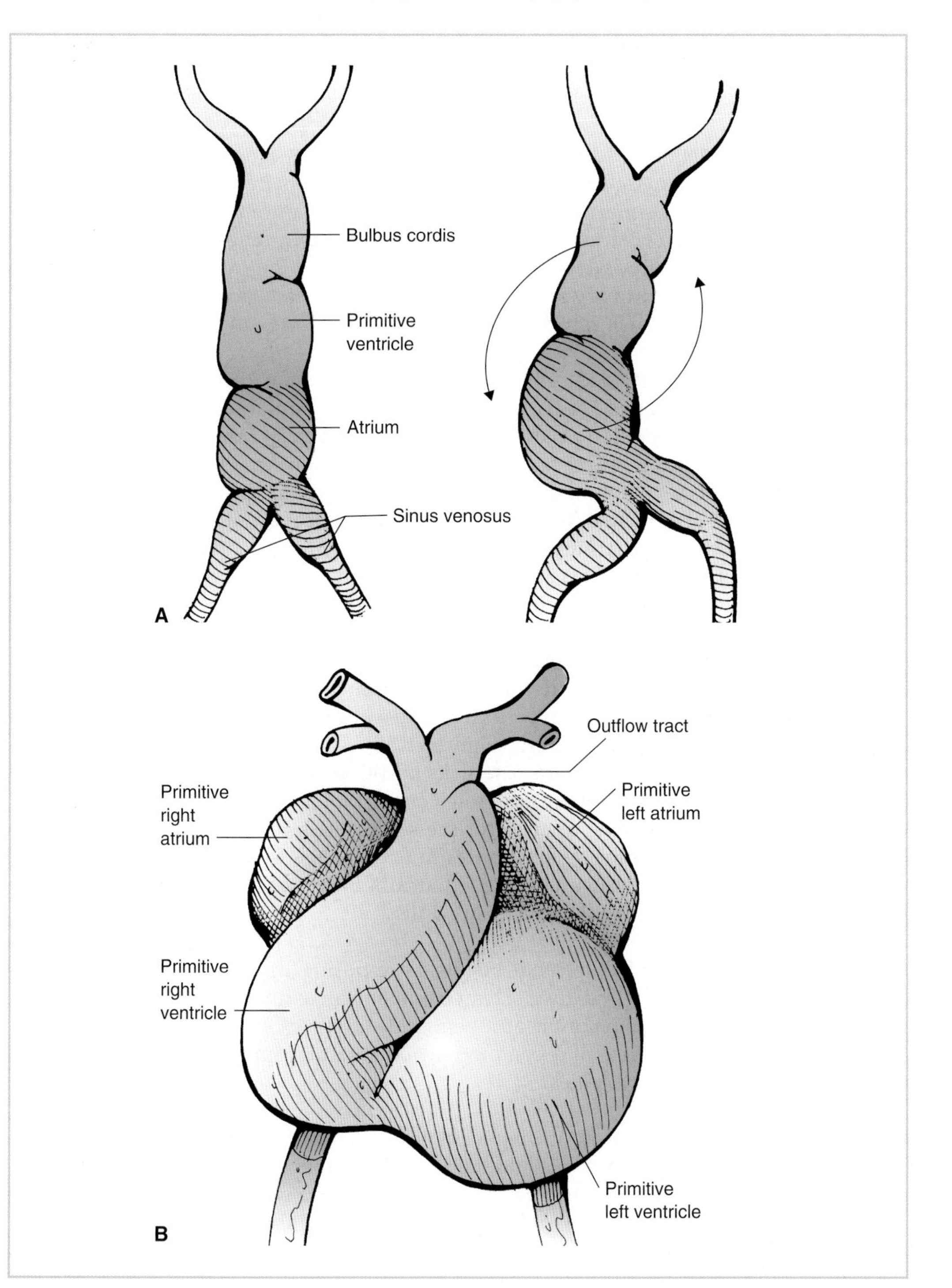

Figure 18.1. A: Differentiation of the single heart tube into components that include the sinus venosus, atrium, primitive ventricle, and bulbus cordis. The illustration on the right indicates the initiation of bending or looping of the heart tube within the pericardial sac. The *arrows* indicate the usual direction of looping. **B:** The heart following completion of looping. Note the cephalad migration of the atria, preseptation common outflow tract, and orientation of the convex surface of the heart to the right.

and the convex surface of the heart is to the right (Figure 18.1B). The reader may be familiar with the term *d-looping*, used by some clinicians to define this aspect of cardiac formation.

Following the completion of looping, the sinus venosus undergoes many changes while developing into the venous system of the heart. It begins as a paired structure and initially fuses to form a transverse sinus with right and left ''horns'' (Figure 18.2A). As development continues, the right horn enlarges and the left horn becomes atretic. Ultimately, the right sinus horn becomes incorporated into the right atrium as the vena cava and the left sinus horn becomes the coronary sinus (Figure 18.2B). *Abnormal persistence of the left horn contributes to persistence of a left superior vena cava (SVC).*

The initial atrium is undivided and communicates with the primitive ventricle that connects to the outlet bulbus cordis. Around 28 days of human embryo development, the process of cardiac septation occurs in the atrium, ventricle, atrioventricular junction and valves, cardiac outflow tracts, and semilunar valves. During septation of the atrium, the septum primum develops in a craniodorsal location and grows inferiorly toward the atrioventricular orifice. Initially the septum primum leaves an opening, the ostium primum, below its free edge. Around 33 days of development a second opening, the ostium secundum, forms in the upper part of the septum primum. This opening provides patency of the interatrial septum to ensure flow of systemic venous blood across the interatrial septum during fetal life. Subsequent to the formation of the ostium secundum, the septum primum extends inferiorly, becomes continuous with developing endocardial cushions of the atrioventricular junction and closes the ostium primum (Figure 18.3A). Around 33 days of development, a second partition, the septum secundum, develops parallel and to the right of the septum primum (Figure 18.3B). The septum secundum covers the ostium secundum but forms an incomplete atrial partition. The formation of an incomplete atrial partition again ensures flow of systemic venous blood across the interatrial septum during fetal life. The remaining opening of the septum secundum is the foramen ovale (Figure 18.3C). Tissue from the septum primum overlies the foramen ovale and forms a valve that closes when the pressure in the left atrium increases following birth. A patent foramen ovale occurs in an estimated 20% of adults.

Septation of the atrioventricular canal begins as apposing masses of tissue known as *endocardial cushions* enlarge and fuse. This occurs concurrently with completion of the septum primum and expansion of the atrioventricular orifice. Defects in this septation are thought to lead to persistence of a common atrioventricular junction and contribute to atrioventricular valve abnormalities.

Septation of the ventricle occurs following formation of a muscular interventricular septum and outgrowths of endocardial tissue and tissue derived from conus and truncal swellings (Figure 18.4). Following fusion, the ventricular septum is comprised of a small membranous and a large muscular component that is divided into inlet, trabecular, and outlet regions. Persistence of a small interventricular communication or incomplete septum formation can lead to interventricular defects.

The outflow tracts of the left and right ventricles are formed following septation of the single truncus arteriosus by the aorticopulmonary septum. Septation includes twisting and ridge fusion with resultant division of the truncus arteriosus into the aortic and pulmonary channels.

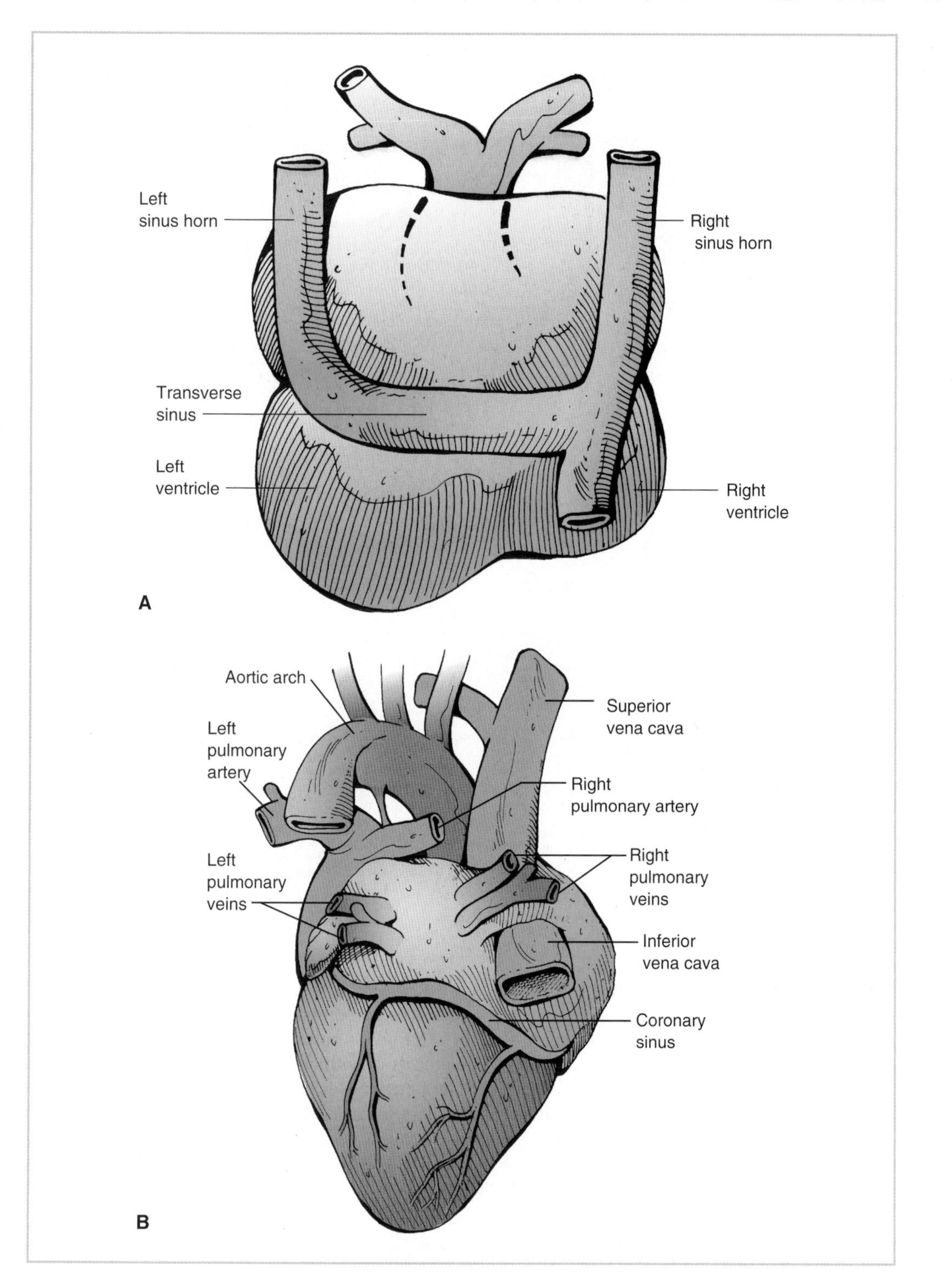

Figure 18.2. **A:** A posterior view of the primitive heart with a transverse sinus and prominent left and right sinus horns. **B:** A posterior view of the formed heart. Note the coronary sinus, a remnant of the left sinus horn, and enlarged right sinus horn, now incorporated into the right atrium as the superior and inferior vena cavae.

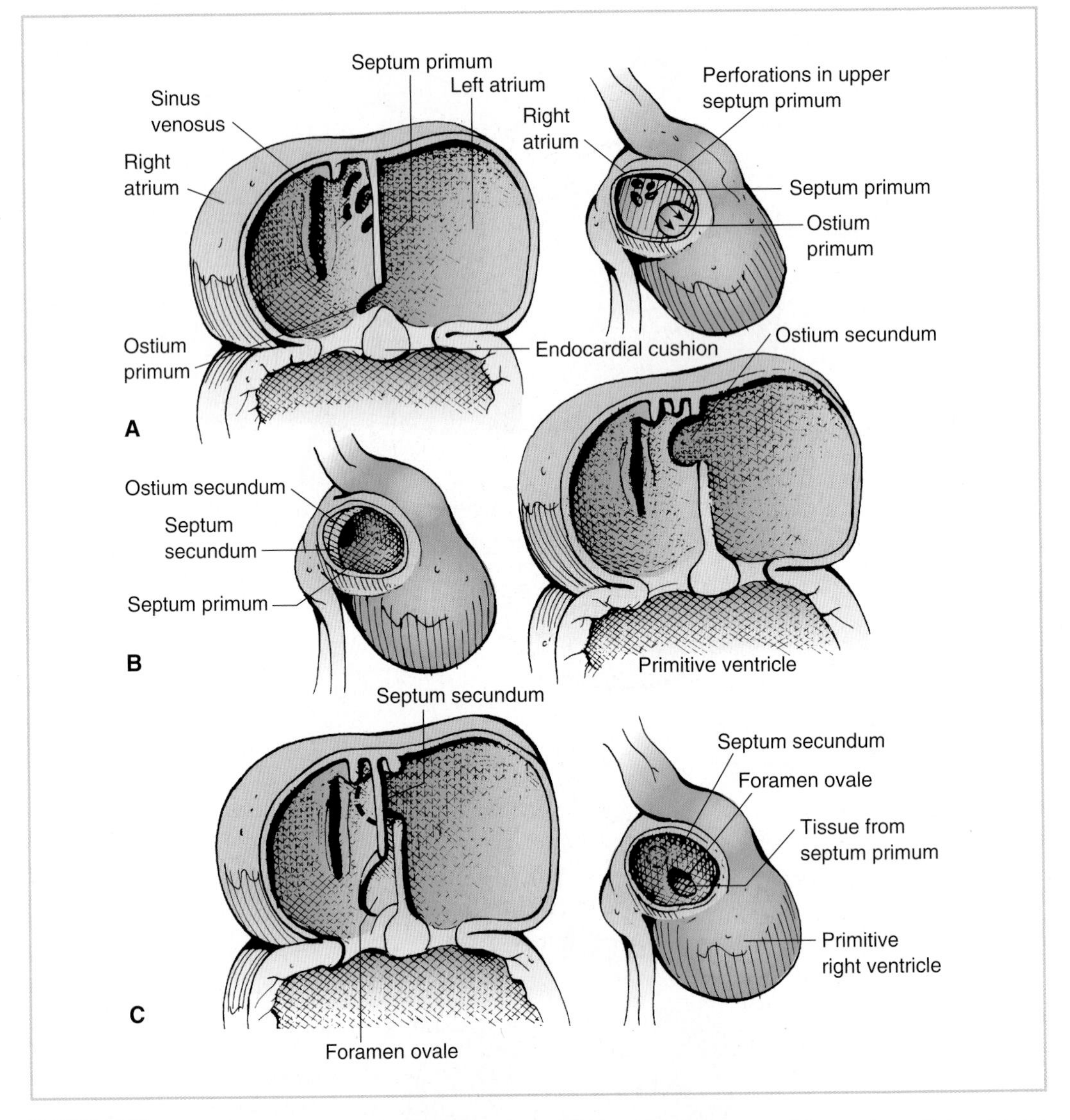

Figure 18.3. **A:** Atrial septation. As the septum primum grows inferiorly toward the endocardial cushions, the ostium secundum, labeled as perforations in upper septum primum, forms in the posterior portion of the septum primum. Once the ostium secundum is formed it ensures the flow of blood across the atrial septum. Thereafter, the septum primum completes its growth and becomes continuous with the developing endocardial cushions of the atrioventricular junction (see *arrows*). **B:** The septum secundum develops parallel and to the right of the septum primum. It forms an incomplete partition. **C:** The remaining opening in the septum secundum is known as the *foramen ovale*. It is covered by a flap-valve formed from tissue from the septum primum. Normally this flap-valve closes when pressure in the left atrium increases following birth and exceeds pressure in the right atrium.

CLASSIFICATION OF CONGENITAL HEART DISEASE

Several classification schemes have been proposed to facilitate the understanding of CHD and the physiologic impact of these defects. Lesions have been characterized according to level of complexity into simple versus complex, presence or absence of cyanosis, and primary physiologic alteration.

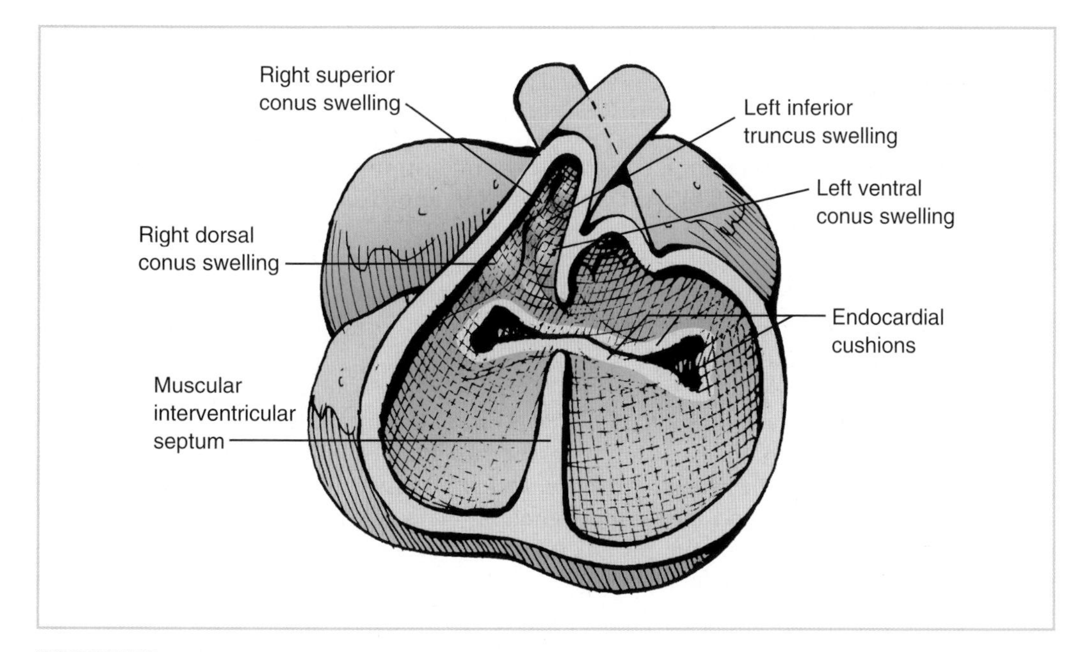

Figure 18.4. Ventricular septation. The muscular interventricular septum grows in a dorsal direction toward the endocardial cushions. Subsequently, the membranous interventricular septum occurs as an outgrowth of endocardial tissue and tissue derived from conus and truncal swellings.

Simple versus Complex Lesions

Isolated defects, such as intracardiac communications (e.g., ASDs), are considered simple lesions. Complex pathology includes lesions associated with multiple concomitant defects and malpositions of the heart and visceral organs (heterotaxy syndromes).

Acyanotic versus Cyanotic Lesions

In this scheme, congenital cardiac malformations are divided into two groups based on whether the primary functional disorder includes cyanosis. Cyanotic conditions are those with restrictive pulmonary blood flow in the presence of intracardiac shunting or complete arterial and venous admixture. Cyanosis is less likely to occur in individuals with pulmonary overcirculation secondary to isolated intracardiac communications.

Shunts, Obstructions, Regurgitant Pathology, and Mixed Lesions

The classification algorithm based on the physiologic spectrum of CHD comprises four major categories: shunts, obstructions to pulmonary or systemic blood flow, regurgitant pathology, and mixed lesions. Shunt lesions may occur within the heart (intracardiac) or outside the heart (extracardiac). The direction and magnitude of the shunt depend on the size of the communication and the relative resistances of the pulmonary and systemic circulations. Obstructive lesions may affect the inflow or outflow of blood and vary widely in severity. Regurgitant lesions are rarely found in isolation. They occur frequently secondary to the primary pathology. In mixed lesions, which account for a significant number of cyanotic heart defects, there is mixing of the systemic and pulmonary venous return.

SPECIFIC DEFECTS

Atrial Septal Defect

ANATOMY

Four types of ASD are ostium secundum, ostium primum, sinus venosus, and coronary sinus defects (Figure 18.5). ASDs account for approximately 30% of all cases of CHD detected in adults.

Ostium secundum defects are located in the central portion of the interatrial septum and account for 70% of all ASDs (Figure 18.6). Associated abnormalities include mitral valve prolapse and mitral regurgitation.

Ostium primum defects (also known as *partial AVSDs*) are located in the inferior portion of the interatrial septum. They account for approximately 20% of ASDs, result from incomplete formation of the septum primum, and are frequently associated with a cleft in the anterior mitral leaflet and mitral regurgitation. (Trisomy 21 is most often associated with a full blown AVSD, not the partial AVSD defined here, and is mentioned in the subsequent text under VSD, inlet defects.)

Sinus venosus defects occur adjacent to the entrance of the SVC (most common) or inferior vena cava (IVC) (Figure 18.5). They account for 5% to 10% of ASDs and are often associated with partial anomalous pulmonary venous drainage.

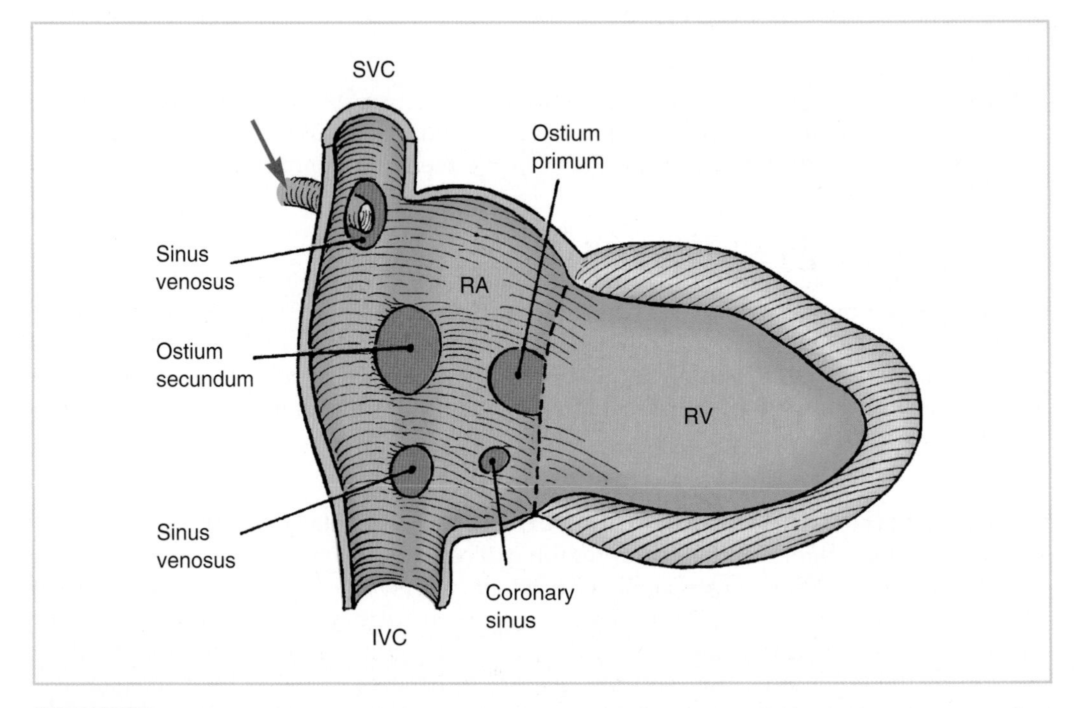

Figure 18.5. Atrial septal defects. Location of atrial septal defects. Centrally located ostium secundum and inferiorly located ostium primum sinus venosus defects near the superior vena cava (*SVC*) or the inferior vena cava (*IVC*), and associated anomalous pulmonary venous connection (*arrow*) and coronary sinus defect. RA, right atrium; RV, right ventricle. (From Perloff JK. *The clinical recognition of congenital heart disease*, fourth ed. Philadelphia: WB Saunders, 1994:295, with permission.)

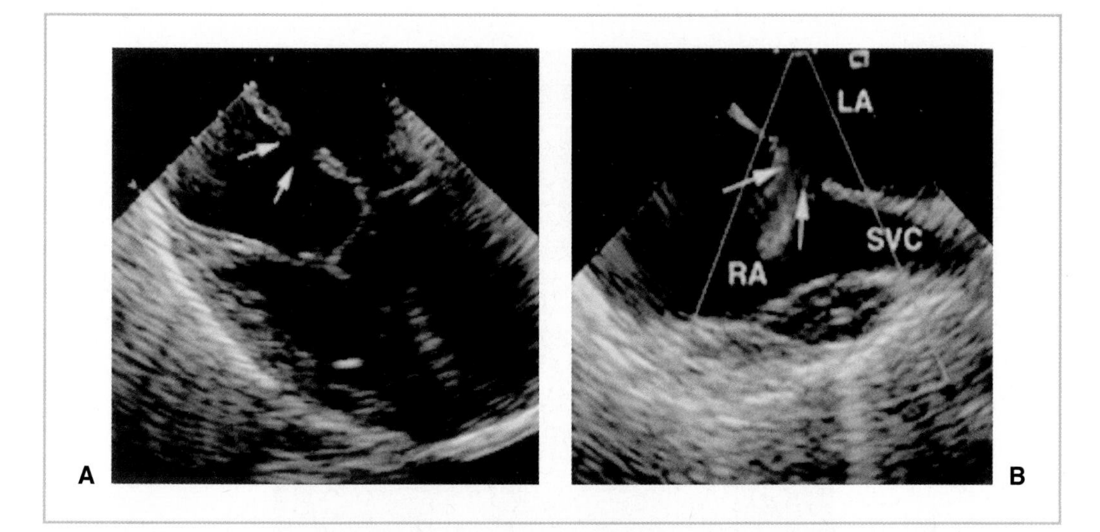

Figure 18.6. Secundum atrial septal defect. **A:** Central defect in the atrial septum (*arrows*), typical of a secundum atrial septal defect, seen in the midesophageal four-chamber view. **B:** Defect in the long-axis plane (midesophageal bicaval view). LA, left atrium; RA, right atrium; SVC, superior vena cava.

Coronary sinus defects are very rare and result from a communication between the left atrium and coronary sinus. They are typically associated with a persistent left SVC and resultant enlarged coronary sinus.

PHYSIOLOGY

The physiologic consequences are determined by the size of the defect and the degree of left-to-right shunting. The defect size, ventricular compliances, and pulmonary artery (PA) pressures determine the magnitude of the shunt. A large defect leading to pulmonary overcirculation results in right-sided volume overload and resultant right atrial, right-ventricular (RV) and PA dilation. Over time the onset of atrial arrhythmias and heart failure can occur. Although most adults with ASDs have mild-to-moderate elevations of PA pressure, severe pulmonary hypertension develops only in 5% to 10% of older patients. *Patients may remain asymptomatic and present with ASD as an incidental finding on intraoperative TEE.*

MANAGEMENT

Most patients with an ASD undergo surgical closure. However, selected ostium secundum defects may be amenable to transcatheter occlusion through device deployment in the cardiac catheterization laboratory (Figure 18.7).

TRANSESOPHAGEAL ECHOCARDIOGRAPHIC EVALUATION

Suggested cross sections for a focused examination: midesophageal (ME) four chamber (4-CH) and ME bicaval (Table 18.1).

Goals of the two-dimensional examination are:

1. Definition of defect location and size
2. Determination of right-sided chambers and vessel dimensions
3. Examination of the mitral valve for prolapse or cleft
4. Evaluation of pulmonary veins

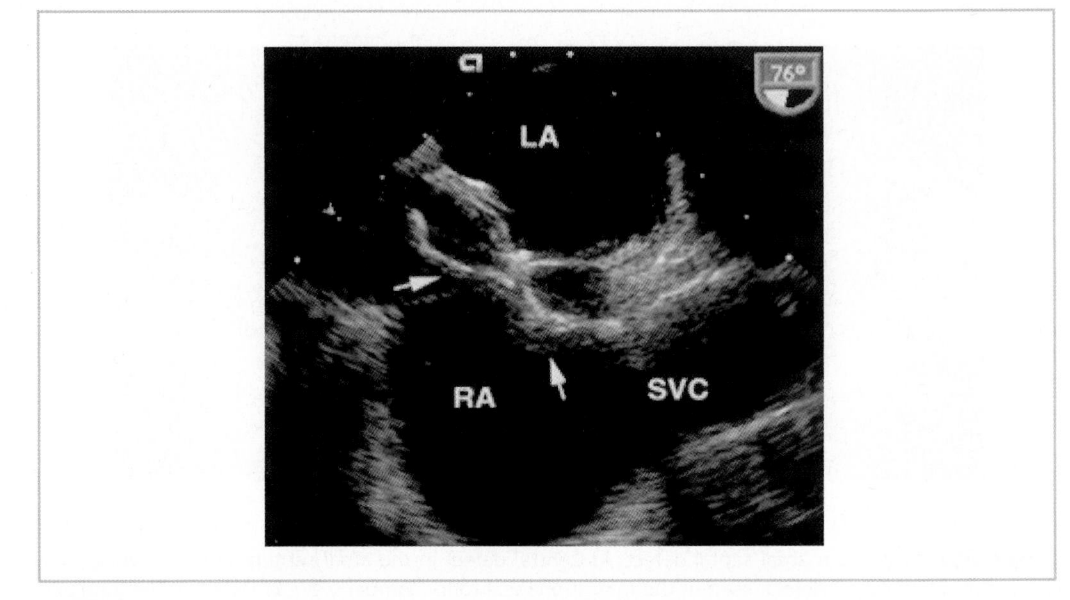

Figure 18.7. Atrial septal defect closure device. Transesophageal imaging (midesophageal bicaval view) during placement of an atrial septal defect closure device (*arrows*). LA, left atrium; RA, right atrium; SVC, superior vena cava.

5. Assessment of ventricular function
6. Detection of an interatrial shunt by the intravenous injection of agitated saline solution or other echocardiography contrast agent

Goals of the Doppler examination are:

1. Assessment of flow across defect (color Doppler)
2. Detection of tricuspid or mitral valve regurgitation (color Doppler)
3. Measurement of tricuspid regurgitant jet velocity to estimate PA systolic pressure (spectral Doppler)
4. Estimation of the magnitude of the shunt (pulmonary and systemic blood flows) in the absence of significant atrioventricular valve regurgitation (spectral Doppler)

Goals of the examination after surgical repair or during/after catheter intervention are:

1. Detection of residual interatrial shunts
2. Evaluation of valve competence
3. Assessment of ventricular function
4. Monitoring during transcatheter interventions
5. Evaluation of proper positioning of closure device and unimpaired flow in SVC, IVC, and pulmonary veins following transcatheter device deployment

Ventricular Septal Defect

ANATOMY

VSDs are classified by location into four major groups: perimembranous, muscular, doubly committed outlet (subarterial), and inlet defects (Figure 18.8). They can occur in isolation

Table 18.1 Transesophageal echocardiography (TEE) in the evaluation of congenital heart disease

Lesion	TEE planes and information provided	Postsurgical evaluation
AS	ME AV SAX: aortic valve morphology	Residual/recurrent obstruction, aortic regurgitation, bioprosthetic/mechanical valve function, perivalvar leak (if prosthetic valve), ventricular function
	ME AV LAX and deep TG LAX: valve morphology and motion, valvar regurgitation, aortic root size, subaortic and supra-aortic anatomy	After Ross procedure: aortic obstruction and regurgitation, function of right ventricular homograft, ventricular function (global and segmental)
	Deep TG LAX: peak gradient across obstruction	
	ME 4-CH: LV hypertrophy and function	
ASD	ME 4-CH: secundum and primum defects, pulmonary venous return, mitral valve anatomy (prolapse)	Residual shunts, ventricular function
	ME bicaval: sinus venosus defect and pulmonary veins	Mitral regurgitation
		Obstruction of pulmonary veins (sinus venosus ASD)
CoA	UE Ao Arch SAX and LAX views of descending thoracic aorta and aortic arch (if visible): posterior shelf, aliased flow by color Doppler and CW Doppler gradient of >2.5 m/s	Residual gradient, recoarctation, aortic aneurysm formation
	ME 4-CH, 2-CH, AV LAX and TG SAX: LV mass and function, mitral valve morphology and function, aortic valve, subvalvular and supravalvular obstruction	
Corrected transposition	ME 4-CH, 2-CH, TG mid SAX: ventricular morphology and function, tricuspid valve function and associated lesions	Following double switch operation:
	ME LAX: RVOT obstruction	Atrial baffle portion: baffle leaks, obstruction of venous pathways, AVV competence, function of systemic ventricle
		Arterial switch portion: outflow obstruction
		Residual intracardiac shunts
***d*-TGA**	ME 4CH: AVV regurgitation, associated intracardiac shunts, ventricular function	After Senning/Mustard procedure: baffle leaks, obstruction of venous pathways, function of systemic (right) ventricle, AVV competence
	ME bicaval: systemic and pulmonary venous baffles	After arterial switch operation: supravalvar (aortic/pulmonary) stenosis or regurgitation, LV function, residual shunts
	TG mid SAX: ventricular function and SWMA	
	Deep TG LAX: ventriculoarterial connections and arterial anastomoses after arterial switch	

(continued)

Table 18.1 *(continued)*

Lesion	TEE planes and information provided	Postsurgical evaluation
PDA	Difficult to visualize by TEE, however ductal flow can be detected in the ME AsAo SAX view by presence of abnormal continuous high velocity aliased flow	Persistent shunt, biventricular function
PS	ME RV inflow–outflow and deep TG LAX: outflow tract evaluation and gradient estimation ME AsAo SAX: evaluation of pulmonic valve, main pulmonary artery and proximal pulmonary artery branches	Residual pulmonary outflow tract obstruction, pulmonary regurgitation, RV size and function
Single ventricle	ME 4-CH, 2-CH, LAX, bicaval, RV inflow–outflow: AV valve morphology and atrioventricular and ventriculoarterial connections	Post-Fontan: cavopulmonary connection, Fontan baffle, aortic regurgitation, systemic outflow tract obstruction, AVV competence, ventricular function, adequacy of ASD
TOF	ME AV LAX and deep TG: VSD and aortic override ME RV inflow–outflow: evaluation of RVOT and estimation of gradient ME 4-CH: location and extension of VSD and other additional VSDs Color Doppler in ME AV SAX and AV LAX: evaluation of coronary artery anomalies	Residual RVOT obstruction, pulmonic or conduit stenosis, residual shunts, ventricular function, aortic regurgitation
VSD	ME 4-CH and AV LAX: perimembranous, inlet and muscular VSDs, chamber sizes, presence of ventricular septal aneurysm ME AV LAX and deep TG LAX: evaluation of aortic valve for regurgitation and herniation	Residual shunts, AVV and semilunar valve competence and ventricular function

AS, aortic stenosis; ME, midesophageal; AV, aortic valve; SAX, short axis; LAX, long axis; TG, transgastric; CH, chamber; LV, left ventricle; ASD, atrial septal defect; CoA, coarctation of the aorta; UE, upper esophageal; Ao, aortic; CW, continuous wave; RVOT, right ventricular outflow tract; d-TGA, d-transposition of the great arteries; AVV, atrioventricular valve; SWMA, segmental wall motion abnormalities; PDA, patent ductus arteriosus; AsAo, ascending aorta; PS, pulmonic stenosis; RV, right ventricle; TOF, tetralogy of Fallot; VSD, ventricular septal defect.
Russell IA, Rouine-Rapp K, Stratmann G, et al. Congenital heart disease in the adult: a review with internet-accessible transesophageal echocardiographic images. *Anesth Analg* 2006;102(3):694–723, with permission.

or as part of complex malformations. An isolated VSD is the most common congenital heart defect diagnosed in infancy. Because larger defects are usually repaired in childhood and up to 60% of smaller defects close spontaneously, VSDs account for only 10% to 15% of defects observed in adults with CHD.

Perimembranous defects account for approximately 70% of VSDs, involve most or all of the membranous septum, and may extend into the muscular septum. Associated findings include a ventricular septal aneurysm, an aneurysm of the membranous septum that is composed of tricuspid valve tissue. This appears as a tissue pouch and most often limits the flow of blood across the defect (Figure 18.9). Another associated finding is aortic valve (AV) cusp herniation with resulting aortic regurgitation.

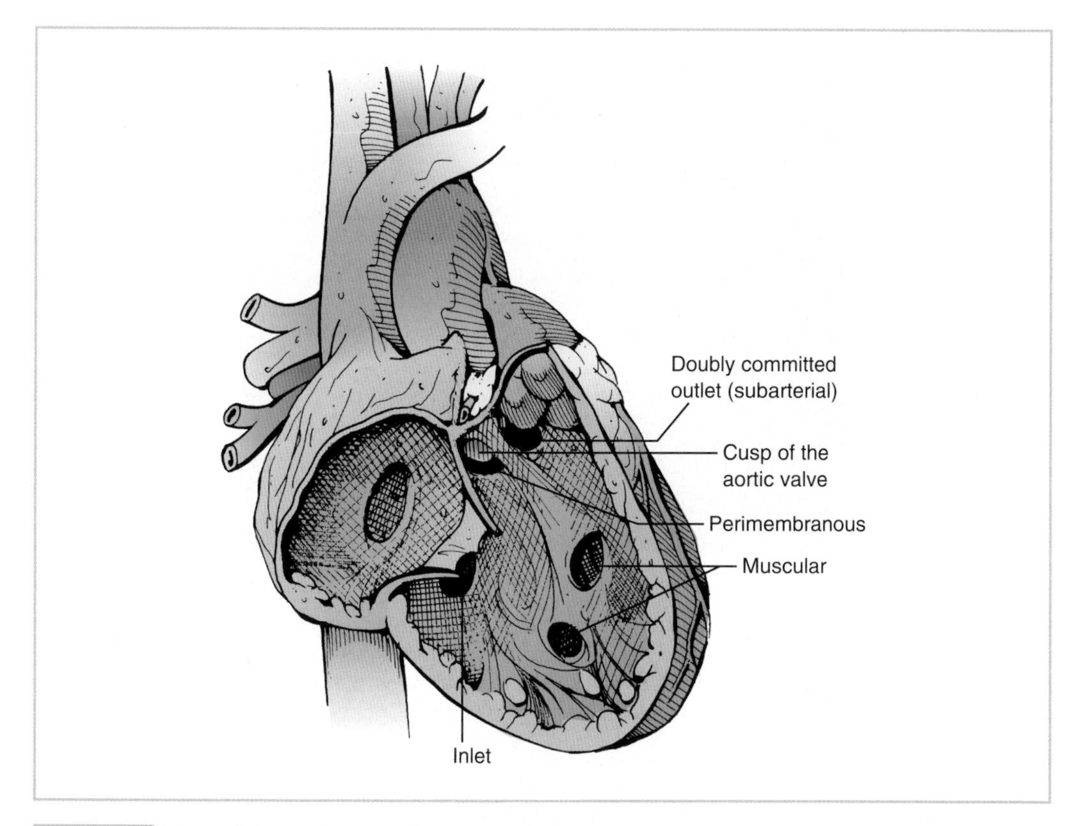

Figure 18.8. View of the interventricular septum from the right ventricle. Ventricular septal defects are classified by location into four major groups: perimembranous, muscular, doubly committed (subarterial) and inlet defects. Muscular defects can occur in the trabecular or inlet portion of the muscular interventricular septum. In this figure, a portion of the aortic valve can be visualized through the perimembranous defect.

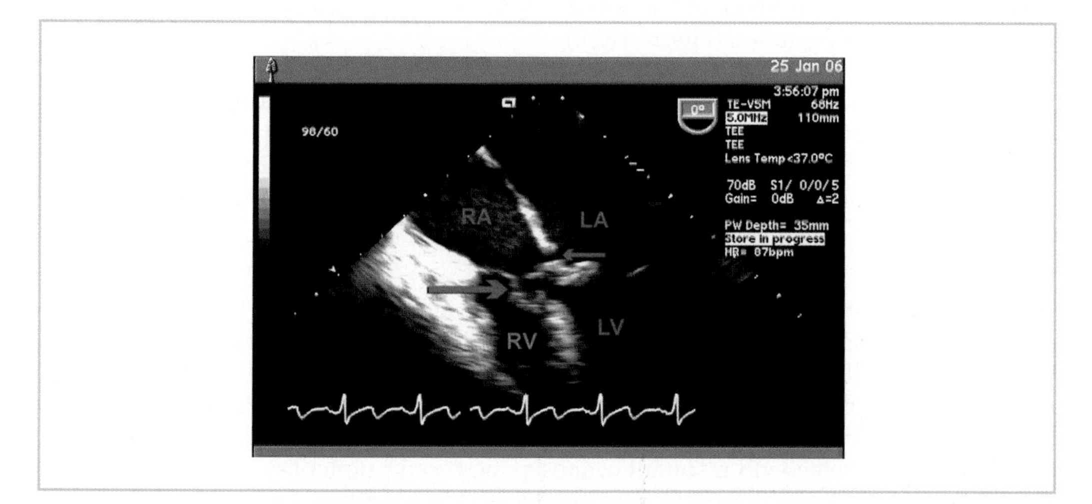

Figure 18.9. Ventricular septal aneurysm. Two-dimensional transesophageal echocardiographic midesophageal four-chamber view demonstrates a tissue pouch (*large arrow*) composed of tricuspid tissue. Note also the small defect (*small arrow*) in the inferior border of the interatrial septum, a primum atrial septal defect. RA, right atrium; LA, left atrium; LV, left ventricle; RV, right ventricle.

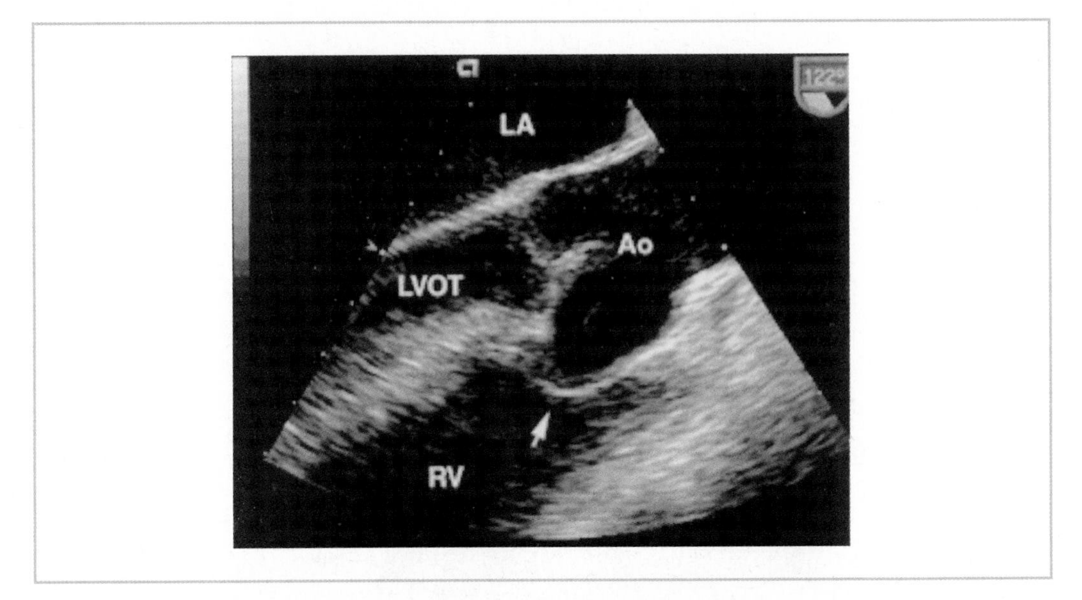

Figure 18.10. Doubly-committed subarterial ventricular septal defect. Two-dimensional transesophageal echocardiographic midesophageal aortic valve long-axis view demonstrates a subarterial ventricular septal defect and herniation of the right coronary aortic valve cusp through the defect (*arrow*). LA, left atrium; LVOT, left ventricular outflow tract; Ao, proximal ascending aorta; RV, right ventricle.

Muscular defects are defined by their location in the muscular portion of the ventricular septum. They account for 20% of VSDs, can be isolated or multiple, and are often located in the central or apical portion of the trabecular septum.

Doubly-committed outlet defects, also known as *supracristal* or *subarterial defects,* are located in the infundibular septum immediately below the pulmonary valve (PV). They account for 5% of VSDs and are frequently associated with AV right coronary cusp prolapse that results in aortic regurgitation (Figure 18.10).

Inlet defects account for approximately 5% of VSDs and are located in close proximity to the atrioventricular valves in the posterior or inlet portion of ventricular septum. An associated primum ASD can be part of a complex defect known as an *AVSD,* or *atrioventricular canal defect*. This defect is present commonly in individuals with trisomy 21 (Down) syndrome (Figure 18.11).

PHYSIOLOGY

The physiologic consequences of a VSD are determined by the size of the defect and the pulmonary vascular resistance. Moderate-to-large defects are associated with significant left-to-right shunting and symptoms of heart failure. Severe pulmonary hypertension can develop in patients with large, long-standing VSDs and substantial pulmonary overcirculation. This in turn can lead to a reversal in the direction (right-to-left) of blood flow through the defect and resultant cyanosis. Increased pulmonary vascular resistance secondary to irreversible vascular changes leads to a condition known as *Eisenmenger syndrome*. Adults in whom Eisenmenger syndrome develops have a decreased survival rate and generally are not considered candidates for surgery.

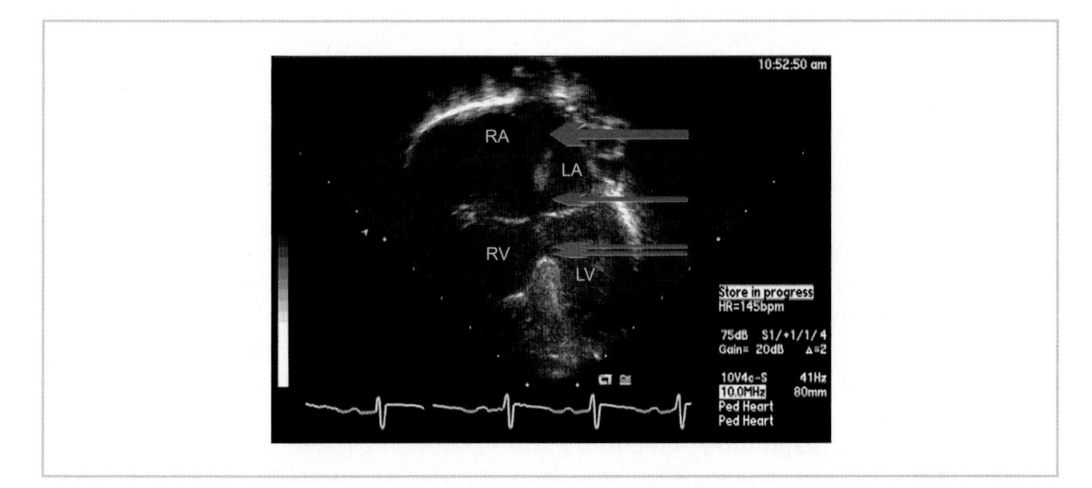

Figure 18.11. Atrioventricular-septal defect. Two-dimensional transesophageal echocardiographic midesophageal four-chamber view demonstrates a ventricular septal defect in the inlet portion of the ventricular septum (*double arrow*), a primum atrial septal defect (*single small arrow*) and a secundum atrial septal defect (*single large arrow*). RA, right atrium; LA, left atrium; RV, right ventricle; LV, left ventricle.

MANAGEMENT

Most defects of moderate-to-large size associated with symptomatology require intervention. Surgical closure of an isolated VSD most commonly is accomplished through the transatrial or transpulmonary approach. In selected cases transcatheter device placement may be an option. A hybrid strategy of periventricular closure using a combination of surgical and interventional techniques has also been described. During a typical hybrid procedure, the surgeon punctures the right-ventricular free wall and together with a cardiologist, uses TEE guidance to introduce a wire to then deploy a closure device across a defect, such as a muscular VSD. Additional corrective surgery can be performed using conventional techniques.

TRANSESOPHAGEAL ECHOCARDIOGRAPHIC EVALUATION

Suggested cross sections for a focused examination: ME 4-CH, ME AV long axis (LAX), and deep transgastric (TG) LAX (Table 18.1).

Goals of two-dimensional examination are:

1. Assessment of defect location, size, and extension
2. Determination of chamber sizes and PA dimensions
3. Inspection for associated abnormalities
4. Identification of ventricular septal aneurysm, if present (Figure 18.9)
5. Evaluation of AV for herniation and prolapse (Figure 18.10)
6. Inspection for findings suggestive of pulmonary hypertension

Goals of Doppler examination are:

1. Detection of tricuspid and/or aortic regurgitation (color Doppler)
2. Enhancement or confirmation of the presence of a defect or additional defects (color Doppler)

3. Determination of the magnitude and direction of shunt flow (color Doppler)
4. Optimization of the alignment of the Doppler beam within the defect jet (color Doppler)
5. Estimation of PA systolic pressure by either of following calculations:
   a. Tricuspid regurgitant jet velocity (TR)
      In the absence of outflow obstruction, PA systolic pressure = RV systolic pressure
      PA pressure = $4(v_{TR})^2 +$ RA pressure
   b. Peak velocity across the VSD (v_{vsd})
      In the absence of outflow obstruction, PA systolic pressure = RV systolic pressure
      RV systolic pressure = Systolic blood pressure—$4(v_{vsd})^2$
6. Distinction between the high-velocity flow of a restrictive VSD and the low-velocity flow of a nonrestrictive lesion with little or no difference in ventricular pressures
7. Estimation of the magnitude of the shunt (pulmonary and systemic blood flows) in the absence of significant atrioventricular valve regurgitation (spectral Doppler)

Goals of the examination after surgical repair or during/after catheter intervention are:

1. Detection of residual shunts
2. Determination of changes in severity of tricuspid or AV regurgitation
3. Monitoring during device placement
4. Assessment of ventricular function

Patent Ductus Arteriosus

ANATOMY

During fetal life, the arterial duct connects the junction of the main and left PAs to the descending aorta adjacent to the origin of the left subclavian artery (Figure 18.12). PDA accounts for approximately 8% of cases of CHD and can be seen in isolation or associated with other cardiac defects.

PHYSIOLOGY

The physiologic consequences of a PDA are determined by the size of the communication and the difference between the systemic and pulmonary vascular resistances. Although a small PDA may have little or no physiologic effect, left-to-right shunting through a moderate-to-large communication leads to pulmonary overcirculation and, if chronic, may result in an increased pulmonary vascular resistance. Most individuals with a large PDA do not survive to late adulthood unless the left-to-right shunt and left ventricular (LV) volume load are limited by an increased pulmonary vascular resistance, a finding associated with the development of Eisenmenger syndrome.

MANAGEMENT

Surgical closure of a PDA in adults may be complicated by the need for the procedure to be done under cardiopulmonary bypass and is contraindicated in those with Eisenmenger syndrome. Smaller communications may be suitable for catheter occlusion.

TRANSESOPHAGEAL ECHOCARDIOGRAPHIC EVALUATION

Examination of a PDA by two-dimensional TEE can be difficult because views of the descending aorta are limited. Suggested cross sections for focused examination: ME ascending aorta short axis (SAX) (Table 18.1).

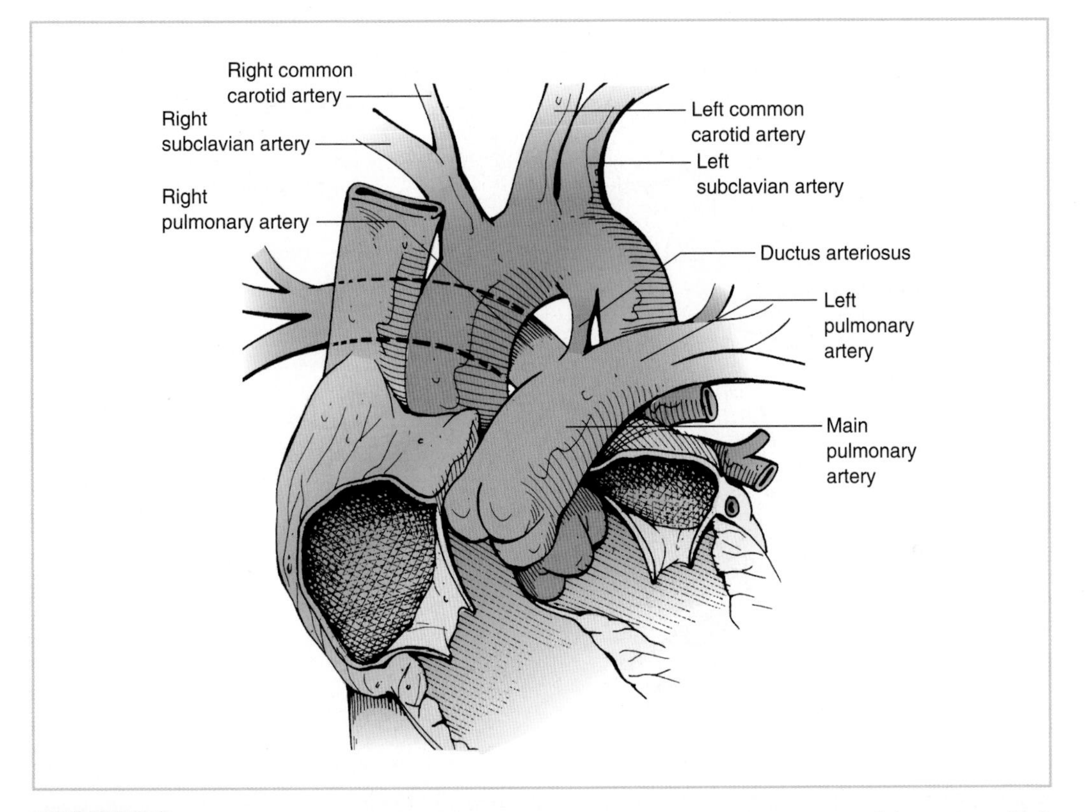

Figure 18.12. Patent ductus arteriosus. The ductus arteriosus connects the junction of the main and left pulmonary arteries to the descending aorta adjacent to the origin of the left subclavian artery.

Goals of two-dimensional examination are:

1. Identification of associated cardiac malformations
2. Detection of left-atrial or ventricular dilation
3. Assessment of LV function

Goals of Doppler examination are:

1. Color-flow mapping to detect ductal flow into the main PA; this increases the diagnostic accuracy but requires the presence of a left-to-right shunt
2. Color-flow Doppler to evaluate tricuspid regurgitation and mitral regurgitation
3. Spectral Doppler to estimate the PA systolic pressure and document retrograde flow in the descending aorta during diastole

Goals of the examination after surgical repair or during/after catheter intervention are:

1. Detection of residual ductal flow that necessitates further intervention

Coarctation of the Aorta

ANATOMY

CoA is characterized by a narrowing of the aorta that typically occurs immediately beyond the origin of the left subclavian artery or just beyond the insertion of the ligamentum

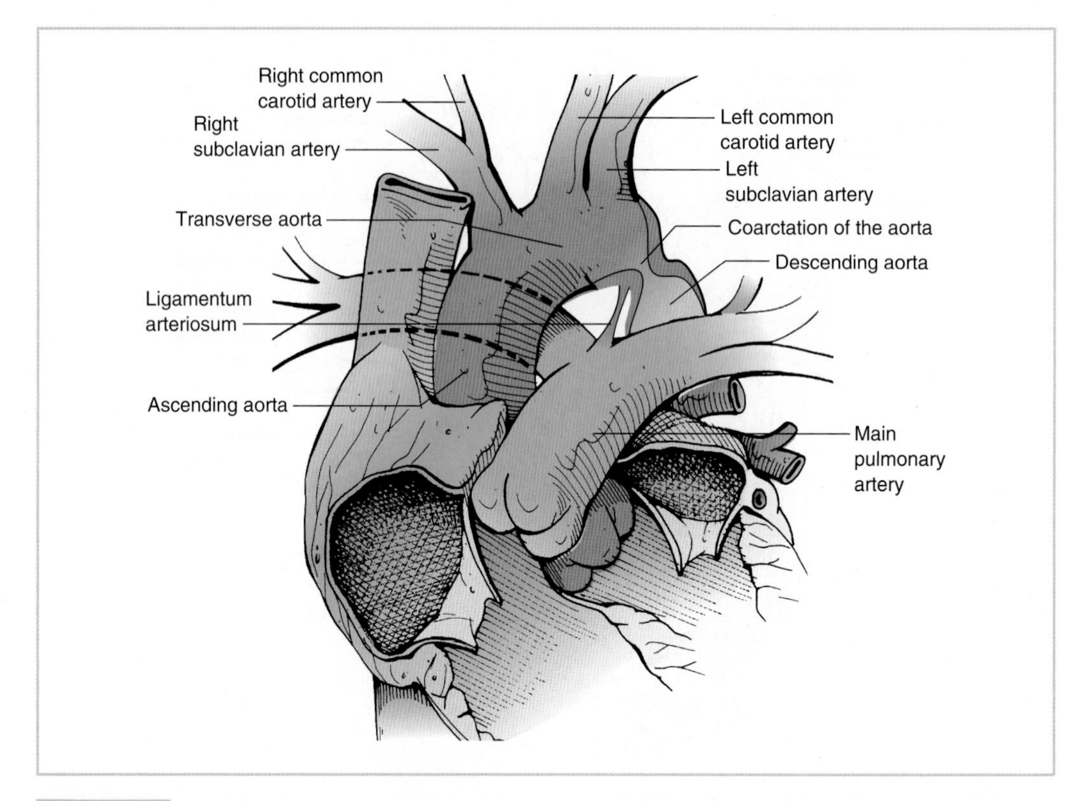

Figure 18.13. Coarctation of the aorta. The aorta is narrowed immediately beyond the left subclavian artery.

arteriosum (juxtaductal) (Figure 18.13). In adults, a discrete obstructing shelf often projects into the aortic lumen. Associated defects may include a PDA, VSD, and in more than 50% of patients, a bicuspid AV. CoA accounts for approximately 6% of all cases of CHD, is more common in males, and 20% of cases are diagnosed in adolescents or adults.

PHYSIOLOGY

The main physiologic consequence of CoA is increased LV afterload. The systolic arterial blood pressure is increased proximal to the coarctation site and decreased distal to it, and systemic hypertension develops subsequently. Most adults with CoA are asymptomatic, although recurrent epistaxis, headache, claudication, dizziness, and palpitations may occur. Major complications include aortic dissection, rupture, or endarteritis of the aorta, cerebral hemorrhage, infective endocarditis, and LV failure.

MANAGEMENT

The severity of the obstruction dictates the need for intervention. Options include surgical management and balloon dilation with or without stent placement.

TRANSESOPHAGEAL ECHOCARDIOGRAPHIC EVALUATION

The anterior position of the air-filled trachea relative to the esophagus limits the TEE examination of the distal ascending aorta and proximal aortic arch, thereby making this a difficult lesion to examine by TEE. Images are obtained most reliably by transthoracic echocardiography (Figure 18.14). Suggested cross sections for focused TEE examination : upper esophageal (UE) Ao Arch SAX and LAX, ME 4-CH, AV LAX, and TG SAX (Table 18.1).

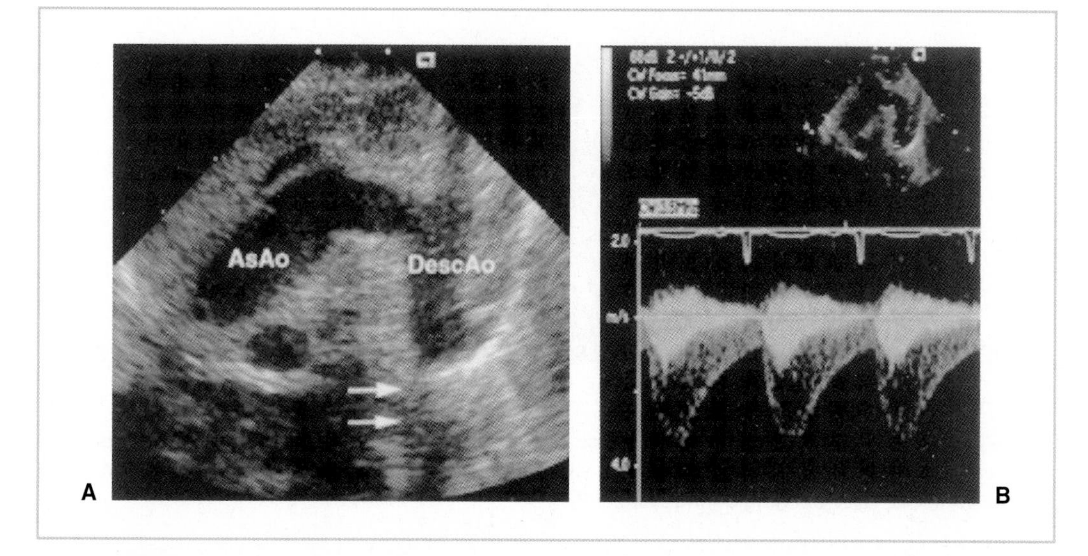

Figure 18.14. Coarctation of the aorta. **A:** Two-dimensional transthoracic image of aortic coarctation. The tight area of obstruction is indicated by the arrows. AsAo, ascending aorta; DescAo, descending aorta. **B:** Typical spectral Doppler flow pattern across the coarctation site. The lighter and darker velocities correspond to the dual population of blood elements across the region. The peak Doppler velocity allows the degree obstruction to be quantified.

Goals of the two-dimensional examination are:

1. Identification of associated lesions and limited evaluation of the aortic arch
2. Monitoring of LV function during aortic-clamp application

Goals of Doppler examination are:

1. Detection of turbulent, eccentric jets or flow acceleration in the descending aorta by color-flow Doppler
2. Determination of flow velocities across the area of narrowing by spectral Doppler; this examination is complicated by the limited ability to align the Doppler beam to the direction of flow

Goals of the examination after surgical repair or during/after catheter intervention are:

1. Detection of residual obstruction

Aortic Valve Stenosis

ANATOMY

Bicuspid AV is the most common malformation of the normally tricuspid AV and frequently results from commissural fusion. After cusp fusion, a raphe or false commissure may remain, and the resultant cusps may be equal or markedly different in size with an eccentric line of closure (Figure 18.15). Aortic stenosis accounts for 6% of all CHD lesions. Bicuspid AV is the most common defect in patients with symptomatic aortic stenosis who are younger than 65 years. In some patients, a weakness in the media of the ascending

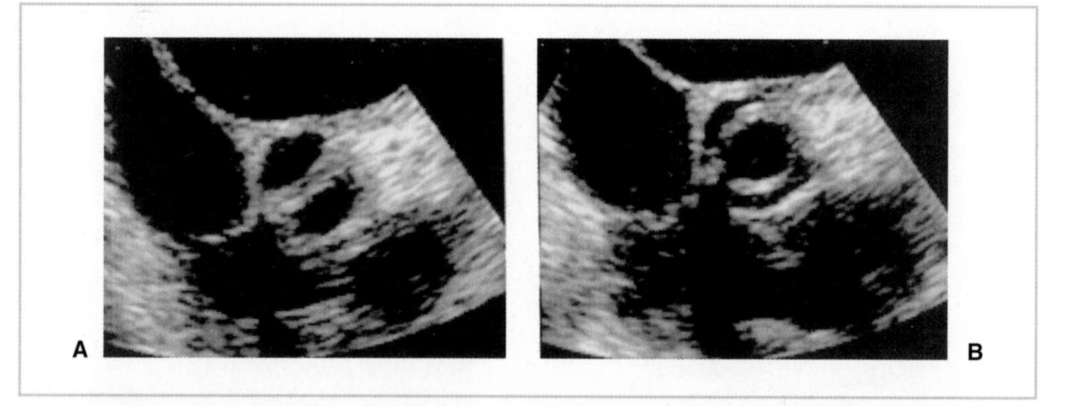

Figure 18.15. Bicuspid aortic valve. Two-dimensional transesophageal echocardiographic midesophageal aortic valve short-axis view of a bicuspid aortic valve demonstrates the single closure line in diastole (**A**) and the abnormal valve opening during systole (**B**).

and transverse aorta predisposes to aneurysm formation. Other associated defects include VSD and CoA.

PHYSIOLOGY

Gradually, the bicuspid AV thickens, calcifies, and looses mobility. As valve stenosis develops, the LV systolic pressure increases and the LV walls hypertrophy. As the area of the valve orifice becomes critical, LV systolic function decreases and heart failure occurs. Aortic regurgitation may develop and lead to an increase in LV preload and dilation.

MANAGEMENT

A number of surgical strategies have been applied in patients with AV obstruction. Patients with a bicuspid AV often require placement of a prosthetic AV. Balloon valvuloplasty may also be effective.

TRANSESOPHAGEAL ECHOCARDIOGRAPHIC EVALUATION

Methods to determine the AV area and severity of the obstruction are discussed elsewhere in this text. The use of planimetry by two-dimensional imaging to estimate AV area is unreliable in patients with a bicuspid AV. Suggested cross sections for focused TEE examination : ME AV SAX, ME AV LAX, deep TG LAX, and ME 4-CH (Table 18.1).

Goals of two-dimensional evaluation are:

1. Determination of AV morphology and motion
2. Measurement of annular size
3. Identification of poststenotic dilation of the ascending aorta
4. Detection of concentric LV hypertrophy or dilation
5. Assessment of global and segmental LV function
6. Identification of associated pathology

Goals of Doppler examination are:

1. Identification of turbulent flow across the AV and/or aortic regurgitation
2. Estimation of peak-instantaneous gradient across the AV with the TG LAX view or the deep TG LAX view by spectral Doppler

Goals of the examination after surgical repair or during/after catheter intervention are:

1. Examination of residual pathology depending on the type of intervention. Aortic regurgitation may be present after valvuloplasty or surgical valvotomy. If AV replacement is accomplished using a pulmonary autograft (Ross procedure), assessment of the autograft function in addition to the pulmonary homograft for stenosis or regurgitation, and assessment of biventricular function are important.
2. Evaluation of prosthetic valve function and the presence of paravalvular leaks following replacement with a prosthetic valve are required.

Pulmonary Stenosis

ANATOMY

PS can occur as an isolated lesion and accounts for approximately 10% of CHD in adults. A domed PV without clear leaflet separation is the most common anatomic pathology that causes congenital PS. The orifice of this lesion ranges from pinhole to several millimeters in diameter (Figure 18.16). Less commonly, PVs are dysplastic with thickened, redundant leaflets, and unfused commissures. Associated lesions include ASD, VSD, and obstructive subpulmonic hypertrophy. Because many authors limit their discussion of PS to patients who have an obstruction of the right-ventricular outflow tract (RVOT) and intact ventricular septum, this discussion will be limited similarly.

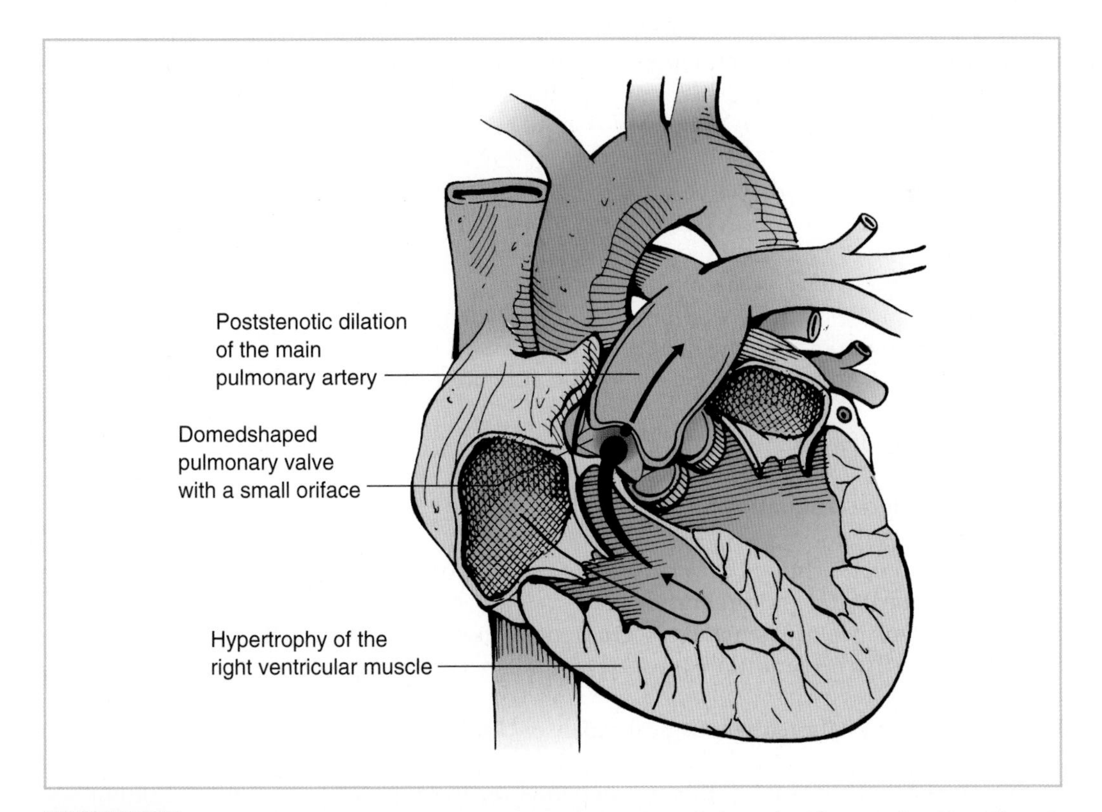

Figure 18.16. Pulmonary stenosis. The pulmonary valve is domed-shaped with a small orifice. There is hypertrophy of the right ventricle and poststenotic dilation of the main pulmonary artery. *Arrows* represent the direction of blood flow on the right side of the heart.

PHYSIOLOGY

The physiologic consequence of PS is elevation of RV pressure and subsequent RV hypertrophy that is proportional to the degree of obstruction. Although patients with mild PS tend to be asymptomatic, those with mild-to-moderate PS likely have mild dyspnea and fatigue during exertion. Recent evidence suggests that a mean gradient across the PV correlates better with a peak-to-peak gradient measured by catheter in these patients, although most severity grading systems use peak-instantaneous gradients. Asymptomatic patients with a gradient across the area of obstruction less than 50 mm Hg are expected to have normal life expectancy. Patients with severe PS have a transvalvular gradient exceeding 80 mm Hg accompanied by RV hypertrophy and can experience RV dilation and failure, although up to 25% may be asymptomatic. The average life expectancy of a patient with severe untreated PS is approximately 30 years. Typically, PS does not progress over time and decisions for intervention are based on symptoms and valve gradient. In 10% to 15% of patients, the PV is dysplastic and the patients are more likely to develop symptoms of fatigue, dyspnea, RV failure, and, in some patients, exertional chest pain and syncope.

MANAGEMENT

Most symptomatic adults are treated with transcatheter balloon valvuloplasty. Pulmonary insufficiency may be present after balloon valvuloplasty but overall, the long-term results are excellent. Adults with a dysplastic PV often require valve replacement. Obstructive subpulmonic hypertrophy can regress after either intervention.

TRANSESOPHAGEAL ECHOCARDIOGRAPHIC EVALUATION

Important aspects of the examination include evaluation of the RVOT above, below, and at the level of the PV. Suggested cross sections for focused TEE examination: ME RV inflow–outflow, deep TG LAX, and ME Asc Ao SAX (Table 18.1).

Goals of two-dimensional evaluation are:

1. Determination of PV morphology and motion
2. Measurement of annular size
3. Evaluation of the main PA and proximal PA branches
4. Identification of poststenotic dilation of the PA
5. Assessment of the RV including systolic function, detection of RV hypertrophy or dilation
6. Identification of associated pathology

Goals of Doppler examination are:

1. Identification of turbulent flow across the PV and/or pulmonary regurgitation
2. Identification of tricuspid regurgitation
3. Estimation of peak-instantaneous gradient across the PV using the ME RV inflow–outflow and TG LAX-outflow tract views and spectral Doppler

Goals of the examination after surgical repair or during/after catheter intervention are:

1. Examination of residual pathology depends on the type of intervention. Pulmonary regurgitation may be present after valvuloplasty or surgical valvotomy. Quantification of a residual gradient should be part of the examination after surgical repair or catheter intervention.

2. Evaluation of prosthetic valve function and the presence of paravalvular leaks following replacement with a prosthetic valve are required.

Tetralogy of Fallot

ANATOMY

The initial description of TOF consisted of a VSD, RVOT obstruction, aortic override, and RV hypertrophy (Figure 18.17). In approximately one third of the cases, an ASD is present. This is one of the most common complex malformations seen in adults. Associated lesions include a right aortic arch, additional VSDs, absence of the pulmonic valve, coronary artery anomalies, systemic venous anomalies, aortopulmonary window, and LV outflow tract obstruction.

PHYSIOLOGY

The clinical findings in patients with TOF are related mainly to the RVOT obstruction and the large, nonrestrictive perimembranous VSD. The degree of ventricular right-to-left

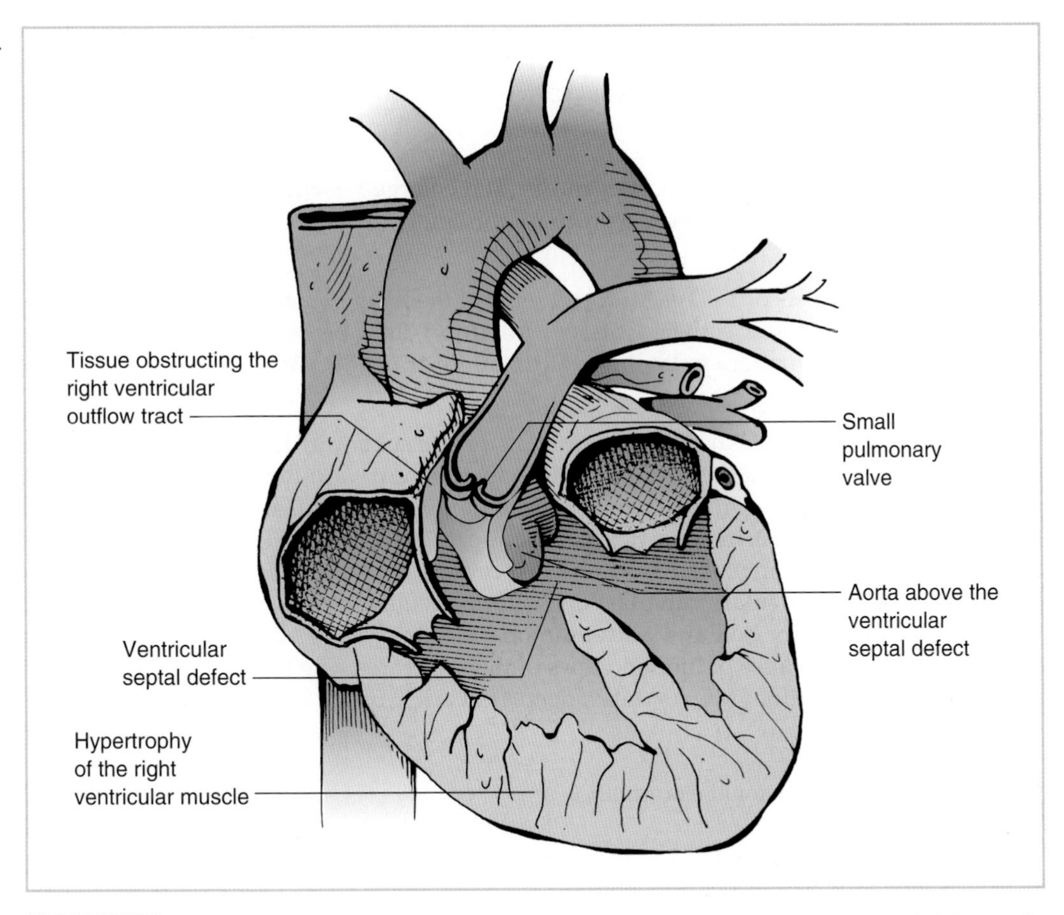

Figure 18.17. Tetralogy of Fallot. Characteristics of this lesion include a ventricular septal defect, right ventricular outflow tract obstruction, right-ventricular hypertrophy, and aortic override, i.e., the aortic position is above the ventricular septal defect. Note the tissue below the pulmonary valve in this figure, it contributes to the right ventricular outflow tract obstruction. The pulmonary valve can be small and dysplastic.

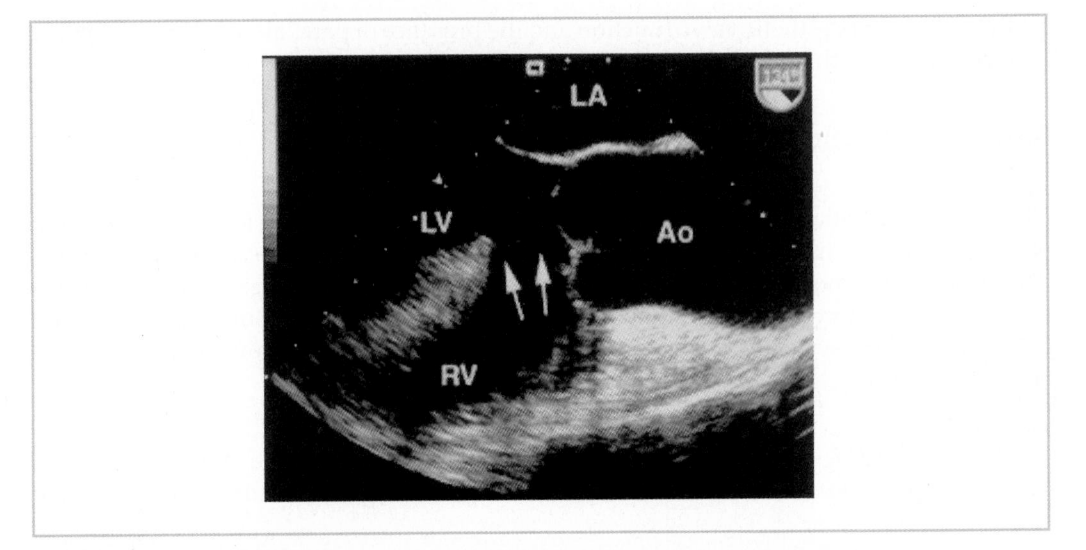

Figure 18.18. Tetralogy of Fallot. Two-dimensional transesophageal echocardiographic midesophageal aortic valve long-axis view demonstrates two features of tetralogy of Fallot: a large ventricular septal defect (*arrows*) and an overriding aorta. LA, left atrium; LV, left ventricle; RV, right ventricle; Ao, proximal ascending aorta.

shunting accounts for the degree of cyanosis. The enlarged aortic root in dextroposition and RV hypertrophy are secondary features of this anomaly.

MANAGEMENT

Surgery in TOF consists of VSD closure and relief of the RVOT obstruction. Reintervention (either surgical or in the catheterization laboratory) may be required for residual or recurrent RVOT obstruction, pulmonic regurgitation, or residual VSD.

TRANSESOPHAGEAL ECHOCARDIOGRAPHIC EVALUATION

The perimembranous VSD in TOF is frequently a large subaortic defect between the right and noncoronary cusps demonstrated in the ME AV short- and long-axis cross-sectional views (Figure 18.18). Additional communications at the atrial and ventricular levels should be considered. Aortic override is best appreciated in the ME AV long-axis view (Figure 18.18). Evaluation of the RVOT and PAs requires a combination of scanning planes that define the subvalvular, valvular, and supravalvular regions. The TEE evaluation of the distal pulmonary bed and aortopulmonary collaterals, if suspected or present, is suboptimal at best because of limited views of the structures. Suggested cross sections for focused TEE examination: ME AV LAX, deep TG LAX, ME RV inflow–outflow, and ME 4-CH (Table 18.1).

Goals of the two-dimensional examination are:

1. Confirmation of diagnosis
2. Characterization of RVOT obstruction
3. Definition of the size and location of the VSD
4. Exclusion of associated pathology
5. Determination of presence of an ASD
6. Definition of coronary artery anatomy
7. Assessment of biventricular function

Goals of Doppler examination are:

1. Assessment of flow across the VSD, including direction and velocity
2. Definition of the severity of the RVOT obstruction using spectral Doppler interrogation
3. Evaluation of the AV for incompetence
4. Detection of tricuspid regurgitation
5. Description of the flow across an ASD

Goals of the examination after surgical repair or during/after catheter intervention are:

1. Evaluation for residual RVOT obstruction and intracardiac shunts
2. Assessment for possible tricuspid, pulmonary, and aortic regurgitation
3. Estimation of ventricular size, wall thickness, and function
4. Evaluation for conduit obstruction and/or regurgitation in patients who require placement of a RV to PA conduit

Dextro-transposition of the Great Arteries

ANATOMY

Dextro-transposition of the great vessels (d-TGA) is characterized by concordance of the atrioventricular connection and discordance of the ventriculoarterial connection. A morphologic right atrium is connected to a morphologic RV, but the RV arterial connection is to the aorta. A morphologic left atrium drains into a morphologic LV that gives rise to the PA (Figure 18.19). Transposition accounts for 4% of all cases of CHD. Associated pathology may include ASD, VSD, PDA, obstruction to pulmonary blood flow, AV abnormalities, variation in the origin and course of the coronary arteries, and aortic arch anomalies.

PHYSIOLOGY

In d-TGA the systemic and pulmonary circulations function in parallel rather than in series, therefore d-TGA is classified as a cyanotic lesion. A communication at the level of the atria, ventricles, or great arteries is essential for survival.

MANAGEMENT

The surgical management of this lesion has changed dramatically through the years. Currently, the favored approach for infants with d-TGA is anatomic correction or arterial switch surgery (Jatene procedure) (Figure 18.20). In this surgery, the great arteries are transected and anastomosed to their appropriate ventricular outflows, and the coronary arteries are translocated to the systemic outflow.

Older adults with d-TGA most likely have undergone palliation or an atrial baffle procedure (Mustard or Senning operation) (Figure 18.21) in which the systemic venous blood is rerouted through the mitral valve, left ventricle, and PA and the pulmonary venous return is diverted into the tricuspid valve, right ventricle, and aorta. This allows for the separation of pulmonary and systemic circulations but maintains the RV as the systemic pump.

TRANSESOPHAGEAL ECHOCARDIOGRAPHIC EVALUATION

The echocardiographic evaluation should include two-dimensional imaging, spectral Doppler examination, color-flow mapping, and possibly contrast echocardiography. Suggested cross sections for focused TEE examination: ME 4-CH, ME bicaval, TG mid SAX, and deep TG LAX (Table 18.1).

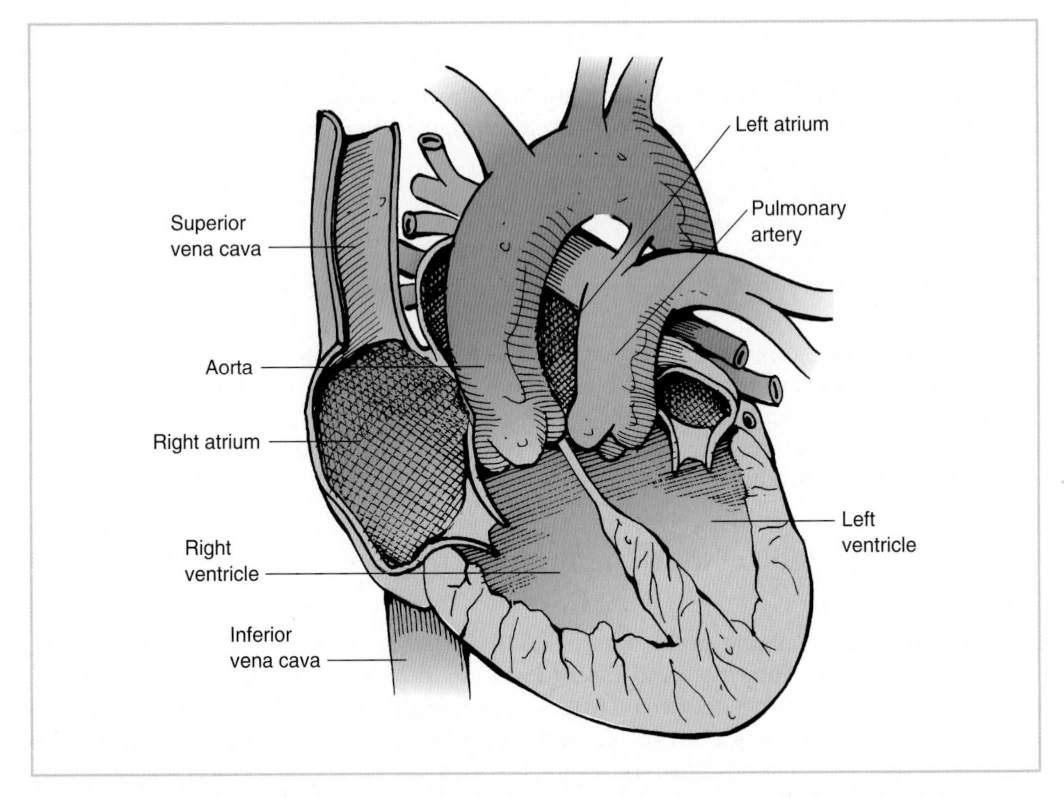

Figure 18.19. Transposition of the great arteries. The right atrium is connected to the right ventricle that gives rise to the aorta. The left atrium is connected to the left ventricle that gives rise to the pulmonary artery. This relationship is defined as atrioventricular concordance and ventriculoarterial discordance. A communication at the level of the atria, ventricles, or great arteries is essential for survival.

Goals of the two-dimensional examination are:

1. Confirmation of diagnosis
2. Assessment of atrioventricular and ventriculoarterial connections
3. Evaluation of associated pathology such as intracardiac communications and outflow tract obstruction
4. Estimation of ventricular sizes and systolic function

Goals of Doppler examination are:

1. Assessment of flow across intracardiac communications
2. Assessment of the peak-instantaneous gradient across an outflow tract obstruction
3. Evaluation of tricuspid or mitral regurgitation

Goals of the examination after surgical repair or during/after catheter intervention are:

1. Visualization of the systemic and pulmonary venous pathways within the atrial baffle and evaluation of obstruction (in atrial baffle procedures)
2. Assessment of baffle leaks in atrial baffle procedures; the administration of agitated saline solution through a peripheral or central vein may assist in the identification of baffle leaks and systemic or pulmonary venous obstruction

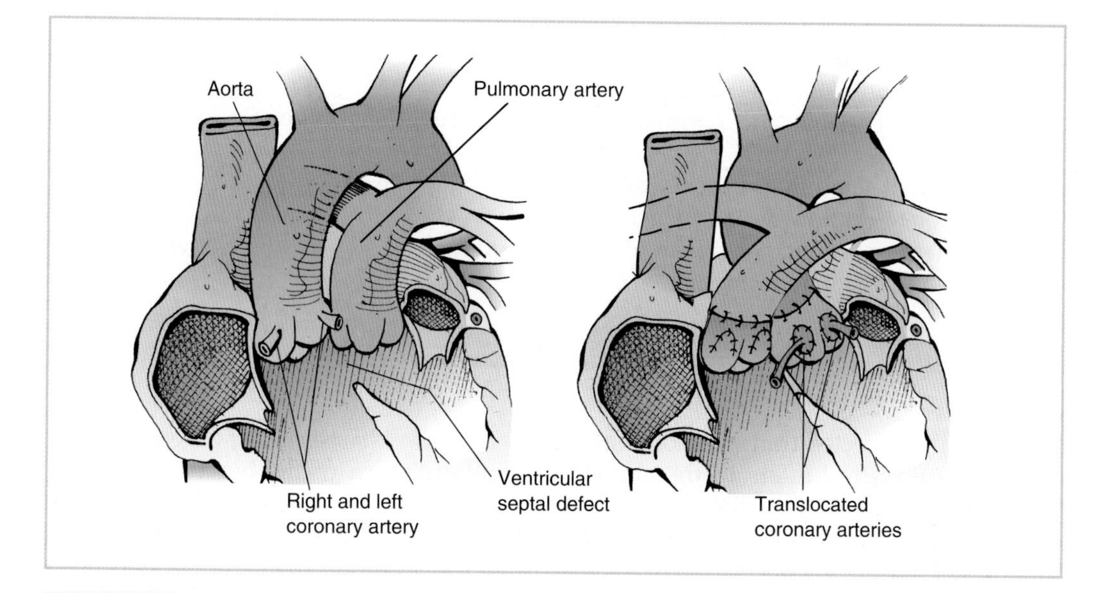

Figure 18.20. Arterial switch procedure. The aorta and pulmonary arteries are transected and anastomosed to their appropriate ventricular outflows. The coronary arteries are excised with surrounding tissue and translocated to the systemic outflow. In this figure, a ventricular septal defect is present. Note that following the arterial switch procedure the pulmonary artery is anterior to the aorta.

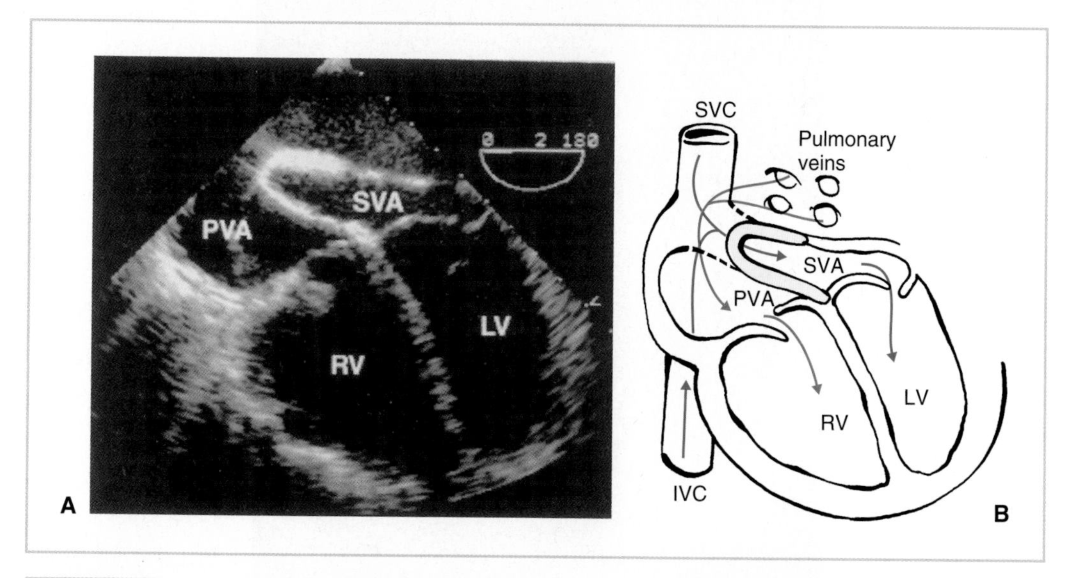

Figure 18.21. Dextro-transposition of the great arteries following an atrial redirection procedure. On the left is a two-dimensional transesophageal echocardiographic midesophageal four-chamber view that demonstrates the features of an atrial redirection procedure. In this procedure, venous return from the systemic and pulmonary circulations is rerouted through a baffle. Following placement of a baffle, desaturated blood from the superior and inferior vena cavae drains into the systemic atrium (*SVA*) then through the mitral valve into the left ventricle (*LV*) then into the pulmonary artery. Blood from the pulmonary veins drains into the pulmonary atrium (*PVA*) then through the tricuspid valve into the right ventricle (*RV*) then into the aorta. The RV remains the systemic ventricle. The illustration on the right is included to clarify the route of blood flow following an atrial redirection procedure. SVC, superior vena cava; IVC, inferior vena cava.

3. Evaluation of the RV (systemic ventricle) for dysfunction (in atrial baffle procedures)
4. Interrogation of the tricuspid valve, which remains the systemic atrioventricular valve, for regurgitation (in atrial baffle procedures)
5. Evaluation of global and segmental ventricular function (following arterial switch operation)
6. Evaluation of semilunar valve regurgitation
7. Evaluation of outflow tract obstruction
8. Assessment of ventricular function following an arterial switch surgery when the LV becomes the systemic ventricle

Congenitally Corrected Transposition (Levo-transposition)

ANATOMY

Congenitally corrected transposition is also known as *levo-transposition of the great arteries* (l-TGA), a term that refers to the abnormal looping pattern of the heart tube during development that results in discordance between the atrioventricular and ventriculoarterial connections. The morphologic LV lies to the right and the morphologic RV to the left in a side-by-side arrangement (Figure 18.22). Corrected transposition frequently is associated

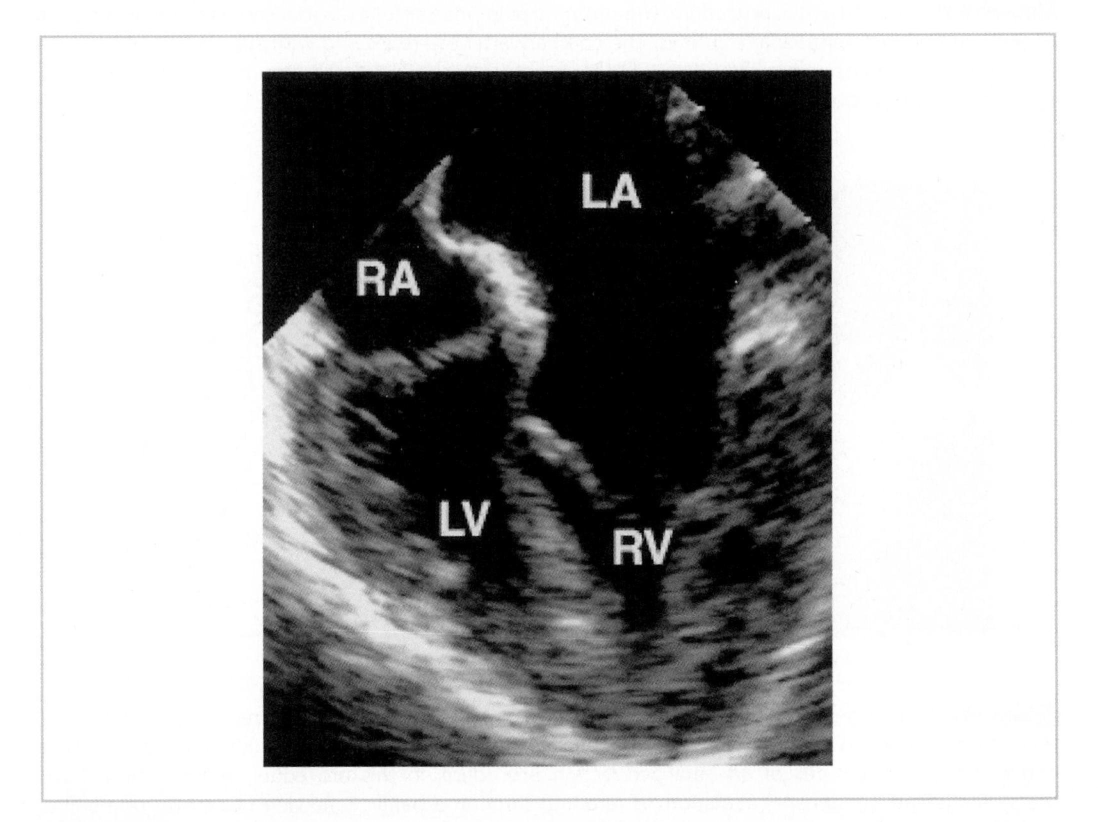

Figure 18.22. Congenitally corrected transposition. Two-dimensional transesophageal echocardiographic midesophageal four-chamber view displays the abnormal (discordant) atrioventricular connection of this lesion. The right atrium empties into the morphologic left ventricle through a mitral valve, and the left atrium empties into the morphologic right ventricle through a tricuspid valve. Note the apical displacement of the tricuspid valve, common in this lesion. RA, right atrium; LA, left atrium; LV, left ventricle; RV, right ventricle.

with other cardiac anomalies, such as VSD, obstruction to pulmonary blood flow, and left atrioventricular (tricuspid) valve anomalies.

PHYSIOLOGY

In this lesion, the systemic veins drain into the anatomic right atrium, which is connected to the morphologic LV then PA. The pulmonary veins drain into the anatomic left atrium and the morphologic RV, which is connected to the aorta. Therefore, the systemic and pulmonary circulations are in series and the physiology is normal—hence the term *corrected*. Note, however, the systemic ventricle in this physiologically corrected lesion is the right ventricle.

MANAGEMENT

Most cases require surgical intervention to address associated defects. These include closure of intracardiac communications, relief of pulmonary outflow tract obstruction, and tricuspid valve repair/replacement. In some cases, more complex interventions such as double switch surgery (atrial redirection and arterial switch) or a modification thereof may be indicated. A high incidence of atrioventricular block is seen in this lesion and therefore the need for pacemaker placement.

TRANSESOPHAGEAL ECHOCARDIOGRAPHIC EVALUATION

Definition of the atrioventricular connections by echocardiography requires identification of the characteristic features that establish ventricular morphology. The atrioventricular valves are associated with their corresponding ventricles, so that the morphologic tricuspid valve will identify the RV and the morphologic mitral valve will identify the LV. In the ME 4-CH view, the morphologic RV is characterized by inferior insertion of the septal leaflet of the tricuspid valve to the ventricular septum and by the moderator band (Figure 18.22). The LV is identified by two distinct papillary muscles in the TG mid short-axis view. Typically, the aorta is anterior and to the left relative to the PA. Suggested cross sections for focused TEE examination: ME 4-CH, 2-CH, TG mid SAX, and ME LAX (Table 18.1).

Goals of the two-dimensional examination are:

1. Confirmation of diagnosis
2. Assessment of atrioventricular and ventriculoarterial connections
3. Evaluation of associated defects such as intracardiac communications, pulmonary outflow tract obstruction, tricuspid valve morphology and competence
4. Estimation of ventricular sizes and systolic function

Goals of Doppler examination are:

1. Characterization of flow across intracardiac communications
2. Assessment of the peak-instantaneous gradient of the pulmonary outflow tract obstruction
3. Evaluation of tricuspid or mitral regurgitation

Goals of the examination after surgical repair or during/after catheter intervention are:

1. Evaluation of residual shunts, outflow obstruction, systemic atrioventricular-valve regurgitation
2. Assessment of progressively decreased function of a morphologic RV in the systemic circulation

Single-Ventricle Lesions or Univentricular Heart

ANATOMY

The spectrum of single ventricle, or univentricular, heart encompasses a wide variety of anatomic arrangements. Most patients have hypoplasia of the right or left ventricle. In some patients with a biventricular heart, a two-ventricle repair may not be feasible, so that a single ventricle management strategy is required. This group of patients may be considered functionally to be in the univentricular category.

PHYSIOLOGY

The major anatomic variants of single ventricle include double-inlet LV, tricuspid atresia, and hypoplastic left heart syndrome. A common feature of these lesions is complete mixing of the systemic and pulmonary venous blood at the atrial or ventricular level. Another frequent finding is systemic or pulmonary outflow obstruction.

MANAGEMENT

Surgical procedures attempt initially to protect the integrity of the pulmonary vascular bed and myocardium. Specific goals are to prevent pulmonary overcirculation, which may lead to elevation of the PA pressure, ventricular overload, and ventricular dysfunction.

Norwood procedure: In infants with LV hypoplasia (hypoplastic left heart syndrome), the initial surgical intervention is a Norwood procedure. This consists of reconstruction of the hypoplastic aorta, creation of an aortopulmonary shunt to provide a source of pulmonary blood flow, and atrial septectomy to ensure the unrestricted return of pulmonary venous blood into the systemic RV. More recently, placement of a conduit from the single ventricle to the PA (Sano procedure) has replaced the aortopulmonary shunt portion of the Norwood procedure in some patients (Figure 18.23).

Modified Blalock-Taussig shunt: In patients whose anatomy is associated with restricted pulmonary blood flow, a systemic-to-pulmonary connection is created (Gore-Tex tube graft) in the form of a modified Blalock-Taussig shunt.

PA band: In patients with excessive pulmonary blood flow, a PA band is placed to limit overcirculation and prevent pulmonary hypertension. The peak systolic pressure gradient across the PA band can be predicted by spectral Doppler with use of the simplified Bernoulli equation (pressure gradient = $4v^2$; Figure 18.24). Ideally, the gradient across the PA band limits the PA systolic pressure to approximately one-third the systemic arterial blood pressure.

Glenn anastomosis and Fontan procedure: The eventual goal of surgical management in the patient with single ventricle physiology is to separate the pulmonary and systemic circulations. At present, the favored approach is sequential diversion of the systemic venous blood directly into the pulmonary vascular bed through the Glenn anastomosis and subsequent Fontan procedure. In the bidirectional Glenn procedure (cavopulmonary anastomosis) the SVC is connected to the PA. The eventual separation of the pulmonary and systemic circulations in patients with single-ventricle physiology requires a Fontan procedure to direct blood from the IVC into the PAs.

TRANSESOPHAGEAL ECHOCARDIOGRAPHIC EVALUATION

Diagnostic assessment of the functional single ventricle requires a combination of multiple imaging planes. The ME 4-CH view is particularly helpful in demonstrating the

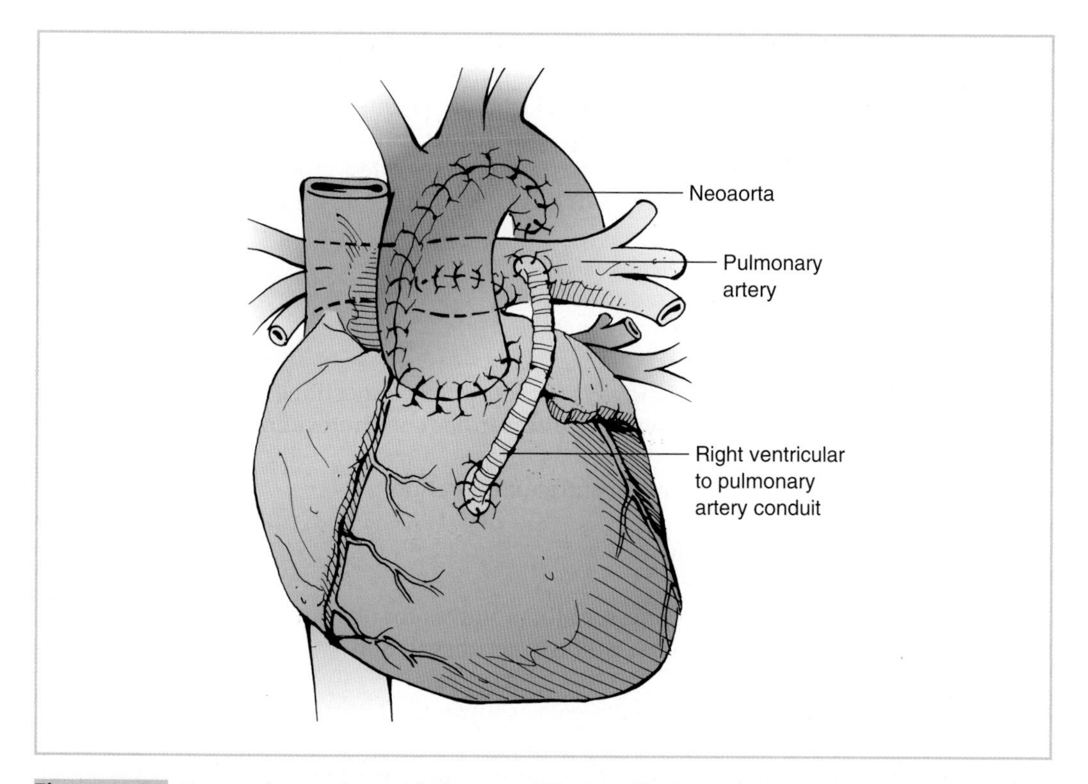

Figure 18.23. Norwood procedure with Sano modification. The hypoplastic aorta is reconstructed and termed *neoaorta*. A conduit is placed from the right ventricle to pulmonary artery to provide pulmonary blood flow.

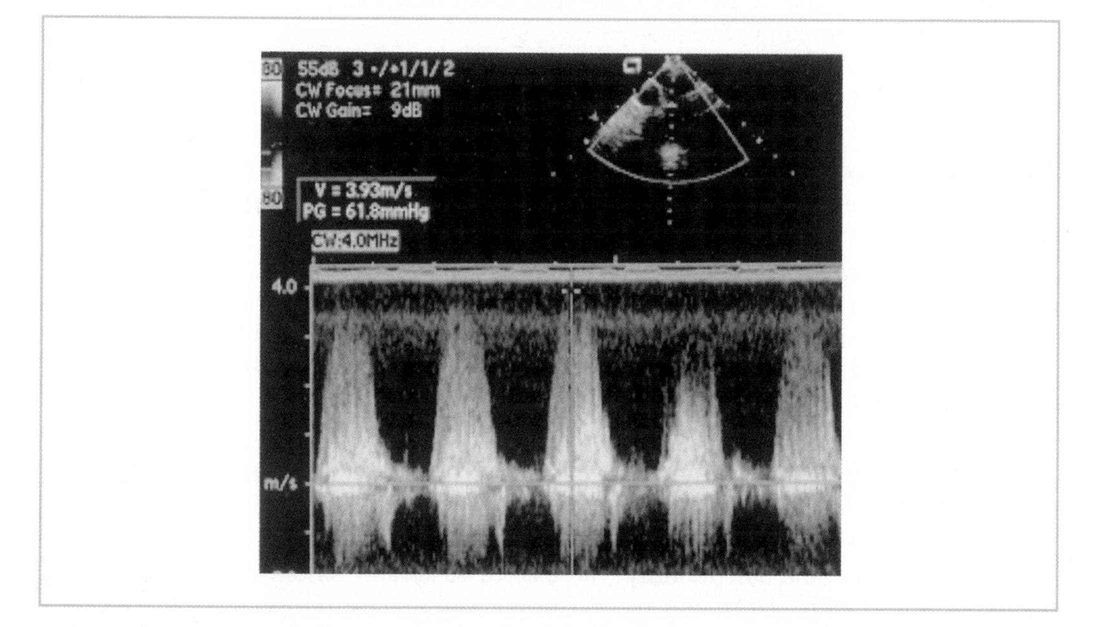

Figure 18.24. Pulmonary artery band. Spectral Doppler interrogation across a pulmonary artery band. The peak velocity obtained by continuous wave Doppler can be used to estimate the right ventricular outflow tract systolic gradient with the modified Bernoulli equation.

crux of the heart and characterizing the atrioventricular connections. Additional views contribute to the segmental analysis by defining the ventriculoarterial connections, ventricular morphology, and location of hypoplastic or rudimentary chambers. Color-flow and spectral-Doppler interrogation is essential to determine AV and semilunar valve competence and inflow/outflow tract obstruction. Suggested cross sections for focused TEE examination: ME 4-CH, 2-CH, ME LAX, ME bicaval, and RV inflow–outflow (Table 18.1).

Goals of the two-dimensional examination are:

1. Confirmation of diagnosis
2. Assessment of atrioventricular and ventriculoarterial connections
3. Evaluation of associated defects such as intracardiac communications and outflow tract obstruction
4. Estimation of size of ventricles and ventricular function

Goals of the Doppler examination are:

1. Assessment of atrioventricular and semilunar valves for obstruction/regurgitation
2. Estimation of gradient across any outflow tract obstruction

Goals of the examination after surgical repair or during/after catheter intervention are:

1. Evaluation of the adequacy of the intervention; imaging of a Blalock-Taussig shunt or Glenn connection is not always possible by TEE because of limited imaging planes
2. Evaluation of valvular competence and ventricular function
3. Exclusion of obstruction of venous pathways
4. Determination of flow through the newly formed right-ventricular to pulmonary-artery conduit and detection of obstruction to flow

TRANSESOPHAGEAL ECHOCARDIOGRAPHY IN THE CARDIAC CATHETERIZATION LABORATORY FOR ADULTS WITH CARDIAC HEART DISEASE

The use of TEE in the cardiac catheterization laboratory to acquire detailed anatomic and hemodynamic data before and during interventions is increasing. TEE provides a real-time evaluation of catheter placement across valves and vessels and immediate assessment of interventional procedures. It is also valuable in monitoring for catheter-induced complications, such as cardiac tamponade.

TRANSESOPHAGEAL ECHOCARDIOGRAPHY FOR NONCARDIAC SURGERY IN ADULTS WITH CARDIAC HEART DISEASE

TEE can be used in this setting to evaluate ventricular volume and function, detect intracardiac shunts and air, identify valvular disease, and assess RV or PA systolic pressures. Adults with CHD may have concurrent acquired heart disease, increasing their risks for additional hemodynamic disturbances. Intraoperative TEE should be considered for patients with poor exercise tolerance and for those considered to be at high perioperative risk during noncardiac procedures.

LIMITATIONS OF TRANSESOPHAGEAL ECHOCARDIOGRAPHY IN CARDIAC HEART DISEASE

Despite the significant contributions of TEE some limitations are recognized. Imaging of certain structures (RV to pulmonary conduits, etc.) may be difficult due to their anterior location with respect to the imaging probe. Other regions of interest may not be amenable to imaging through the transesophageal window. With respect to the perioperative setting, it is recognized that a variety of perioperative factors (level of inotropic support, high level of catecholamines immediately after bypass, loading conditions, functional state of the myocardium) may influence the echocardiographic findings and lead to an underestimate or overestimate of the hemodynamic severity of the condition in question. Therefore, decisions regarding return to bypass to address residual lesions must be made within the context of the hemodynamic state, with the understanding that for an optimal hemodynamic assessment, conditions that reflect the patient's baseline state are required.

SUMMARY

TEE is known to provide anatomic and hemodynamic information beyond that acquired with conventional transthoracic imaging in the adult patient with suboptimal acoustic windows. In the operating room, TEE allows for confirmation of preoperative diagnoses and modification of the surgical approach as appropriate. TEE assists in the formulation of anesthetic plans by guiding the management of fluids, inotropes, and vasodilators, and allows for continuous monitoring of myocardial function and the detection of intracavitary/intravascular air and myocardial ischemia. Suboptimal surgical interventions and significant postoperative residue can be identified immediately by this imaging modality. TEE is also of benefit in evaluating factors that may contribute to difficulties in weaning from cardiopulmonary bypass. In several series, the reinstitution of cardiopulmonary bypass and reoperation were prompted by TEE in as many as 5% to 7% of cases. In surgical situations such as these, TEE can provide substantial cost-saving benefits as well. The benefits of TEE have also been documented in the cardiac catheterization laboratory during monitoring of interventions in addition to reducing exposure to ionizing radiation and allowing for the immediate identification of complications.

SUGGESTED READINGS

Brickner ME, Hillis LD, Lange RA. Congenital heart disease in adults, part I. *N Engl J Med* 2000;342:256–263.

Brickner ME, Hillis LD, Lange RA. Congenital heart disease in adults, part II. *N Engl J Med* 2000;342:334–342.

Child JS, Perloff JK. *Congenital heart disease in adults*. Philadelphia: Harcourt Health Sciences, 1998.

Gatzoulis MA, Webb GD, Daubeney PEF. *Diagnosis and management of adult congenital heart disease*. London: Churchill Livingstone, 2003.

International Society for Adult Congenital Heart Disease. www.isaccd.org. Accessed 2006.

Miller-Hance WC, Silverman NH. Transesophageal echocardiography in congenital heart disease with focus on the adult. *Cardiol Clin* 2000;18:861–892.

Russell IA, Rouine-Rapp K, Stratman G, et al. Congenital heart disease in the adult: a review with internet-accesible transesophageal echocardiographic images. *Anesth Analg* 2006;102(3):694–723.

Shanewise JS, Cheung AT, Aronson S, et al. ASE/SCA guidelines for performing a comprehensive intraoperative multiplane echocardiography examination: recommendations of the American Society of Echocardiography Council for Intraoperative Echocardiography and the Society of Cardiovascular Anesthesiologists Task Force for Certification in Perioperative Transesophageal Echocardiography. *Anesth Analg* 1999;89:870–884.

Silverman NH. *Pediatric echocardiography*. Baltimore: Williams & Wilkins, 1992.

Silvilairat S, Cabalka AK, Cetta F, et al. Echocardiographic assessment of isolated pulmonary valve stenosis: which outpatient Doppler gradient has the most clinical validity? *J Am Soc Echocardiogr* 2005;18(11):1137–1142.

Stumper O, Sutherland R. *Transesophageal echocardiography in congenital heart disease*. London: Hodder Headline Group, 1994.

Therrien J, Dore A, Gersony W, et al. CCS Consensus Conference 2001 update: recommendations for the management of adults with congenital heart disease, part I. *Can J Cardiol* 2001;17:943–959.

Therrien J, Dore A, Gersony W, et al. CCS Consensus Conference 2001 update: recommendations for the management of adults with congenital heart disease, part II. *Can J Cardiol* 2001;17:1029–1050.

Therrien J, Dore A, Gersony W, et al. CCS Consensus Conference 2001 update: recommendations for the management of adults with congenital heart disease, part III. *Can J Cardiol* 2001;17:1135–1158.

Warnes CA, Liberthson R, Danielson GK, et al. Task force 1: the changing profile of congenital heart disease in adult Life. *J Am Coll Cardiol* 2001;37:1170–1175.

Webb GD, Harrison DA, Connelly MS. Challenges posed by the adult with congenital heart disease. *Adv Intern Med* 1996;41:437–495.

Webb GD, Williams RG. Care of the adult with congenital heart disease: introduction. *J Am Coll Cardiol* 2001;37:1166.

Yale University School of Medicine. http://info.med.yale.edu/intmed/cardio/chd/contents/index.html. Accessed 2006.

QUESTIONS

1. A common transesophageal echocardiography (TEE) finding in an adult with a substantial shunt from a large secundum atrial septal defect (ASD) is
   a. Bicuspid aortic valve
   b. Mitral valve stenosis
   c. Abnormal pulmonary venous connections
   d. Dilation of the right ventricle (RV)

2. Eisenmenger syndrome
   a. Is common in adults with tetralogy of Fallot
   b. Is associated with coarctation of the aorta
   c. Does not alter patient survival
   d. Can occur in adults with a large patent ductus arteriosus

3. A previously undiagnosed perimembranous ventricular septal defect (VSD) in an adult is likely to be associated with
   a. Tricuspid valve stenosis
   b. Mitral valve regurgitation
   c. Aortic valve cusp herniation
   d. Doubly-committed outlet VSD

4. TEE evaluation of an adult with a large patent ductus arteriosus is likely to
   a. Define the size, length, and position of the patent ductus arteriosus
   b. Detect left ventricular (LV) hypertrophy
   c. Estimate pulmonary artery (PA) pressure within the normal range
   d. Document retrograde flow in the descending aorta during diastole

5. Adults with a bicuspid aortic valve
   a. Often have a primum ASD
   b. Are at risk for aneurysm formation in the ascending aorta
   c. Also have a patent ductus arteriosus in approximately 40% of cases
   d. Have a central line of valve closure detected by TEE

6. Preoperative TEE assessment in tetralogy of Fallot includes all the following except
   a. Evaluation of the size of the VSD
   b. Doppler interrogation of the right ventricular outflow tract (RVOT)
   c. Functional evaluation of the aortic valve
   d. Two-dimensional definition of the transverse aorta

7. Classic anatomic findings in dextro-transposition of the great arteries include
   a. Bicuspid aortic valve (AV)
   b. Discordance of the AV connections
   c. Aorta originating from the RV
   d. Single-chamber heart

8. Contributions of TEE in patients with a univentricular heart include all of the following except
   a. Evaluation of ventricular function
   b. Assessment of valvular regurgitation
   c. Detailed inspection of the distal pulmonary bed
   d. Exclusion of venous pathway pathology

9. Which of the following statements regarding the use of TEE in congenital heart disease (CHD) is true

a. It may modify the intraoperative surgical plan
b. It plays no role in the catheterization laboratory
c. It may document pathology after surgery, in which case a return to bypass is always required
d. It is too expensive for its use in selective noncardiac surgery to be justified

10. A 19-year-old patient is undergoing closure of a VSD. A TEE probe is placed for the procedure. In the post-bypass examination, a residual defect is noted with left-to-right shunting. The following hemodynamic and echocardiographic data are obtained:

Heart rate, 90 beats/min
Blood pressure (BP), 112/76 mm Hg
Body surface area (BSA), 1.8 m^2
Main PA (MPA) diameter, 2.1 cm
MPA time-velocity integral (TVI), 15.3 cm/s
Left ventricular outflow tract (LVOT) diameter, 1.9 cm
LVOT TVI, 14.8 cm/s
Peak Doppler velocity across the VSD, 4.6 m/s

Calculate the following: LV stroke volume, RV SV, cardiac output (CO), cardiac index (CI), Q_p/Q_s, and RV systolic pressure (RVSP).

Answers appear at the back of the book.

19 Cardiac Masses and Embolic Sources

Farid Jadbabaie

Transesophageal echocardiography (TEE) is an extremely useful imaging modality for assessment of cardiac masses and sources of emboli. Enhanced resolution of TEE and proximity of the transducer to posterior cardiac structures enables visualization of small masses or thrombi in the left atrium or the left atrial appendage (LAA) that would otherwise be missed on transthoracic echocardiography. It is essential to identify and distinguish normal cardiac structures and image artifacts that can be mistaken for a cardiac mass or thrombus (1,2). Normal structures such as pectinate muscle in the LAA or the tissue fold between LAA and left upper pulmonary vein (Coumadin ridge) can be mistaken for a thrombus or a small tumor. Similarly, a prominent Chiary network in the right atrium can be mistaken for a right atrial mass (Figure 19.1).

CARDIAC TUMORS

Primary cardiac tumors are very rare and comprise 25% of all cardiac neoplasms in pathologic studies (3). Metastatic tumors involve the heart or pericardium through local invasion or hematogeneous spread. Tumors that invade the heart locally can at times be seen on TEE.

Myxoma

Myxoma is the most common primary cardiac tumor in adults and accounts for 30% of all primary cardiac neoplasms. Cardiac myxomas commonly arise from the left atrium but can also originate from right atrium or the ventricles. These tumors are usually pedunculated and have a smooth surface. The most common attachment site is the fossa ovalis on the left side of atrial septum. Myxoma is a slow growing tumor and can remain asymptomatic for a long period of time. It can grow in size and occupy a significant portion of the left atrium, causing obstruction of the flow across the mitral valve (Figure 19.2). Cardiac myxomas are friable and can often result in systemic embolization.

Lipoma

Lipomas are the second most common cardiac tumors in adults and account for 10% of all benign cardiac neoplasms (3). These tumors usually originate from ventricular myocardium and less commonly from atrial myocardium. They are often sessile with increased echogenicity and a smooth surface. Lipomas are slow-growing tumors and can become large and cause blood flow obstruction (Figure 19.3). Cardiac lipomas should be distinguished from lipomatous hypertrophy of interatrial septum. A condition in which there is infiltration of mature fat cells without a distinct capsule and a characteristic appearance of dumbell-shaped thickening of atrial septum with sparing of fossa ovalis (4) (Figure 19.4). Lipomatous hypertrophy is more commonly seen in older adults, especially older women and usually has a benign clinical course.

Papillary Fibroelastoma

Papillary fibroelastoma is the third most common primary cardiac tumor in adults. Fibroelastomas are small mobile tumors that commonly originate from valvular leaflets

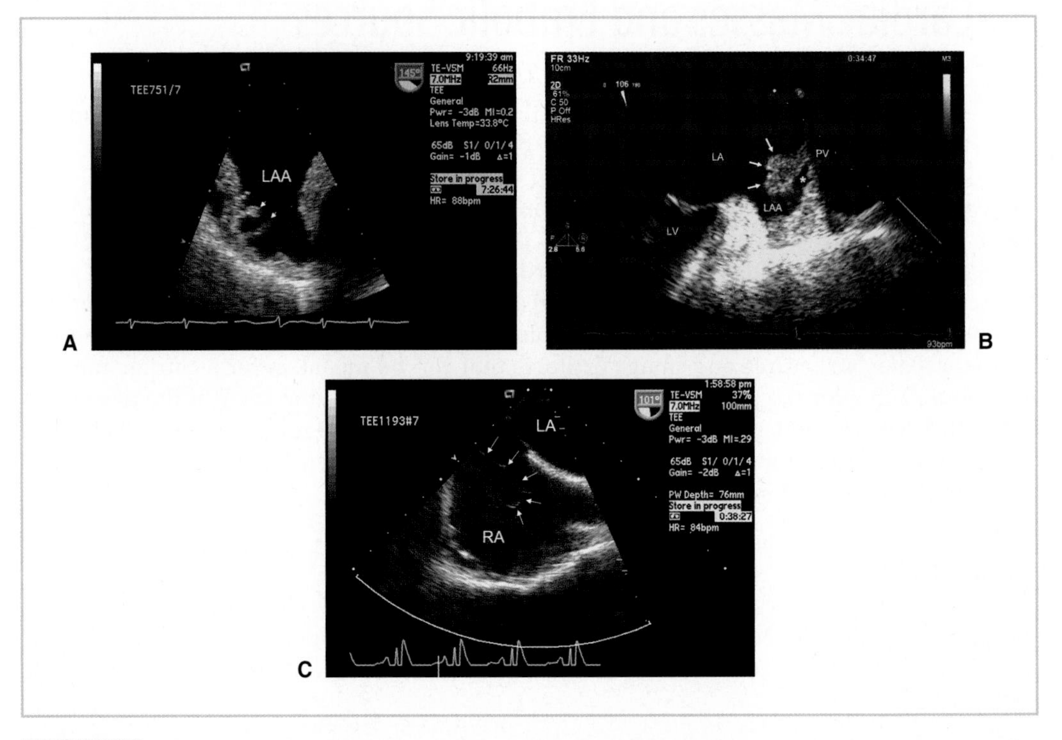

Figure 19.1. Normal cardiac structures can often be mistaken for cardiac masses or thrombus. Panel **A** shows prominent pectinate muscle in left atrial appendage mimicking a thrombus. An example of a prominent Coumadin ridge is shown in panel **B** and an example of a prominent Chiary network is shown in panel **C.** LAA, left atrial appendage; LA, left atrium; PV, pulmonary vein; LV, left ventricle; RA, right atrium.

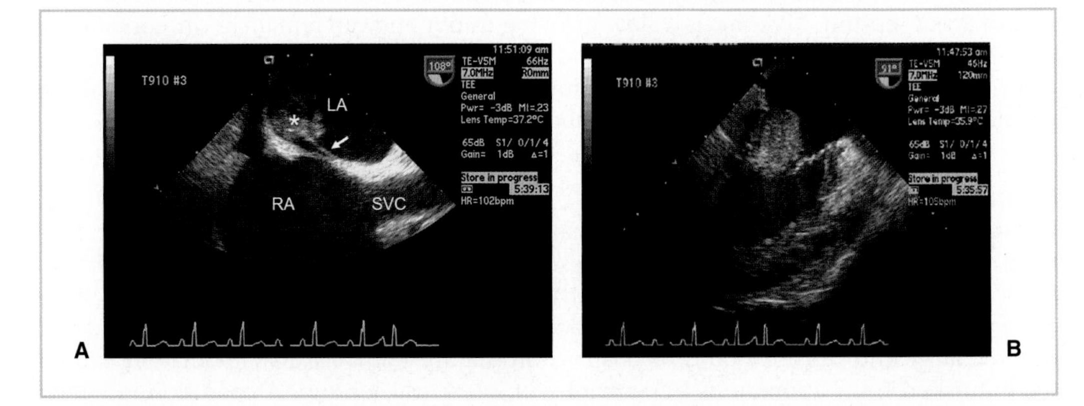

Figure 19.2. Example of a large myxoma in the left atrium with a stalk attached to atrial septum (panel **A**). Tumor prolapses into left ventricle during diastole (panel **B**). LA, left atrium; RA, right atrium; SVC, superior vena cava.

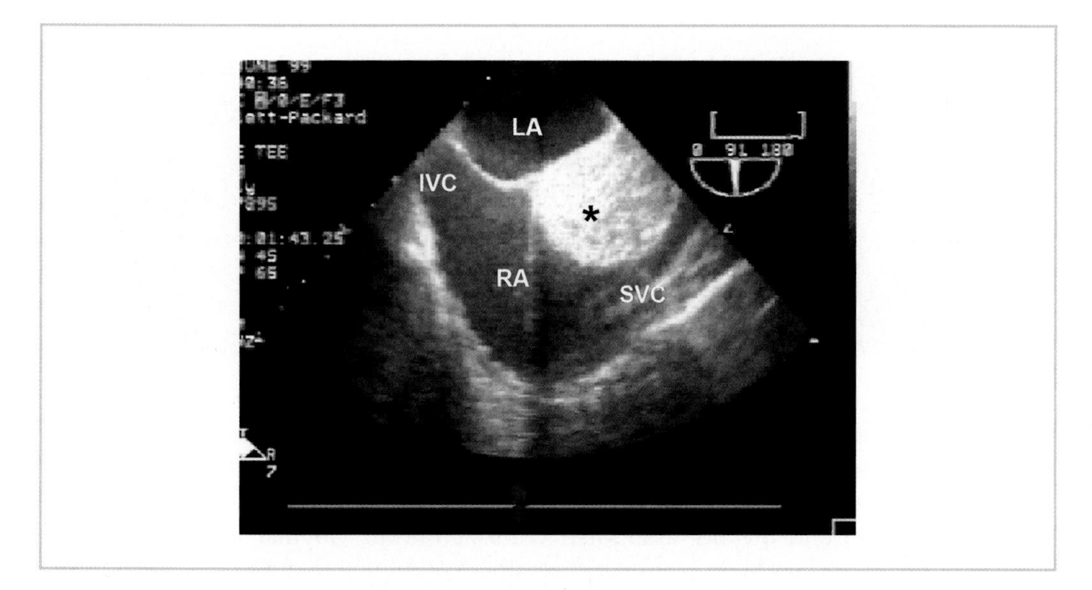

Figure 19.3. Example of a large lipoma (*) involving the interatrial septum. LA, left atrium; IVC, inferior vena cava; RA, right atrium; SVC, superior vena cava.

but can also arise from other endocardial surfaces. Aortic valve is the most common site of origin followed by the mitral valve. These tumors appear as a small (0.5–2 cm) pedunculated echo density, often with multiple mobile fibrillar projections, that is attached to the valve leaflets (5–7) (Figure 19.5) Fibroblastomas also have high potential for embolization, which is thought to be from embolization of tumor fragments or associated thrombi. Risk of embolization is higher as the tumor grows larger. Valvular fibroelastomas are often confused with vegetations given the size, location, and potential for embolization. In contrast to vegetations, fibroelastoma mostly arise from the aortic side of aortic

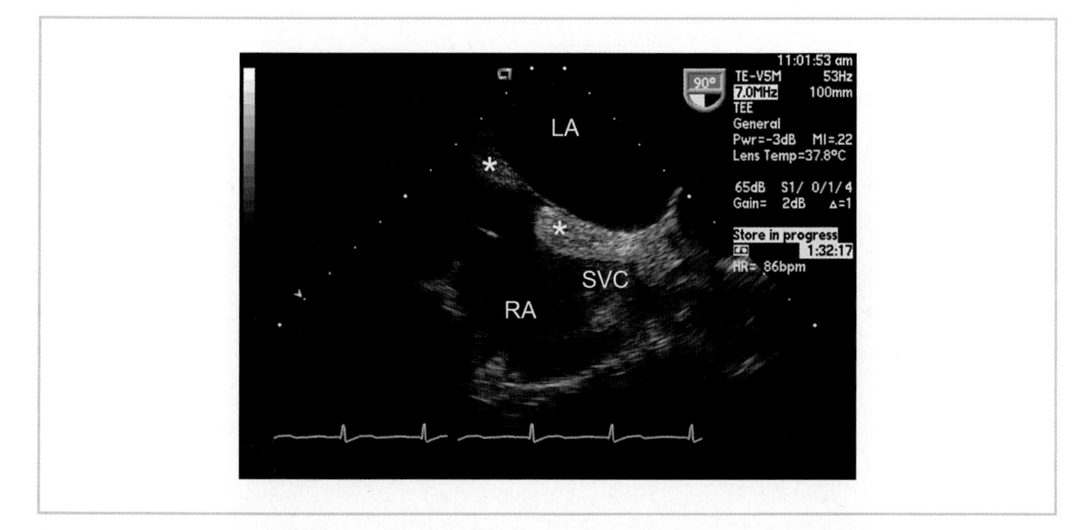

Figure 19.4. Example of lipomatous hypertrophy of interatrial septum (*) is depicted. Note the characteristic "dumbell-shape" appearance and sparing of fossa ovalis. Pacemaker wire is seen in the right atrium. LA, left atrium; SVC, superior vena cava; RA, right atrium.

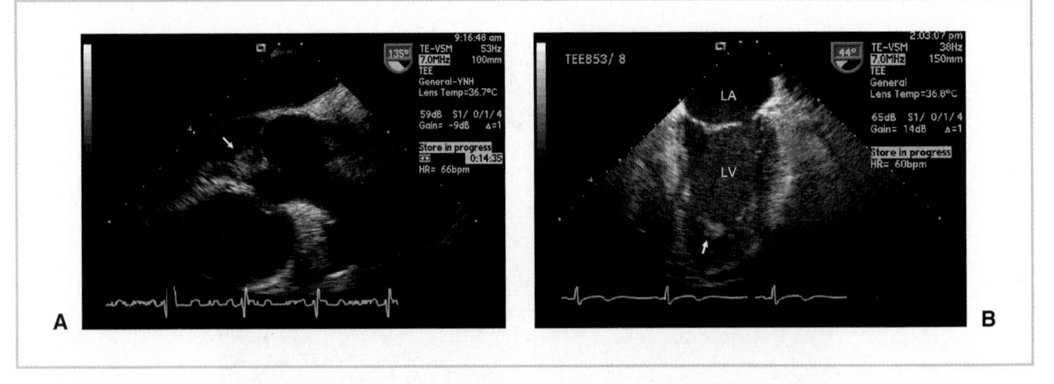

Figure 19.5. **A:** Example of a papillary fibroelastoma on aortic valve (*arrow*). **B:** Example of a papillary fibroelastoma arising from cordae tendinae in the left ventricle (*arrow*). LA, left atrium; LV, left ventricle.

valve leaflets (5,6) and are not associated with significant valvular abnormalities (7). Prominent valvular (Lambl) excrescences are other conditions that can also be confused with fibroelastomas (6). Valvular excrescences are commonly seen on commissural edges of the valve leaflets and are comprised of a small fibrous core covered by endothelial cells. These densities are commonly seen on TEE in all groups and are usually not associated with embolic events (8). An example of a prominent Lambl excrescence on aortic valve is shown in Figure 19.6.

Rhabdomyoma

Rhabdomyomas are the most common primary cardiac tumor in children (2,3) Rhabdomyomas are almost always associated with tuberous sclerosis. They usually originate from ventricles and are often multiple. These tumors can become large and cause valvular or outflow tract obstruction. Asymptomatic rhabdomyomas are usually observed as some of these tumors can spontaneously resolve.

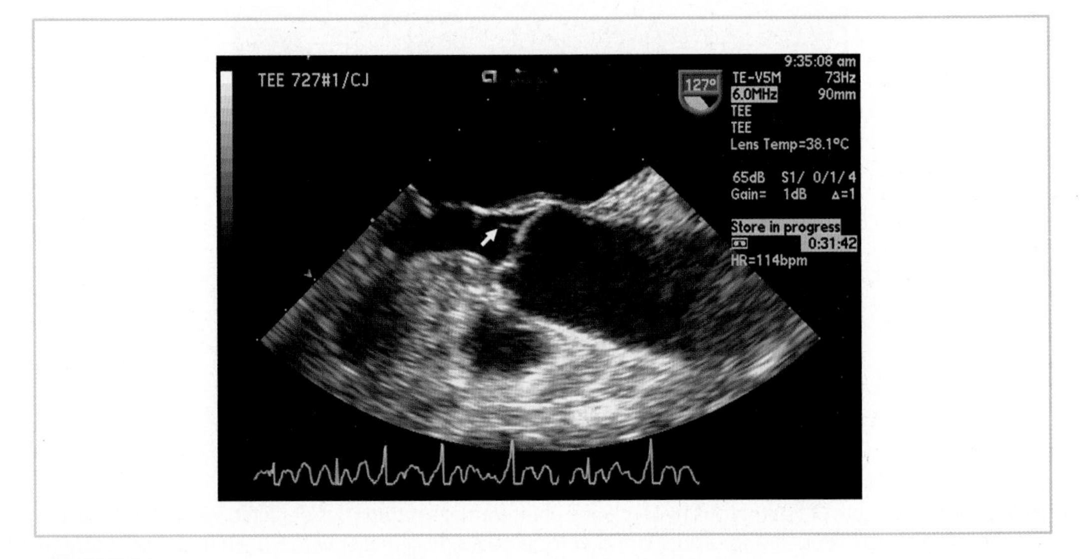

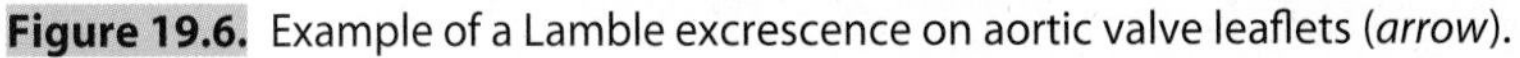
Figure 19.6. Example of a Lamble excrescence on aortic valve leaflets (*arrow*).

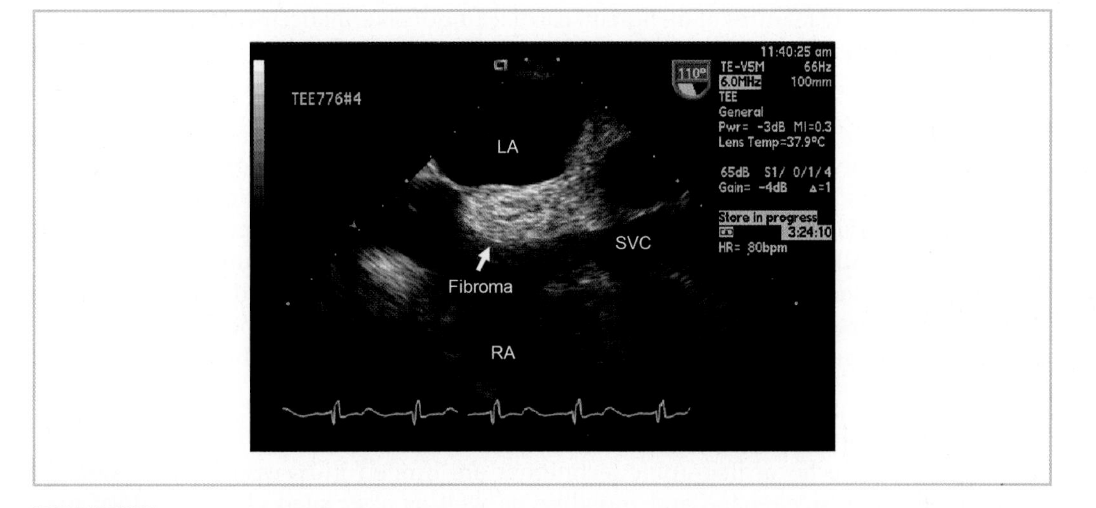

Figure 19.7. Example of a fibroma involving medial left atrial wall (*arrowheads*) and atrial septum (*arrow*). LA, left atrium; SVC, superior vena cava; RA, right atrium.

Fibroma

Fibromas are the second most common benign cardiac tumor in children. Fibromas usually originate from the ventricles or atrioventricular groves. A characteristic feature of fibroma is the presence of central calcification. They usually appear as a large single intramural mass with multiple central densities. Singularity and presence of central calcification are key factors in differentiating fibromas from rhabdomyomas (Figure 19.7).

MALIGNANT TUMORS

Cardiac Sarcomas

Sarcomas are rare causes of cardiac tumors and usually originate from the ventricular myocardium. These tumors can become large and invade into cavity and surrounding structures with protruding mobile components and attached thrombus (Figure 19.8). One

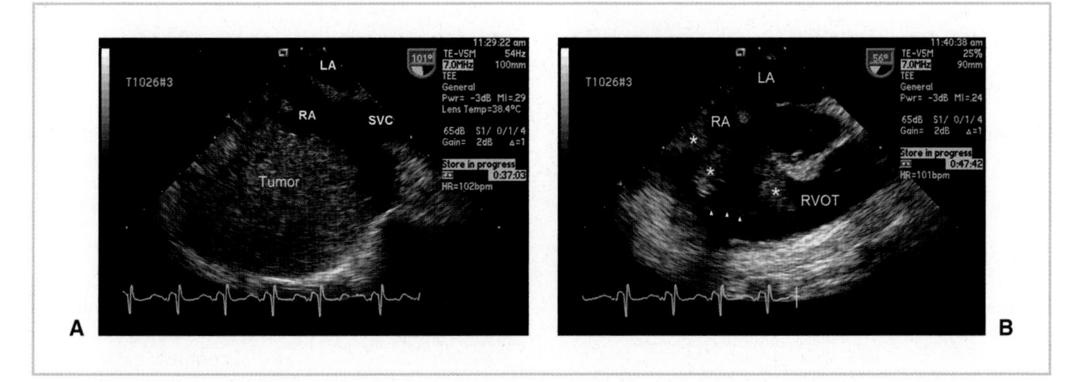

Figure 19.8. Midesophageal bicaval view of angiosarcoma of right atrium is depicted. In this image, a large mass is occupying entire right atrium (panel **A**) with prolapse across the tricuspid valve into right ventricle and ventricular outflow tract (panel **B**). LA, left atrium; RA, right atrium; SVC, superior vena cava; RVOT, right ventricular outflow tract.

of the distinguishing features of malignant cardiac tumors is enhancement with ultrasound contrast given extensive vascularity.

Embolization

Most cardiac tumors have the potential for embolization. Certain tumors, such as fibroelastoma and myxoma, are associated with higher rates of embolization. In one study, 30% of patients with incidental finding of fibroelastoma had symptoms consistent with systemic embolization on clinical follow-up (5). Emboli can be from tumor fragments or dissociation of attached thrombus. Rarely large tumor fragments from distant sites can be seen in transit through vena cava and the right heart. Renal cell carcinoma is commonly associated with embolization and transit of tumor fragments through the right heart.

Technical Consideration in Evaluation of Cardiac Masses

Although current echocardiographic techniques are limited in assessment of histology, anatomic location, size, shape and mobility, as well as associated clinical history may offer clues to origin and type of the mass. In addition, use of ultrasound contrast agents can provide further information on vascularity of the suspected mass. Malignant tumors with high vascularity are enhanced with ultrasound contrast whereas thrombi and benign stromal tumors with low vascularity appear as filling defects (9). Echocardiographic characteristics of different cardiac masses are summarized in Table 19.1.

Thrombus

Thrombi can be formed within any cardiac chambers and are mostly associated with underlying wall motion abnormality or low flow states leading to stasis of blood. The most common site for intracardiac thrombus is the LAA and left atrium in patients with atrial fibrillation or rheumatic mitral disease (Figure 19.9). Thrombus can be formed on intracardiac devices such as pacemaker wires or septal closure devices or be attached to indwelling catheters in the right heart (Figure 19.10). Thrombus in the ventricles is almost always associated with underlying wall motion abnormality. Fresh thrombi tend to be round and mobile whereas chronic thrombi appear flat and laminated and are less mobile. Size and mobility are important predictors of systemic embolization.

Table 19.1 Echocardiographic characteristics of common cardiac masses

Mass type	Appearance	Size and location	Other
Myxoma	Large, smooth surface, mobile and pedunculated	Left atrium, right atrium	Minimal enhancement with echo contrast
Papillary fibroelastoma	Mobile pedunculated, multiple fibrillar projections	Small (<1 cm), attached to valvular structures/cords	No significant valvular regurgitation
Lipoma	Smooth surface, large	Ventricular and atrial myocardium	Minimal enhancement with ultrasound contrast
Thrombus	Stagnation, prior instrumentation, often mobile	Any size, commonly in low flow areas such as atrial appendage or apex with wall motion abnormalities	No enhancement with contrast

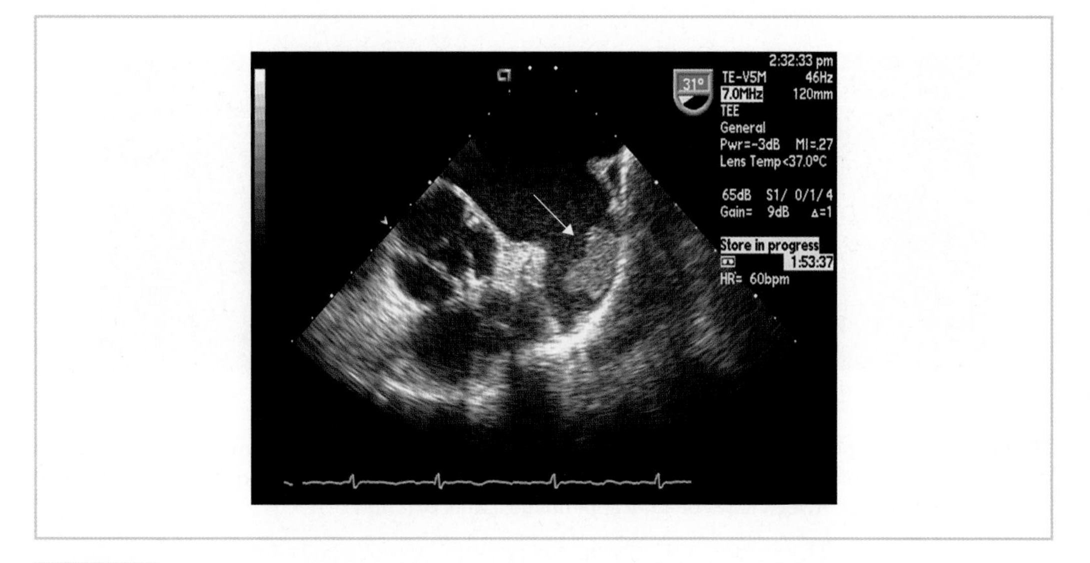

Figure 19.9. Midesophageal image of left atrial appendage at 30 degrees is depicted. A large thrombus is seen in the appendage (*arrow head*).

Transesophageal Echocardiography in Assessment of Cardiac Sources of Emboli

Emboli originating from heart or great vessels are common etiologic factors in stroke and peripheral arterial occlusions. More than 20% of all cases of ischemic stroke are embolic in origin. In as many as 40% of stroke patients, despite intense clinical work up, the etiology is not identified. These patients with cryptogenic stroke are younger, with less evidence of generalized atherosclerosis (10,11). It has been shown that the incidence of patent foramen ovale (PFO) is higher in this population, suggesting a potential role of paradoxical embolism as the etiologic factor. Atherosclerotic disease of ascending aorta and aortic arch is another potential source of embolus in older patients.

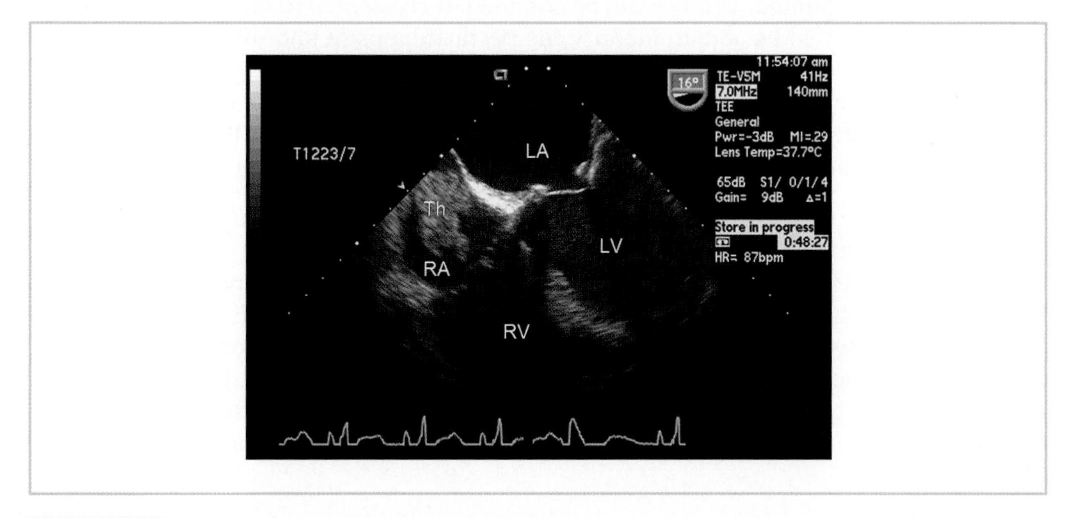

Figure 19.10. Example of a large thrombus in the right atrium is shown in a patient with pulmonary emboli after removal of a pacemaker wire. LA, left atrium; Th, thrombus; RA, right atrium; LV, left ventricle; RV, right ventricle.

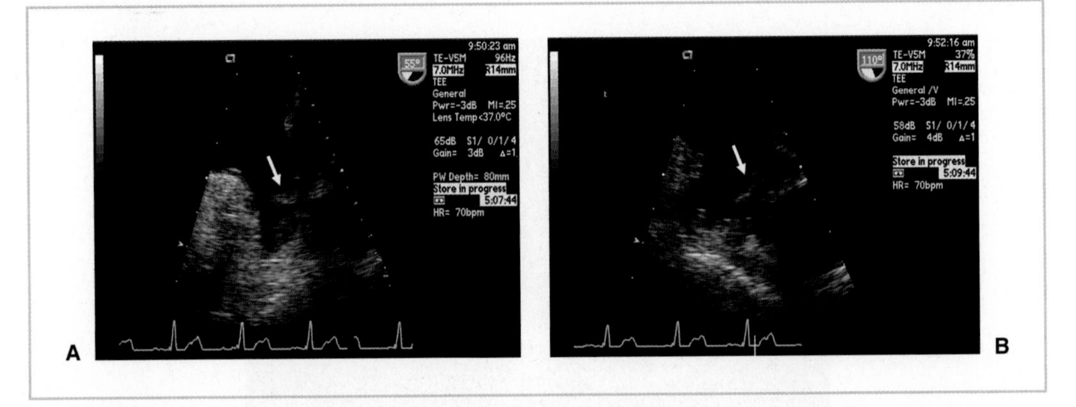

Figure 19.11. Example of prominent pectinate muscle in left atrial appendage mimicking a thrombus is depicted (panel **A**). Images obtained at an orthogonal plane from the same patient demonstrates that the density is a septation between lobes of atrial appendage (panel **B**) (*arrow*).

Cardiac sources of emboli can be further divided into probable and possible sources based on the strength of association.

PROBABLE SOURCES OF EMBOLI

Thrombus in the Left Atrial Appendage

Thrombus in left atrium or LAA is a common source of systemic embolization especially in patients with atrial fibrillation (Figure 19.9). Left atrial clot is usually an extension of existing thrombus in the LAA. LAA is an extension of left atrial cavity and originates from superior aspect of the left atrium anterior to insertion site of left upper pulmonary vein. It is lined with pectinate muscles and in majority of cases has two or more lobes. LAA is best visualized in the midesophageal position with transducer at 30- to 60-degree rotation. With gradual increase in the transducer rotation up to 150 degrees, detailed views of the wall structure and number of lobes can be obtained. It is essential to image the appendage in orthogonal views to be able to identify the pectinate muscle and distinguish it from a potential thrombus (Figure 19.11). In addition to two-dimensional (2-D) images, a detailed examination of the atrial appendage should include assessment of blood flow velocity by pulse wave Doppler. Decreased blood flow velocity (<40 cm/sec) in the LAA has been shown to be associated with increased risk of thromboembolic events.

Thrombus in Left Ventricle

Thrombus in the ventricle is usually associated with regional wall motion abnormalities. Majority of thrombi in the left ventricle (LV) are located in the apex. TEE is often limited in visualizing the apex given its anterior location and relative distance from the transducer. LV apex is best seen on midesophageal long-axis views with slight retroflexion of the probe. In contrast to TEE, transthoracic echocardiography is a better technique to assess of the LV apex.

Endocarditis

Vegetation on cardiac valves can also be a source of embolic events. Vegetation size (size >10 mm) and mobility on TEE are independent risk factors for embolic events (12).

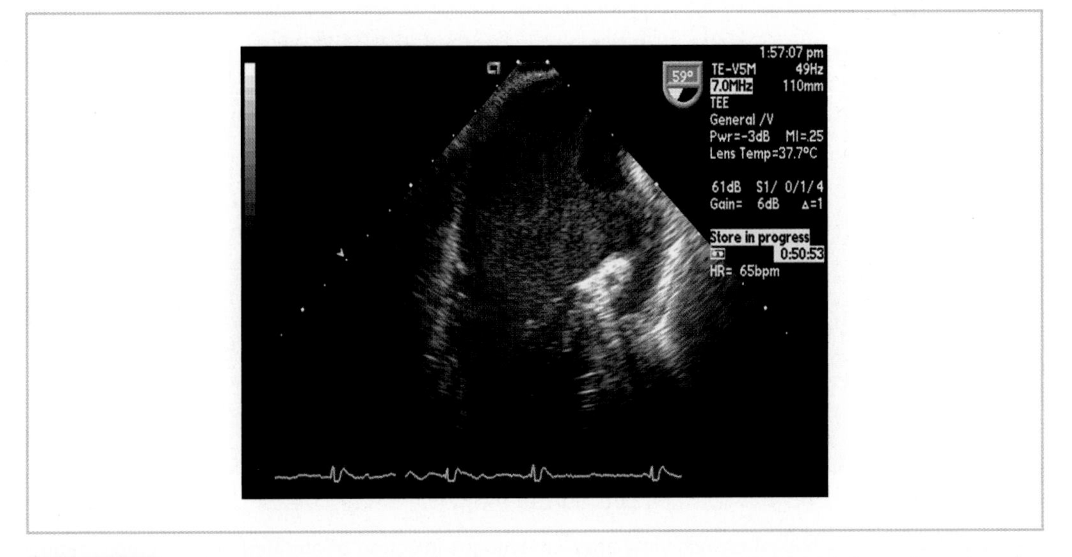

Figure 19.12. Midesophageal image of left atrium demonstrating increased left atrial size and spontaneous echo contrast.

Spontaneous Echo Contrast (Smoke)

Spontaneous echo contrast (SEC) or smoke is an echogenic swirling pattern of blood flow in the left atrium associated with stagnation (Figure 19.12). The exact mechanism of SEC is not well understood but it is thought to be due to aggregation of red blood cells. The presence of SEC in the left atrium or LAA is associated with increased risk of thromboembolism (13).

Paradoxical Embolus Through Patent Foramen Ovale

Transit of a venous embolus through a PFO across the atrial septum can lead to systemic embolization. This theory is further supported by anecdotal reports of paradoxical embolus caught in transit across the septum (Figure 19.13) and higher incidence of PFOs in young

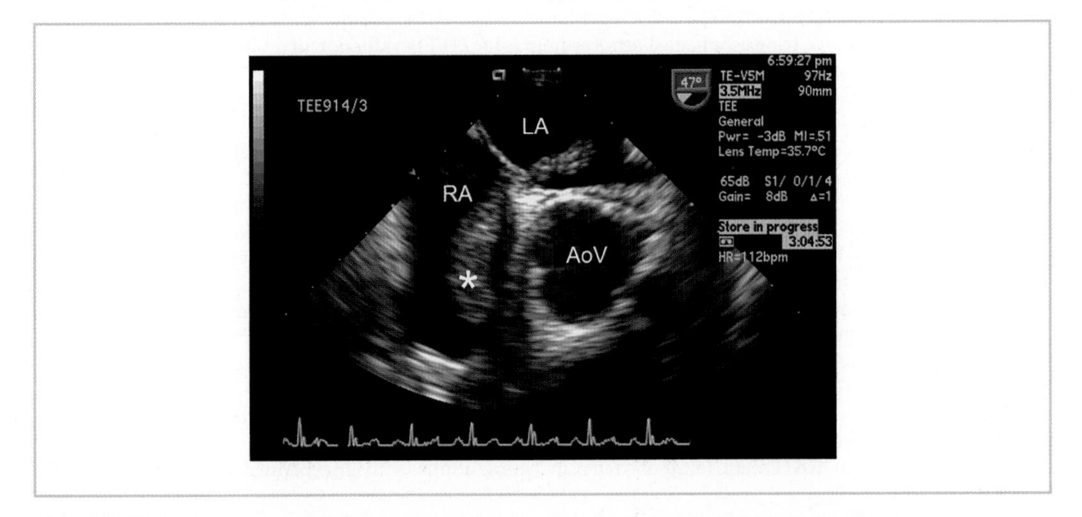

Figure 19.13. Midesophageal short-axis image at the level of atrial septum demonstrating passage of a paradoxical embolus across a patent foramen ovale. LA, left atrium; RA, right atrium; AoV, aortic valve.

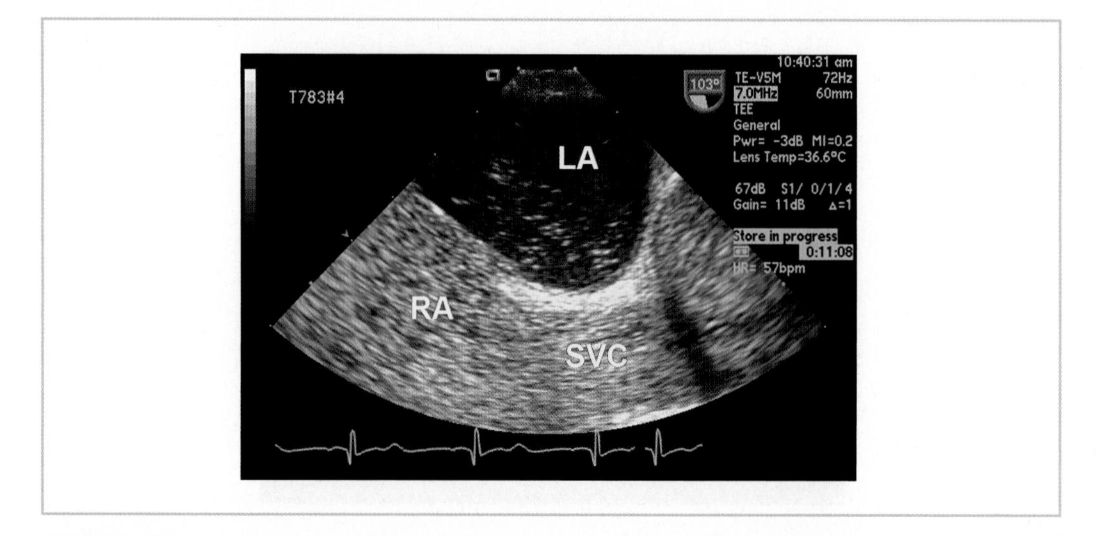

Figure 19.14. Midesophageal bicaval view after intravenous injection of agitated saline demonstrating passage of saline bubbles across patent foramen ovale into left atrium. LA, left atrium; RA, right atrium; SVC, superior vena cava.

patients with cryptogenic stroke (10,14). Therefore, a TEE for evaluation of sources of embolus should include detailed evaluation of atrial septum for presence of a PFO including color Doppler interrogation and performance of agitated saline bubble study. The atrial septum is best seen in the midesophagus with a transducer angle of 100 to 120 degrees (ME bicaval LAX view). PFO can be seen by color Doppler demonstrating flow across foramen ovale or by early appearance of agitated saline bubbles in the left atrium after intravenous injection of agitated saline contrast (Figure 19.14).

REFERENCES

1 Priscilla J, Peters PJ, Reinhardt S. The echocardiographic evaluation of intracardiac masses: a review. *J Am Soc Echocardiogr* 2006;19:230–240.
2 Goldman JH, Foster E. Transesophageal echocardiographic (TEE) evaluation of intracardiac and pericardial masses. *Cardiol Clin* 2000;18(4):849.
3 Feigenbaum H, Armstrong WF, Ryan T. Masses, tumors, and source of embolus. *Feigenbaum's echocardiography*, 6th ed. Philadelphia: Lippincott Williams & Wilkins, 2005.
4 O'Connor S, Recavarren R, Nichols LC, et al. Lipomatous hypertrophy of the interatrial septum: an overview. *Arch Pathol Lab Med* 2006;130(3):397–399.
5 Sun JP, Asher CR, Yang XS, et al. Clinical and echocardiographic characteristics of papillary fibroelastomas. A retrospective and prospective study in 162 patients. *Circulation* 2001;103:2687–2693.
6 Gowda RM, Khan IA, Nair CK, et al. Cardiac papillary fibroelastoma: a comprehensive analysis of 725 cases. *Am Heart J* 2003;146(3):404–410.
7 Klarich KW, Enriquez-Sarano M, Gura GM. Papillary fibroelastoma: Echocardiographic characteristics for diagnosis and pathologic correlation. *J Am Coll Cardiol* 1997;30:784–790.
8 Roldan CA, Shivley BK, Crawford MH. Valve excrescences: prevalence, evolution and risk for cardioembolism. *J Am Coll Cardiol* 1997;30(5):1308–1314.
9 Kirkpatrick JN, Wong T, Bednarz JE, et al. Differential diagnosis of cardiac masses using contrast echocardiographic perfusion imaging. *J Am Coll Cardiol* 2004;43:1412–1419.
10 Kizer JR, Devereux RB. Patent foramen ovale in young adults with unexplained stroke. *N Engl J Med* 2005;353:2361–2372.
11 Wu LA, Malouf JF, Dearani JA, et al. Patent foramen ovale in cryptogenic stroke: current understanding and management options. *Arch Intern Med* 2004;164(9):950–956.

12 Thuny F, Disalvo G, Belliard O, et al. Risk of embolism and death in infective endocarditis: prognostic value of echocardiography: a prospective multicenter study. *Circulation* 2005;112(1):69–75.
13 Bernhardt P, Schmidt H, Hammerstingl C, et al. Patients with atrial fibrillation and dense spontaneous echo contrast at high risk a prospective and serial follow-up over 12 months with transesophageal echocardiography and cerebral magnetic resonance imaging. *J Am Coll Cardiol* 2005;45(11):1807–1812.
14 Cramer SC. Patent foramen ovale and its relationship to stroke. *Cardiol Clin* 2005;23(1):7–11.

QUESTIONS

1. **All of the following statements regarding utility of transesophageal echocardiography in assessment of cardiac masses are true except:**
   a. Transesophageal echocardiography is very useful in assessment of small masses given high image resolution and proximity to posterior cardiac structures.
   b. Normal variant cardiac structures at times can be mistaken for cardiac masses.
   c. Echocardiographic brightness and density of backscattered signal can assist in identification of histology of cardiac masses.
   d. Location, size, and mobility of the mass are important clues in identification of type of the mass.

2. **Which of the following best describes cardiac myxoma?**
   a. Myxoma is the most common benign primary cardiac tumor in adults.
   b. Myxoma is usually pedunculated with a stalk attached to fossa ovalis in the left atrium.
   c. Myxoma is associated with systemic embolization.
   d. All of the above.

3. **Which of the following statements is true regarding the utility of intravenous ultrasound contrast in evaluation of cardiac masses?**
   a. Malignant tumors with high vascularity are enhanced with ultrasound contrast agents.
   b. Thrombus will appear as a filling defect with ultrasound contrast.
   c. Benign stromal tumors will not enhance with ultrasound contrast.
   d. All of the above.

4. **Which of the following statements is true regarding lipomatous hypertrophy of atrial septum?**
   a. Lipomatous hypertrophy is a condition with fatty infiltration of atrial septum without a capsule and should be distinguished from lipoma.
   b. Lipomatous hypertrophy is a common finding in young males.
   c. Characteristic echocardiographic feature is isolated thickening of atrial septum at the fossa ovalis.
   d. Lipomatous hypertrophy often involves the AV node and causes bradyarrhythmias.

5. **Which one of the following statements is true regarding fibroelastomas?**
   a. Papillary fibroelastomas are often small and pedunculated with multiple fibrillar projections and commonly arise from cardiac valves.
   b. Aortic valve is the most common site of origin followed by the mitral valve.
   c. Fibroelastomas are associated with increased risk of systemic embolization.
   d. All of the above.

6. **Which statement is true regarding cardiac tumors in children?**
   a. Rhabdomyoma is the most common primary cardiac tumor in children and is almost always associated with tuberous sclerosis.
   b. Fibroma is the second most common cardiac tumor and is characterized by central calcifications.
   c. Spontaneous resolution is common in rhabdomyoma.
   d. All of the above.

7. **Which of the following statements regarding cardiac sources of emboli is true?**
   a. In as many as 40% of patients with ischemic stroke, etiology is not identified despite intense clinical workup.
   b. Thrombus in left atrial appendage in patients with atrial fibrillation is associated with an increased risk of systemic embolic events.
   c. There is increased incidence of patent foramen ovale among young patients with cryptogenic stroke suggesting that paradoxical embolous may be a potential source.
   d. All of the above.

8. **Which of the following is an independent predictor of systemic embolization in patients with endocarditis?**
   a. Vegetation size greater than 10 mm
   b. Vegetation mobility
   c. Vegetations on recently placed prosthetic valves
   d. **a** and **b**

9. **In which of the following conditions is an etiologic link to stroke is well established?**
   a. Spontaneous echo contrast
   b. Thrombus in left atrial appendage
   c. Patent foramen ovale
   d. All of the above

10. **Which of the following cardiac structures is most likely to be mistaken for left atrial thrombus on transesophageal echocardiography?**
    a. Pectinate muscle
    b. Papillary muscle
    c. Crista terminalis
    d. Moderator band

Answers appear at the back of the book.

V

Man and Machine

20 Common Artifacts and Pitfalls of Clinical Echocardiography

Joseph P. Miller, Albert C. Perrino, Jr., and Zak Hillel[1]

Clinically important imaging artifacts result from the interplay of the ultrasound system, the patient, and the interpreting echocardiographer. The most common artifacts seen in clinical practice are the result of (a) normal or variant anatomic structures that are misdiagnosed, (b) the physical limitations of ultrasound imaging, and (c) undesirable interactions of ultrasound with tissues or medical devices. Accordingly, this chapter is organized into three sections. First, we review common false interpretations of normal anatomy. Second, we discuss the artifacts commonly encountered in two-dimensional imaging, and finally, we discuss the artifacts commonly encountered in Doppler examinations.

NORMAL ANATOMIC VARIANTS IN TWO-DIMENSIONAL IMAGING

Both novice and experienced echocardiographers may call normal structures abnormal. These normal variants can affect the intraoperative diagnosis and lead to inappropriate surgery, which can have a devastating impact on outcome. Careful evaluation and a consideration of the common variants discussed in the subsequent text can help limit problems related to misdiagnosis.

Crista Terminalis

The crista terminalis has been misinterpreted as a right atrial tumor or thrombus. This prominent muscular ridge can be differentiated from an anomaly by its characteristic appearance and position. The crista terminalis originates at the junction of the right atrium and superior vena cava junction and runs longitudinally toward the inferior vena cava. The trabeculations of the appendage originate from the crista terminalis. The crista terminalis separates the trabeculated appendage of the atrium from the smooth tubular portion. The structure is best visualized in the midesophageal (ME) bicaval view (Figure 20.1).

Eustachian Valve or Chiari Network

The eustachian valve is often misdiagnosed as an intra-atrial thrombus. The eustachian valve (called a *Chiari network* when fenestrated) is the remnant of the embryologic right venous valve, which is important *in utero* to direct inferior vena cava blood flow across the fossa ovalis. The filamentous structures can be differentiated from thrombus by their characteristic "insertion" into the atrial wall. They are best visualized in the ME bicaval view, in which they can be seen originating from the junction of the right atrium and inferior vena cava (Figure 20.1).

Lipomatous Hypertrophy of the Atrial Septum

Myxomas, the most common cardiac tumors, often originate from the interatrial septum and typically involve the fossa ovalis. Lipomatous hypertrophy of the atrial septum can

[1]The opinions or assertions contained herein are the private views of the author(s) and are not to be construed as official or as reflecting the views of the Department of Defense.

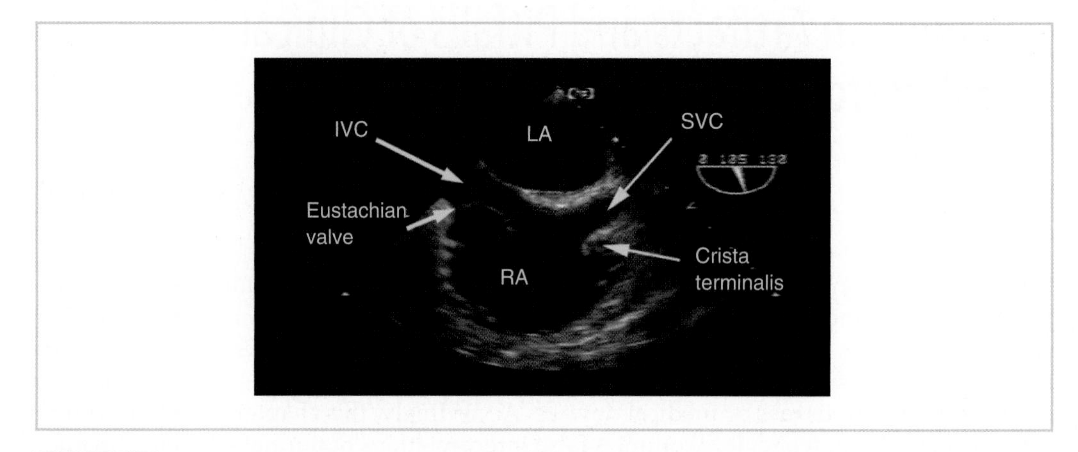

Figure 20.1. The **crista terminalis** and **eustachian valve** are easily seen in this midesophageal bicaval view. IVC, inferior vena cava; LA, left atrium; SVC, superior vena cava; RA, right atrium.

mimic atrial masses such as myxomas. The characteristic "dumbbell" shape seen in the ME four-chamber or ME bicaval view differentiates lipomatous hypertrophy from other structures. The appearance is caused by fatty infiltration of the atrial septum with *sparing* of the fossa ovalis (Figure 20.2).

Coumadin Ridge

A prominent muscle ridge is formed between the left atrial appendage and the atrial insertion of the left upper pulmonary vein. This prominence is often misdiagnosed as thrombus and is referred to as the *coumadin ridge* or *"Q-tip" sign*. The lack of mobility and characteristic location, best seen in the ME two-chamber view; help distinguish it from an abnormal structure (Figure 20.3).

Pericardial Sinuses

Pericardial sinuses (or folds) between the atria and great vessels can give rise to echolucent spaces despite only minimal amounts of pericardial fluid. The transverse and oblique sinuses of the pericardium can easily mimic pericardial cysts or abscesses. Pericardial fat seen in these extracardiac structures can also mimic intracardiac thrombus (Figure 20.4).

Lambl Excrescences

Fine filamentous strands, Lambl excrescences, can be seen originating from the aortic valve of elderly patients. These structures can be differentiated from valvular vegetations by their characteristic "delicate" appearance in the absence of any clinical evidence of endocarditis (Figure 20.5).

Moderator Band

The moderator band of the right ventricle has been misinterpreted as an intracardiac mass. This specialized cardiac trabeculation runs from the right ventricular free wall to the interventricular septum. It is often best seen in the ME four-chamber view (Figure 20.6).

Pleural Effusion

Pleural effusions of the left side of the chest can mimic aortic dissection. In the descending aorta long-axis view, a pleural effusion will parallel the course of the aorta and have the

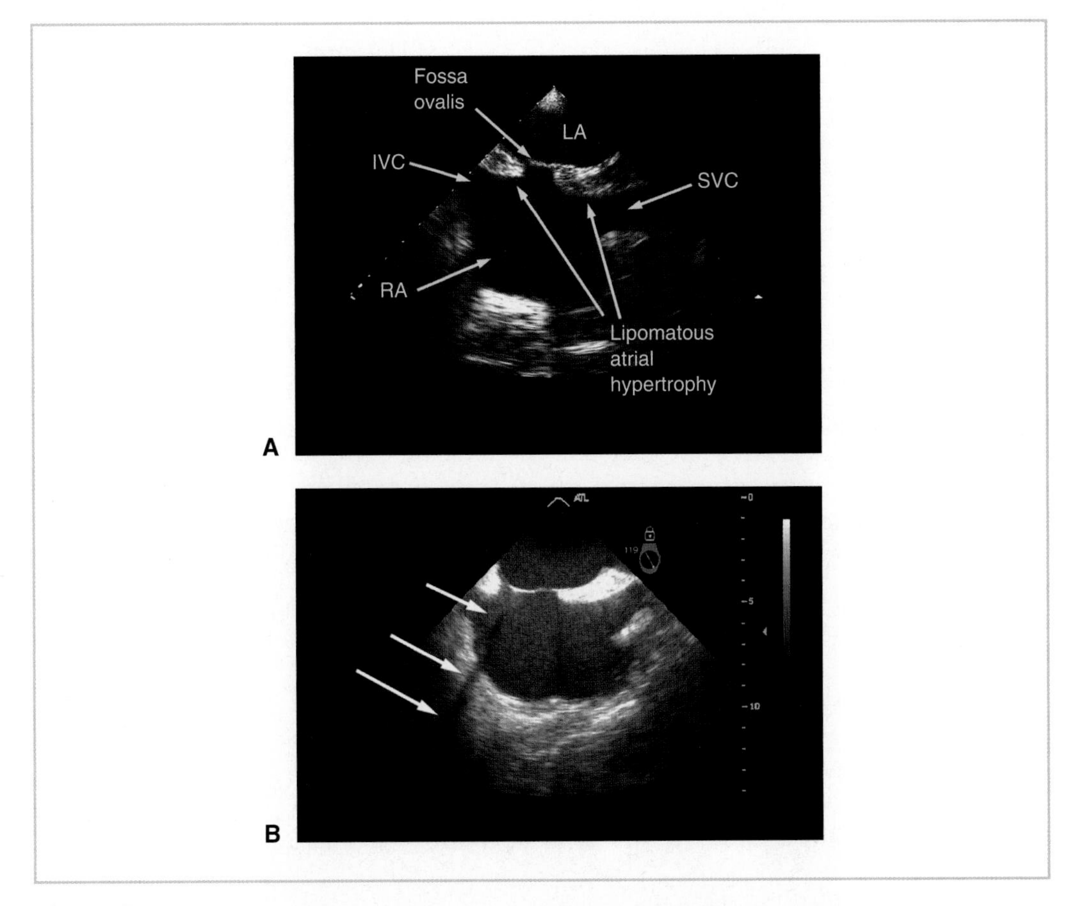

Figure 20.2. **A:** The characteristic dumbbell shape of a **lipomatous atrial septum** with sparing of the fossa ovalis is seen in this midesophageal bicaval view. **B:** This is a different cross section of a lipomatous atrial septum. Note the shadowing from a pulmonary artery catheter that is not visible in this plane. This is an example of both a side lobe and shadowing artifact (see text for description). LA, left atrium; IVC, inferior vena cava; SVC, superior vena cava; RA, right atrium.

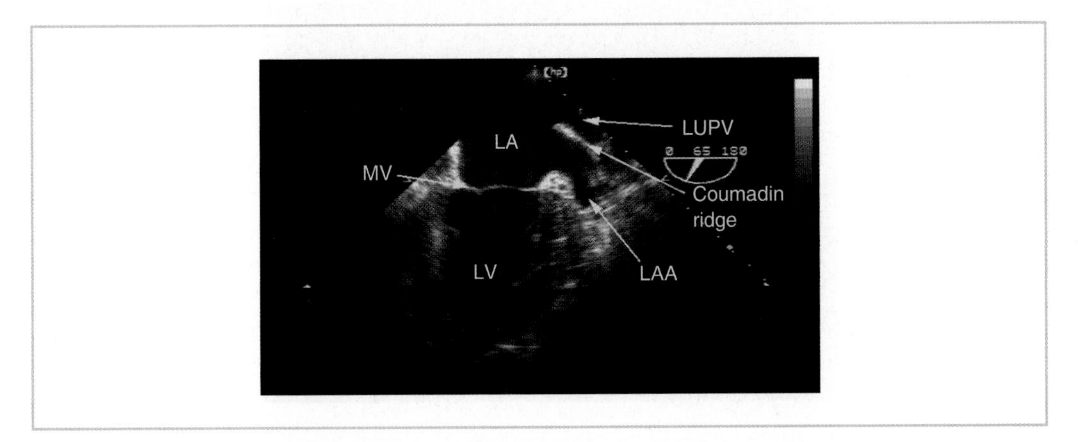

Figure 20.3. A **Coumadin ridge** is seen between the left atrial appendage and the left upper pulmonary vein (LUPV). Notably, the parallel arcs of electrocautery interference are also seen in this midesophageal (ME) two-chamber view. LA, left atrium; MV, mitral valve; LV, left ventricle; LAA, left atrial appendage.

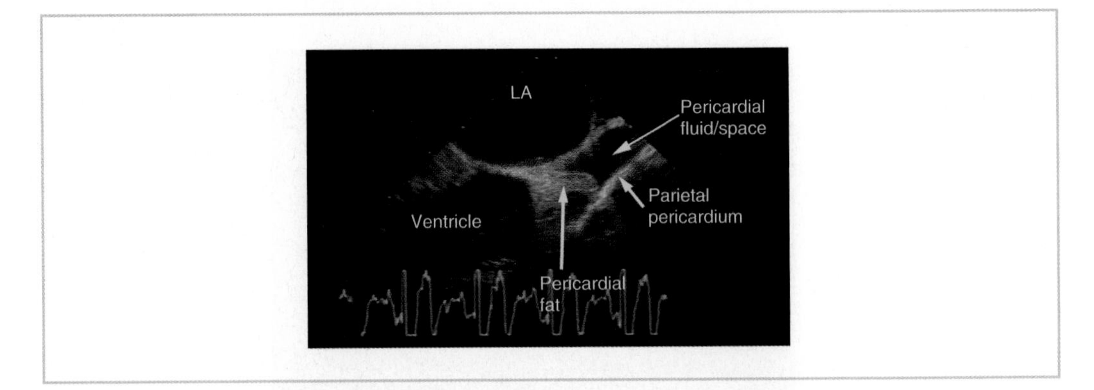

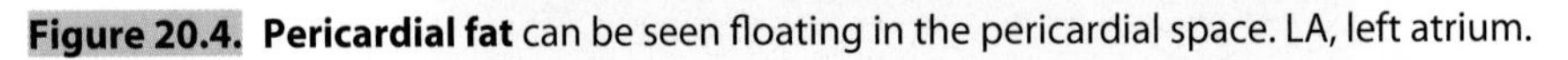

Figure 20.4. **Pericardial fat** can be seen floating in the pericardial space. LA, left atrium.

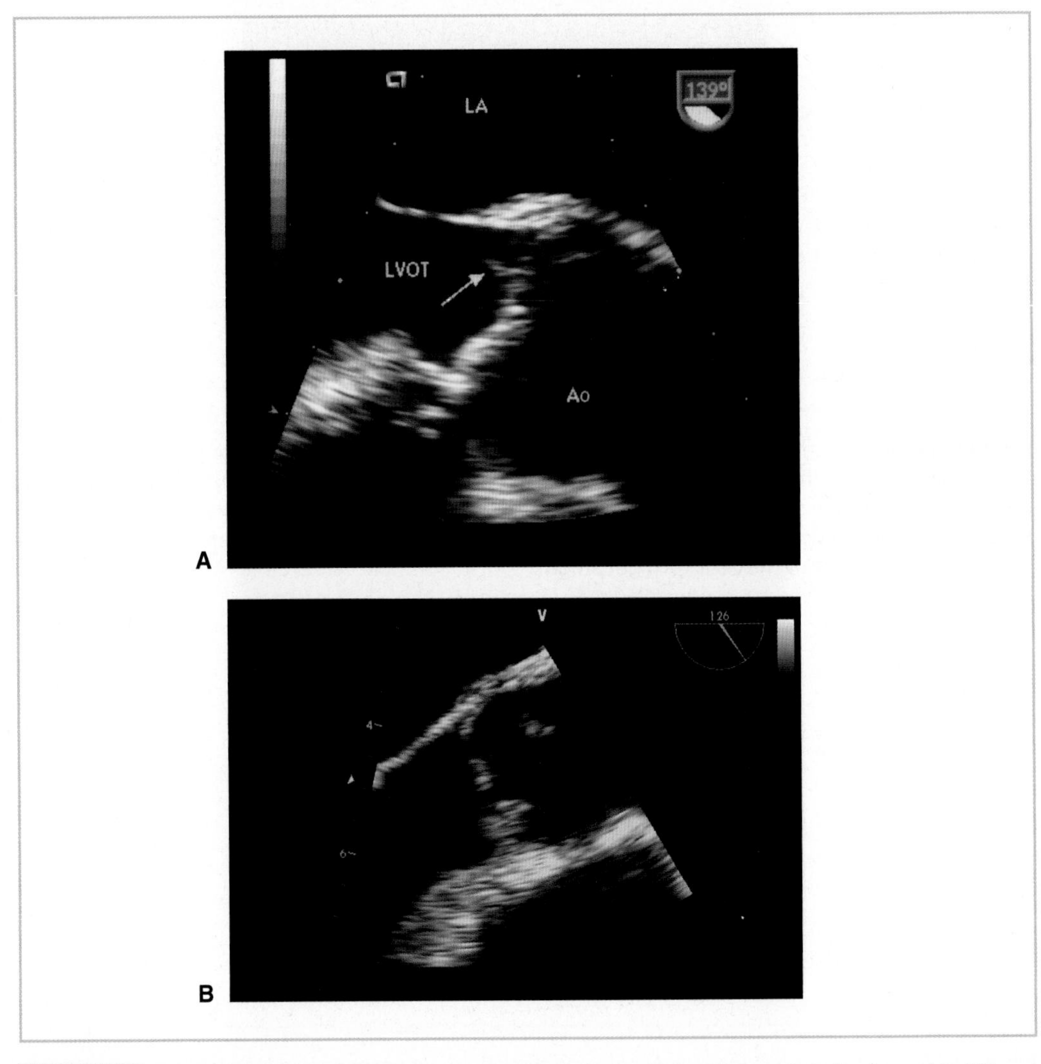

Figure 20.5. A **Lambl excrescence** is seen on the ventricular surface of the aortic valve (*arrow*) in **(A)** and on the aortic surface in **(B)**. LA, left atrium; LVOT, left ventricular outflow tract; Ao, aorta; V, ventricle.

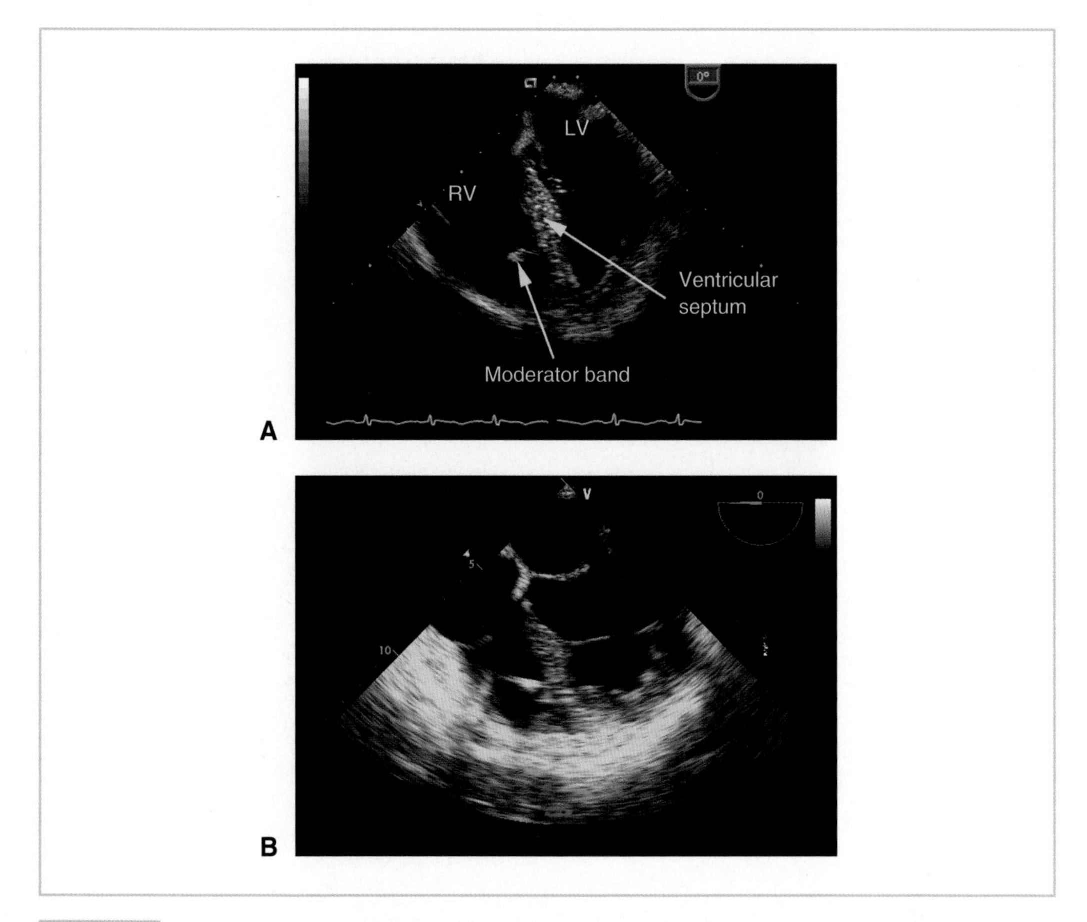

Figure 20.6. **A:** The **moderator band** of the right ventricle is seen in this midesophageal four-chamber view. This is in contrast to (**B**) where the structure seen crossing the left ventricle is a false chord. LV, left ventricle; RV, right ventricle; V, ventricle.

appearance of a true lumen–false lumen dissection. Changing to the descending aorta short-axis view and identifying the characteristic triangular shape of a left-sided pleural effusion easily confirms the diagnosis of effusion versus dissection (Figure 20.7).

TWO-DIMENSIONAL ECHOCARDIOGRAPHIC IMAGING ARTIFACTS

Suboptimal Image Quality

The inability to visualize cardiac structures because of suboptimal image quality remains a challenge in transesophageal echocardiographic diagnosis. Most commonly, improper settings of the ultrasound unit are to blame, but patient anatomy, acoustic interfaces (e.g., air between the probe and the stomach or esophageal wall, hiatal hernia), and sonographer skill play a definite role. Surprisingly, adjustments in machine settings coupled with minor manipulations of the ultrasound probe can lead to substantial improvement in the quality of images that are difficult to obtain. This topic is discussed further in Chapter 21.

Air between the transducer surface and tissue, encountered in transesophageal views more often than in transgastric (TG) views, causes severe image degradation to the point

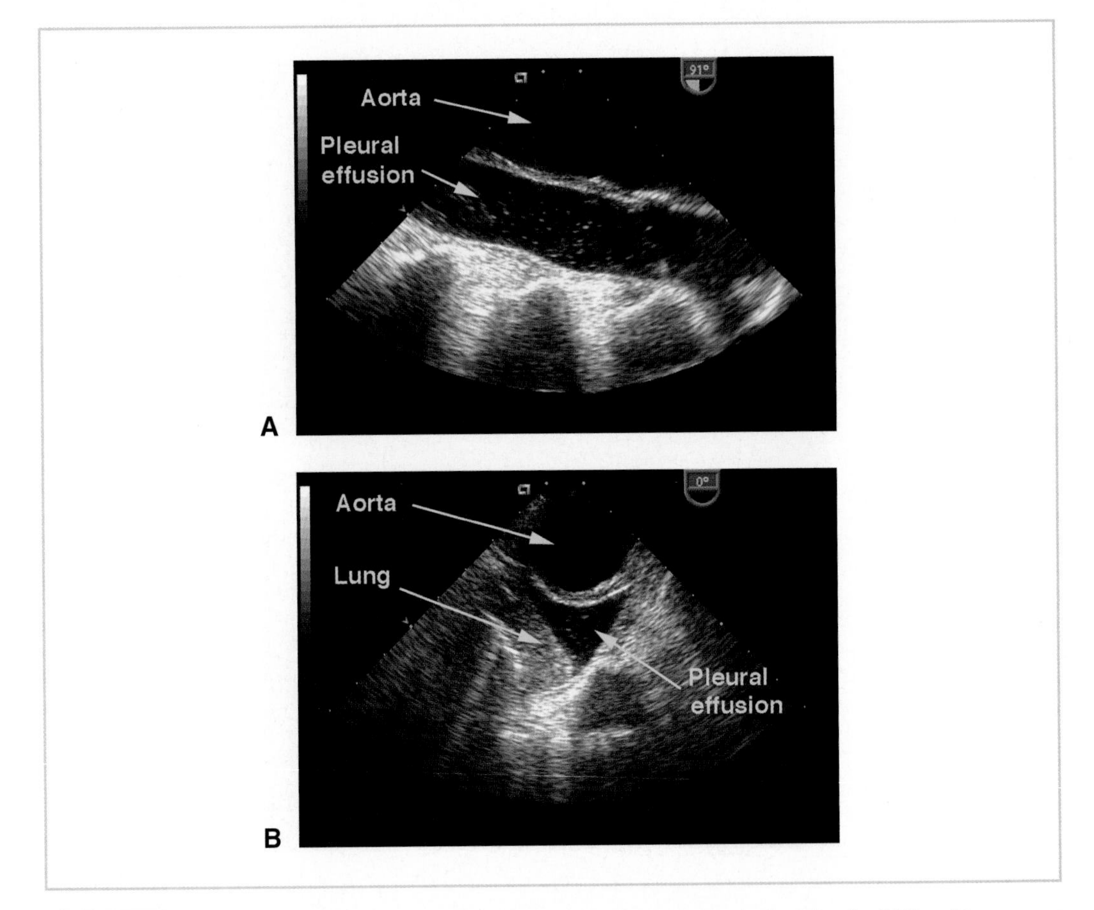

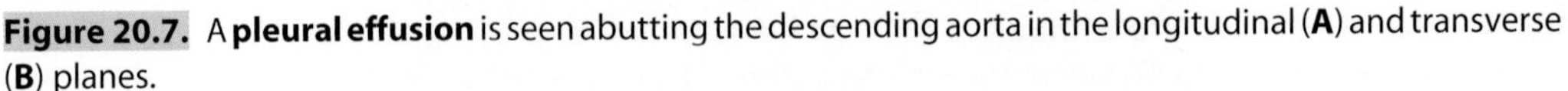

Figure 20.7. A **pleural effusion** is seen abutting the descending aorta in the longitudinal (**A**) and transverse (**B**) planes.

of complete inability to image. *Gastric suctioning before the transesophageal echocardiographic examination can reduce the poor acoustic contact caused by an air–tissue interface.*

Imaging is also frequently suboptimal when the cardiac structure of interest is parallel to the ultrasound beam. A common example of this artifact is "dropout" of the lateral and septal walls in the TG mid short-axis and ME four-chamber views (Figure 20.8). Specular reflections are maximized when tissue interfaces lie perpendicular to the ultrasound beam, and this artifact is overcome by repositioning the ultrasound probe to a more favorable vantage point. An example of this phenomenon is the impaired ability to visualize thin linear structures, such as the chordae tendineae of the mitral valve, when they are parallel to the ultrasound beam (ME five-chamber view) (Figure 20.9A). However, when these structures are perpendicular to the beam (TG two-chamber view), they are easily visualized (Figure 20.9B).

Acoustic Shadowing

Acoustic shadowing occurs when the ultrasound beam meets an interface of two structures with marked differences in acoustic impedance. Common examples include structures with a high level of acoustic impedance, such as calcific aortic or mitral valves (Figure 20.10A).

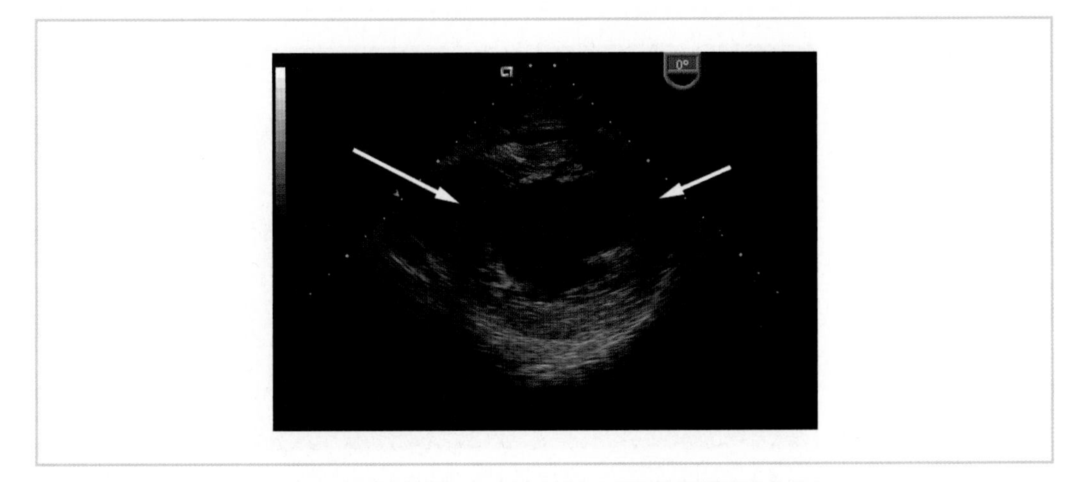

Figure 20.8. **Transgastric** mid short-axis view demonstrating septal and lateral wall dropout (*arrowheads*).

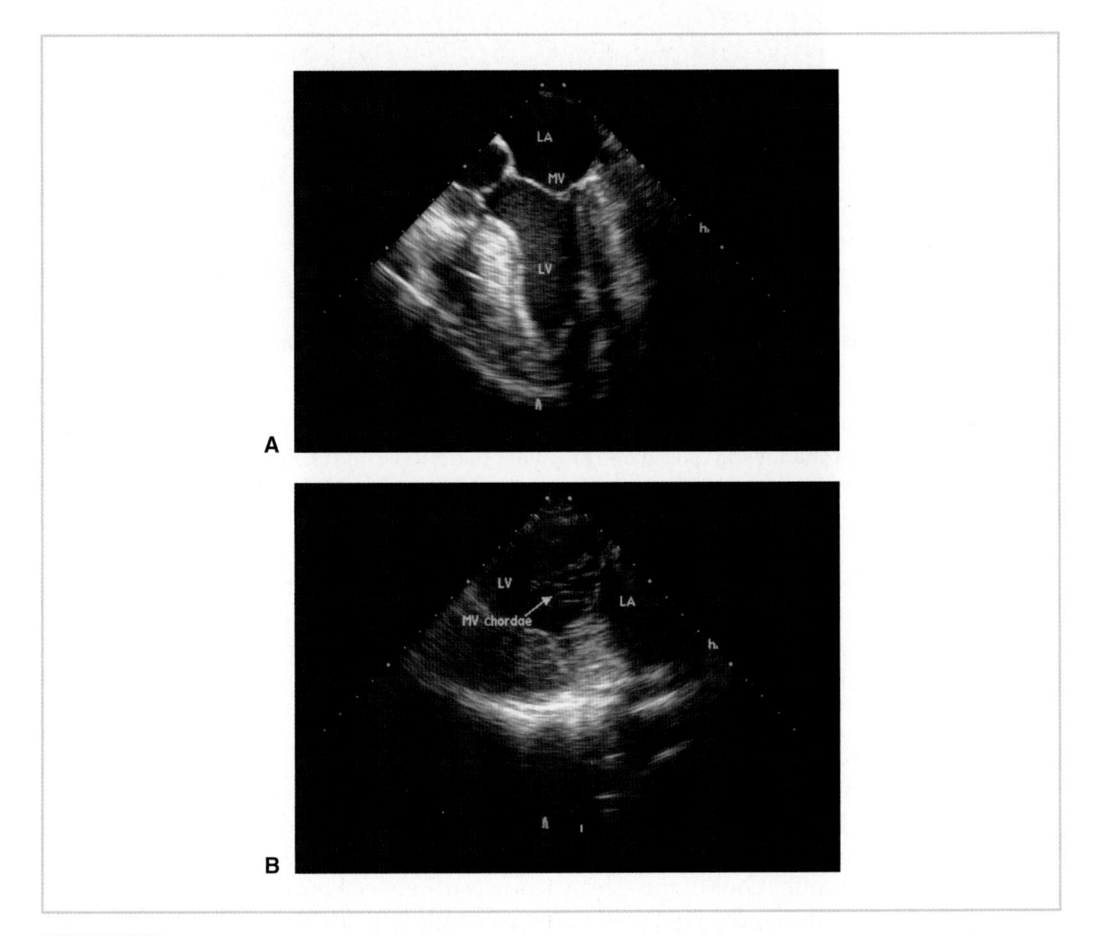

Figure 20.9. **A:** Mitral valve and apparatus imaged with chordae tendineae parallel to the ultrasound beam (midesophageal five-chamber view). **B:** Markedly improved delineation of the chordae tendineae with the ultrasound beam perpendicular to the chordae tendineae (transgastric long-axis view). LA, left atrium; MV, mitral valve; LV, left ventricle.

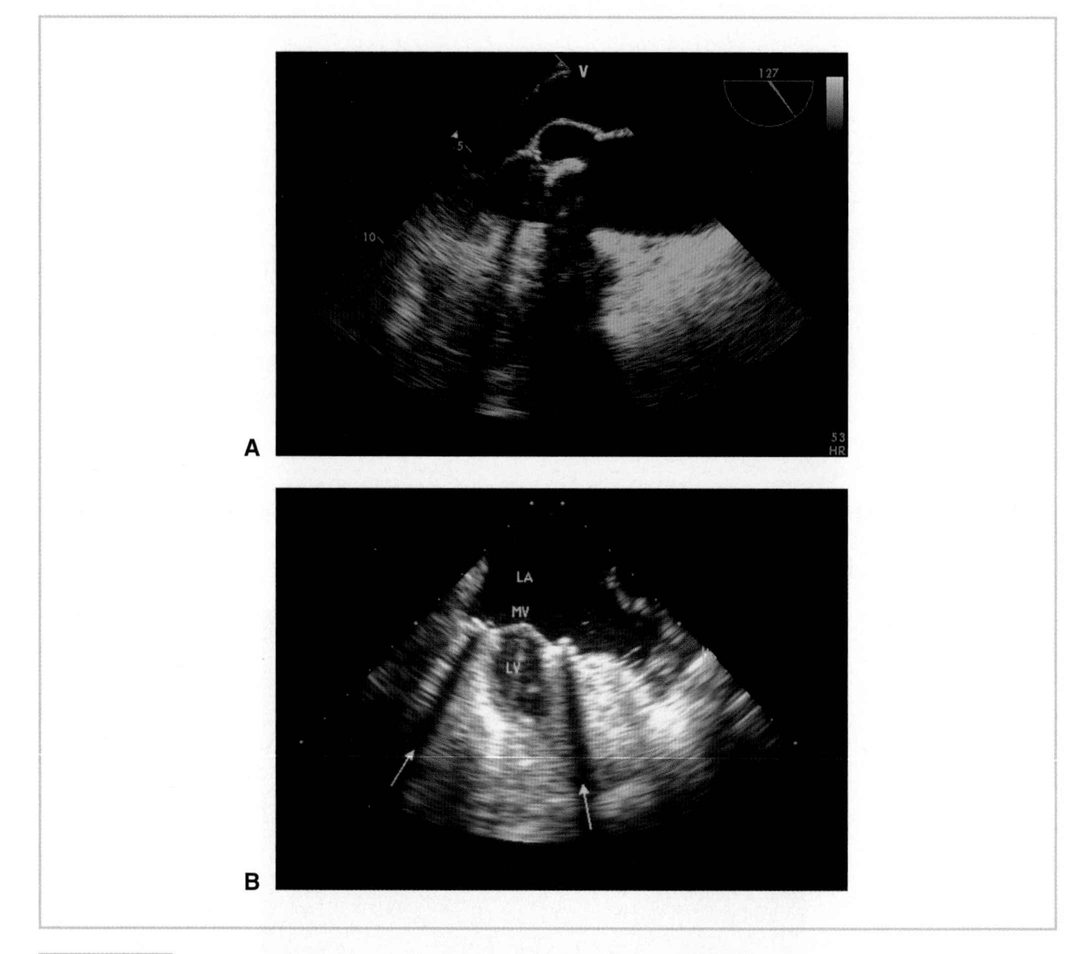

Figure 20.10. **A:** In this view a broad area of the distal scan is not visible due to shadowing from a calcific aortic valve. **B: Acoustic shadowing** caused by a prosthetic mitral valve ring imaged in the midesophageal commissural view. The *arrow* points to the long axial shadows. V, ventricle; LA, left atrium; MV, mitral valve; LV, left ventricle.

These strongly reflect and scatter the ultrasound signal, thereby limiting distal penetration of the sound waves. Similarly, mechanical prostheses and the struts of bioprosthetic valves produce shadowing. The resultant image reveals an echo-dense structure with a lack of signal in the sector beyond the structure (Figure 20.10B).

Lateral Resolution

The two-dimensional image is created from a series of individual ultrasound beams. Because structures lying between any two beams are not interrogated, the machine creates their display by averaging information received from the adjacent beams. This causes two problems. First, determinations of the size of a structure between beams (lateral resolution) are never as good as measurements made down a single beam (axial resolution). In most systems, axial resolution is at least twice lateral resolution. Second, the ultrasound beam fans out as it travels farther from the transducer, so that the distance between individual scan lines increases. This differential resolution of two-dimensional echocardiography can produce shape distortion. Lateral stretching of small but strongly echogenic objects, such

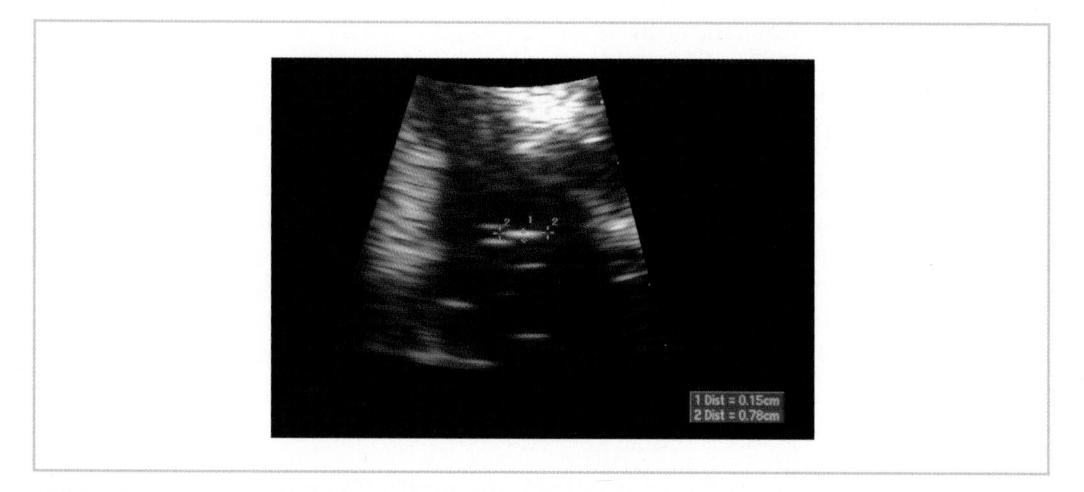

Figure 20.11. Discrepancy between **axial** and **lateral** sizes of microbubbles as a consequence of resolution artifact. *1 Dist* and *2 Dist* indicate axial and lateral sizes, respectively.

as intracardiac catheters or wires, may occur. The images may show a markedly elongated shape instead of the true round cross-sectional shape. Similarly, intracardiac contrast (very small air bubbles at times) may incorrectly appear elongated laterally instead of round (Figure 20.11).

Side Lobe and Beam Width

Side lobes are weak "beam leaks" outside the path of the main ultrasound beam. Although weak, when they encounter an echo-dense structure, such as a calcified aorta, mitral valve ring, any prosthetic material, or a catheter (Figure 20.12), they cause reflections strong enough to be detected. The scanner misplaces these echoes in the image, incorrectly assuming that they have been generated by structures lying in the path of the main beam. The artifact is displayed at the appropriate distance from the transducer but at the wrong

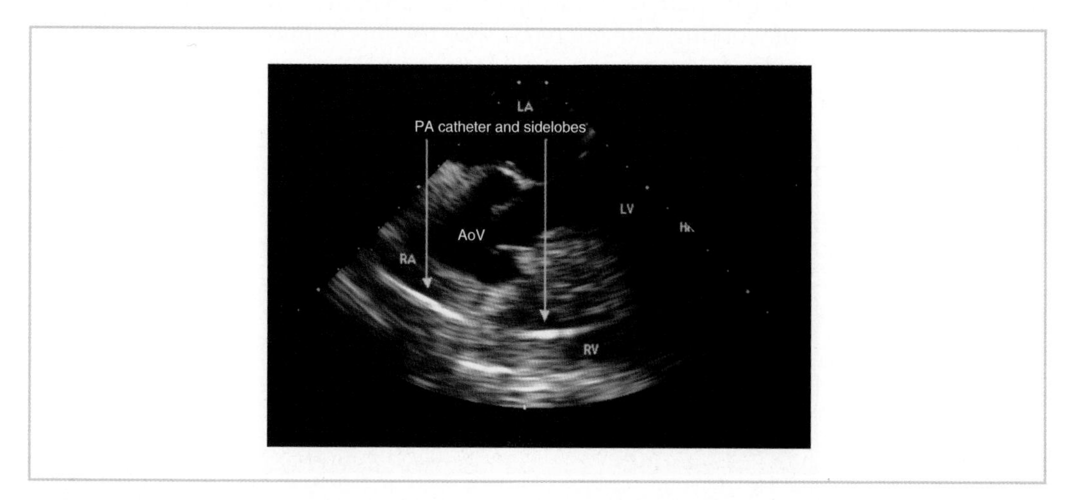

Figure 20.12. **Side lobe** artifact of a pulmonary artery catheter imaged in the right atrium and right ventricle demonstrated in the midesophageal five-chamber view. LA, left atrium; PA, pulmonary artery; LV, left ventricle; AoV, aortic valve; RA, right atrium; RV, right ventricle.

lateral position. Some dramatic artifacts are produced when the examiner sees the image of a structure that is physically outside the scan sector overlying the two-dimensional image from the main beam! Because the main beam sweeps the entire scan sector, side lobe artifacts may appear as narrow, curvilinear densities smeared over its entire width.

Beam width artifacts occur because ultrasound waves are three-dimensional, cone-shaped structures, not just two-dimensional planar structures. Structures adjacent to the imaging plane but still within the imaging cone can be displayed in the imaging plane. The result varies depending on the location of the structures outside the imaging plane. They can appear as flaps in the aorta, structures or catheters in the wrong position (Figure 20.12), or elongated structures. Beam width artifacts also occur with spectral Doppler and are discussed later.

Reverberation

Reverberations are caused by the repeated back-and-forth reflection of an ultrasound wave between two strong specular reflectors. This phenomenon leads to two types of imaging artifacts. In the first, multiple linear densities are produced in the area of the imaging sector distal to the reflecting structures (Figure 20.13). The second type of artifact occurs when the strong echoes are reflected from the transducer itself. The reflection then travels back to the same target, where it is echoed a second time toward the detecting transducer. As a result, an artifact is produced that appears as a duplication of the structure in the far field. Because this second trip doubles the travel distance, and hence the travel time, the target structure is imaged once at the correct distance and a second time at twice the distance from the transducer. The descending thoracic aorta in both the transverse and longitudinal scans is a common source of this type of reverberation artifact. The vessel is imaged correctly in the near field and falsely duplicated immediately below. The duplicating reverberation artifact also extends in this case to color flow imaging (Figure 20.14).

Electronic Noise

Electronic noise, of which electrocautery is the major source, cause an imaging artifact that resembles a "snowed image" pattern. Viewing cardiac anatomy through this snowstorm is an annoying reality of working with surgeons who use this technology (Figure 20.15).

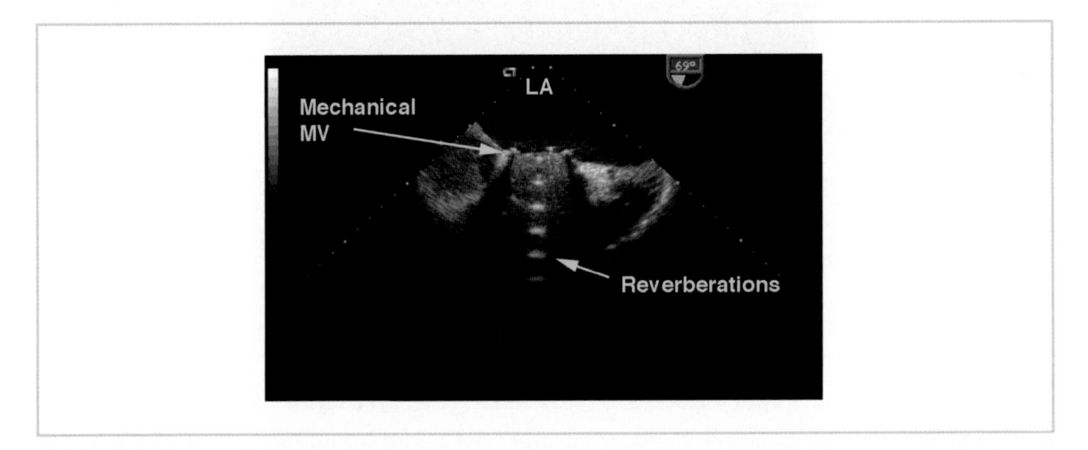

Figure 20.13. Reverberation artifact resulting from a mechanical mitral valve is easily seen distal to the valve. LA, left atrium.

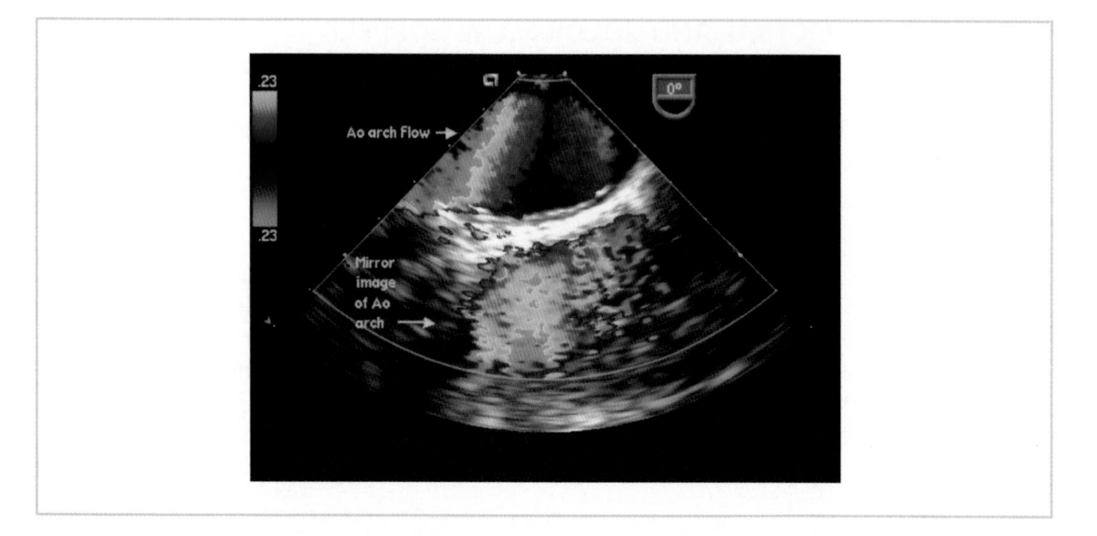

Figure 20.14. A **mirror image** of the true aortic arch is seen in the far field. Note that the false arch is the same size as the true structure. The color flow Doppler signals are also duplicated. Ao, aortic.

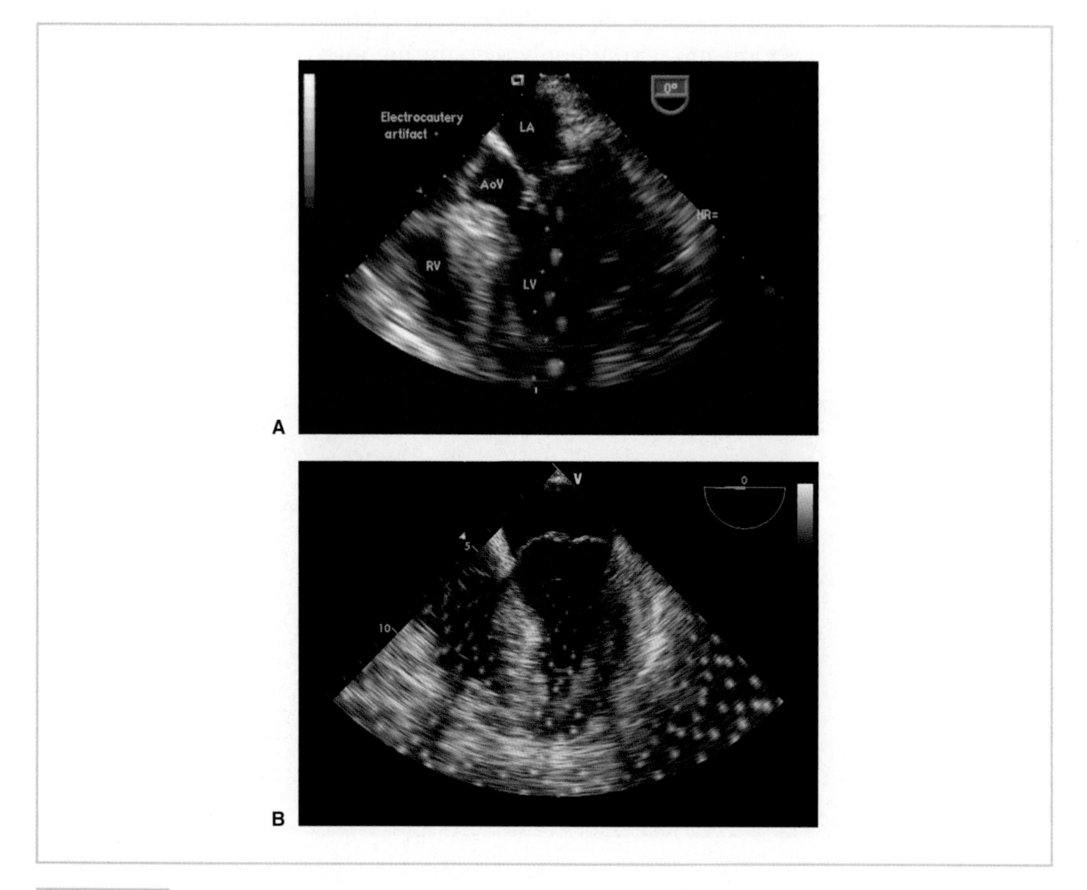

Figure 20.15. **A: Electrocautery** artifacts are indicated by *asterisks* in the midesophageal five-chamber view. **B:** Electrocautery interference can be localized as seen in (**A**) or diffuse as seen in this view. LA, left atrium; AoV, aortic valve; RV, right ventricle; LV, left ventricle; V, ventricle.

ARTIFACTS IN SPECTRAL AND COLOR FLOW DOPPLER

Spectral and color flow Doppler are susceptible to several of the mechanisms of artifact production that occur in two-dimensional imaging; however, the appearance of the artifacts is quite different. In addition, the Doppler examinations are susceptible to a number of artifacts unique to this method.

Aliasing

A shortcoming of pulsed wave Doppler systems, which includes color flow Doppler, is that the maximal blood velocities that can be accurately quantified are limited by the pulse repetition frequency. Specifically, any Doppler frequency shift greater than one half the pulse repetition frequency, known as the *Nyquist limit,* results in a distorted spectral signal. The distortion in the Doppler signal, called *aliasing,* causes several types of artifacts in the pulse wave spectral signal or color flow map. Common examples include "wraparound" of the spectral signal (see Figure 5.10) and red-blue stippling on the color flow map (see Figure 5.14).

Acoustic Shadowing in Color Flow

Strong specular reflectors result in acoustic shadowing not only with two-dimensional imaging but also with Doppler modes. This artifact can be misinterpreted as a lack of blood flow in the shadowed region and is commonly seen during interrogation of prosthetic or heavily calcified valves (Figure 20.16).

Nonparallel Beam Angle

Because the Doppler shift is proportional to the cosine of the angle between the path of the ultrasound beam and that of the blood flow, blood flow velocities are underestimated when the orientation of the ultrasound beam is not parallel to blood flow. With color flow Doppler, this artifact typically occurs when the course of a vessel is oblique to

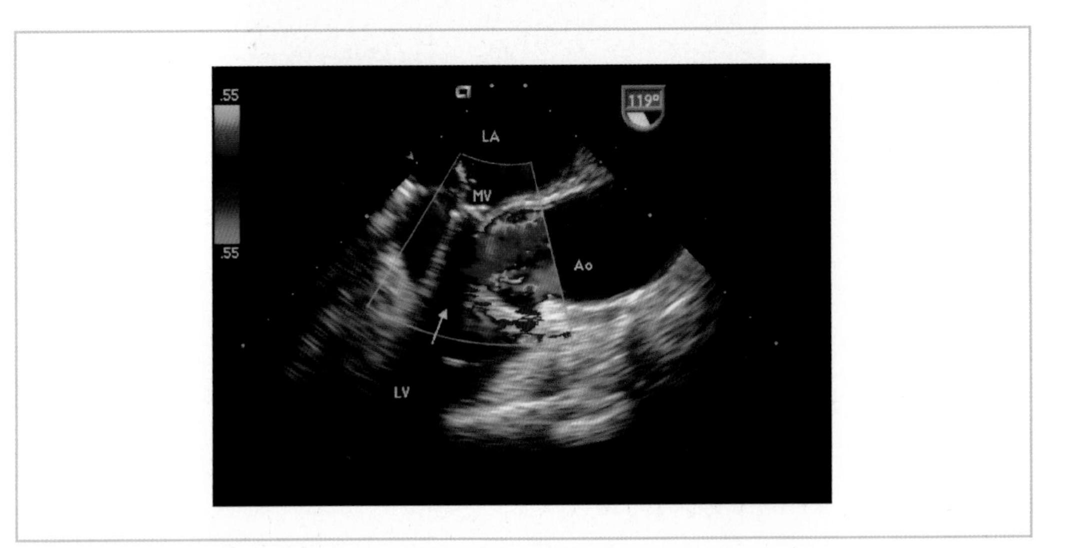

Figure 20.16. Acoustic shadowing in color flow Doppler caused by a prosthetic mitral valve ring in the midesophageal aortic valve long-axis view. The *arrow* points to the long axial shadow. LA, left atrium; MV, mitral valve; Ao, aorta; LV, left ventricle.

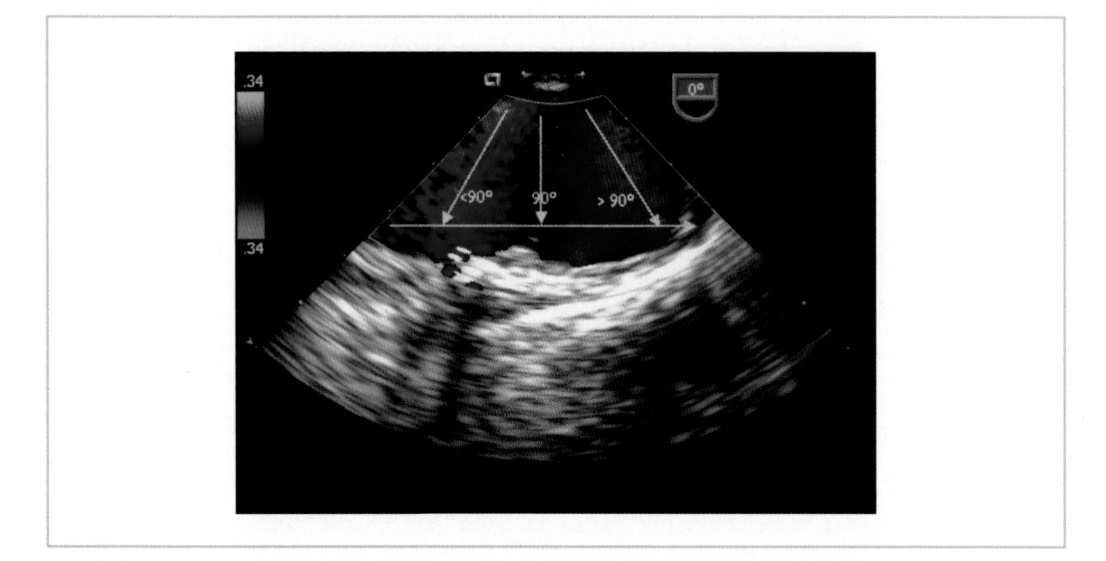

Figure 20.17. Nonparallel beam angle color flow Doppler artifact in the aortic arch. The direction of blood flow is indicated by the *horizontal arrow*. The *angled arrows* indicate the direction of the Doppler ultrasound interrogating beam.

the ultrasound beam. The blood flow perpendicular to the path of the Doppler beam is color-coded black (i.e., no flow). Also, as the Doppler beam sweeps across the imaging sector, it intersects the blood path at varying angles, causing a peculiar artifact in the color flow map. For example, if the blood flow in an artery is directed from left to right across the ultrasound sector, the color mapper will characterize the flow in the left side of the sector red (i.e., directed toward the transducer) and the blood flow in the right side of the sector blue (i.e., moving away from the transducer). Therefore, an image is created in which it appears as if the blood were colliding in the middle portion of the vessel (Figure 20.17).

Mirroring

This artifact appears in the spectral display as a symmetric duplication of the actual flow signal, but in the opposite direction (Figure 20.18). It is related to a process known as *quadrature phase demodulation,* which allows the echo system to separate the Doppler-shifted signal from the complex returning signal. The demodulation procedure uses a weaker signal that is generated out of phase with the broadcast signal. Excessive gain in the system causes the weak but incompletely canceled signal to be displayed as a mirror image of the actual flow signal.

Color Flow Reverberation and Gain-Related Anomalies

Reverberations are secondary reflections that occur when ultrasound is reflected a second time, typically from the transducer, highly reflective tissue, or intracardiac materials (e.g., a pulmonary artery catheter). The secondary reflection creates a ghost of the primary image that often appears at twice the distance of the actual target from the transducer. With Doppler reverberation, the reflected signal from a moving target is stronger than the original signal, so that the color intensity of the ghost is increased in comparison with that of the primary target (Figures 20.14 and 20.19).

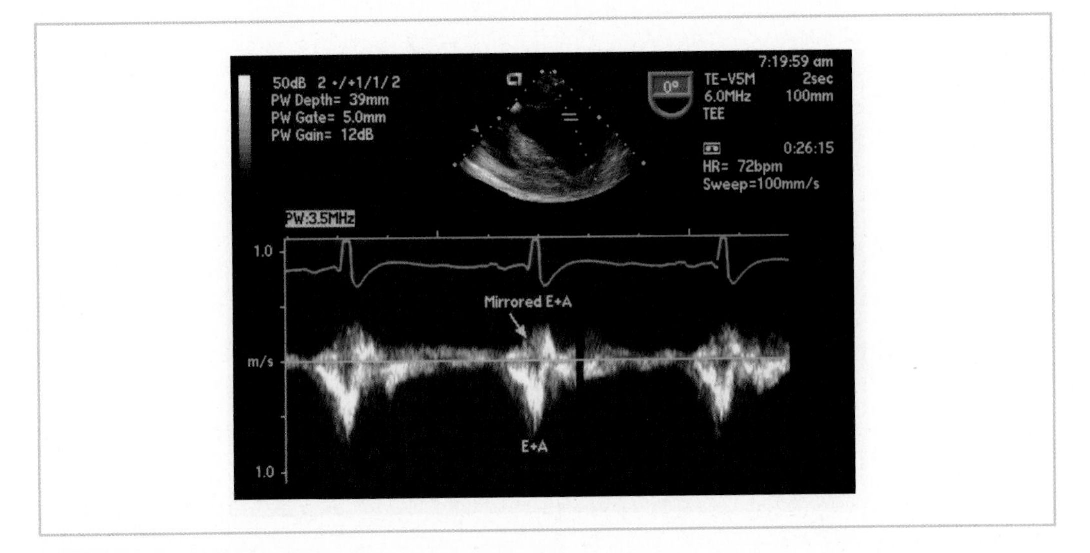

Figure 20.18. Pulsed wave Doppler mirroring artifact. Transmitral flow and its weaker mirrored signal.

Beam Width Flow Artifacts

Although we view the heart with echocardiography as a two-dimensional image, the image is actually created by three-dimensional ultrasound signals. Because the width of the ultrasound signal increases with the distance from the transducer, it becomes possible to detect structures or blood flow outside the displayed two-dimensional image. An example of this phenomenon is shown in Figure 20.20A, in which interrogation of the interventricular septum reveals high-velocity flow. This is not the result of a ventricular septal defect but an artifact caused by blood flow in the left ventricular outflow tract, which lies in a plane just anterior to the TG short-axis view seen in Figure 20.20B.

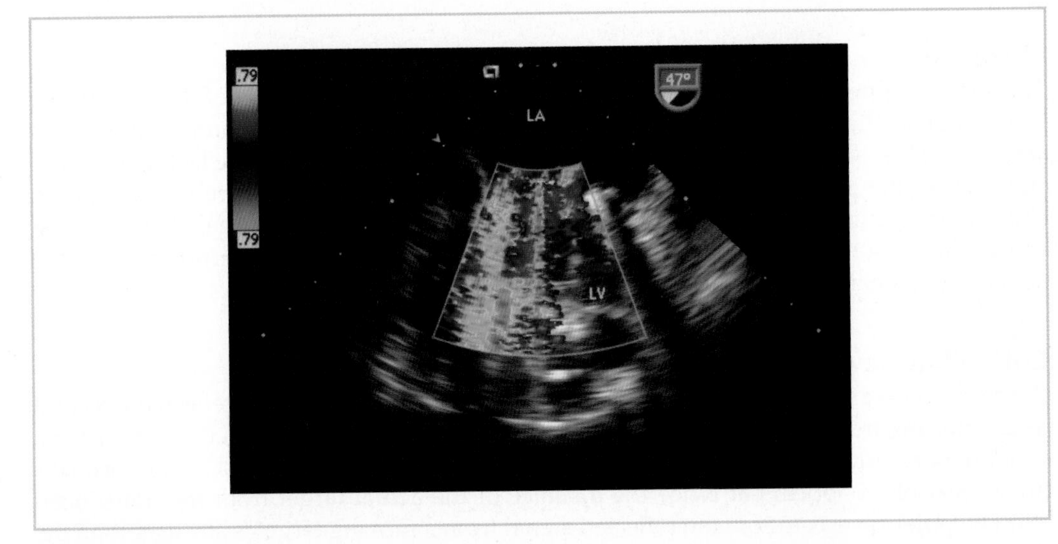

Figure 20.19. Color flow Doppler **reverberations** are seen distal to a mechanical mitral valve in this midesophageal commissural view. LA, left atrium; LV, left ventricle.

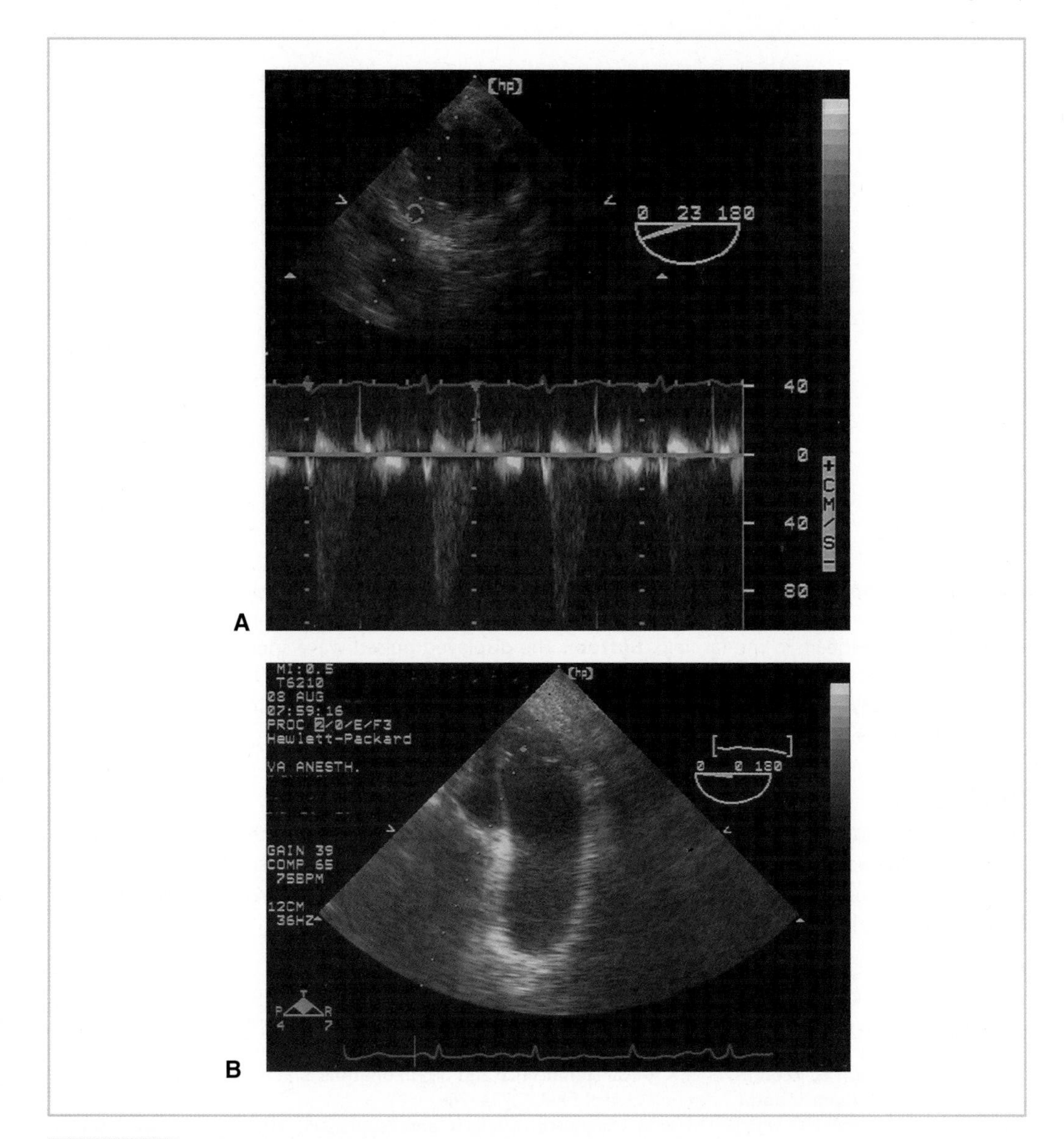

Figure 20.20. A: From the transgastric (TG) mid short-axis view, the pulsed wave sample volume is shown placed on the interventricular septum. Spectral signals show high-velocity flow during systole. This is not caused by an interventricular septal defect; rather, it is an artifact of blood flow from the adjacent left ventricular outflow tract (LVOT), which lies just anterior to the imaged plane. With slight anteroflexion of the probe, the LVOT is visualized in the deep TG long axis (**B**).

Range Ambiguity with Pulsed Wave Doppler

One of the main advantages of pulsed wave Doppler is the ability to range-gate a sample volume. However, strong reflected signals originating from blood flow at two or three times the depth of the pulsed wave sample volume arrive at the transducer simultaneously with those from the target. These signals are displayed and can be misinterpreted as blood flow within the target volume (Figure 20.21). Range ambiguity is particularly problematic with high pulse repetition frequency Doppler.

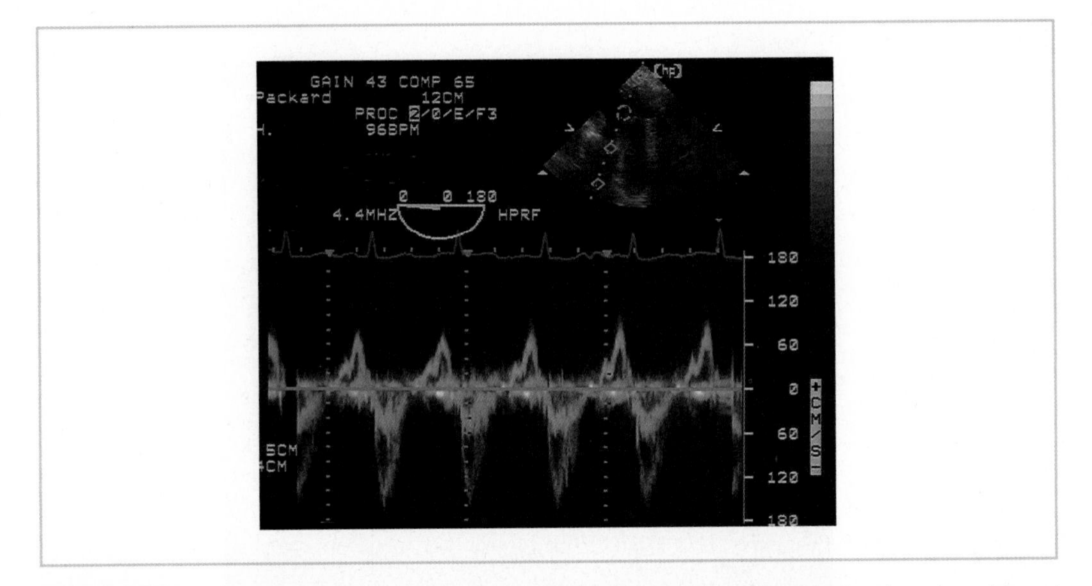

Figure 20.21. Top: In the deep transgastric long axis, the pulsed wave Doppler sample volume is positioned at the tips of the mitral valve leaflets. Note that the left ventricular outflow tract and ascending aorta lie in the path of the beam in the far field. **Bottom:** The displayed pulsed wave spectral signal shows not only diastolic flow through the mitral valve but also the left ventricular outflow tract and aortic blood flow velocities during systole. These measurements of the far field velocities are at exactly two and three times the distance to the primary measurement.

SUMMARY

An appreciation of cardiac embryology and anatomy will enable the echocardiographer to interpret cardiac structures with an unusual appearance accurately, so that unnecessary surgical intervention is prevented. A thorough understanding of two-dimensional and Doppler technologies is required to minimize misinterpretation.

SUGGESTED READINGS

Appelbe AF, Walker PG, Yeoh JK, et al. Clinical significance and origin of artifacts in transesophageal echocardiography of the thoracic aorta. *J Am Coll Cardiol* 1993;21:754–760.

Blanchard DG, Dittrich HC, Mitchell M, et al. Diagnostic pitfalls in transesophageal echocardiography. *J Am Soc Echocardiogr* 1992;5:525–540.

Cahalan MK. *Intraoperative transesophageal echocardiography. An interactive text and atlas*. New York: Churchill Livingstone, 1997.

Ducart AR, Broka SM, Collard EL. Linear reverberation in the ascending aorta: a cause of multiplane transesophageal echocardiographic artifact. *Anesthesiology* 1996;85:1497–1498.

Freeman WK, Seward JB, Khandheria BJ, et al. *Transesophageal echocardiography*. Boston: Little, Brown and Company, 1994.

Otto CM, Pearlman AS. *Textbook of clinical echocardiography*. Philadelphia: WB Saunders, 1995.

Seward JB, Khandheria BJ, Oh JK, et al. Critical appraisal of transesophageal echocardiography: limitations, pitfalls and complications. *J Am Soc Echocardiogr* 1992;5:288–305.

St. John Sutton MG, Oldershaw PJ, Kotler MN. *Textbook of echocardiography and Doppler in adults and children*, 2nd ed. Boston: Blackwell Science, 1996.

Stoddard MF, Liddell NE, Longaker RA, et al. Transesophageal echocardiography: normal variants and mimickers. *Am Heart J* 1992;124:1587–1598.

Weyman AE. *Principles and practice of echocardiography*, 2nd ed. Philadelphia: Lea & Febiger, 1994.

QUESTIONS

1. **What is the most common type of imaging artifact?**
   a. Acoustic shadowing
   b. Reverberation
   c. Suboptimal image quality
   d. Mirroring

2. **Acoustic shadowing will produce a dark area**
   a. Proximal to the strong reflector
   b. Distal to the strong reflector
   c. Left of the strong reflector
   d. Right of the strong reflector

3. **In most imaging systems, axial resolution is at least**
   a. Equal to lateral resolution
   b. Twice lateral resolution
   c. Ten times lateral resolution
   d. Half of lateral resolution

4. **Which of the following factors is not related to aliasing in spectral Doppler imaging?**
   a. Pulse repetition frequency
   b. Nyquist limit
   c. "Wraparound"
   d. Lateral resolution

5. **The crista terminalis is located in the**
   a. Right atrium
   b. Left atrium
   c. Right ventricle
   d. Left ventricle

6. **The moderator band is in the**
   a. Right atrium
   b. Left atrium
   c. Right ventricle
   d. Left ventricle

7. **Which of the following statements is not true of a lipomatous atrial septum?**
   a. It has a dumbbell shape.
   b. The fatty infiltration is echo-dense.
   c. The fossa ovalis is thickened.
   d. The fossa ovalis is spared.

8. **In an interrogation of flow with spectral Doppler, a nonparallel beam angle will**
   a. Overestimate the true velocity
   b. Underestimate the true velocity
   c. Correctly measure the velocity
   d. Spectral Doppler does not measure velocities

9. **Side lobe artifacts**
   a. Are true structures outside the path of the main beam
   b. Are incorrectly displayed in the two-dimensional sector

c. Are true structures in the path of the main beam
d. **a** and **b**

10. Reverberation artifacts will not produce
a. Multiple linear densities
b. Dual structures in an axial orientation
c. Dual structures in a left-right orientation
d. A duplication that is the same size as the original

Answers appear at the back of the book.

21 Techniques and Tricks for Optimizing Transesophageal Images

Herbert W. Dyal II, Michael D. Frith, and Scott T. Reeves

The accuracy and diagnostic confidence of a transesophageal echocardiographic (TEE) study depend greatly on the quality of the ultrasound image. Image quality is affected by several factors, including patient anatomy, the quality of the ultrasound system, and the skill of the echocardiographer. This chapter discusses the controls on the echocardiography machine and the process of optimizing their settings to obtain images of the highest quality.

TWO-DIMENSIONAL CONTROLS

Preprocessing versus Postprocessing Controls

Preprocessing controls adjust the transmission and acquisition of the ultrasound signals. Preprocessing settings control the formatting of the ultrasound signal for conversion into an electric signal. Changes in the preprocessing controls affect the information that the scanner will access to create an image (1), and this formatted information is the basis on which an image is created. Postprocessing settings affect the manner in which the formatted information is displayed on the monitor. Simply put, postprocessing defines the "cosmetic appearance" of the ultrasound data displayed on the monitor.

Transmit Power

Transmit power controls the amplitude (acoustic power) of the transmitted ultrasound signal. Modern echocardiography systems default to a high-power setting to maximize the signal-to-noise ratio. A theoretic concern is that high-power ultrasound can have deleterious effects on tissue, particularly in fetal echocardiography. Federal standards restrict the maximal intensities allowed for transmit power settings on commercially available ultrasound systems. Typically, echocardiography systems default to the maximum transmit power; however, proper adjustment of transmit power becomes critical when echo contrast studies are performed.

Gain

Increasing the gain increases the amplitude of the electric signal generated by returning ultrasound signals received at all depths. Unfortunately, any noise present is also amplified. Setting the gain too high or too low affects the ability to read the image correctly. When the gain is set too high, the image appears quite bright, and linear structures, such as the mitral valve, appear thickened. Increases in the gain also increase the amount of visible noise. For instance, with moderately excessive gain settings, the left ventricular (LV) cavity acquires a speckled appearance, which can make it difficult to differentiate the LV cavity from the myocardium. With further increases in the gain, the entire LV takes on a whitened appearance, and the ability to differentiate structures is lost.

When the gain is set too low, only bright signals, such as those from the pericardium, are visible, and very low-amplitude signals, such as the signal from an LV thrombus or

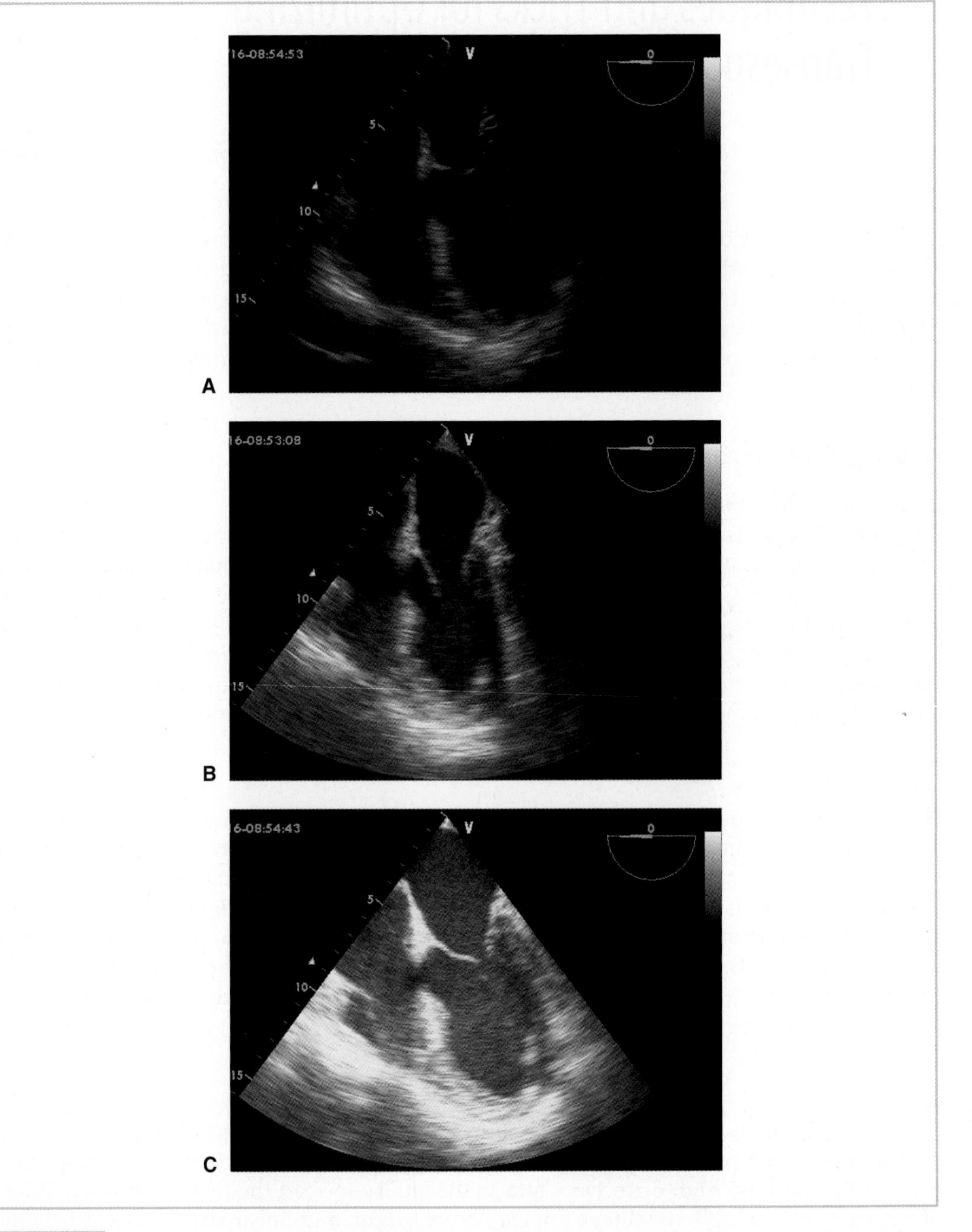

Figure 21.1. The midesophageal four-chamber view with the gain setting too low (**A**), normal (**B**), and too high (**C**).

"smoke" in the LV, are lost (2). Therefore, the gain should be adjusted to obtain an image with a gray scale ranging from low-amplitude (dark gray) to high-amplitude (white) signals. The gray scale, displayed as a bar graph on the right side of the image, is useful for guiding adjustments. Figure 21.1 demonstrates the effect of three separate gain settings on the same midesophageal (ME) four-chamber view.

CLINICAL PEARL

The bright ambient lighting of the operating room often misleads the echocardiographer to use excessive gain settings. This problem can be overcome by eliminating the operating room lights briefly during the examination or shielding the screen with a hood.

Time Gain Compensation

Because the amplitude of the reflected ultrasound depends on the distance traveled (depth) and the echogenicity of the tissue, the ability to adjust the gain setting selectively at each depth is essential to optimize the image. Time gain compensation allows the operator to adjust the gain at specific depths (3). For example, the echocardiographer can use the time gain compensation to amplify the weaker signals returning from the far field more than the signals returning from shallower depths (near field). The echocardiographer should be careful when adjusting the time gain compensation. If it is set too low, the elimination of true tissue signals is a risk. The time gain compensation should be used to eliminate gain-related artifacts and optimize far field structures. The effects of time gain compensation settings on image quality are shown in Figure 21.2.

CLINICAL PEARL

In a normal examination, the time gain compensation controls are set lower in the near field and higher in the far field. However, for imaging pathology in the near field with low echogenicity (e.g., thrombus in the aorta or left atrium), the near field time gain compensation should be increased.

Depth

This control selects the maximal distance to be displayed. Increasing depth beyond the structure of interest has several negative consequences.

1. ***The image size is reduced.*** The most obvious consequence is that the image size is reduced because a larger area of the cardiac anatomy must be displayed on a screen of fixed size. The display of the cardiac structure of interest will be smaller and therefore more difficult to evaluate.
2. ***The frame rate is lower.*** In addition, as the depth is increased, the frame rate of the two-dimensional ultrasound is slowed because the system must wait longer for signals to be received. Doubling the depth of penetration doubles the wait time before another pulse can be sent, so that the pulse repetition frequency and subsequently the frame rate are decreased (4).

Therefore, to optimize image display and temporal resolution, the depth should be set just beyond the structure of interest, as shown in Figure 21.3.

It must also be appreciated that the lateral resolution of the ultrasound system is inversely proportional to the depth. Therefore, it is practical to have the position of the probe as close as possible to the structure of interest. For example, when the leaflets of the aortic valve are being evaluated, the ME aortic valve short-axis view is preferable to the deep transgastric (TG) long-axis view because the probe is closer to the aortic valve and lateral resolution is improved.

CLINICAL PEARL

Resist increasing the depth beyond the setting that displays the structure of interest.

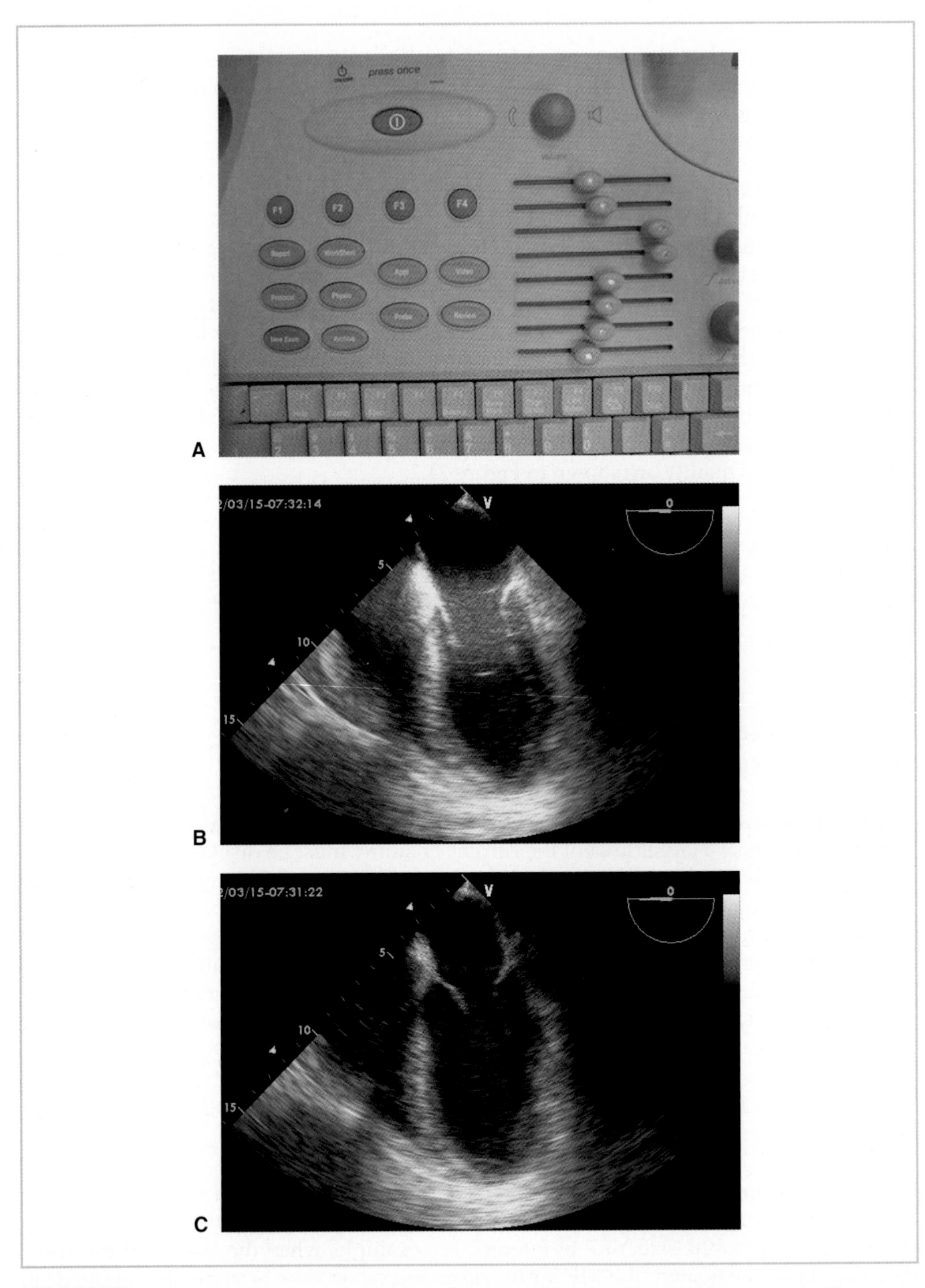

Figure 21.2. A: The time gain compensation is determined by a series of sliding controls. The upper controls affect the near field and the lower controls the far field. Note the high settings of the third and fourth controls and their effects on the midfield in **B**. **B:** The mitral valve apparatus is obscured by specular noise. **C:** The time gain compensation controls were subsequently reduced, after which the image quality improved markedly.

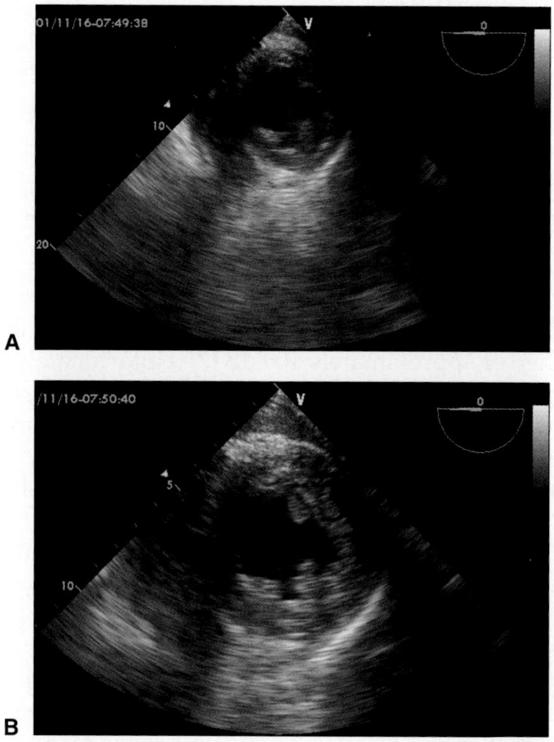

A

B

Figure 21.3. The transgastric mid short-axis view with too much depth **(A)** and with the depth correctly set **(B)**. Note that the focal point in image **(B)** is located at 5 cm, exactly in the center of the left ventricle. The focal point is marked with a *solid arrowhead.*

Focus

The focus control enables the operator to focus the ultrasound beam at a selected distance from the transducer. This is achieved by altering the sequences of electric impulses sent to the transducer elements. The goal of focusing is to have the beam narrowest at the location of the structure being evaluated because a thinner beam improves lateral resolution (5). The user must be cognizant of the focus depth of the system, which is typically marked on the edge of the sector (Figure 21.3). If the focal zone is located too far from the area of interest, the image resolution may not be sufficient for proper evaluation. When the atrial septum is being evaluated for a patent foramen ovale, the focus should be placed at this level. Remember that structures distal to the focal point lie in the far field and may appear "fuzzy" or abnormally thick. Avoid evaluating small structures distal to the focal point until the focal point is moved to that level.

CLINICAL PEARL

Adjust the focus point to the level of the structure of interest for high-resolution imaging.

Frequency

A feature of modern TEE systems is that they are capable of multiple frequencies, so that the transmitted ultrasound frequency can be adjusted. This can be especially important in TEE applications. When the structures being evaluated are in close proximity to the transducer (atria, aorta), higher frequencies are used to optimize resolution (6). When the structures being evaluated are farther from the transducer (deep TG views), higher frequencies may not be adequate because penetration is poor. In these situations, the frequency should be reduced until a satisfactory image is produced.

CLINICAL PEARL

Use higher frequencies when evaluating shallow structures and lower frequencies when evaluating deep structures (i.e., TG views).

Dynamic Range

Modern ultrasound transducers are capable of detecting reflected ultrasound signals with amplitudes over a range of approximately 100 dB (7). Unfortunately, the monitors used in these systems are capable of displaying only a much smaller range (~30 dB). Therefore, to display the range of ultrasound signals detected by the transducer, the dynamic range control allows the wide spectrum of ultrasound amplitudes to be compressed. The compressed signals are then displayed on the monitor as varying shades of gray.

Ultrasound systems have both a fixed dynamic range, which is limited by the hardware of the system, and a selectable dynamic range, which can be changed according to the echocardiographer's preference. Increasing the dynamic range of the system increases the number of shades of gray between black and white within the image and therefore increases image detail, so that a smoother image appears on the display screen. Decreasing the dynamic range of the system increases the contrast of the image, with more black and white areas than shades of gray. The effect of dynamic range on image quality is shown in Figure 21.4.

Compression

Compression is a postprocessing tool that in conjunction with the preprocessing dynamic range control setting alters the range of the displayed gray scale (8). The compression control changes how the given dynamic range of ultrasound data is displayed. When the compression control is reduced, the given dynamic range is displayed with the largest range of allowable shades of gray. The lowest-intensity signal is displayed as black, and the highest-intensity signal is displayed as white. As the compression control is increased, the range of shades of gray used to produce the image is reduced to produce a softer, smoother image. The gray scale is therefore compressed by eliminating the display of shades of gray at each end of the spectrum. Compression settings are a personal preference of the echocardiographer.

Reject

In the early stages of ultrasound development, it was discovered that ultrasound transducers detect many sources of low-level interference from within the body. Examples include movement artifacts, the electronic noise of equipment, such as ventilators, and aberrant ultrasound resulting from refraction of the ultrasound signal. These low-level signals are detected by the scanner and displayed in the image as "noise." To eliminate such signals, all ultrasound systems have a fixed or default "filter" that removes any signal below a certain amplitude threshold (the lower limit of the displayed dynamic range) (9). Sometimes, the default filter is not enough to remove the noise in an image. The reject control is an adjustable control that enables the user to eliminate a greater number of

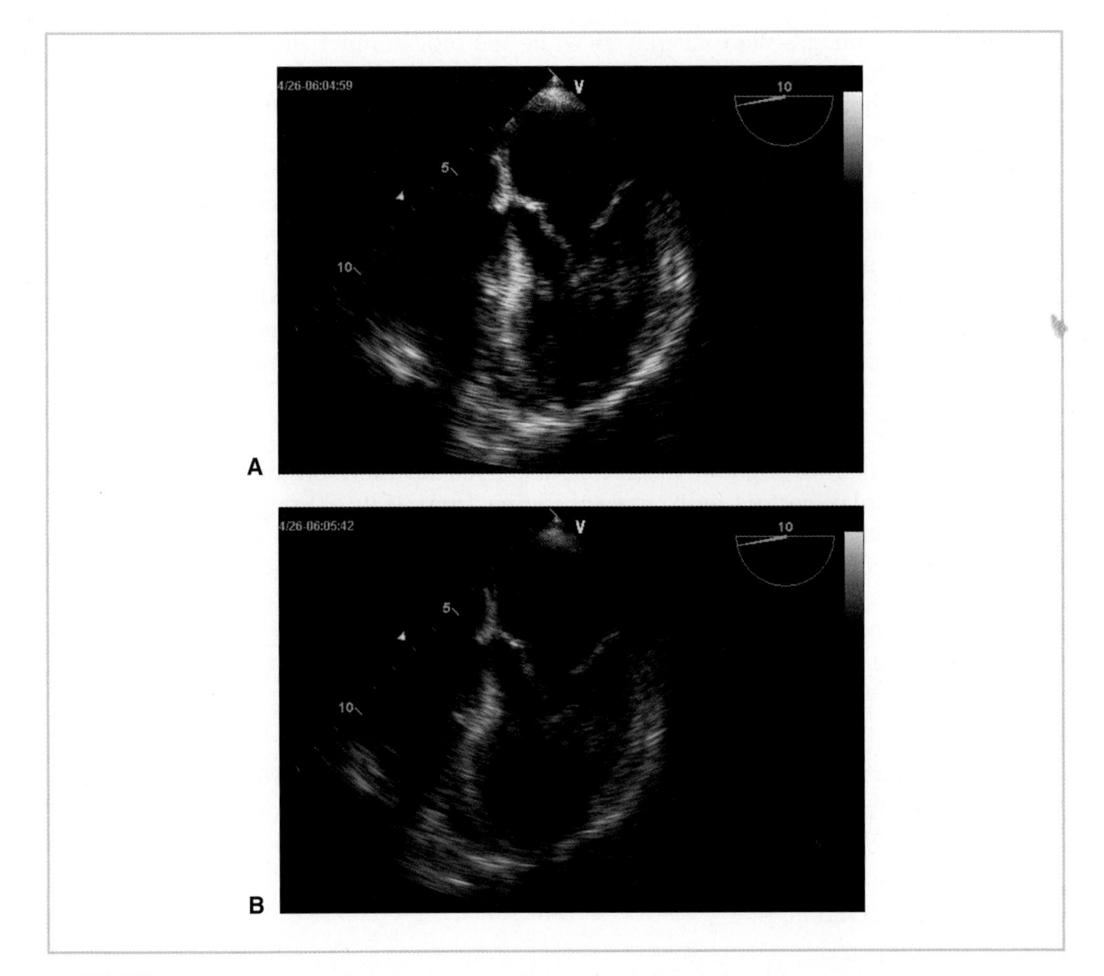

Figure 21.4. A partial midesophageal four-chamber view concentrating on the left atrium and left ventricle. **A:** The dynamic range is set too low. Note the increased contrast in the image, with more black and white than shades of gray. **B:** The same image with the proper dynamic range setting.

low-intensity signals. The reject control is used to eliminate signals that are usually located in blood pools and are a result of artifacts. When the reject control is adjusted, care must be taken not to eliminate important low-intensity echoes from certain pathologic conditions. Specifically, fresh thrombi within a cardiac chamber or vessel have a low-intensity (dark) signal that may be eliminated from the image if the reject is set too high.

CLINICAL PEARL

Increase the reject control to eliminate noise (random echoes often found in blood pools and other low-intensity areas). Do not use excessive reject because low-intensity echoes such as thrombi may be removed from the image.

Persistence

Persistence is a postprocessing control that can best be described as signal averaging or image blending. The term is derived from earlier ultrasound systems that used cathode ray tubes for display. After the phosphor elements in the tube were illuminated to form an image, rather than disappearing instantly, the luminescence faded gradually (or persisted).

As a result, new images were displayed while the old, dimmer image was still on the screen (10). With the advent of digital scan converters and the replacement of cathode ray tubes with modern monitors, the term *persistence* is now used for frame averaging in the digital scan converter. As incoming signals are processed by the system, images are displayed as they are created in their purest form (no persistence), or the system can average one image with the next and display the averaged image. Persistence is used to smooth the appearance of the heart in motion. As the persistence control is increased, more images are used to create the averaged image, and temporal and spatial resolution is decreased. If the persistence is set too high, the image is often described as appearing to be in "slow motion." Because valvular structures move rapidly, persistence is usually set low in echocardiographic applications to retain temporal resolution and a real-time appearance.

Sector Size

Sector size controls the angle of the sector displayed on the monitor. Most ultrasound scanners can display sectors with angles ranging from 15 to 90 degrees. Wide angles allow the operator to survey a broad array of cardiac structures in a single view. The most important effect of the sector size is on the frame rate. The wider the sector size, the lower the frame rate and the temporal resolution. For a proper evaluation of fast-moving structures, the sector size should be kept small to allow for higher frame rates. Some scanning systems do not depend on sector size for high frame rates and can achieve adequate frame rates with a full 90-degree sector.

CLINICAL PEARL

Larger sector sizes result in lower frame rates and a lower level of temporal resolution. When valvular structures are evaluated, it is helpful to decrease the sector size (or use motion mode [M-mode]) to improve the frame rates.

COLOR CONTROLS

Region of Interest

The region of interest is the area that defines where the color will be displayed. There are certain limitations to setting the size of the region of interest. As the width of the region of interest increases, the frame rate decreases (11). The goal is to optimize the frame rate to improve temporal resolution and the assessment of blood flow. The depth also affects the color frame rate. As the depth increases, the system must wait longer for the returning signal; therefore, the frame rate is slower.

Color Gain

Color gain is similar to two-dimensional gain in that it increases or amplifies the signal generated by the returning echoes. It is very important to have the color gain set properly. If the gain is set too low, a small jet, such as a small atrial septal defect or patent foramen ovale, can be missed. If the gain is set too high, the size of a regurgitant jet is frequently overestimated. The color gain is adjusted simply by increasing the color gain control until speckles of color lay outside the blood pools and then decreasing the gain one to two settings until the speckles go away. Figure 21.5 shows different color gain settings.

Color Scale

The color scale is the range of color velocities displayed. To optimize the color scale, one must be cognizant of the general velocities of the blood flow being evaluated. For example,

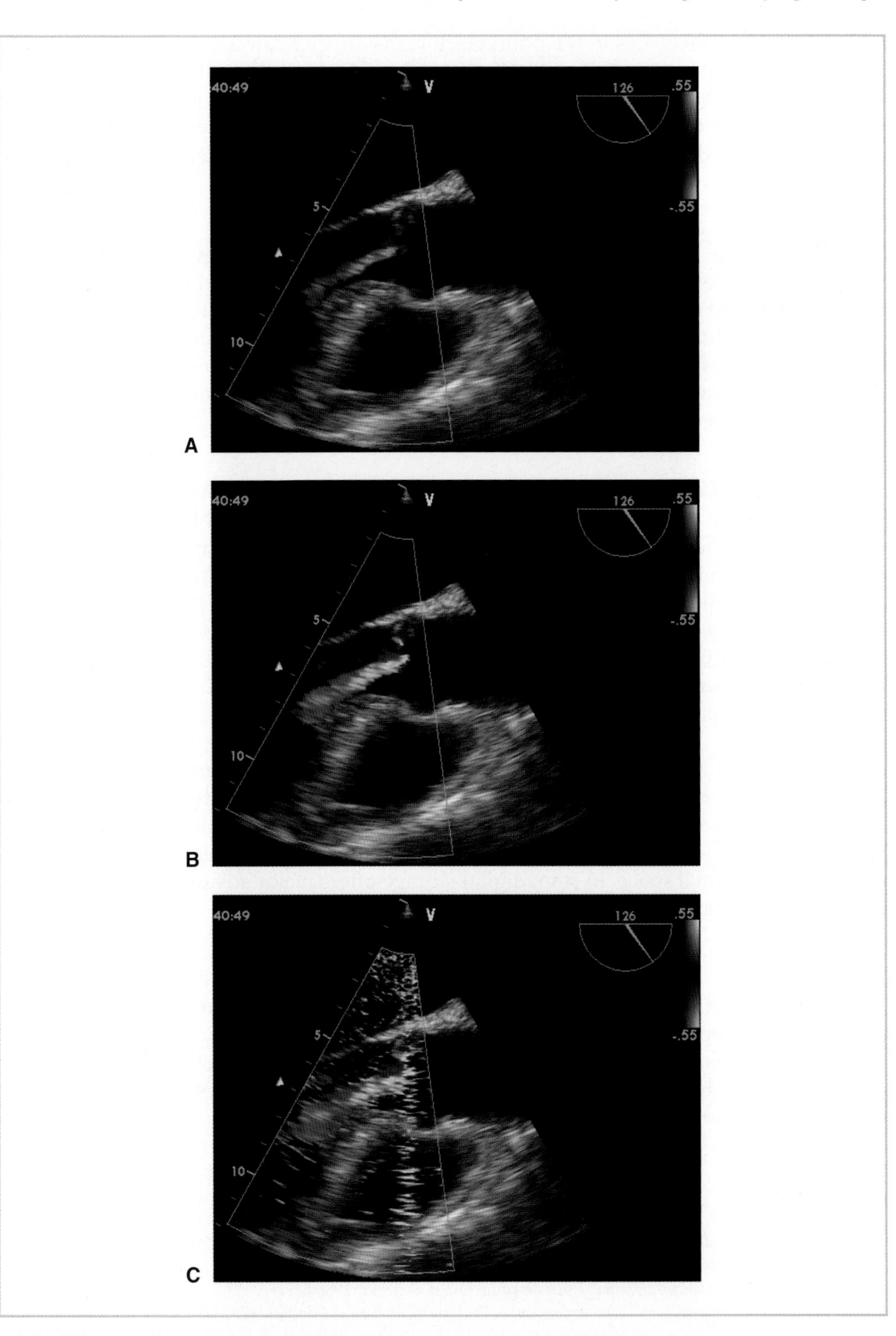

Figure 21.5. Midesophageal aortic valve long-axis view in a patient with aortic insufficiency. **A:** The color gain is set too low, so that the width of the aortic insufficiency jet is underestimated. **B:** The color gain is correctly set. **C:** The color gain is too high.

when lower-flow velocities in the pulmonary veins are evaluated, one must decrease the color scale. Adjusting the scale will affect the Nyquist limit. Velocities sampled outside this range cause aliasing within the color display. In certain applications, such as when the proximal isovelocity surface area (PISA) is calculated, adjusting the color scale to produce aliasing is required to create an adequate flow convergence hemisphere for measurement.

Variance

The variance color flow map displays the range of velocities in any given sample volume. The variance in flow is displayed as shades of green, whereas normal flows are displayed with the standard red-blue color flow map. In laminar flow, the range of velocities in a given sample volume is relatively small, and laminar flow appears color-coded as red or blue. In turbulent flow, the number of velocities is increased (i.e., increased variance) such that turbulent flow is color-coded as green (12). A variance map may help to identify a small turbulent jet by tagging it with a different (i.e., green) color.

STORAGE SYSTEMS: ANALOG VIDEOTAPE VERSUS DIGITAL STORAGE

The advantages of videotape storage are its availability and reasonable cost. It is the most common storage format used currently. A patient's study can be reviewed anywhere a videocassette recorder is available. A shortcoming is that it is difficult to archive and retrieve studies, and to directly compare different studies of the same patient. For example, if a patient has an LV ejection fraction of 40% on one examination and on a subsequent examination a value of 30% is reported, it is essential to determine whether this represents deterioration in function or differences in interpretation. With digital technology, a direct side-by-side comparison can be performed.

Current digital technology also allows the study data to be manipulated. The reviewer can adjust the *postprocessing* controls, including contrast, brightness, and two-dimensional and Doppler gain. It is also possible to make measurements from stored images without having to recalibrate the system. Finally, optical storage media make it practical to house large databases in minimal space. In sum, digital storage offers major advantages for archiving, retrieving, and sharing echocardiographic studies.

SUMMARY

The extensive control options of modern full-platform echocardiography systems provide the echocardiographer with tools for reliably obtaining high-quality images under a broad range of conditions. With a firm understanding of the control settings available, the examiner can optimize image acquisition and display and detect pathology that might otherwise be missed.

REFERENCES

1 Marcus ML, Schelbert HR, Skorton DJ, et al., *Cardiac imaging—a companion to Braunwald's "heart disease"*. Philadelphia: WB Saunders, 1991:363.
2 Feigenbaum H. *Echocardiography*. Philadelphia: Lea & Febiger, 1986:57.
3 Weyman AE. *Cross-sectional echocardiography*. Philadelphia: Lea & Febiger, 1982:26.
4 Weyman AE. *Principles and practice of echocardiography*. Philadelphia: Lea & Febiger, 1994:219.
5 Thrush A, Hartshorne T. *Peripheral vascular ultrasound how, why, and when*. London: Churchill Livingstone, 1999:17–18.
6 Weyman AE. *Cross-sectional echocardiography*. Philadelphia: Lea & Febiger, 1982:17.

7 Weyman AE. *Principles and practice of echocardiography*. Philadelphia: Lea & Febiger, 1994:49–50.
8 Hagen-Ansert SL. *Textbook of diagnostic ultrasonography*. St. Louis: Mosby, 1989:38–39.
9 Feigenbaum H. *Echocardiography*. Philadelphia: Lea & Febiger, 1986:23.
10 Weyman AE. *Cross-sectional echocardiography*. Philadelphia: Lea & Febiger, 1982:55.
11 Thrush A, Hartshorne T. *Peripheral vascular ultrasound how, why, and when*. London: Churchill Livingstone, 1999:42.
12 Weyman AE. *Principles and practice of echocardiography*. Philadelphia: Lea & Febiger, 1994:225–226.

QUESTIONS

1. The left ventricle (LV) appears very small on the screen. Which control would you adjust to make it appear larger on the screen?

a. Increase frequency
b. Decrease frequency
c. Increase depth
d. Decrease depth

2. When obtaining a deep transgastric (TG) long-axis view, how would you adjust the frequency of the transducer to increase the penetration?

a. Increase frequency
b. Decrease frequency
c. The frequency does not affect penetration

3. What effect does increasing the sector size have on an image?

a. Increases the resolution
b. Increases the frame rate
c. Decreases the frame rate
d. Has no effect

4. There is too much aliasing in the color Doppler display. Which control would you adjust to decrease the amount of aliasing in the display?

a. Increase depth
b. Decrease depth
c. Increase the scale/pulse repetition frequency
d. Decrease the scale/pulse repetition frequency

5. Which control is best used to adjust the brightness of the image at a specific depth?

a. Time gain compensation
b. Gain
c. Depth
d. Power

6. Which color map will help to identify a turbulent flow pattern?

a. Red-blue
b. Low flow
c. Mosaic
d. Variance

7. Which control is best used to filter out low-level noise from the two-dimensional or Doppler image?

a. Reject
b. Gain
c. Dynamic range
d. Compression

8. Which method of storage best allows the user to manipulate data after the study?

a. Videocassette recorder tape
b. Digital storage
c. It is not possible to manipulate an image after it has been saved

9. Which of the following is a preprocessing control?

a. Persistence
b. Transmit power

c. Contrast
d. Color gain

10. When reviewing a study obtained in the operating room, your colleagues in the echocardiography laboratory comment that the image is too bright. What can be done in the future to optimize image quality?

a. Decrease the gain settings.
b. Turn off the operating room lights briefly while the transesophageal echocardiographic (TEE) examination is performed.
c. Shield the monitor with a hood.
d. All of the above.

Answers appear at the back of the book.

Appendices

A Transesophageal Echocardiographic Anatomy

ME Asc aortic SAX	Probe adjustment: neutral	Sector depth: ~6 cm
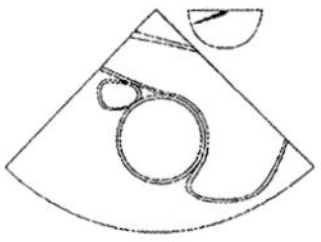	**Primary diagnostic issues** Aortic atherosclerosis Aortic dissection Pulmonary artery pathology (emboli, dilation, other)	**Required structures** Aorta in cross section in transverse plane (0 degree) Pulmonary artery (main and proximal right)
ME Asc aortic LAX	Probe adjustment: neutral	Sector depth: ~6 cm
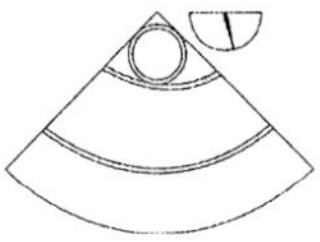	**Primary diagnostic issues** Aortic atherosclerosis Aortic dissection	**Required structures** Ascending aorta in long axis Right pulmonary artery in cross section
UE aortic arch SAX	Probe adjustment: neutral	Sector depth: ~6 cm
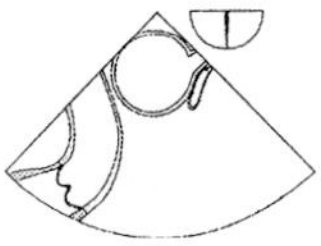	**Primary diagnostic issues** Aortic atherosclerosis Aortic dissection Pulmonic valve	**Required structures** Aortic arch in cross section Main pulmonary artery (often not well seen)
UE aortic arch LAX	Probe adjustment: rightward	Sector depth: ~6 cm
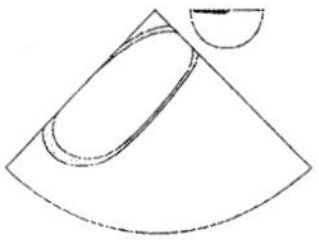	**Primary diagnostic issues** Aortic atherosclerosis Aortic dissection Visualization of aortic cannulation site	**Required structures** Distal ascending aortal/aortic arch
Desc aortic SAX	Probe adjustment: neutral	Sector depth: ~6 cm
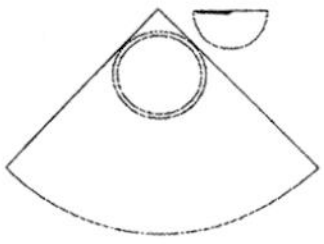	**Primary diagnostic issue** Aortic atherosclerosis Aortic dissection	**Required structures** Descending aorta in cross section in transverse plane (0 degree)
Desc aortic LAX	Probe adjustment: neutral	Sector depth: ~6 cm
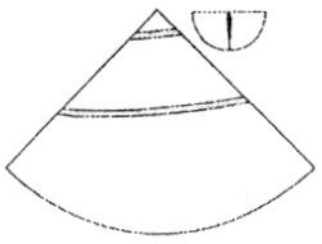	**Primary diagnostic issues** Aortic atherosclerosis Aortic dissection	**Required structures** Descending aorta in long axis in longitudinal plane (90 degrees)

(continued)

ME AV SAX	Probe adjustment: neutral	Sector depth: ~10 cm
	Primary diagnostic issue Aortic stenosis Valvular morphology	**Required structures** Three leaflets Commissures Coaptation point
ME RV inflow–outflow	Probe adjustment: neutral	Sector depth: ~10 cm
	Primary diagnostic issues Pulmonic valve disease Pulmonary artery pathology RVOT pathology Doppler evaluation of tricuspid valve	**Required structures** Pulmonic valve Tricuspid valve Main pulmonary artery (at least 1 cm distal to the pulmonic valve) RVOT (at least 1 cm proximal to the pulmonic valve)
ME AV LAX	Probe adjustment: neutral	Sector depth: ~10 cm
	Primary diagnostic issues Aortic valve pathology Aortic pathology (ascending and root) LVOT pathology Anterior leaflet mitral valve	**Required structures** LVOT (at least 1 cm proximal to the aortic valve) Aortic valve (visualized cusps approximately equal in size) Ascending aorta (at least 1 cm distal to the sinotubular junction)
ME bicaval	Probe adjustment: neutral	Sector depth: ~10 cm
	Primary diagnostic issues Atrial septal defect Tumor Retrograde venous cannula positioning	**Required structures** RA free wall (or appendage) Superior vena cava (at least its entry into the RA) Interatrial septum
ME four-chamber	Probe adjustment: neutral-retroflex	Sector depth: ~14 cm
	Primary diagnostic issues Atrial septal defect Chamber enlargement dysfunction Mitral disease Tricuspid disease Detection of intracardiac air	**Required structures** LA LV Mitral valve Tricuspid valve (maximal annular dimension)

ME two-chamber	Probe adjustment: neutral	Sector depth: ~14 cm
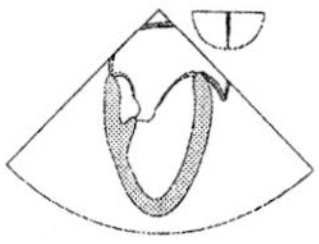	**Primary diagnostic issues** LA appendage Mass/thrombus LV apex pathology LV systolic dysfunction (apical segments)	**Required structures** LA appendage Mitral valve LV apex (i.e., maximal LV length)
ME LAX	Probe adjustment: neutral	Sector depth: ~12 cm
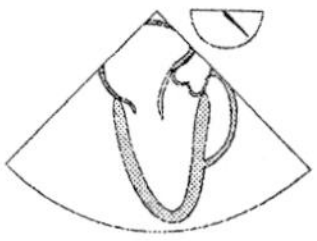	**Primary diagnostic issues** Mitral valve pathology LVOT pathology	**Required structures** LV Mitral valve LVOT
ME mitral commissural	Probe adjustment: neutral	Sector depth: ~12 cm
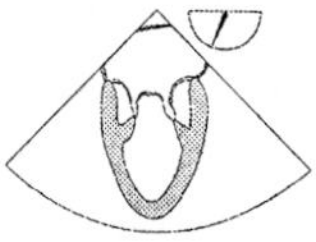	**Primary diagnostic issues** Localization of mitral valve pathology	**Required structures** Mitral valve (P_1, P_3, and A_2 scallops) Papillary muscles/chordae tendineae LA LV
TG mid-SAX	Probe adjustment: neutral	Sector depth: ~12 cm
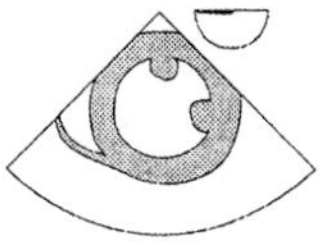	**Primary diagnostic issues** Hemodynamic instability LV enlargement LV hypertrophy LV systolic dysfunction (global and regional)	**Required structures** LV cavity LV walls (at least 50% of circumference with visible endocardium) Papillary muscles (approximately equal in size and distinct from ventricular wall)
TG two-chamber	Probe adjustment: neutral	Sector depth: ~12 cm
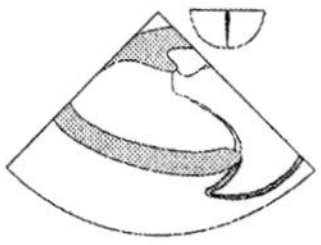	**Primary diagnostic issues** LV systolic dysfunction (anterior and inferior basal segments)	**Required structures** Mitral leaflets Mitral subvalvular apparatus LV (anterior and inferior: basal plus mild segments)

(continued)

TG RV inflow	Probe adjustment: neutral-rightward	Sector depth: ~12 cm
	Primary diagnostic issues RV systolic dysfunction Tricuspid valve pathology	**Required structures** Tricuspid leaflets Tricuspid subvalvular apparatus
TG RV inflow–outflow	Probe adjustment: neutral-rightward	Sector depth: ~14 cm
	Primary diagnostic issues RV systolic dysfunction RVOT pathology Pulmonary artery pathology Pulmonic valve evaluation	**Required structures** RA RV Main pulmonary artery Pulmonic valve
TG basal SAX	Probe adjustment: neutral	Sector depth: ~12 cm
	Primary diagnostic issues LV systolic dysfunction (basal segments) Mitral valve pathology	**Required structures** Mitral leaflets Mitral subvalvular apparatus LV (basal segments)
TG LAX	Probe adjustment: neutral-leftward	Sector depth: ~12 cm
	Primary diagnostic issues LV systolic dysfunction (anteroseptal and posterior: basal segments) Doppler evaluation of aortic valve	**Required structures** Mitral leaflets Mitral subvalvular apparatus LV (anteroseptal and posterior: basal plus midsegments) Aortic valve
Deep TG LAX	Probe adjustment: neutral	Sector depth: ~16 cm
	Primary diagnostic issues Aortic valve pathology LVOT pathology Doppler evaluation of aortic valve	**Required structures** LV Aortic valve Aorta

ME, midesophageal; Asc, ascending; SAX, short axis; LAX, long axis; UE, upper esophageal; Desc, descending; AV, aortic valve; RV, right ventricular; LVOT, left ventricular outflow tract; RA, right atrium; LA, left atrium; LV, left ventricular; RVOT, right ventricular outflow tract; TG, transgastric.

Modified from Miller JP, Lambert SA, Shapiro WA, et al. The adequacy of basic intraoperative transesophageal echocardiography performed by experienced anesthesiologists. *Anesth Analg* 2001;92:1103–1110, with permission.

B Cardiac Dimensions

Table B.1 Reference values for normal adult TEE measurements

Parameter		Mean ± SD (mm)	Range (mm)
	Right pulmonary artery diameter[a]	17 ± 3	12–22
	Left upper pulmonary vein diameter	11 ± 2	7–16
Left atrial appendage	Length	28 ± 5	15–43
	Diameter	16 ± 5	10–28
	Superior vena cava diameter	15 ± 3	8–20
	Right ventricular outflow tract diameter[b]	27 ± 4	16–36
Left atrium[c]	Anteroposterior diameter	38 ± 6	20–52
	Medial-lateral diameter	39 ± 7	24–52
Right atrium[c]	Anteroposterior diameter	38 ± 5	28–52
	Medial-lateral diameter	38 ± 6	29–53
	Tricuspid annular diameter[c]	28 ± 5	20–40
	Mitral annular diameter[c]	29 ± 4	20–38
	Coronary sinus diameter	6.6 ± 1.5	4–10
Left ventricle[d]	Anteroposterior diameter (diastole)	43 ± 7	33–55
	Medial-lateral diameter (diastole)	42 ± 7	23–54
	Anteroposterior diameter (systole)	28 ± 6	18–40
	Medial-lateral diameter (systole)	27 ± 6	18–42
	Aortic root diameter[b]	28 ± 3	21–34
Descending thoracic aorta diameter	Proximal	21 ± 4	14–30
	Distal	20 ± 4	13–28

[a]Right pulmonary artery diameter measured in midesophageal ascending aorta short-axis view.
[b]Aortic root and right ventricular outflow tract diameters measured in the midesophageal right ventricular inflow/outflow tract view.
[c]Atrial (end-systole) and both mitral and tricuspid annular (mid-diastole) diameters measured in the midesophageal four-chamber view.
[d]Left ventricular dimensions measured in transgastric mid short-axis view.
SD, standard deviation.
Adapted from Cohen G, White M, Sochowski R, et al. Reference values for normal transesophageal measurements. *J Am Soc Echocardiogr* 1995;8:221–230.

Hemodyamic Calculations

Table C.1 Estimation of hemodynamic pressures

Pressure estimated	Required measurement	Formula	Normal values (mm Hg)
CVP	Respiratory IVC collapse (spontaneously breathing)	$\geq$40% $<$10 mm Hg	
Right ventricular systolic pressure (RVSP)	Peak $velocity_{TR}$ CVP estimated or measured	$RVSP = 4(v_{TR})^2 + CVP$ (No PS)	16–30 mm Hg
RV systolic pressure (with VSD)	Systemic systolic blood pressure (SBP) Peak v_{LV-RV}	$RVSP = SBP - 4(v_{LV-RV})^2$ (No AS or LVOT obstruction)	Usually $>$50 mm Hg
Pulmonary artery systolic (PASP)	Peak $velocity_{TR}$ CVP estimated or measured)	$PASP = 4(v_{TR})^2 + CVP$ (no PS)	16–30 mm Hg
Pulmonary artery diastolic (PAD)	End diastolic $Velocity_{PR}$ CVP estimated or measured	$PAEDP = 4(v_{PR\ ED})^2 + CVP$	0–8 mm Hg
Pulmonary artery mean (PAM)	Acceleration time (AT) to peak V_{PA} (in m/s)	$PAM = (-0.45)\ AT + 79$	10–16 mm Hg
RV dP/dt	TR spectral envelope $T_{TR\ (2\ m/s)} - T_{TR\ (1\ m/s)}$	$RV\ dP = 4v^2_{TR\ (2\ m/s)} - 4v^2_{TR\ (1\ m/s)}$ $RV\ dP/dt = dP/T_{TR\ (2\ m/s)} - T_{TR\ (1\ m/s)}$	$>$150 mm Hg/ms
Left atrial systolic (LASP)	Peak v_{MR} SBP	$LASP = SBP - 4(v_{MR})^2$ (No AS or LVOT obstruction)	3–15 mm Hg
LA (PFO)	$Velocity_{PFO}$ CVP estimated or measured	$LAP = 4(v_{PFO})^2 + CVP$	3–15 mm Hg
LV diastolic (LVEDP)	End diastolic $Velocity_{AR}$ Diastolic blood pressure (DBP)	$LVEDP = DBP - 4(v_{AR})^2$	3–12 mm Hg
LV dP/dt	MR spectral envelope $T_{MR\ (3\ m/s)} - T_{MR\ (1\ m/s)}$	$LV\ dP = 4v^2_{MR\ (3\ m/s)} - 4v^2_{MR\ (1\ m/s)}$ $LV\ dP/dt = dP/T_{MR\ (3\ m/s)} - T_{MR\ (1\ m/s)}$	$>$1000 mm Hg/ms

CVP, central venous pressure; IVC, inferior vena cava; RV, right ventricle; Dysfx, dysfunction; TR, tricuspid regurgitation; PS, pulmonary stenosis; VSD, ventricular septal defect; LV, left ventricle; AS, atrial stenosis; LVOT, left ventricular outflow tract; PAEDP, pulmonary artery end-diastolic pressure; PR ED, pulmonary regurgitation end diastolic; PA, pulmonary artery; MR, mitral regurgitation; LA, left atrium; PFO, patent foramen ovale; AR, aortic regurgitation.

D Valve Prostheses

Table D.1 Normal Doppler echocardiographic values of aortic valve prosthesis

Valve	Size	n	Peak gradient (mm Hg)	Mean gradient (mm Hg)	Peak velocity (m/s)	Effective orifice area (cm^2)
ATS open pivot AP	16	6	47.7 ± 12	27 ± 7.3	3.44 ± 0.47	0.61 ± 0.09
ATS open pivot	19	9	47 ± 12.6	26.2 ± 7.9	3.41 ± 0.43	0.96 ± 0.18
(bileaflet)	21	15	25.5 ± 6.1	14.4 ± 3.5	2.4 ± 0.39	1.58 ± 0.37
	23	8	19 ± 7	12 ± 4		1.8 ± 0.2
	25	12	17 ± 8	11 ± 4		2.2 ± 0.4
	27	10	14 ± 4	9 ± 2		2.5 ± 0.3
	29	5	11 ± 3	8 ± 2		3.1 ± 0.3
Biocor stentless	21	45	35.97 ± 4.06	18 ± 4		
(stentless	23	115	29.15 ± 8.28	18.64 ± 7.14	3 ± 0.6	1.4 ± 0.5
bioprosthesis)	25	100	28.65 ± 6.6	17.72 ± 6.99	2.8 ± 0.5	1.6 ± 0.38
	27	55	25.87 ± 2.81	18 ± 2.8	2.7 ± 0.2	1.9 ± 0.46
	≥29	16	24 ± 2			
Biocor extended	19–21	12	17.5 ± 5.8	9.7 ± 3.5		1.3 ± 0.4
stentless (stentless	23	18	14.8 ± 5.9	8.1 ± 3.1		1.6 ± 0.3
bioprosthesis)	25	20	14.2 ± 3.5	7.7 ± 1.9		1.8 ± 0.3
Bioflo pericardial	19	16	37.25 ± 8.65	24.15 ± 5.1		0.77 ± 0.11
(stented	21	9	28.7 ± 6.2	18.7 ± 5.5		1.1 ± 0.1
bioprosthesis)	23	4	20.7 ± 4	12.5 ± 3		1.3 ± 0.09
Björk-Shiley	19	37	46.0	26.67 ± 7.87	3.3 ± 0.6	0.94 ± 0.19
monostrut (tilting	21	161	32.41 ± 9.73	18.64 ± 6.09	2.9 ± 0.4	
disk)	23	153	26.52 ± 9.67	14.5 ± 6.2	2.7 ± 0.5	
	25	89	22.33 ± 7	13.3 ± 4.96	2.5 ± 0.4	
	27	61	18.31 ± 8	10.41 ± 4.38	2.1 ± 0.4	
	29	9	12 ± 8	7.67 ± 4.36	1.9 ± 0.2	
Björk-Shiley spherical	17	1			4.1	
(tilting disk) or not	19	2	27.0	21.8 ± 3.4	3.8	1.1
specified	21	18	38.94 ± 11.93	17.34 ± 6.86	2.92 ± 0.88	1.1 ± 0.25
	23	41	33.86 ± 11	11.5 ± 4.55	2.42 ± 0.4	1.22 ± 0.23
	25	39	20.39 ± 7.07	10.67 ± 4.31	2.06 ± 0.28	1.8 ± 0.32
	27	23	19.44 ± 7.99		1.77 ± 0.12	2.6
	29	5	21.1 ± 7.1		1.87 ± 0.18	2.52 ± 0.69
	31	2			2.1 ± 0.14	
Carbomedics	17	7	33.4 ± 13.2	20.1 ± 7.1		1.02 ± 0.2
(bileaflet)	19	63	33.3 ± 11.19	11.61 ± 5.08	3.09 ± 0.38	1.25 ± 0.36
	21	111	26.31 ± 10.25	12.68 ± 4.29	2.61 ± 0.51	1.42 ± 0.36
	23	120	24.61 ± 6.93	11.33 ± 3.8	2.42 ± 0.37	1.69 ± 0.29
	25	103	20.25 ± 8.69	9.34 ± 4.65	2.25 ± 0.34	2.04 ± 0.37
	27	57	19.05 ± 7.04	8.41 ± 2.83	2.18 ± 0.36	2.55 ± 0.34
	29	6	12.53 ± 4.69	5.8 ± 3.2	1.93 ± 0.25	2.63 ± 0.38

(Continued)

Table D.1 *(Continued)*

Valve	Size	*n*	Peak gradient (mm Hg)	Mean gradient (mm Hg)	Peak velocity (m/s)	Effective orifice area (cm^2)
Carbomedics reduced (bileaflet)	19	10	43.4 ± 1.8	24.4 ± 1.2		1.22 ± 0.08
Carbomedics supraannular top hat (bileaflet)	19	4	29.04 ± 10.1	19.5 ± 2.12	1.8	1 ± 0.18
	21	30	29.61 ± 8.93	16.59 ± 5.79	2.62 ± 0.35	1.18 ± 0.33
	23	30	24.38 ± 7.53	13.29 ± 3.73	2.36 ± 0.55	1.37 ± 0.37
	25	1	22.0	11.0	2.4	
Carpentier-Edwards (stented bioprosthesis)	19	56	43.48 ± 12.72	25.6 ± 8.02		0.85 ± 0.17
	21	73	27.73 ± 7.6	17.25 ± 6.24	2.37 ± 0.54	1.48 ± 0.3
	23	100	28.93 ± 7.49	15.92 ± 6.43	2.76 ± 0.4	1.69 ± 0.45
	25	85	23.95 ± 7.05	12.76 ± 4.43	2.38 ± 0.47	1.94 ± 0.45
	27	50	22.14 ± 8.24	12.33 ± 5.59	2.31 ± 0.39	2.25 ± 0.55
	29	24	22.0	9.92 ± 2.9	2.44 ± 0.43	2.84 ± 0.51
	31	4			2.41 ± 0.13	
Carpentier-Edwards pericardial (stented prothesis)	19	14	32.13 ± 3.35	24.19 ± 8.6	2.83 ± 0.14	1.21 ± 0.31
	21	34	25.69 ± 9.9	20.3 ± 9.08	2.59 ± 0.42	1.47 ± 0.36
	23	20	21.72 ± 8.57	13.01 ± 5.27	2.29 ± 0.45	1.75 ± 0.28
	25	5	16.46 ± 5.41	9.04 ± 2.27	2.02 ± 0.31	
	27	1	19.2	5.6	1.6	
	29	1	17.6	11.6	2.1	
Carpentier-Edwards supraannular AV (stented bioprosthesis)	19	15	34.1 ± 2.7			1.1 ± 0.09
	21	8	25 ± 8	14 ± 5		1.06 ± 0.16
CryoLife O'Brien stentless (stentless prothesis)	19	47		12 ± 4.8		1.25 ± 0.1
	21	163		10.33 ± 2		1.57 ± 0.6
	23	40		8.5		2.2
	25	40		7.9		2.3
	27	39		7.4		2.7
Duromedics (Tekna; bileaflet)	19	1			3.6	
	21	3	19.08 ± 16	8.98 ± 5		1.3
	23	12	19.87 ± 7	7 ± 2	2.64 ± 0.27	
	25	18	21 ± 9	5 ± 2	2.34 ± 0.38	
	27	15	22.5 ± 12	6 ± 3	1.88 ± 0.6	
	29	1	13.0	3.4	2.1	
Edwards Prima stentless (stentless bioprosthesis)	19	7	30.9 ± 11.7	15.4 ± 7.4		1 ± 0.3
	21	30	31.22 ± 17.35	16.36 ± 11.36		1.25 ± 0.29
	23	62	23.39 ± 10.17	11.52 ± 5.26	2.8 ± 0.4	1.49 ± 0.46
	25	97	19.74 ± 10.36	10.77 ± 9.32	2.7 ± 0.3	1.7 ± 0.55
	27	46	15.9 ± 7.3	7.1 ± 3.7		2 ± 0.6
	29	11	11.21 ± 8.6	5.03 ± 4.53		2.49 ± 0.52
Hancock I (stented bioprosthesis)	21	1			3.5	
	23	14	19.09 ± 4.35	12.36 ± 3.82	2.94 ± 0.24	
	25	26	17.61 ± 3.13	11 ± 2.85	2.36 ± 0.37	
	27	20	18.11 ± 6.92	10 ± 3.46	2.4 ± 0.36	
	29	2			2.23 ± 0.04	
	31	1			2.0	

Table D.1 ***(Continued)***

Valve	Size	n	Peak gradient (mm Hg)	Mean gradient (mm Hg)	Peak velocity (m/s)	Effective orifice area (cm^2)
Hancock II (stented bioprosthesis)	21	39	20 ± 4	14.8 ± 4.1		1.23 ± 0.27
	23	119	24.72 ± 5.73	16.64 ± 6.91		1.39 ± 0.23
	25	114	20 ± 2	10.7 ± 3		1.47 ± 0.19
	27	133	14 ± 3			1.55 ± 0.18
	29	35	15 ± 3			1.6 ± 0.15
Ionescu-Shiley (stented bioprosthesis)	17	11	42.0	21.1 ± 3.21		0.86 ± 0.1
	19	63	23.17 ± 6.58	20.44 ± 8.47	2.63 ± 0.32	1.15 ± 0.18
	21	11	27.63 ± 8.34	15.1 ± 1.56	2.75 ± 0.25	
	23	5	18.09 ± 6.49	9.9 ± 2.85	2.1 ± 0.38	
	25	1	18.0			
	27	3	14.75 ± 2.17	8.97 ± 0.57	1.92 ± 0.14	
	29	1	16.0	7.3	2.0	
Jyros bileaflet (bileaflet)	22	4	17.3	10.8		1.5
	24	7	18.6	11.4		1.5
	26	8	14.4	8.4		1.7
	28	3	10.0	5.7		1.9
	30	1	8.0	6.0		1.6
Lillehei-Kaster (tilting disk)	14	1			2.7	
	16	2			3.43 ± 0.39	
	18	2			2.85 ± 0.21	
	20	1			1.7	
Medtronic Freestyle stentless (stentless bioprosthesis)	19	11		13.0		
	21	85		7.99 ± 2.6		1.6 ± 0.32
	23	141		7.24 ± 2.5		1.9 ± 0.5
	25	164		5.35 ± 1.5		2.03 ± 0.41
	27	105		4.72 ± 1.6		2.5 ± 0.47
Medtronic-Hall (tilting disk)	20	24	34.37 ± 13.06	17.08 ± 5.28	2.9 ± 0.4	1.21 ± 0.45
	21	30	26.86 ± 10.54	14.1 ± 5.93	2.42 ± 0.36	1.08 ± 0.17
	23	27	26.85 ± 8.85	13.5 ± 4.79	2.43 ± 0.59	1.36 ± 0.39
	25	17	17.13 ± 7.04	9.53 ± 4.26	2.29 ± 0.5	1.9 ± 0.47
	27	8	18.66 ± 9.71	8.66 ± 5.56	2.07 ± 0.53	1.9 ± 0.16
	29	1			1.6	
Medtronic intact (stented bioprosthesis)	19	16	39.43 ± 15.4	23.71 ± 9.3	2.5	
	21	55	33.9 ± 12.69	18.74 ± 8.03	2.73 ± 0.44	1.55 ± 0.39
	23	110	31.27 ± 9.62	18.88 ± 6.17	2.74 ± 0.37	1.64 ± 0.37
	25	41	27.34 ± 10.59	16.4 ± 6.05	2.6 ± 0.44	1.85 ± 0.25
	27	16	25.27 ± 7.58	15 ± 3.94	2.51 ± 0.38	2.2 ± 0.17
	29	5	31.0	15.6 ± 2.1	2.8	2.38 ± 0.54
Medtronic Mosaic, porcine (stented bioprosthesis)	21	51		12.43 ± 7.3		1.6 ± 0.7
	23	121		12.47 ± 7.4		2.1 ± 0.8
	25	71		10.08 ± 5.1		2.1 ± 1.6
	27	30		9.0		
	29	6		9.0		
Mitroflow (stented bioprosthesis)	19	4	18.7 ± 5.1	10.3 ± 3		1.13 ± 0.17
	21	7	20.2	15.4	2.3	
	23	5	14.04 ± 4.91	7.56 ± 3.38	1.85 ± 0.34	
	25	2	17 ± 11.31	10.8 ± 6.51	2 ± 0.71	
	27	3	13 ± 3	6.57 ± 1.7	1.8 ± 0.2	

(Continued)

Table D.1 *(Continued)*

Valve	Size	n	Peak gradient (mm Hg)	Mean gradient (mm Hg)	Peak velocity (m/s)	Effective orifice area (cm^2)
O'Brien-Angell stentless (annular position; stentless bioprosthesis)	23			14.5 ± 7.77		1.15 ± 0.07
	25	50		19 ± 12.72		1.12 ± 0.25
	27			18 ± 12.72		1.55 ± 0.21
	29			12 ± 7.07		2.05 ± 1.2
O'Brien-Angell stentless (supraannular position; stentless bioprosthesis)	23			9 ± 1.4		1.58 ± 0.58
	25	50		7.5 ± 0.7		2.37 ± 0.18
	27			8.5 ± 0.7		2.85 ± 0.87
	29			7 ± 1.4		2.7 ± 0.42
Omnicarbon (tilting disk)	21	71	36.79 ± 12.59	19.41 ± 5.46	2.93 ± 0.47	1.25 ± 0.43
	23	83	29.33 ± 9.67	17.98 ± 6.06	2.66 ± 0.44	1.49 ± 0.34
	25	81	24.29 ± 7.71	13.51 ± 3.85	2.32 ± 0.38	1.94 ± 0.52
	27	40	19.63 ± 4.34	12.06 ± 2.98	2.08 ± 0.35	2.11 ± 0.46
	29	5	17.12 ± 1.53	10 ± 1.53	1.9 ± 0.06	2.27 ± 0.23
Omniscience (tilting disk)	19	2	47.5 ± 3.5	28 ± 1.4		0.81 ± 0.01
	21	5	50.8 ± 2.8	28.2 ± 2.17		0.87 ± 0.13
	23	8	39.8 ± 8.7	20.1 ± 5.1		0.98 ± 0.07
On-X (bileaflet)	19	6	21.3 ± 10.8	11.8 ± 3.4		1.5 ± 0.2
	21	11	16.4 ± 5.9	9.9 ± 3.6		1.7 ± 0.4
	23	23	15.9 ± 6.4	8.5 ± 3.3		2 ± 0.6
	25	12	16.5 ± 10.2	9 ± 5.3		2.4 ± 0.8
	27-29	8	11.4 ± 4.6	5.6 ± 2.7		3.2 ± 0.6
Sorin Allcarbon (tilting disk)	19	7	44 ± 7	29 ± 8	3.3 ± 0.3	0.9 ± 0.1
	21	25	36.52 ± 9.61	21.07 ± 6.72	2.93 ± 0.2	1.08 ± 0.19
	23	37	34.97 ± 10.97	18.72 ± 6.49	2.9 ± 0.41	1.31 ± 0.2
	25	23	22 ± 4.68	13.85 ± 3.97	2.37 ± 0.23	1.96 ± 0.71
	27	13	16.3 ± 3.3	10.15 ± 3.76	2 ± 0.25	2.51 ± 0.57
	29	4	13 ± 4	8 ± 2	1.8 ± 0.3	4.1 ± 0.7
Sorin Bicarbon (bileaflet)	19	19	29.53 ± 4.46	16.35 ± 1.99	2.5 ± 0.1	1.36 ± 0.13
	21	70	24.52 ± 7.1	12.54 ± 3.3	2.46 ± 0.31	1.46 ± 0.2
	23	71	17.79 ± 6.1	9.61 ± 3.3	2.11 ± 0.24	1.98 ± 0.23
	25	40	18.46 ± 3.1	10.05 ± 1.6	2.25 ± 0.19	2.39 ± 0.29
	27	8	12 ± 3.25	7 ± 1.5	1.73 ± 0.21	3.06 ± 0.47
	29	4	9 ± 1.25	5 ± 0.5	1.51 ± 0.1	3.45 ± 0.02
Sorin Pericarbon (stentless bioprosthesis)	23	15	39 ± 13	25 ± 8		2.0
St. Jude Medical (bileaflet)	19	100	35.17 ± 11.16	18.96 ± 6.27	2.86 ± 0.48	1.01 ± 0.24
	21	207	28.34 ± 9.94	15.82 ± 5.67	2.63 ± 0.48	1.33 ± 0.32
	23	236	25.28 ± 7.89	13.77 ± 5.33	2.57 ± 0.44	1.6 ± 0.43
	25	169	22.57 ± 7.68	12.65 ± 5.14	2.4 ± 0.45	1.93 ± 0.45
	27	82	19.85 ± 7.55	11.18 ± 4.82	2.24 ± 0.42	2.35 ± 0.59
	29	18	17.72 ± 6.42	9.86 ± 2.9	2 ± 0.1	2.81 ± 0.57
	31	4	16.0	10 ± 6	2.1 ± 0.6	3.08 ± 1.09
St. Jude Medical Hemodynamic Plus (bileaflet)	19	19	25.81 ± 7.52	16.44 ± 3.57		1.65 ± 0.2
	21	30	18.9 ± 7.31	9.62 ± 3.37		2.15 ± 0.29

Table D.1 *(Continued)*

Valve	Size	*n*	Peak gradient (mm Hg)	Mean gradient (mm Hg)	Peak velocity (m/s)	Effective orifice area (cm^2)
Starr-Edwards (ball-and-cage)	21	5	29.0			1.0
	22	2			4	
	23	22	32.6 ± 12.79	21.98 ± 8.8	3.5 ± 0.5	1.1
	24	43	34.13 ± 10.33	22.09 ± 7.54	3.35 ± 0.48	
	26	29	31.83 ± 9.01	19.69 ± 6.05	3.18 ± 0.35	
	27	14	30.82 ± 6.3	18.5± 3.7		1.8
	29	8	29 ± 9.3	16.3 ± 5.5		
Stentless porcine xenograft (stentless bioprosthesis)	21	3	14 ± 5	8.7 ± 3.5		1.33 ± 0.38
	22	3	16 ± 5.6	9.7 ± 3.7		1.32 ± 0.48
	23	4	13 ± 4.8	7.7 ± 2.3		1.59 ± 0.6
	24	3	13 ± 3.8	7.7 ± 2.2		1.4 ± 0.01
	25	6	11.5 ± 7.1	7.4 ± 4.5		2.13 ± 0.7
	26	3	10.7	7 ± 2.1		2.15 ± 0.2
	27	1	9.2	5.5		3.2
	28	1	7.5	4.1		2.3
Toronto stentless, porcine (stentless bioprosthesis)	20	1	10.9	4.6		1.3
	21	9	18.64 ± 11.8	7.56 ± 4.4		1.21 ± 0.7
	22	1	23.0			1.2
	23	84	13.55 ± 7.28	7.08 ± 4.33		1.59 ± 0.84
	25	190	12.17 ± 5.75	6.2 ± 3.05		1.62 ± 0.4
	27	240	9.96 ± 4.56	4.8 ± 2.33		1.95 ± 0.42
	29	200	7.91 ± 4.17	3.94 ± 2.15		2.37 ± 0.67

Table D.2 Normal Doppler echocardiographic values for mitral valve prosthesis

Valve	Size	*n*	Peak gradient (mm Hg)	Mean gradient (mm Hg)	Peak velocity (m/s)	Pressure half-time (ms)	Effective orifice area (cm^2)
Biocor (stentless bioprosthesis)	27	3	13 ± 1				
	29	3	14 ± 2.5				
	31	8	11.5 ± 0.5				
	33	9	12 ± 0.5				
Bioflo pericardial (stented bioprosthesis)	25	3	10 ± 2	6.3 ± 1.5			2 ± 0.1
	27	7	9.5 ± 2.6	5.4 ± 1.2			2 ± 0.3
	29	8	5 ± 2.8	3.6 ± 1			2.4 ± 0.2
	31	1	4.0	2.0			2.3
Björk-Shiley (tilting disk)	23	1			1.7	115	
	25	14	12 ± 4	6 ± 2	1.75 ± 0.38	99 ± 27	1.72 ± 0.6
	27	34	10 ± 4	5 ± 2	1.6 ± 0.49	89 ± 28	1.81 ± 0.54
	29	21	7.83 ± 2.93	2.83 ± 1.27	1.37 ± 0.25	79 ± 17	2.1 ± 0.43
	31	21	6 ± 3	2 ± 1.9	1.41 ± 0.26	70 ± 14	2.2 ± 0.3
Björk-Shiley monostrut (tilting disk)	23	1		5.0	1.9		
	25	102	13 ± 2.5	5.57 ± 2.3	1.8 ± 0.3		
	27	83	12 ± 2.5	4.53 ± 2.2	1.7 ± 0.4		
	29	26	13 ± 3	4.26 ± 1.6	1.6 ± 0.3		
	31	25	14 ± 4.5	4.9 ± 1.6	1.7 ± 0.3		
Carbomedics (bileaflet)	23	2			1.9 ± 0.1	126 ± 7	
	25	12	10.3 ± 2.3	3.6 ± 0.6	1.3 ± 0.1	93 ± 8	2.9 ± 0.8
	27	78	8.79 ± 3.46	3.46 ± 1.03	1.61 ± 0.3	89 ± 20	2.9 ± 0.75
	29	46	8.78 ± 2.9	3.39 ± 0.97	1.52 ± 0.3	88 ± 17	2.3 ± 0.4
	31	57	8.87 ± 2.34	3.32 ± 0.87	1.61 ± 0.29	92 ± 24	2.8 ± 1.14
	33	33	8.8 ± 2.2	4.8 ± 2.5	1.5 ± 0.2	93 ± 12	
Carpentier-Edwards (stented bioprosthesis)	27	16		6 ± 2	1.7 ± 0.3	98 ± 28	
	29	22		4.7 ± 2	1.76 ± 0.27	92 ± 14	
	31	22		4.4 ± 2	1.54 ± 0.15	92 ± 19	
	33	6		6 ± 3		93 ± 12	
Carpentier-Edwards pericardial (stented bioprosthesis)	27	1		3.6	1.6	100	
	29	6		5.25 ± 2.36	1.67 ± 0.3	110 ± 15	
	31	4		4.05 ± 0.83	1.53 ± 0.1	90 ± 11	
	33	1		1.0	0.8	80	
Duromedics (bileaflet)	27	8	13 ± 6	5 ± 3		75 ± 12	
	29	14	10 ± 4	3 ± 1	161 ± 40	85 ± 22	
	31	21	10.5 ± 4.37	3.3 ± 1.36	140 ± 25	81 ± 12	
	33	1	11.2	2.5	138 ± 27	85	
Hancock I or not specified (stented bioprosthesis)	27	3	10 ± 4	5 ± 2			1.3 ± 0.8
	29	13	7 ± 3	2.46 ± 0.79		115 ± 20	1.5 ± 0.2
	31	22	4 ± 0.86	4.86 ± 1.69		95 ± 17	1.6 ± 0.2
	33	8	3 ± 2	3.87 ± 2		90 ± 12	1.9 ± 0.2
Hancock II (stented bioprosthesis)	27	16					2.21 ± 0.14
	29	64					2.77 ± 0.11
	31	90					2.84 ± 0.1
	33	25					3.15 ± 0.22

Table D.2 ***(Continued)***

Valve	Size	*n*	Peak gradient (mm Hg)	Mean gradient (mm Hg)	Peak velocity (m/s)	Pressure half-time (ms)	Effective orifice area (cm^2)
Hancock pericardial (stented bioprosthesis)	29	14		2.61 ± 1.39	1.42 ± 0.14	105 ± 36	
	31	8		3.57 ± 1.02	1.51 ± 0.27	81 ± 23	
Ionescu-Shiley (stented bioprosthesis)	25	3		4.87 ± 1.08	1.43 ± 0.15	93 ± 11	
	27	4		3.21 ± 0.82	1.31 ± 0.24	100 ± 28	
	29	6		3.22 ± 0.57	1.38 ± 0.2	85 ± 8	
	31	4		3.63 ± 0.9	1.45 ± 0.06	100 ± 36	
Ionescu-Shiley low profile (stented bioprosthesis)	29	13		3.31 ± 0.96	1.36 ± 0.25	80 ± 30	
	31	10		2.74 ± 0.37	1.33 ± 0.14	79 ± 15	
Labcor-Santiago pericardial (stented bioprosthesis)	25	1	8.7	4.5		97	2.2
	27	16	5.6 ± 2.3	2.8 ± 1.5		85 ± 18	2.12 ± 0.48
	29	20	6.2 ± 2.1	3 ± 1.3		80 ± 34	2.11 ± 0.73
Lillehei- Kaster (tilting disk)	18	1			1.7	140	
	20	1			1.7	67	
	22	4			1.56 ± 0.09	94 ± 22	
	25	5			1.38 ± 0.27	124 ± 46	
Medtronic-Hall (tilting disk)	27	1			1.4	78	
	29	5			1.57 ± 0.1	69 ± 15	
	31	7			1.45 ± 0.12	77 ± 17	
Medtronic Intact, porcine (stented prosthesis)	29	3		3.5 ± 0.51	1.6 ± 0.22		
	31	14		4.2 ± 1.44	1.6 ± 0.26		
	33	13		4 ± 1.3	1.4 ± 0.24		
	35	2		3.2 ± 1.77	1.3 ± 0.5		
Mitroflow (stented bioprosthesis)	25	1		6.9	2.0	90	
	27	3		3.07 ± 0.91	1.5	90 ± 20	
	29	15		3.5 ± 1.65	1.43 ± 0.29	102 ± 21	
	31	5		3.85 ± 0.81	1.32 ± 0.26	91 ± 22	
Omnicarbon (tilting disk)	23	1		8.0			
	25	16		6.05 ± 1.81	1.77 ± 0.24	102 ± 16	
	27	29		4.89 ± 2.05	1.63 ± 0.36	105 ± 33	
	29	34		4.93 ± 2.16	1.56 ± 0.27	120 ± 40	
	31	58		4.18 ± 1.4	1.3 ± 0.23	134 ± 31	
	33	2		4 ± 2			
On-X (bileaflet)	25	3	11.5 ± 3.2	5.3 ± 2.1			1.9 ± 1.1
	27–29	16	10.3 ± 4.5	4.5 ± 1.6			2.2 ± 0.5
	31–33	14	9.8 ± 3.8	4.8 ± 2.4			2.5 ± 1.1
Sorin Allcarbon (tilting disk)	25	8	15 ± 3	5 ± 1	2 ± 0.2	105 ± 29	2.2 ± 0.6
	27	20	13 ± 2	4 ± 1	1.8 ± 0.1	89 ± 14	2.5 ± 0.5
	29	34	10 ± 2	4 ± 1	1.6 ± 0.2	85 ± 23	2.8 ± 0.7
	31	11	9 ± 1	4 ± 1	1.6 ± 0.1	88 ± 27	2.8 ± 0.9
Sorin Bicarbon (bileaflet)	25	3	15 ± 0.25	4 ± 0.5	1.95 ± 0.02	70 ± 1	
	27	25	11 ± 2.75	4 ± 0.5	1.65 ± 0.21	82 ± 20	
	29	30	12 ± 3	4 ± 1.25	1.73 ± 0.22	80 ± 14	
	31	9	10 ± 1.5	4 ± 1	1.66 ± 0.11	83 ± 14	

(Continued)

Table D.2 *(Continued)*

Valve	Size	*n*	Peak gradient (mm Hg)	Mean gradient (mm Hg)	Peak velocity (m/s)	Pressure half-time (ms)	Effective orifice area (cm^2)
St Jude Medical (bileaflet)	23	1		4.0	1.5	160	1.0
	25	4		2.5 ± 1	1.34 ± 1.12	75 ± 4	1.35 ± 0.17
	27	16	11 ± 4	5 ± 1.82	1.61 ± 0.29	75 ± 10	1.67 ± 0.17
	29	40	10 ± 3	4.15 ± 1.8	1.57 ± 0.29	85 ± 10	1.75 ± 0.24
	31	41	12 ± 6	4.46 ± 2.22	1.59 ± 0.33	74 ± 13	2.03 ± 0.32
Starr-Edwards (ball-and-cage)	26	1		10.0			1.4
	28	27		7 ± 2.75			1.9 ± 0.57
	30	25	12.2 ± 4.6	6.99 ± 2.5	1.7 ± 0.3	125 ± 25	1.65 ± 0.4
	32	17	11.5 ± 4.2	5.08 ± 2.5	1.7 ± 0.3	110 ± 25	1.98 ± 0.4
	34	1		5.0			2.6
Stentless quadrileaflet bovine pericardial (stentless bioprosthesis)	26	2		2.2 ± 1.7	1.6	103 ± 31	1.7
	28	14			1.58 ± 0.25		1.7 ± 0.6
	30	6			1.42 ± 0.32		2.3 ± 0.4
Wessex (stented bioprosthesis)	29	9		3.69 ± 0.61	1.66 ± 0.17	83 ± 19	
	31	22		3.31 ± 0.83	1.41 ± 0.25	80 ± 21	

Table D.3 Normal Doppler echocardiographic values for tricuspid prosthesis

Valve type	Examples	Peak velocity (m/s)	Mean pressure gradient (mm Hg)
Caged ball	Starr-Edwards	1.3 ± 0.2	3.2 ± 0.8
Tilting disk	Björk-Shiley	1.3	2.2
Bileaflet	St. Jude	1.2 ± 0.3	2.7 ± 1.1
Porcine	Carpentier-Edwards	1.3 ± 0.2	3.2 ± 0.8

Adapted from Rosenhek R, Binder T, Maurer G, et al. Normal values for Doppler echocardiographic assessment of heart valve prostheses. *J Am Soc Echocardiogr* 2003;16:116.

E Classification of the Severity of Valvular Disease

Table E.1 Aortic regurgitation

Parameter	Caveats	Mild	Moderate	Severe
2-D Imaging LV size (at end of diastole)	Enlarged in other conditions Normal in acute	Normal (chronic)	Variable	Dilated (chronic)
Aortic leaflets	Inaccurate Anatomic defect not reflective of severity	Variable	Variable	Abnormal (flail coaptation defect)
Doppler Jet diameter in LVOT (aliasing velocity 50–60 cm/s)	Inaccurate for eccentric jets	Small	Medium	Large (central) Variable (eccentric)
Diastolic flow reversal descending aorta	Stiff aorta Brief reversal is normal	Brief early diastolic reversal	Variable	Holodiastolic reversal
CW Doppler spectral density	Qualitative Moderate-severe overlap	Faint	Variable	Dense
Pressure half-time (m/s)	Dependent on aortic-LV gradient	Slow >500	Medium 500–200	Steep <200
Vena contracta width (cm)	Multiple jets	<0.3	0.3–0.6	>0.6
Jet width/LVOT width (%) (aliasing velocity 50–60 cm/s)	Eccentric jets	<25	25–64	>65
Jet CSA/LVOT CSA (%)	Eccentric jets	<5	5–59	>60
Regurgitant volume (mL/beat)	Combined MR and AR	<30	30–59	>60
Regurgitant volume (mL/beat)	Maximum	<30	30–59	≥60
Regurgitant fraction (%)	Maximum	<30	30–49	≥50
ROA (cm^2)	Maximum RVA	<0.10	0.10–0.29	≥0.30

LV, left ventricle; CF, color flow; LVOT, left ventricular outflow tract; PW, pulse wave; CW, continuous wave; CSA, cross-sectional area; MR, mitral regurgitation; AR, aortic regurgitation; PISA, proximal isovelocity surface area; ROA, regurgitant orifice area; RVA, right ventricular area.

Table E.2 Aortic stenosis

Parameter	Caveats	Mild	Moderate	Severe
2-D imaging	Qualitative	>20 mm	10–20 mm	<10 mm
M-mode maximum cusp separation	Cursor must be perpendicular			
Aortic valve leaflets	Qualitative estimation	≤1 leaflet immobility	2 leaflet immobility	3 leaflet immobility
Planimetered valve area: normal = 3–4 cm^2	Inaccurate with Ca^{2+} Image plane must be perpendicular	>1.5 cm^2	0.75–1.5 cm^2	<0.75 cm^2
Doppler				
Peak velocity (assumes nl CO)	Increased with AR	≤2.3 m/s	3.0–4.0 m/s	>4.0 m/s
Mean gradient (assumes nl CO)	Cardiac output dependent	<25 mm Hg[a]	25–40 mm Hg[a]	>40 mm Hg[a]
Continuity equation AoV area = $\frac{TVI_{LVOT} \times area_{LVOT}}{TVI_{AoV}}$	Squared diameter (introduces large error) Regurgitation in reference valve LVOT obstruction	1.5–2.0 cm^2	1.0–1.5 cm^2	≤1.0 cm^2
Dimensionless index TVI_{LVOT}/TVI_{AV}	Less quantitative			<0.25

[a]If gradient less than 30 mm Hg with poor left ventricle function, dobutamine may clarify even with AR; gradient greater than 50 mm Hg suggestive of significant AS.

M-mode, motion mode; CW, continuous wave; CO, cardiac output; AR, aortic regurgitation; AoV, aortic valve; TVI, time-velocity integral; LVOT, left ventricular outflow tract.

Table E.3 Mitral regurgitation

Parameter		Caveats	Mild	Moderate	Severe
2-D imaging	LA size	LAE may be caused by other conditions Acute MR may have normal LA size	Usually normal	Variable	LA enlargement
	LV size	—	Usually normal	Variable	Often enlarged (chronic MR)
	MV apparatus	May have severe MR with structurally normal MV	Normal or abnormal	Normal or abnormal	Often visible coaptation defect
Color flow Doppler (CFD)	Maximum jet area	Technical (power, aliasing velocity, color gain, frequency) Load dependent Wall impingement	<4 cm^2	—	>8 cm^2 Wall jet Circumferential LA jet
	Jet area/LA area	—	—	—	$>40\%$
	Visible flow convergence area	Dependent on gain and aliasing velocity	Rarely present	Sometimes present	Often present
Vena contracta width (cm)		Not useful for multiple jets Cannot add diameters	<0.3	0.3–0.69	≥ 0.7
Spectral Doppler	PW mitral Inflow	Dependent on load, diastolic fx, MVA, AF	A dominant	Variable	Restrictive pattern
	PW PV flow	Increased LAP, AF	—	Often systolic blunting	Systolic flow reversal
	CW spectral density	—	Faint	—	Dense
Regurgitant volume (mL/beat)	—		<30	30–59	≥ 60
Regurgitant fraction (%)	—		<30	30–49	≥ 50
ROA (cm^2)	—		<0.20	0.20–0.39	≥ 0.40

LA, left atrium; LAE, left atrial enlargement; LV, left ventricle; MV, mitral valve; MR, mitral regurgitation; PW, pulse wave; PV, pulmonary valve; fx, function; MVA, mitral valve area; AF, atrial fibrillation; PISA, proximal isovelocity surface area; ROA, regurgitant orifice area.

Table E.4 Mitral valve stenosis

Parameter		Caveats	Mild	Moderate	Severe
2-D imaging	LA size (LAE >45 mm anteroposterior diameter exclude LAA thrombi)	Nonspecific	Normal excludes chronic MS		>60 mm in chronic MS
	Spontaneous contrast	Nonspecific	Usually absent	May be present	Present
	Planimetered MV area	Inaccurate with Ca^{2+} or previous commissurotomy	1.5–2.0 cm^2	1.0–1.5 cm^2	≤0.9 cm^2
Doppler	CF Doppler proximal flow convergence (aliasing velocity 50–60 cm/s)	Nondiagnostic Present following MVrep MVR	Not present	Usually present	Always present Absence excludes
Mean gradient[a]		Severe AR decreases Heart rate dependent Dependent on LA–LV compliance	<6 mm Hg	6–12 mm Hg	>12 mm Hg
Pressure half-time[a] MVA = 220/PHT (use longer slope if two present)		Severe AR decreases PHT Heart rate dependent Dependent on LA–LV compliance	<150 ms	150–220 ms	>220 ms
Deceleration time[a] MVA = 759/DT PHT = 0.29 × DT		Severe AR decreases Heart rate dependent Dependent on LA–LV compliance	<517 ms	517–759 ms	>759 ms
Continuity equation[a] MVA = $(Area_{LVOT} \times TVI_{LVOT})/TVI_{MV}$		Time consuming	1.5–2.0 cm^2	1.0–1.5 cm^2	≤0.9 cm^2
Proximal isovelocity[a] surface area MVA = $2\pi r^2 \times V_{Aliasing}/\text{peak } V_{MS} \times \alpha/180$ degrees		Funnel angle Subvalve stenosis Time consuming	1.5–2.0 cm^2	1.0–1.5 cm^2	≤0.9 cm^2

[a]With atrial fibrillation, average five consecutive diastoles.

LA, left atrium; LAE, left atrial enlargement; LAA, left atrial appendage; MS, mitral stenosis; MV, mitral valve; CF, color flow; Mvrep, mitral valve repair; MVR, mitral valve replacement; PW, pulmonary wave; PV, pulmonary venous; AR, aortic regurgitation; LV, left ventricle; CW, continuous wave; MVA, mitral valve area; PHT, pressure half time.

Table E.5 Tricuspid regurgitation

Parameter		Caveats	Mild	Moderate	Severe
2-D imaging	RA/RV/IVC size RA diameter <4.6 cm RV diameter <4.3 cm	Not specific Normal in acute TR	Normal	Variable	Usually dilated
	Tricuspid valve structure	Nonspecific	Normal	Variable	Flail poor coaptation
Doppler	Maximum jet area (Nyquist limit 50–60 cm/s)	Technical factors Loading Underestimates (eccentric jets)	<5 cm^2	5–10 cm^2	>10 cm^2
	Hepatic vein flow	Blunting multiple causes	Systolic dominance	Systolic blunting	Systolic reversal
	CW Doppler jet density-contour	Qualitative, complimentary data	Soft parabolic	Dense variable contour	Dense triangular with early peaking
	Vena contracta diameter (VCD) (cm)	Directs need of further confirmation	Not defined	<0.7	>0.7
	PISA radius (cm) baseline shift with (Nyquist 28 cm/s)	Validation lacking	<0.5	0.6–0.9	>0.9

RA, right atrium; RV, right ventricle; IVC, inferior vena cava; CF, color flow; PW, pulse wave; CW, continuous wave; PISA, proximal isovelocity surface area.

Table E.6 Tricuspid stenosis

Parameter		Caveats	Mild	Moderate	Severe
2-D imaging	Tricuspid valve (thickness, reduced mobility, Ca^{2+})	Nonspecific	Normal	Normal or abnormal	Abnormal
	RA size	Nonspecific	—	—	>4 cm
	RV size RV diameter <4.3 cm RV ED area ≤35.5 cm^2	Nonspecific	Normal	Normal or dilated	Dilated
Doppler	Color flow Proximal flow convergence (Nyquist limit 50–60 cm/s)	Qualitative Poor correlation with severity of PR	—	—	—
	Continuous wave Jet density and deceleration	Slow deceleration rate caused by PR and left right shunt	Faint Steep deceleration	Dense Variable deceleration	Dense Delayed deceleration
	Continuous wave	Correct alignment	<1 m/s	1–2.5 m/s	>2.5 m/s
	Peak gradient	Compliance RA RV	<4 mm Hg	4–25 mm Hg	>25 mm Hg
	Mean gradient	Flow and HR dependent	<2 mm Hg	2–7 mm Hg	>7 mm Hg
	(TVA = 190/PHT)	Inaccurate with abnormal Compliance (RA, RV) PR reduces PHT and overestimates area			>190 ms

RA, right atrium; RV, right ventricle; ED, end diastolic; IVC, inferior vena cava; TR, tricuspid regurgitation; CF, color flow; PW, pulse wave; CW, continuous wave; PISA, proximal isovelocity surface area.

Table E.7 Pulmonary regurgitation (PR) severity

Parameter		Caveats	Mild	Moderate	Severe
2-D imaging	Pulmonic valve		Normal	Variable	Abnormal
	RV size				
	RV diameter <4.3 cm	Nonspecific	Normal	Variable	Dilated (except acute)
	RVED area ≤35.5 cm^2				
	Paradoxical septal motion (volume overload pattern)	Not specific for PR	Normal	Variable	Flail and poor coaptation
Doppler	Color flow Doppler Jet size	Poor correlation with severity of PR	Small <10 mm length	Variable	Large
	Vena contracta (Nyquist limit 50–60 cm/s)	Not validated	<small	Variable	Wide origin
	CW Doppler jet density and deceleration	Qualitative	Faint Slow deceleration	Variable density and deceleration	Dense Steep deceleration Short
	Pulmonic systolic flow compared to systemic	Time consuming	Slight increase	Intermediate	Great increase

RA, right atrium; RV, right ventricle; RVED, right ventricular end diastolic; CW, continuous wave.

Adapted from Zoghbi WA, Enriquez-Sarano M, Foster E, et al. Recommendations for evaluation of the severity of native valvular regurgitation with two-dimentional and Doppler echocardiography. *J Am Soc Echocardiogr* 2003;16(7):777–802.

Bonow RO. Carabello BA. Chatterjee K. et al. ACC/AHA 2006 guidelines for the management of patients with valvular heart disease: a report of the American College of Cardiology/American Heart Association Task Force on Practice Guidelines (writing Committee to Revise the 1998 guidelines for the management of patients with valvular heart disease) developed in collaboration with the Society of Cardiovascular Anesthesiologists endorsed by the Society for Cardiovascular Angiography and Interventions and the Society of Thoracic Surgeons. 2006;48(3):e1–148.

Adapted from Hatle L. Noninvasive assessment of valve lesions with Doppler ultrasound. *Herz* 1984;9:213–221; Fawzy ME, Mercer EN, Dunn B, et al. Doppler echocardiography in the evaluation of tricuspid stenosis. *Eur Heart J* 1989;10(11):985–990.

Answers to End-of-Chapter Questions

Chapter 1

1. d
2. e
3. d
4. d
5. b
6. b
7. e
8. b
9. c
10. c

Chapter 2

1. a
2. b
3. a
4. c
5. d
6. b
7. d
8. d
9. d
10. b

Chapter 3

1. b and d
2. Fractional shortening = {(5.2 – 3.1)/5.2} × 100 = 40%, which is normal.
3. e
4. c
5. a
6. a
7. c. All four chambers are often dilated.
8. e.
9. d.
10. e.
11. c.
12. a
13. a, b, c, e.
14. Negative.
15. Negative.

Chapter 4

1. d
2. a
3. c
4. b
5. c
6. d
7. d
8. b
9. e
10. b

Chapter 5

1. c
2. b
3. d
4. c
5. a
6. c
7. c
8. a
9. b
10. d

Chapter 6

1. d
2. c
3. d
4. c
5. d
6. c
7. a
8. d
9. e
10. e

Chapter 7

1. d
2. a
3. d
4. c
5. a
6. b
7. d
8. c
9. a
10. b
11. b

Chapter 8

1. e
2. a
3. d
4. d
5. b
6. c
7. d
8. a
9. d
10. b

Chapter 9

1. c
2. c
3. d
4. c
5. b
6. a
7. c
8. c
9. d
10. d

Chapter 10

1. c
2. b
3. b
4. a
5. e
6. b
7. c
8. a
9. e
10. b

Chapter 11

1. d
2. d
3. e
4. d
5. e
6. b
7. e
8. a
9. e
10. a

Chapter 12

1. c
2. c
3. d
4. b
5. a
6. f
7. b
8. d
9. a
10. d

Chapter 13

1. b
2. c
3. a
4. d
5. d
6. a
7. c
8. a
9. b
10. a

Chapter 14

1. d
2. a
3. d
4. b
5. b
6. b
7. d
8. b
9. b
10. d

Chapter 15

1. d
2. b
3. c
4. d
5. c
6. d
7. a
8. b
9. c
10. b

Chapter 16

1. b
2. c
3. d
4. a
5. c
6. e
7. d
8. c
9. b
10. a
11. c
12. d
13. e
14. c
15. e
16. b
17. b
18. e
19. e
20. d

Chapter 17

1. d
2. d
3. e
4. d
5. c
6. c
7. d
8. d
9. c
10. a

Chapter 18

1. d
2. d
3. c
4. d
5. b
6. d
7. c
8. c
9. a
10.

$$\begin{aligned} \text{LVOT SV} &= \text{Area}_{\text{LVOT}} \times \text{TVI}_{\text{LVOT}} \\ &= 3.14(1.9/2)^2 \times 14.8 \\ &= 41.9 \text{ cc} \end{aligned}$$

$$\begin{aligned} \text{RV SV} &= \text{Area}_{\text{MPA}} \times \text{TVI}_{\text{MPA}} \\ &= 3.14(2.1/2)^2 \times 15.3 \\ &= 53 \text{ mL} \end{aligned}$$

$$\begin{aligned} \text{CO} &= \text{LVOT-SV} \times \text{HR} \\ &= 41.9 \times 90 \\ &= 3.8 \text{ L/ min} \end{aligned}$$

$$\begin{aligned} \text{CI} &= \text{CO/BSA} \\ &= 3.8/1.8 \\ &= 2.1 \text{ L/ min /m}^2 \end{aligned}$$

$$\begin{aligned} Q_p/Q_s &= \text{SV of the pulmonary circuit/SV of the systemic arterial circuit} \\ Q_p &= \text{SV from RV} \\ Q_s &= \text{SV from LVOT} \end{aligned}$$

$$\begin{aligned} Q_p/Q_s &= 53 \text{ mL}/42 \text{ mL} \\ &= 1.3 : 1 \end{aligned}$$

$$\begin{aligned} \text{RVSP} &= \text{BP—4}(v_{\text{vsd}})2 \\ &= 112\text{—}4(4.6)^2 \\ &= 27 \text{ mm Hg} \end{aligned}$$

Chapter 19

1. c
2. d
3. d
4. a
5. d
6. d
7. d
8. d
9. b
10. a

Chapter 20

1. c
2. b
3. b
4. d
5. a
6. c
7. c
8. b
9. d
10. c

Chapter 21

1. d
2. b
3. c
4. c
5. a
6. d
7. a
8. b
9. b
10. d

Index

Note: Page numbers followed by f indicate figures; those followed by t indicate tables.